IMAGING OF THE LIVER,
PANCREAS AND SPLEEN

Imaging of the Liver, Pancreas and Spleen

EDITED BY

ROBERT A. WILKINS

BSc MB ChB FRCR
Consultant Radiologist
Northwick Park Hospital
London

HEATHER B. NUNNERLEY

MB ChB DCH DObst DRCOG DMRD FRCR
Director of Radiology
King's College Hospital
London

FOREWORD BY

E. RHYS DAVIES

President
The Royal College of Radiologists

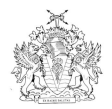

PUBLISHED FOR THE

ROYAL COLLEGE OF RADIOLOGISTS BY

BLACKWELL SCIENTIFIC PUBLICATIONS

OXFORD LONDON

EDINBURGH BOSTON MELBOURNE

© 1990 by
Blackwell Scientific Publications
Editorial offices:
Osney Mead, Oxford OX2 0EL
25 John Street, London WC1N 2BL
23 Ainslie Place, Edinburgh EH3 6AJ
3 Cambridge Center, Suite 208
   Cambridge, Massachusetts 02142, USA
107 Barry Street, Carlton
   Victoria 3053, Australia

First published 1990

Set by Setrite Typesetters, Hong Kong
Printed and bound in Great Britain
by William Clowes Ltd, Beccles and London

DISTRIBUTORS

Marston Book Services Ltd
PO Box 87
Oxford OX2 0DT
(*Orders*: Tel: 0865 791155
        Fax: 0865 791927
        Telex: 837515)

USA
Year Book Medical Publishers
200 North LaSalle Street
Chicago, Illinois 60601
(*Orders*: Tel: (312) 726−9733)

Canada
The C.V. Mosby Company
5240 Finch Avenue East
Scarborough, Ontario
(*Orders*: Tel: (416) 298−1588)

Australia
Blackwell Scientific Publications
(Australia) Pty Ltd
107 Barry Street
Carlton, Victoria 3053
(*Orders*: Tel: (03) 347−0300)

British Library
Cataloguing in Publication Data

Imaging of the liver, pancreas and spleen.
1. Man. Radiology. Biliary tract
I. Wilkins, Robert A.   II. Nunnerley,
H. B.   616.3'60757

ISBN 0−632−02609−X

Contents

v

List of Contributors

D.M. ACKERY MA, MB, BChir, MSc, FRCR, *Professor of Nuclear Medicine, Southampton General Hospital, Southampton SO9 4XY*

D.J. ALLISON BSc, MB, BS, MD, FRCR, *Director and Professor of Diagnostic Radiology, Royal Postgraduate Medical School, Hammersmith Hospital, Du Cane Road, London W12 0HS*

V.B. BATTY MB, BS, MSc, DMRD, FRCR, *Consultant in Radiology and Nuclear Medicine, Southampton General Hospital, Southampton SO9 4XY*

L.A. BERGER MB, BS, FRACP, DMRD, FRCR, *Consultant Radiologist, Royal Free Hospital, London NW3 2QG*

G.M. BYDDER FRCR, *Professor of Diagnostic Radiology, Department of Radiology, Hammersmith Hospital, Du Cane Road, London W12 0HS*

H. CARTY MB, ChB, FRCPI, FRCR, *Consultant Radiologist, Alder Hey Children's Hospital, Eaton Road, Liverpool L12 2AP*

A.H. CHALMERS MA, FRCP, FRCR, *Consultant Radiologist, Royal United Hospital, Combe Park, Bath BA1 3NG*

D.O. COSGROVE MA, FRCP, FRCR, *Consultant in Nuclear Medicine and Ultrasound, Royal Marsden Hospital, Fulham Road, London SW3 6JJ*

K.C. DEWBURY BSc, MB, BS, FRCR, *Consultant Radiologist, Southampton General Hospital, Southampton SO9 4XY*

R. DICK MB, BS, MRACR, FRCR, *Consultant Radiologist, Royal Free Hospital, London NW3 2QG*

A.K. DIXON MD, MRCP, FRCR, *University Lecturer, Department of Radiology, University of Cambridge; Honorary Consultant Radiologist, Addenbrooke's Hospital, Hills Road, Cambridge CB2 2QQ*

P.A. DUBBINS MB, BS, FRCR, *Consultant Radiologist, Plymouth General Hospital, Freedom Fields, Plymouth, PO4 7JJ*

E.W.L. FLETCHER MA, MB, BChir, FRCR, *Consultant Radiologist, John Radcliffe Hospital, Oxford; Fellow, Green College, Oxford, OX2 6HG*

S.J. GOLDING MB, BS, FRCR, *Lecturer in Radiology, University of Oxford; Director, Oxford Regional Computed Tomography Unit, Oxford*

A. GRUNDY MB, ChB, DCH, FRCR, *Consultant and Senior Lecturer, Diagnostic Radiology, St George's Hospital and Medical School, London SW17*

A.P. HEMINGWAY BSc, FRCS, LRCP, MB, BS, MRCP, DMRD, FRCR, *Academic Department of Radiology, Royal Hallamshire Hospital, Glossop Road, Sheffield S10 2JF*

E.R. HOWARD MS, FRCS, *Consultant Surgeon, King's College Hospital, Denmark Hill, London SE5 9RS*

A.E.A. JOSEPH MB, MSc, FRCR, *Consultant Radiologist and Honorary Senior Lecturer, St George's Hospital and Medical School, London SW17*

A.D. JOYCE MB, FRCS, *Registror, King's College Hospital, Denmark Hill, London SE5 9RS*

J. KARANI MB, BS, BSc, FRCR, *Consultant Radiologist, King's College Hospital, Denmark Hill, London SE5 9RS*

D.E. KATZ MB, BCh, FRCR, *Consultant Radiologist, Northwick Park Hospital, Watford Road, Harrow HA1 3UJ*

A. KENNEDY MB, BCH, BAO, BA, MRCP *Registrar in Radiology, Hammersmith Hospital, Du Cane Road, London W12 0HS*

D.M. KING MB, BS, DMRD, FRCR, *Consultant Radiologist, Westminster Hospital, Dean Ryle Street, London SW1; Royal Marsden Hospital, Fulham Road, London SW3*

J.W. LAWS CBE, FRCP, FRCR, *Consultant Radiologist, 5 Frank Dixon Way, Dulwich, London SE21 7BB*

W.R. LEES MB, BS, FRCR, *Consultant Radiologist, The Middlesex Hospital, Mortimer Street, London W1N 8AA*

D.J. LINTOTT MB, BS, FRCR, *Consultant Radiologist, The General Infirmary at Leeds, Great George Street, Leeds LS1 3EX*

E.M. McILRATH MB, BCh, FRCR, FFR, RCSI, *Consultant Radiologist, Royal Victoria Hospital, Grosvenor Road, Belfast BT12 6BA*

H.B. MEIRE MB, BS, FRCR, *Consultant Radiologist, King's College Hospital, Denmark Hill, London SE5 9RS*

H.B. NUNNERLEY MB, ChB, DCH, DObst, RCOG, DMRD, FRCR, *Director of Radiology, King's College Hospital, Denmark Hill, London SE5 9RS*

F.W. SMITH MO, FFRRCS(1), DMRD, *Consultant Radiologist, Aberdeen Royal Infirmary, Foresterhill, Aberdeen AB9 2ZB*

K.C. TAN FRCS, *Consultant Surgeon, King's College Hospital, Denmark Hill, London SE5 9RS*

P.S. THOMAS MB, BCh, FRCR, *Consultant Radiologist, Royal Belfast Hospital for Sick Children, Belfast BT12 6BE*

R.A. WILKINS BSc, MB, ChB, FRCR, *Consultant Radiologist, Northwick Park Hospital, Watford Road, Harrow HA1 3UJ*

Foreword

The Royal College of Radiologists has extended its interest in postgraduate education during the last decade by encouraging and commissioning a number of textbooks, each devoted to a clearly identified theme or system. This entirely new volume was specifically aimed to incorporate the rapid recent advances that are taking place in this particular field. It reflects the current state of practice of clinical radiology in the United Kingdom and we are certain it will find favour amongst English speaking radiologists worldwide.

We welcome Blackwell Scientific Publications as the publishers of this textbook, for the quality of their work is already well known to readers of the College journal, *Clinical Radiology*. We wish to express our deep gratitude to the editor and contributors to this volume and look forward to the possibility of other volumes in this series.

E. RHYS DAVIES
President and Council of
The Royal College of Radiologists

Part 1
The Normal Liver

1: The Liver — General Considerations

R.A. WILKINS

Introduction

It will come as no surprise to readers of this text that the liver is the largest single organ in the body and lies in the right upper quadrant of the abdomen. The fact that the liver is not only a large organ but an important one has been recognized through the ages.

In fact, in past ages the liver was considered the seat of life, hence its name — liver, the thing we live with. Shakespeare recognized this on more than one occasion: for instance in *Love's Labour's Lost* (IV, iii), Berowne, as an aside whilst Longaville reads verses, says 'This is the liver-vein, which makes flesh a deity'. The Ancient Greeks and Romans saw the importance of the liver in more practical terms. In the auspices considered before a battle, the liver of the sacrificed animal if red and healthy was a good omen, whereas if pale, defeat was forecast. Advances in medical knowledge have confirmed the vital place of the liver, though understanding of its precise role has been somewhat modified with time.

Anatomy

Gross anatomy of the liver can be viewed in various ways. The anatomy of the isolated liver is well established (Fig. 1.1). The liver is traditionally divided into four lobes: the right and left lobes, and two lesser subdivisions of the right lobe, the quadrate and caudate lobes. The right and left lobes are separated by the falciform ligament. This is a peritoneal fold and, as well as containing two layers of peritoneum, it also contains strands of fibrous tissue which help to stabilize the liver by attaching it to the diaphragm and the anterior abdominal wall. The ligamentum teres, a remnant of the umbilical vein of the fetus, runs in the free edge of the falciform ligament from the umbilicus. Perhaps more important in the adult is the persistence of some para-umbilical veins in this 'ligament' which may dilate in certain diseases of the liver. These veins are also occasionally of considerable value as an access route to the portal system, as they may be cannulated either at the time of abdominal surgery, or as a primary procedure through a small skin incision. An example of this usage is the placement of catheters at the time of colorectal cancer surgery for the perfusion of the liver with cytotoxins.

The liver is also anchored by several other 'ligaments'. The coronary ligament or bare area is an irregular triangle-shaped area on the posterior surface of the liver where the peritoneal covering of the liver is deficient and the posterior surface of the liver is applied directly to the diaphragm, separated only by some loose areolar tissue. A

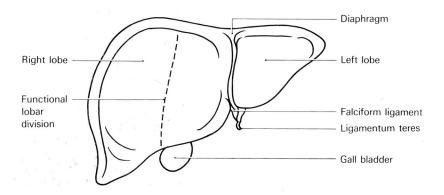

Fig. 1.1 Anatomy of the liver. Anterior aspect.

substantial part of the inferior vena cava and hepatic veins lie within this area. It also forms another potential pathway for collateral vessels. The inferior extension of the bare area is sometimes referred to as the hepatorenal ligament. This is a layer of peritoneum and fibrous tissue which extends to the anterior surface of the right kidney as a slightly thickened band. Perhaps more important than its anchoring role is the observation that this fold of peritoneum often contains small vessels.

Viewed anteriorly, the liver appears as a wedged-shaped block of tissue with a slight indentation at the point at which the falciform ligament crosses the anterior surface. This is in contrast to many other mammals in which the liver is a multi-lobulated structure.

Viewed posteriorly, the two accessory lobes can be seen (Fig. 1.2). The caudate lobe lies between the inferior vena cava (IVC), which forms its lateral border, and the porta hepatis. The caudate lobe is particularly of note as the venous drainage of this lobe is frequently distinct from the rest of the liver. This separate drainage, direct to the IVC rather than through the hepatic veins, may allow the caudate lobe to be spared from the fibrosis which ensues elsewhere secondary to hepatic-vein

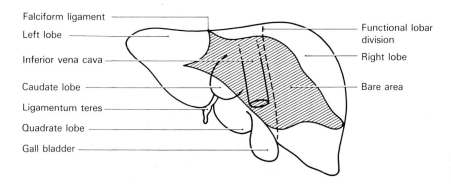

Falciform ligament

Left lobe

Inferior vena cava

Caudate lobe

Ligamentum teres

Quadrate lobe

Gall bladder

Functional lobar division

Right lobe

Bare area

Fig. 1.2 Anatomy of the liver. Posterior aspect.

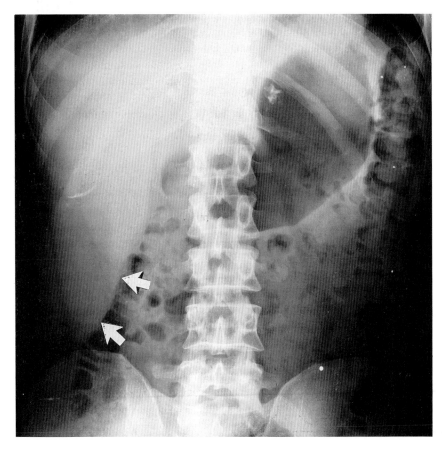

Fig. 1.3 Riedel's lobe (*arrows*) may extend to the pelvic brim. A normal anatomic variant.

occlusion in the Budd—Chiari syndrome. The quadrate lobe lies inferiorly and is bordered by the ligamentum teres (or round ligament, the remnant of the fetal umbilical vein) and the bed of the gall bladder.

Viewed from below the liver presents an undulating surface as it is closely applied to the adjacent abdominal organs. The stomach, duodenum, hepatic flexure of the colon, the right kidney and the right adrenal gland are all in contact with the inferior surface of the liver and may cause impressions on it. The porta hepatis, also visible on the inferior surface, is the gateway to the liver for the portal vein and the hepatic artery, and the way out for the bile ducts.

Accessory lobes

The most important accessory lobe as far as the radiologist is concerned is the so-called Riedel's lobe, which is not truly an accessory lobe at all but simply a downward extension of the lateral aspect of the right lobe (Fig. 1.3). It is a fairly common variation of normal anatomy and may extend as far as the iliac crest. It has no pathological significance.

True accessory lobes may rarely be seen; in these cases the human liver follows a pattern more commonly seen in other mammals, being a multilobulated organ. Up to 16 lobes have been recorded.

Surface anatomy

The majority of the liver is contained within the protection of the rib cage. The right border of the liver is closely applied to the lateral abdominal wall and the inferior costal margin at mid-inspiration. The tip of the left lobe lies beneath the left diaphragm in about the mid-clavicular line and in its mid-section the liver is often palpable in the epigastrium (roughly mid-way between the

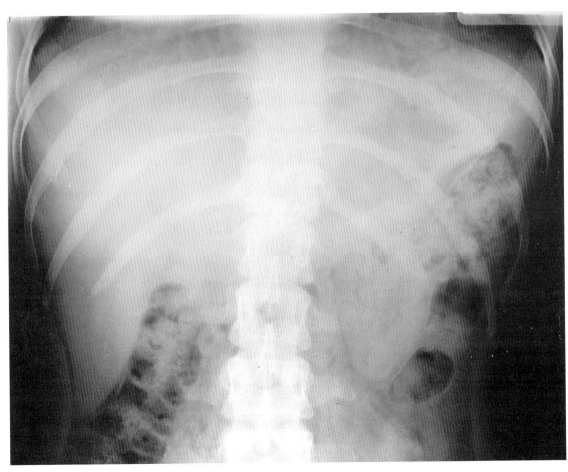

Fig. 1.4 Plain abdominal radiograph showing the soft-tissue shadow of the liver. Note how well the tip of the right lobe may be seen silhouetted against peritoneal fat.

xiphoid and the umbilicus). The liver moves on respiration some 1–3 cm with the diaphragm to which it is closely applied. The free edge of the right lobe may frequently be felt in normal subjects just below the costal margin. Extension more than 3 cm below the costal margin is considered clinical hepatomegaly, though Blendis *et al.* (1970) showed wide observer variation in this assessment. Others have confirmed this and demonstrated a within-observer error of 15–20% and a between-observer error of 20–25% in the clinical estimation of liver size. In patients in whom for some reason the lungs are hypervolaemic the normal liver may be displaced downwards and be readily palpable. The volume of the liver also exhibits a diurnal variation of some 17% (Leung *et al.*, 1986).

The liver is relatively larger in infants than in adults, in whom it is half the relative size. This is principally due to the prominence of the left lobe, which accounts for the protuberant epigastrium in young children.

Radiographic anatomy (plain films)

The radiographic anatomy is dependent upon the morphology of the organ and the radiographic features of the adjacent organs. The plain radiograph of the liver is of a homogeneous structure of soft-tissue density. The superior margin is clearly demarcated by the diaphragm, or rather the lung above it, but the inferior margin is less easily defined. The tip of the right lobe, whether it be a Riedel's lobe or not, frequently lies in a small indentation in the peritoneal fat layers and can thus be seen as a silhouette against the low-density fat (Fig. 1.4). The rest of the inferior surface tends to blend with the soft-tissue structures of other organs in the abdomen, and the edge can usually only be defined by identifying other structures of lower density which impinge on the liver. This is frequently the gas contained within hollow organs.

It has been shown (Blendis *et al.*, 1970) that the inferior margin detected radiographically is the anterior edge of the liver. Radiological and clinical assessment of this edge correlates rather poorly in the small liver but quite well the liver is enlarged. The confines of the left lobe, unless enlarged, are very difficult to judge radiographically. Radiographic estimation of hepatomegaly is almost as inaccurate as clinical evaluation (Riemenschneider & Whalen, 1965). Ultrasound is probably more accurate (Rasmussen, 1972), and SPECT scanning

the most accurate imaging technique (Strauss *et al.*, 1984) for this purpose.

Surgical anatomy

Although the gross anatomy would imply that the liver is readily separated into two or four lobes, the surgical reality does not bear this out. The liver is a uniform mass of parenchyma, not divided into septa or lobes by fibrous strands or vascular grooves. Nevertheless, a line of demarcation between a functional right and left side of the liver can be identified. This line runs obliquely from a point just to the right of the falciform ligament towards the bed of the gall bladder (Figs 1.1 and 1.2).

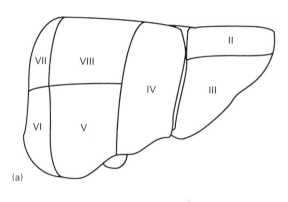
(a)

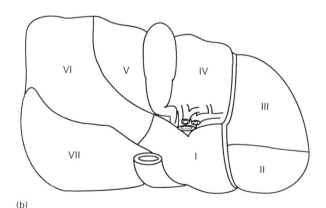
(b)

Fig. 1.5 The surgical segments of the liver. (a) Diaphragmatic surface. (b) Visceral surface.

  I Caudate lobe
 II Lateral superior segment, left lobe
III Lateral inferior segment, left lobe
IV Medial segment, left lobe
 V Anterior inferior segment, right lobe
VI Posterior inferior segment, right lobe
VII Posterior superior segment, right lobe
VIII Anterior superior segment, right lobe

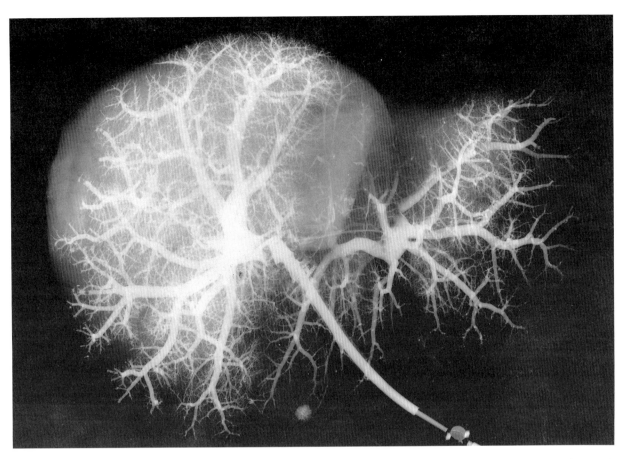

Fig. 1.6 Autopsy specimen. The portal vein is opacified. Note the branching pattern and orientation of the vessels.

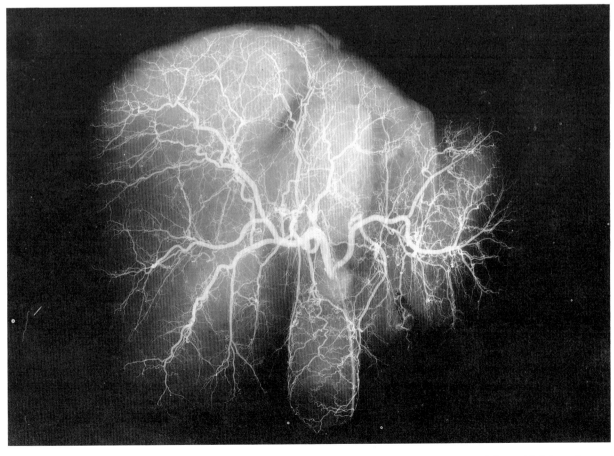

Fig. 1.7 Autopsy specimen. The hepatic artery has been opacified. Note the main division into right and left branches and the supply to the gall bladder.

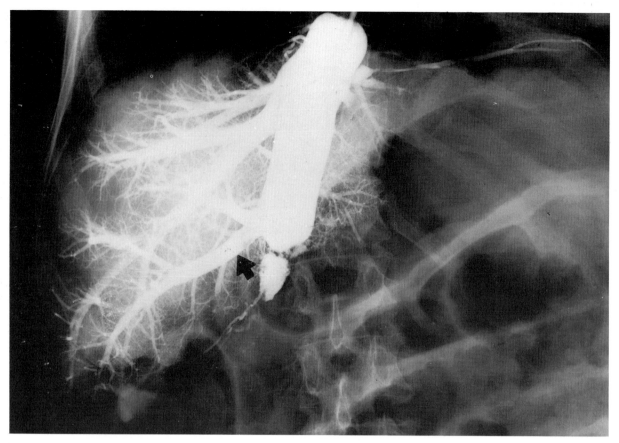

Fig. 1.8 Autopsy specimen. The IVC and hepatic veins have been opacified. Note the drainage of the caudate lobe (*arrow*).

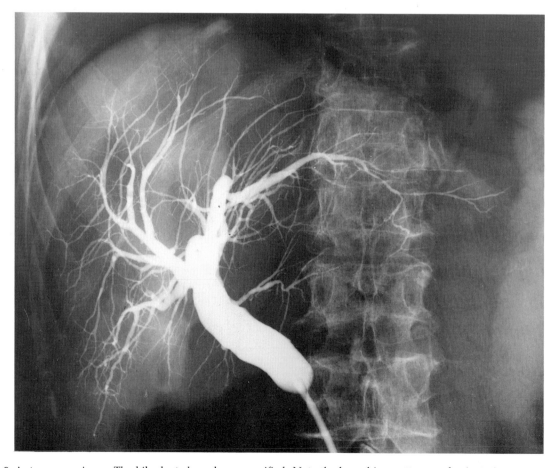

Fig. 1.9 Autopsy specimen. The bile ducts have been opacified. Note the branching pattern and orientation.

The line extends through the liver to the inferior vena cava. This division corresponds to the functional division of the right and left hepatic artery, portal vein and bile duct. This functional separation of the right and left segments of the liver is becoming increasingly important as surgical techniques, including partial resection, become more commonplace.

Despite the fact that no clear anatomical septation occurs, contemporary surgical technique has perfected segmental hepatic resection. This management may be used in liver trauma and in malignancy, both primary and secondary. The liver is divided into eight segments, four in the right and four in the left lobe (Fig. 1.5). The segments conform largely to the branching pattern of the portal vein (Goldsmith & Woodburne, 1957) (Fig. 1.6).

Vascular anatomy

This will largely be covered in subsequent sections, but some brief reference here is important in relation to the previous section. The portal vein formed by the union of the superior mesenteric and the splenic vein runs through the porta hepatis and divides just within the liver substance into the right and left branches (Fig. 1.5). They are fairly closely accompanied by the equivalent branches of the hepatic artery (Fig. 1.7), which arises in most cases from the coeliac axis although frequent variations are found. It is well known that the liver is thus a beneficiary of a double vascular supply.

The hepatic veins follow the general anatomical form of the hepatic artery and portal vein less closely, as shown in Fig. 1.8. They normally come together as a single large hepatic vein that drains into the inferior vena cava immediately proximal to the inflow into the right atrium. Hepatic veins are usually subdivided into three sections, the left,

middle and right groups of veins. The caudate lobe frequently drains separately, directly to the IVC. This fact is of clinical significance in the Budd–Chiari syndrome.

The lymphatic drainage is towards the hilum of the liver, where there is a large collection of nodes at the porta hepatis. A second and accessory pathway for the lymphatic channels is around the hepatic veins where they drain into nodes at the inferior vena cava.

The bile ducts follow fairly closely the anatomical structure of the hepatic artery and form distinct right and left duct systems that unite to form the common hepatic duct (Fig. 1.9). The cystic duct enters the common hepatic duct at or below the hilum of the liver to form the common bile duct. Many variations exist in these basic vascular and duct outlines, and they will be described in later chapters.

References

Blendis, L.M., McNeilly, W.J., Sheppard L., Williams, R. & Laws, J.W. (1970) Observer variation in the clinical and radiological assessment of hepatosplenomegaly. *British Medical Journal*, **1**, 727–730.

Goldsmith N.A. & Woodburne R.T. (1957) Surgical anatomy pertaining to liver resection. *Surgery Gynecology and Obstetrics*, **105**, 310–318.

Leung, N.W.Y., Farrant, P. & Peters, T.J. (1986) Liver volume measurement by ultrasonography in normal subjects and alcoholic patients. *Journal of Hepatology*, **2**, 157–164.

Rasmussen, S.N. (1972) Liver volume determination by ultrasonic scanning. *British Journal of Radiology*, **45**, 579–585.

Riemenschneider, P.A. & Whalen, J.P. (1965) The relative accuracy of estimation of enlargement of the liver and spleen by radiologic and clinical methods. *American Journal of Roentgenology*, **94**, 462–468.

Strauss, L.G., Clorius, J.H., Frank, T. & Van Kaick, G. (1984). Single photon emission computerized tomography (SPECT) for estimates of liver and spleen volume. *Journal of Nuclear Medicine*, **25**, 81–85.

2: Ultrasound of the Liver

H.B. MEIRE

Introduction

The purpose of this chapter is to introduce the reader to the capability and limitations of ultrasound imaging for the diagnosis of liver disease, to indicate the preferred technique, and to suggest what features of the liver should be specifically evaluated in order to optimize the chances of diagnosing liver disease.

During the past 10 years ultrasound has become a widely accepted technique for imaging the liver, and its role in the diagnosis and management of hepatic disorders has become fairly clear. Diagnostic ultrasound is essentially an anatomical imaging technique and does not depend for its success upon any aspect of organ function. These features dictate both the advantages and limitations of the technique, namely that it is very successful for detecting localized abnormalities of structure but is inappropriate for and unsuccessful at the diagnosis of diffuse liver disease.

Attempts have been made over a number of years to enhance the ability of ultrasound to detect diffuse liver disorders by utilizing sophisticated computerized analyses of the ultrasound signal. These techniques have been misnamed ultrasound 'tissue characterization'. They have fallen short of characterizing tissue and have failed to become incorporated into routine clinical investigation. An alternative approach has been the evaluation of the Doppler signals obtained from within the hepatic artery, portal vein, and hepatic veins. This particular application of diagnostic ultrasound is still in its infancy but does appear to offer rather more clinically relevant information than tissue characterization.

Equipment

In the early and mid 1970s the majority of ultrasound scanners in clinical use were relatively cumbersome, manually operated, static compound scanners. A high degree of operator expertise was necessary to achieve diagnostic imaging with such a system, and a considerable degree of patient cooperation was also essential. The images obtained could be of very high quality and had the major advantage of covering a large anatomical area. However, the disadvantages of these systems led to a decline in their use when the modern automatic 'real-time' scanners were developed and the 'static scanners' have now fallen almost completely into disuse.

There is now a wide range of different types of real-time scanner and whilst all can be used for imaging the liver, the configurations and mechanical properties of the different systems give them both advantages and disadvantages in different clinical areas. Modern real-time scanners can be divided into two basic groups, mechanical and electronic. The mechanical systems comprise one or more transducers that are either oscillated or rotated by electromechanical mechanisms. These scanners produce an image of a sector of the patient which is very narrow near the surface and rapidly widens out with increasing depth (see Fig. 2.1). The major advantages of the mechanical sector scanners are the small area of contact and the consequent ease with which the probe can be directed into relatively inaccessible areas such as between the ribs. The major disadvantage of the mechanical systems is potential wear in the mechanical components. In practice this is seldom a significant consideration.

The solid-state electronic scanners are divided into two main groups, the linear and curvilinear arrays, and the phased arrays. The transducers of the linear and curvilinear arrays are typically 10–12 cm in length and require that the whole of the length of the transducer is maintained in good contact with the patient during imaging. The field of view of the linear array is a rectangle, the width of which is the same as the length of the transducer. This format of display, combined with the

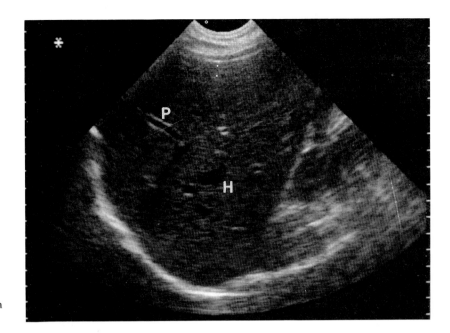

Fig. 2.1 Longitudinal scan of the right lobe of the liver to show the normal appearance of the portal vein walls (P) and hepatic veins (H).

size of the transducer, makes the linear array less than optimal for examination of the liver. The curvilinear array transducer tends to be rather shorter in length and its truncated sector field of view is rather better for liver imaging than the straight linear array. The phased array transducer comprises an extremely small solid-state transducer from which the beam is steered electronically through a sector of up to 90°. These systems combine the advantages of the mechanical sector scanners with the absence of mechanical components. The quality of images obtained from a phased array system can be very high, but unfortunately are seriously degraded in the more obese patients. Although all of the above systems can be used for liver diagnosis, the best compromise is currently achieved by the mechanical sector scanners.

The frequency of the interrogating ultrasound beam determines the depth to which it penetrates within the patient. The lower frequencies penetrate more readily but generally have a wider beam width and therefore worse resolution. Higher frequency probes produce better resolution but with less penetration. The choice of transducer will of course be determined by the size and shape of the patient to be examined. The majority of adults will require a frequency of 3.5 MHz, whilst children can be examined with 5 MHz, and neonates with 7.5 MHz.

Technique

No preparation of the patient is necessary for ultrasound examination of the liver, but since the biliary system will almost invariably be examined at the same time it is advisable to have the patients fasted. The success of the subcostal approach to the liver may be impaired by excessive gaseous distension of the stomach, and patients should therefore be asked to avoid the consumption of fizzy drinks prior to ultrasound investigation.

As with all other special radiological techniques it is useful but not essential for the operator to have a simple protocol for the examination of his patient to ensure that no anatomical area or structure is overlooked. The protocol used is a question of personal preference, but the one outlined below ensures examination of as much of the liver volume as possible.

Patients are placed comfortably in the supine position. Generous quantities of contact medium are placed on the skin and the transducer applied lightly in the left subcostal region to perform longitudinal scans of the left lobe of the liver. Visualization of the liver may be assisted by asking the patient to inhale briefly. The organ is then examined from the extreme left lateral extremity of the left lobe, passing towards the mid-line, taking care to identify the caudate lobe. The plane of examination is extended across, towards the right side of the abdomen until passage of the transducer to the right is impeded by the right costal margin. This technique should permit examination of the whole of the volume of the left lobe in the longitudinal plane; this lobe should now be briefly examined in the transverse plane, again during suspended inspiration, starting with the transducer immediately inferior to the xiphisternum and sweeping inferiorly. In cases where extreme difficulty in imaging the left lobe is experienced, it may be helpful to examine the patient in the sitting or standing position, when gravity will bring the liver into a more readily accessible position.

The exact shape of the patient's subcostal margin will determine the degree to which the right lobe of the liver can be imaged from beneath the costal margin. The combination of deep inspiration and angling the probe superiorly and laterally beneath the costal margin will permit the examination of most of the right lobe in most patients. The superolateral aspect of the right lobe is the area most likely to be overlooked by this approach, and this area should be examined by a series of intercostal scans taken with the scanner orientated along the long axis of the lateral intercostal spaces. It is not necessary to request the patient to breathe in for these views and they are therefore particularly helpful in very ill and unco-operative patients. In the small proportion of patients where these approaches fail to demonstrate the majority of the right lobe of the liver, two further approaches can be used. The first of these is the erect approach as for the left lobe, and the second is the left lateral decubitus position. With the patient lying on his or her left side the right lobe of the liver tends to fall medially, and if this position is combined with deep inspiration remarkably good views can often be obtained in difficult patients. This view is also particularly helpful for identifying the gall bladder and porta hepatis structures.

The equipment control settings will be determined by the patient's body habitus. Correct setting of the equipment controls is more critical for liver imaging than for any other organ. It is important that sufficient power is used to enable the sound to penetrate to the deepest portion of the liver and the depth-gain or time-gain compensation controls should be adjusted to ensure that the liver is displayed with even brightness from the most superficial to the deepest portions. The commonest error made by ultrasound operators is inadequate depth-gain compensation, which leads to lack of information from the most distal portion of the liver.

Normal appearances

PARENCHYMA

The appearance of the liver parenchyma will be determined by the make of equipment in use, the characteristics of the transducers selected, and the settings of the equipment controls. The combination of these factors together with the complex nature of the structure of the liver make it impossible to describe the typical appearance of a normal liver. However, most operators regularly performing ultrasound investigations rapidly become accustomed to the normal appearances for their particular equipment and transducers. The parenchymal echoes received from the normal liver should be roughly even in brightness and texture and should be interrupted only by the major hepatic veins and the portal vein and its branches. In the majority of images these vessels will be cut in oblique sections and can usually be differentiated from each other by the relatively highly reflective walls of the portal veins compared with the normal complete absence of any obvious wall echo from hepatic veins (Fig. 2.1). When a hepatic vein is cut in cross section it will appear circular and could be mistaken for a spherical filling defect. It is important for the operator to be aware of this problem and to examine adjacent slices carefully to confirm that the structure is indeed tubular, rotating the plane of imaging to identify the structure along its long axis.

The reflectivity of the liver parenchyma should be assessed in each patient, since this may be modified by various diffuse processes. As a general rule the reflectivity is decreased by acute hepatitis and acute heart failure (Kurtz et al., 1980) and may be increased in some forms of cirrhosis (Dewbury & Clarke, 1979). The parenchymal reflectivity is most markedly increased by fat deposits either as a result of obesity or fatty liver disease (Foster et al., 1980). Unfortunately the overall brightness of the displayed liver parenchymal echoes is entirely dependent upon the selection of equipment and the control settings. It is therefore essential to have internal references for the parenchymal reflectivity. As a general rule, one or more of the following three structures are used, the portal vein walls, the body of the pancreas, and the cortex of the right kidney. The brightness of the displayed echoes from the portal vein walls should be noticeably greater than that of the background parenchyma,

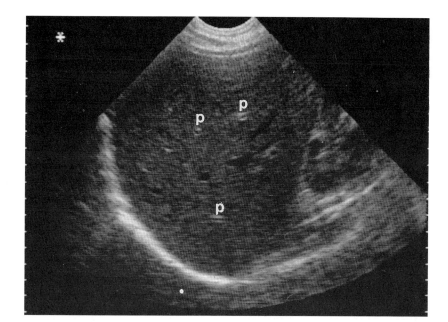

Fig. 2.2 Longitudinal scan of the right lobe lateral to Fig. 2.1 to show the appearance of the small portal vein radicals (p) within the normal parenchyma.

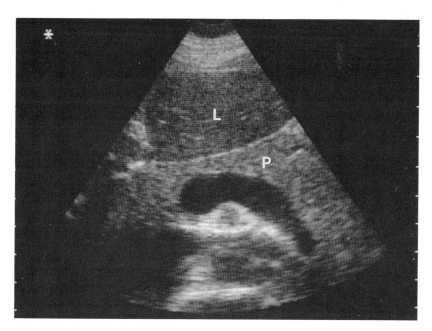

Fig. 2.3 Transverse scan in the mid-line comparing the reflectivity of the left lobe of the liver (L) with the normal pancreas (P).

thereby permitting easy identification of even the small portal vein radicals (Fig. 2.2).

The normal liver parenchyma can be compared most easily with the pancreas on longitudinal or transverse scans in the mid-line. It is important that the depth-gain control settings are correct and do not give rise to inappropriate overamplification of the pancreatic echoes. With this proviso it is normal for the pancreatic parenchyma, assuming this to be normal, to be of roughly similar reflectivity to the liver in young adults, slightly brighter than the liver in the 40–60 years age group, and of markedly greater brightness with increasing age

(Fig. 2.3). In the paediatric age group the pancreas may sometimes be seen to be of slightly lower reflectivity than the adjacent normal liver. The normal right kidney can be most readily compared with the liver on a lateral coronal scan. Ideally the brightness of the displayed liver parenchyma should be compared with an area of renal cortex at the same depth from the transducer in order to avoid artefacts due to incorrect equipment control settings. The normal renal parenchyma should be slightly less reflective than the adjacent liver (Fig. 2.4).

As mentioned in the Introduction, ultrasound is

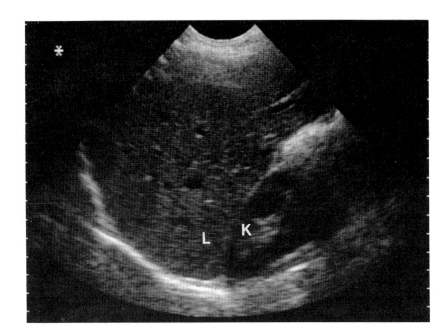

Fig. 2.4 Longitudinal scan of the right lobe showing the slightly greater reflectivity in the normal liver parenchyma (L) compared with the cortex of the right kidney (K).

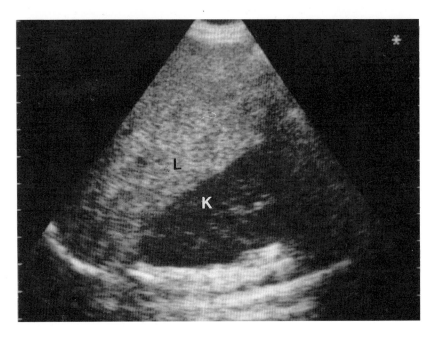

Fig. 2.5 Longitudinal scan of the right lobe in a patient with excessive glycogen deposits within the liver. The liver parenchyma (L) is much brighter than the adjacent kidney (K).

not an ideal technique for the diagnosis of diffuse liver diseases, but attention to the above points may enable the astute ultrasound operator to identify both increases and decreases in parenchymal reflectivity. Increased reflectivity is much more readily identified because of the loss of the portal vein walls and the marked increase in brightness of the liver compared with the right kidney (Fig. 2.5).

Cirrhosis and other diffuse disorders may give rise to alteration in the parenchymal architecture of the liver, but these are necessarily subjective changes, which will vary according to the equipment in use, and are difficult to describe. These features underline the limitations of ultrasound for diagnosis of diffuse liver disorders.

The surface texture of the liver is normally not available for ultrasound assessment, but in the presence of ascites the surface may be clearly seen, and choice of an appropriately focused transducer may permit assessment of the detailed texture of the liver surface. The liver surface should normally be smooth but may become irregularly nodular in the presence of multifocal metastases, and regu-

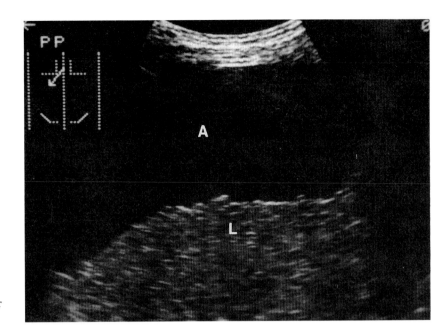

Fig. 2.6 Anterior scan of the right upper quadrant in a patient with ascites and hepatic cirrhosis. The presence of the ascites (A) enables the ultrasound scan to demonstrate the finely nodular surface of the liver (L).

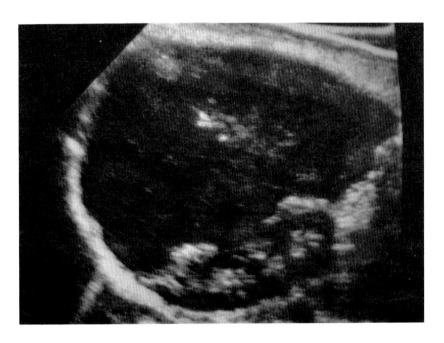

Fig. 2.7 Multiple hepatic metastases causing irregularity of the inferior margin of the right lobe of the liver.

larly nodular in the presence of cirrhosis (Fig. 2.6). Coarse nodularity can sometimes be detected in the absence of ascites by inspection of the inferior margin of the right lobe in patients with metastases (Fig. 2.7).

Ultrasound is especially valuable for the identification of focal changes within the liver parenchyma, and it is therefore important for the equipment operator to be certain that the parenchymal echo pattern has been surveyed throughout the entire liver volume. The different focal pathologies within the liver may give rise to areas of either increased or decreased reflectivity with clearly or poorly defined borders, and thus all forms of departure from the normal pattern of reflectivity and architecture should be carefully sought.

THE HEPATIC VESSELS

Hepatic artery

The intrahepatic branches of the hepatic artery are too small to be readily identified in the majority of

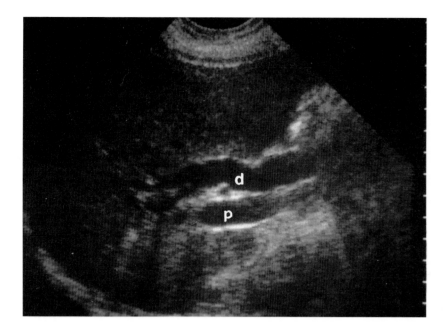

Fig. 2.8 Scan along the long axis of a dilated common hepatic duct (d). The hepatic artery can be seen end on between the duct and the portal vein (p).

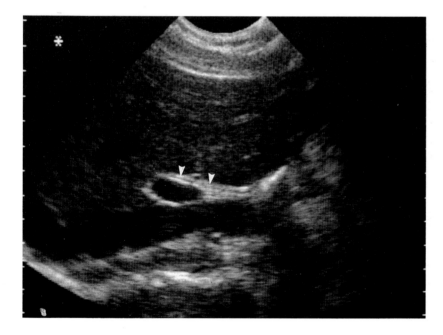

Fig. 2.9 Scan at the porta hepatis showing the normal non-dilated common hepatic duct (*arrows*) running posterior to the hepatic artery.

patients. Localized areas of arterial pulsation may be evident in real-time images, but it is seldom possible to identify any sections other than the main hepatic artery and its primary divisions. The most commonly identified segment is the main trunk of the right hepatic artery, which normally passes posterior to the common hepatic duct and anterior to the portal vein (Fig. 2.8). In a minority of patients the artery may be placed anterior to the common hepatic duct (Fig. 2.9). Awareness of this potential anomaly will avoid misinterpretation of the anatomy in the subjects and may occasionally be of value to the surgeon who may have to operate in this region.

Portal vein

The major components of the extrahepatic portal venous system are readily identifiable and their diameters can be measured if necessary. However, the ranges of normal for the diameters of the splenic, superior mesenteric, and portal veins are extremely wide; the diameters of these vessels will be seen to have increased after a meal (Bellamy *et*

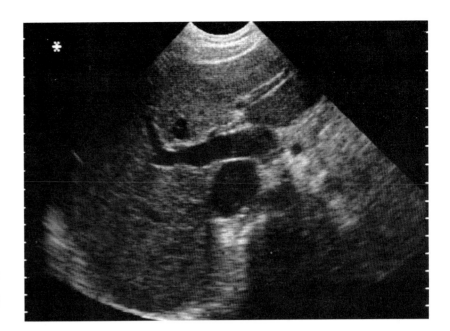

Fig. 2.10 Transverse scan of the right upper quadrant showing the portal vein entering the liver. The lumen of the portal vein is virtually echo free.

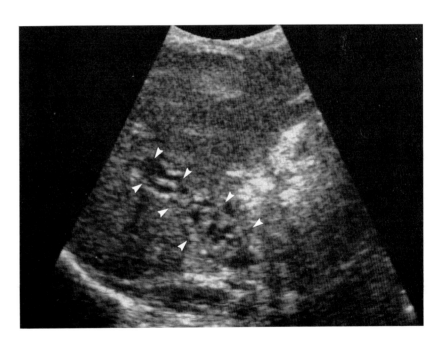

Fig. 2.11 Cavernous transformation of the portal vein. The portal vein (*arrows*) has been replaced by numerous irregular channels.

al., 1984) and there is a very poor correlation between vessel diameter and the intraluminal pressure. The large majority of patients with proven portal hypertension have normal diameter portal veins. In those patients with large extra-hepatic portal collaterals, these may be well demonstrated both in the region of the porta hepatis and near the splenic hilum (Kane & Katz, 1982).

The main portal vein can be identified in every patient as it enters the liver and divides into its left and right branches (Fig. 2.10). Again the diam-

eter of the vessel is not very helpful in the diagnosis of disease, but its patency should be noted. Occlusion of the portal vein may occur as a result of portal pyaemia, invasion from both primary and secondary intrahepatic malignancies (Meire *et al.*, 1987), and as a primary condition, often in childhood. Childhood portal vein obstruction usually gives rise to cavernous transformation and in this situation the single major channel is replaced by numerous small serpiginous channels (Fig. 2.11) (Kauzlaric *et al.*, 1984). Occasionally one or more of

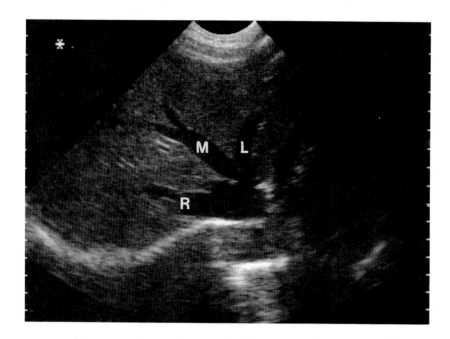

Fig. 2.12 Transverse scan in the midline showing the left (L) middle (M) and right (R) hepatic veins in a normal subject.

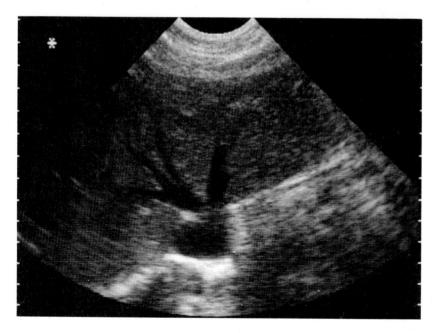

Fig. 2.13 Transverse scan showing the hepatic veins in a different subject from Fig. 2.13. The middle hepatic vein is represented by two separate trunks.

these may be sufficiently large to masquerade as a portal vein and mislead the unwary investigator (Dewbury *et al.*, 1988).

Hepatic veins

There are normally three major hepatic veins, the right, middle, and left but any one of these major veins may be represented by two or more channels (Fig. 2.12, 2.13).

Identification of the hepatic veins is of relevance to confirm their presence, to exclude a diagnosis of Budd–Chiari syndrome, and to assess the vessels' diameters. The diameters are extremely variable, being particularly large in young females. In addition, if the examinations are performed during suspended inspiration, patients may involuntarily perform a Valsalva manoeuvre, causing further distension of the hepatic veins. Pathological distension of the hepatic veins occurs in patients with raised right-sided cardiac pressures and may be a clue to cardiac disease as a cause of hepatic decompensation in some patients.

The hepatic veins are rarely invaded by tumour

but this possibility should always be borne in mind when investigating patients with focal liver tumours in whom possible resection is being considered. More importantly the hepatic veins should be identified in tumour patients as a means of assessing the feasibility of segmentectomy. The major hepatic veins identify the margins between the hepatic segments and may permit the ultrasonographer to help the surgeon in planning his surgical approach.

THE LIVER LOBES

Surgeons divide the liver into two major lobes, the left and the right, and each of these into four segments (Dawson, 1985). Many of these divisions, particularly that between the superior and inferior segments of both lobes, are not discernible to the ultrasonologist. However, a full knowledge of the segmental anatomy of the liver is very important, both to help the surgeon in planning partial resections and to avoid misinterpretation caused by asymmetrical atrophy or hypertrophy of the various liver segments which may occur in different disease processes.

The major lobar anatomy of the liver is best seen on transverse ultrasound scans. The lateral segment of the left lobe lies to the left of the mid-line and is not difficult to identify. It is separated from the medial segment by the umbilical fissure, which is usually readily identified by the presence of the thick ligamentum teres within it (Fig. 2.14). The division between the right lobe and the medial segment of the left lobe is marked by the plane of the middle hepatic vein. This plane may be difficult to identify in those patients with more than one such vein. It should be noted that this division is always well to the right of the mid-line and that in most patients the entire medial segment of the left lobe is to the right of the patient's mid-line. A significant proportion of the lateral segment may also lie to the right of the mid-line.

The caudate lobe lies in the mid-line posterior to the left lobe, and anatomically it is a component of the left lobe. The caudate lobe is separated from the lateral segment of the left lobe by the fissure for the ligamentum venosum, which can almost invariably be seen clearly on transverse scans. Reference to Fig. 2.15 and 2.16 shows that the plane of the fissure for the ligamentum venosum may vary considerably from one patient to another, as indeed may the size and shape of the caudate lobe. If the fissure lies in the coronal plane it may also be well seen on longitudinal anterior mid-line scans (see Fig. 2.17), whereas if it lies obliquely to the coronal plane it may be difficult or impossible to detect in this view. In patients in whom the caudate lobe is well seen on anterior longitudinal scans it is important to identify it as a component of the liver and not to misinterpret it as a pathological mass. The apparent reflectivity of the parenchyma within the caudate lobe may sometimes be different from that of the adjacent liver. This is almost certainly due to some attenuation of the ultrasound beam within the fissure for the ligamentum venosum. This appearance must be dif-

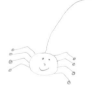

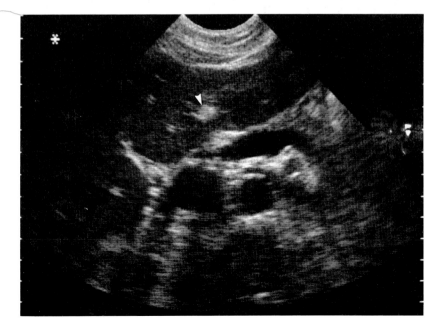

Fig. 2.14 Transverse scan in the mid-line showing the ligamentum teres (*arrow*), seen in cross-section within the left lobe of the liver.

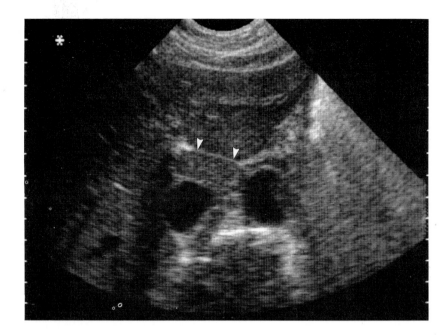

Fig. 2.15 Transverse scan in the midline showing the fissure for the ligamentum venosum (*arrows*) separating the lateral segment of the left lobe of the liver from the caudate lobe.

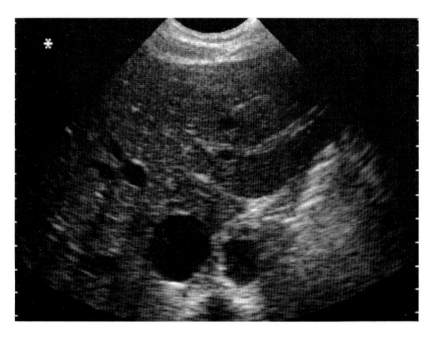

Fig. 2.16 Transverse scan showing the fissure for the ligamentum venosum. In this patient the fissure lies more obliquely to the transverse plane than that shown in Fig. 2.15, and would be difficult to image on longitudinal scans.

ferentiated from focal disease processes confined to the caudate lobe. This is seldom a major problem, as the majority of infiltrative processes also cause enlargement of the lobe. Disproportionate enlargement of the caudate lobe may also occur in patients with cirrhosis from different causes. In the Budd–Chiari syndrome the venous drainage of the caudate lobe may be preserved and the lobe may hypertrophy massively to more than 10 times its normal volume. In these circumstances the normal anatomy will be greatly distorted and care must be exercised to identify the lobe correctly and not misinterpret the finding as a pathological space-occupying lesion.

The right lobe of the liver is divided anatomically into anterior and posterior segments, each of which is subdivided into superior and inferior segments. The margins between these segments cannot be identified by clearly defined landmarks on ultrasound imaging. The quadrate lobe is really a lobule on the anterior inferior border of the right lobe of the liver. Pathologically it is not of any great significance but it is important for the ultrasonologist to be aware of its existence, since on some oc-

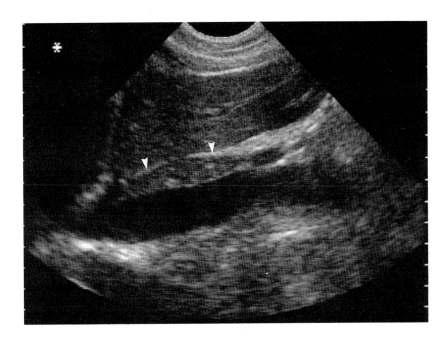

Fig. 2.17 Longitudinal scan over the IVC showing the fissure for the ligamentum venosum (*arrows*) throughout its length.

casions on longitudinal scans of the right lobe the quadrate may appear as an apparently separate subhepatic structure. Scans in two planes should always be performed in order to identify the area of attachment of the quadrate lobe to the right lobe and thus correctly identify its true nature. The quadrate lobe is also of importance to the diagnostic ultrasonologist, since it may be spared from generalized fatty infiltration of the liver and may therefore appear to be of much lower reflectivity than the remainder of the organ. Once again, careful surveying of the anatomy, together with knowledge of this phenomenon, will prevent an erroneous diagnosis.

Anatomists divide the liver slightly differently from surgeons; the surgical definition of the lobes has been used in this chapter, as the only indication for identifying the lobes and their segments is to advise the surgeon concerning resectability of focal lesions. Anatomists divide the left and right lobes at the plane of the umbilical fissure, thus making both the surgical medial segment of the left lobe and also the caudate lobe components of the right lobe rather than the left.

In a minority of patients there is an additional tongue-like process of liver extending inferiorly from the lateral margin of the right lobe, the so-called Riedel's lobe. This anatomical variant is commoner in females, and patients with this lobe may have an unusually small left lobe. The presence of a Riedel's lobe is of no pathological significance, but it may give rise to an incorrect clinical diag-

nosis of hepatomegaly, and on longitudinal scans may give a false impression of an enlarged right lobe. Ultrasound can usually correctly identify a Riedel's lobe by detecting the Riedel's branch of the right branch of the portal vein, which extends in a longitudinal direction inferiorly into the Riedel's lobe (Fig. 2.18).

Estimation of liver size

Patients are commonly referred for ultrasound for assessment of liver size. Unfortunately, in view of the variable size and shape of both liver and patients, the ultrasound assessment of liver size is entirely subjective, there being no single measurement which accurately reflects the size of the organ, although some have been proposed (Gosink & Leymaster, 1981).

Ultrasound may occasionally identify the presence of a very low right diaphragm, causing a normal sized liver to extend well down into the subcostal region and giving an erroneous clinical impression of hepatomegaly.

Although there is no dimensional measurement to indicate absolute liver size, several observations may indicate abnormal enlargement of the lobes (Cosgrove & Bark, 1983). Enlargement of the left lobe can be assessed by observing the angle at its inferior border and noting the shape of the inferior margin. The inferior angle should be sharp and less than 45°, and in the majority of patients the inferior border should be straight or concave (Fig.

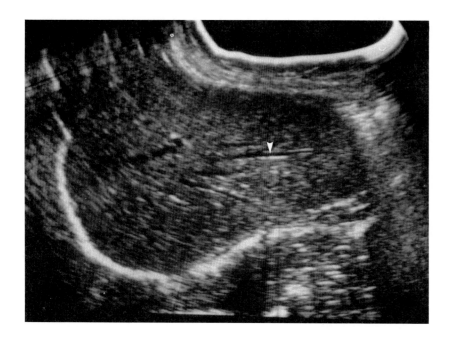

Fig. 2.18 Longitudinal scan along the long axis of a Riedel's lobe. The lobe appears as an inferior prolongation of the right lobe of the liver. The Riedel's lobe vein is well shown in this example (*arrow*).

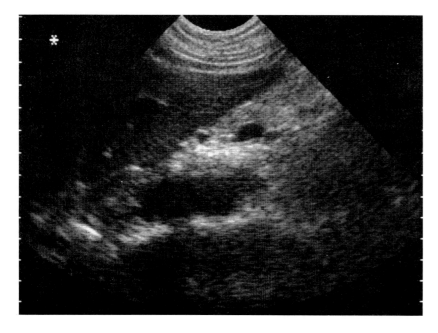

Fig. 2.19 Longitudinal scan to the left of the mid-line showing the acute inferior angle of the left lobe of the liver and the slightly concave inferior margin to the left lobe in this normal subject.

2.19). The caudate lobe, as seen on both longitudinal and transverse scans, should have a diameter no more than 50% of that of the AP diameter of the left lobe, anterior to it in the mid-line.

The size of the right lobe of the liver is more difficult to assess. The inferior angle should be sharp and less than 90°. The shape of the inferior border is very variable, but enlargement of the right lobe can sometimes be judged by observing the area of contact between the right lobe and the right kidney on longitudinal anterior scans. If the liver is normal in size the two organs will be in close apposition along approximately two-thirds of the anterior border of the right kidney (Fig. 2.20). If the liver is abnormally enlarged the area of contact extends inferiorly (Fig. 2.21).

It is possible, using the parallel planimetric method, to measure the liver size accurately with an error of significantly less than 5%. This technique requires the use of a manually operated static scanner, but although the method is accurate its main use has been in the research environment and it cannot realistically be applied in normal diagnostic practice (Leung *et al.*, 1986).

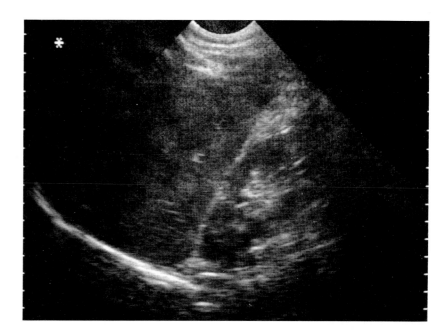

Fig. 2.20 Longitudinal scan of the right lobe showing the area of contact between the right lobe and the upper two-thirds of the right kidney.

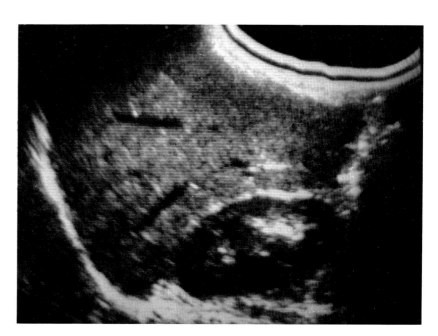

Fig. 2.21 Longitudinal scan of the right lobe of an enlarged liver that is in contact with the right kidney throughout approximately 95% of the renal length.

Conclusion

Careful attention to equipment selection, control of settings, and the normal shape and appearances of the organ should enable the experienced ultrasound equipment operator to survey close to 100% of the liver volume, to make a subjective assessment of size, and to diagnose or exclude focal lesions. Diffuse liver disease is more difficult to diagnose, but abnormal parenchymal architecture, with or without an increase in parenchymal reflec-

tivity, may be a useful guide to the presence of diffuse disease.

References

Bellamy, E.H., Bossi, M.C. & Cosgrove, D.O. (1984) Ultrasound demonstration of changes in the normal portal venous system following a meal. *British Journal of Radiology*, **57**, 147–149.

Cosgrove, D.O. & Bark, M. (1983) Ultrasound in the diagnosis of liver disease. In Herlinger, H. *et al.* (eds.) *Clinical Radiology of the Liver*, p. 193. Marcel Dekker, New York.

Dawson, J.L. (1985) In Wright, R. *et al.* (ed.) *Liver and Biliary Disease*, pp. 6–8. Baillieré Tindall, London.

Dewbury, K.C. & Clark, B.E. (1979) The accuracy of ultrasound diagnosis in the detection of cirrhosis of the liver. *British Journal of Radiology*, **52**, 945.

Dewbury, K.C., Meire, H.B. & Cosgrove, D.O. (1988) In Farrant, P. (ed) *Ultrasound Teaching Cases*, Vol. 2, pp. 25, 39. Wiley, Chichester.

Foster, K.J., Dewbury, K.C., Griffith, A.H. & Wright, R. (1980) The accuracy of ultrasound in the detection of fatty infiltration of the liver. *British Journal of Radiology*, **53**, 440.

Gosink, B.B. & Leymaster, C.E. (1981) Ultrasonic determination of hepatomegaly. *Journal of Clinical Ultrasound*, **9**, 37–41.

Kane, R.A. & Katz, S.G. (1982) The spectrum of sonographic findings in portal hypertension: a subject review and new observations. *Radiology*, **142**, 453–458.

Kauzlaric, D., Petrovic, M. & Barmeir, E. (1984) Sonography of cavernous transformation of the portal vein. *American Journal of Roentgenology*, **142**, 383–384.

Kurtz, A.B., Rubin, C.S., Cooper H.S. Nisenbaum, H.L., Cole-Beuglet, C., Medoff, J. & Goldberg, B.B. (1980) Ultrasonic findings in hepatitis. *Radiology*, **136**, 717–723.

Leung, N.W.Y., Farrant, P. & Peters, T.J. (1986) Liver volume measurements by ultrasonography in normal subjects and alcoholic patients. *Journal of Hepatology*, **2**, 157–164.

Meire, H.B., Dewbury, K.C. & Cosgrove, D.O. (1987) In Farrant, P. (ed) *Ultrasound Teaching Cases*, 2nd edn. Vol. 1, p. 11. Wiley, Chichester.

3: Computerized Tomography Scanning of the Normal Liver

D.E. KATZ

Introduction

The reliability and accuracy of computerized tomography (CT) in the detection of liver lesions may be greatly influenced by the technique of scanning, available equipment and the expertise of the radiologist. For optimum results each scan should be tailored to the individual patient's needs and scans should be planned, monitored and checked by the radiologist as the examination progresses. Active monitoring with all the clinical details available provides the flexibility to modify, extend or terminate examinations at the optimum time.

Technique

In general when the liver is of primary interest, slices of 10 mm thickness are taken at 8 mm intervals from the dome of the diaphragm to beyond the inferior margin. Decisions are made about contrast enhancement after review of the unenhanced scans. Scans should be viewed and imaged at a viewing console that allows manipulation of the image. It is important to view liver images at narrow window widths (80−200 Hounsfield units) to increase the contrast and accentuate the relative attenuation differences between normal and abnormal liver tissue.

Plain CT

The liver parenchyma is normally homogenous, with attenuation values varying between 40 and 70 Hounsfield units on unenhanced scans (Baert *et al.*, 1980). Normal liver parenchyma is at least as dense, and usually denser, than blood and other solid organs. The vessels are seen as low-attenuation areas within the liver substance. Vessels can be recognized by their characteristic shape, distribution and density. Depending on their axis relative to the CT plane, vessels may be linear, ovoid, circular, or branching. Hepatic veins

may be recognized in the superior portion of the liver, converging towards the inferior vena cava. Most of the vessels seen are portal branches arising from the porta hepatis. Hepatic arteries and bile ducts are smaller and make only a minor contribution to recorded images (Haaga & Alfidi, 1983).

Dilated intrahepatic bile ducts may be difficult to distinguish from portal veins on plain scans. When contrast is given it is taken up by vessels and the vessels become homogenous or denser than the rest of the liver parenchyma. Bile ducts are unaffected by contrast and remain as low-density areas in a liver increased in density by the contrast (Fig. 3.1).

The density and homogeneity of the liver parenchyma may be altered by a number of extraneous causes and artefacts. The density of the most superior part of the liver may be artificially reduced by a contribution from the overlying lung tissue in the section: the partial volume effect. Streak artefacts may be superimposed on the liver and may arise from the interface between gas and contrast material in the stomach, from materials of very high or low density, especially when associated with movement during the exposure, or from inconsistencies in the X-ray beam as it is attenuated through the body tissue (McCullough, 1977).

Radiologists must be familiar with the appearance of these artefacts so that they are not misinterpreted as liver lesions.

Contrast

The effects of contrast on the liver image depend on the concentration of contrast in the various liver compartments at the time of scanning. This is plainly directly related to the quantity, concentration of iodine, and rate of delivery of the intravenous fluid. Injected blood arrives at the liver initially via the hepatic artery and portal vein. Scans taken very soon after injection show the vessels to be considerably denser than the rest of

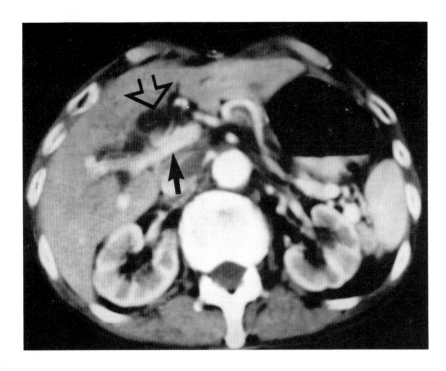

Fig. 3.1 Bolus injection of contrast allows easy differentiation between vessels (*closed arrow*) and dilated ducts (*open arrow*).

the hepatic parenchyma. Maximum arterial opacification lasts for about 20 s and maximum venous opacification occurs later in the first minute. There is rapid accumulation of contrast in both vascular and extravascular compartments, and overall maximum enhancement is seen in the first minute. Over the next few minutes the vascular density declines, while the parenchymal density remains relatively stable. Eventually vessels become isodense with the liver substance and opacification is largely due to extravascular contrast.

There has been much debate about which CT technique is most accurate when evaluating focal liver lesions. Opinion has been divided as to whether i.v. contrast should be used at all, and if so how much iodine should be injected. Various techniques of administration (bolus, drip infusion, or a combination of both) and times of scanning (immediately or delayed) have been tried. Early reports indicated that many lesions seen on unenhanced scans could be missed after contrast (Moss *et al.*, 1979). These results were almost certainly due to the time taken for scanning and the equipment limitations. Several authors have suggested that rapid administration of a large volume of contrast coupled with rapid sequential CT provides a very accurate method for the detection of liver lesions (Foley *et al.*, 1983; Moss *et al.*, 1982). This technique is probably the most practical for general evaluation.

Although only a small percentage of lesions not

seen on unenhanced scans will become visible, a significant percentage are more clearly displayed, improving the diagnostic confidence (Berland *et al.*, 1982) (Fig. 3.2). The key to the technique is the evaluation of the whole of the liver within 3–4 min after injection. This is the time when the greatest concentration of iodine is present within the intravascular spaces of the liver, creating the largest contrast–density difference between normal and diseased tissue. At longer times and with slow rates of injection, renal excretion of iodine and loss into the extravascular spaces decreases the contrast between normal and abnormal tissue.

There are techniques that have been shown to be more accurate than dynamic sequential hepatic CT but these are not practical for routine use. CT angiography with direct intra-arterial injection appears to show more lesions but is cumbersome, invasive, and expensive. While the routine use of this technique is obviously limited, it may be considered prior to hepatic resections (Freeny & Marks, 1983). Delayed-interval CT scanning has also been used to detect hepatic lesions. The liver secretes some (1–2%) of the iodine load into the biliary system. Delayed-interval CT requires at least 60 g of iodine to obtain a 20-Hounsfield density difference between pre- and post-contrast scans done 4–6 h after injection. Focal liver lesions do not secrete iodine and are seen as areas of reduced attenuation in a liver of increased density. When there is biliary obstruction however, the

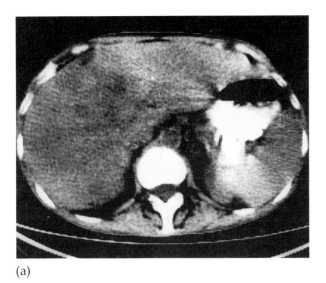 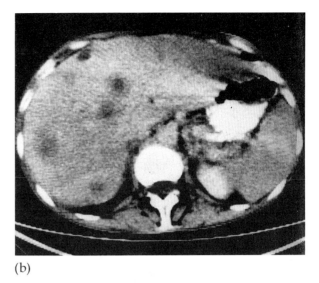

(a)   (b)

Fig. 3.2 Metastasis shown much more clearly after contrast administration.

technique is less useful, as normal liver function has been altered. Increases in detection of focal lesions of up to 25% have been reported with this technique (Bernardino *et al.*, 1986).

Other techniques using hepatic-specific contrast agents such as iodinated lipid compounds and colloid-based agents such as ethiodized oil emulsion (EOE−13) have also demonstrated increased sensitivity for focal lesion detection. Intravenous administration of these agents, which are phagocytosed by the reticuloendothelial cells of the liver and spleen, opacifies the normal parenchyma without affecting the abnormal foci. At the time of writing, these agents are not commercially available for routine clinical use, although they hold promise for the future not only in the detection of hepatic metastases but especially in the staging of lymphomas, which hitherto have been a relatively blind spot for CT assessment (Vermess *et al.*, 1980; Lamarque *et al.*, 1979).

Disorders detected by CT

Focal lesions

The true accuracy of CT in detection of focal lesions cannot be established because it is not possible to conduct pathological examinations on all livers. Available evidence suggests that CT is highly accurate but not infallible in detecting focal lesions when modern scanners, careful technique and skilled interpretation are employed.

Since the introduction of CT, several attempts have been made to evaluate its efficiency compared with other procedures. Technical advances have been so rapid in all imaging modalities that studies comparing the various methods of hepatic imaging tend to be out of date as soon as they are published. (Biello *et al.*, 1978, Bryan *et al.*, 1977, Snow *et al.*, 1979, Petasnick *et al.*, 1979). Variations in equipment, technical ability, interpretative skill, and enthusiasm for a particular technique are such that results obtained are often variable between different institutions. The inherent limitations of the various modalities are well known and practical consideration will often determine the choice of modality. Nuclear medicine, ultrasound, magnetic resonance imaging, and CT all derive their images from different properties of tissue, and it is often worthwhile to obtain complementary information from more than one method (Fig. 3.3).

No criteria allow absolute distinction of benign from malignant or primary from secondary liver disease. Experience with bolus techniques has allowed characteristic patterns of enhancement to be recognized in both benign and malignant liver tumours, which help in their differentiation (Barrett *et al.*, 1980, Itai *et al.*, 1981, Marchal *et al.*, 1980) (Fig. 3.4). As with ultrasound, CT is usually accurate in the differentiation of benign cysts from other focal liver disease. A visibly thick wall, diffuse or focal in extent, mural nodules, septations or non-homogenous fluid content, or enhancement of the wall post-contrast, should alert one to the possibility that something other than benign disease may be present.

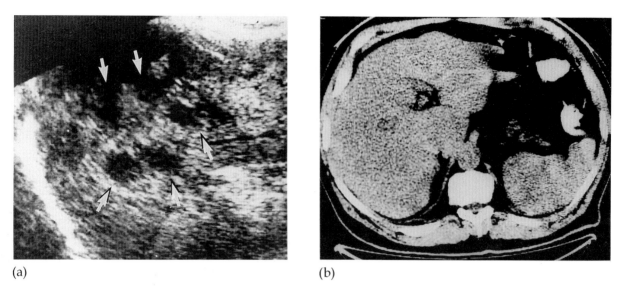

(a)   (b)

Fig. 3.3 Obvious metastases on ultrasound (a) (*arrowed*) may be difficult to appreciate on unenhanced CT scans (b). The liver margins are irregular, however.

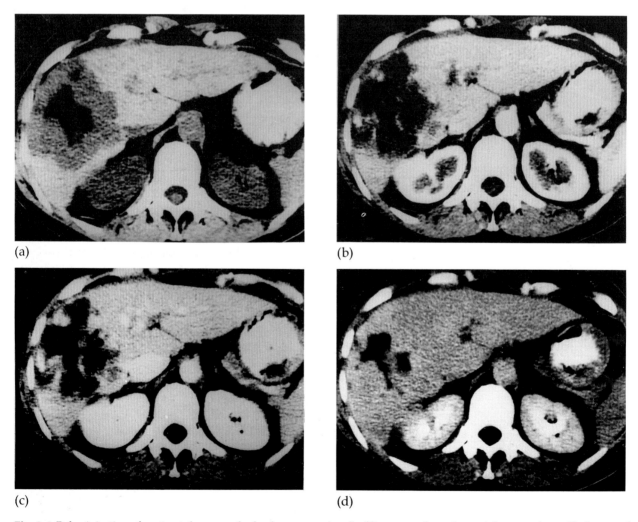

(a)   (b)

(c)   (d)

Fig. 3.4 Bolus injection of contrast shows gradual enhancement (a–d) of liver mass from the periphery, and opacified parts of tumour eventually become isodense with the uninvolved hepatic parenchyma. This type of enhancement is specific for cavernous haemangioma.

Diffuse disease

As a rule, CT is of less value in assessing diffuse parenchymal liver disease than focal lesions. The appearance of diffuse parenchymal disease is very variable, depending on the aetiology and severity of involvement. Acute hepatitis for example will produce no change in density or contour of the liver, although varying degrees of hepatomegaly may be present. Generalized alteration in size and configuration is readily appreciated on CT. The late stages of post-hepatic cirrhosis for example are usually quite apparent, showing marked alterations in contour as well as segmental areas of atrophy or regeneration (Lee *et al.*, 1983).

Disorders that alter the density (attenuation) values of the liver are easily assessed. Reduced attenuation due to fatty infiltration is seen in a variety of conditions and the infiltrate may affect the whole liver or only parts of it (Fig. 3.5). With

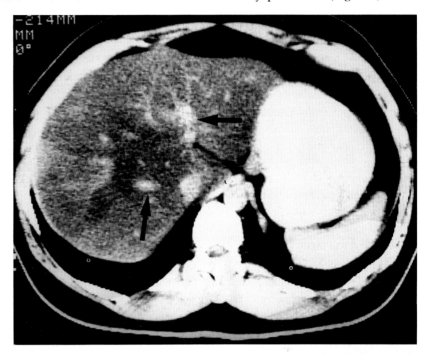

Fig. 3.5 Diffuse fatty infiltration of the liver. The vessels are seen as areas of increased density in the liver parenchyma, which is a reverse of the normal.

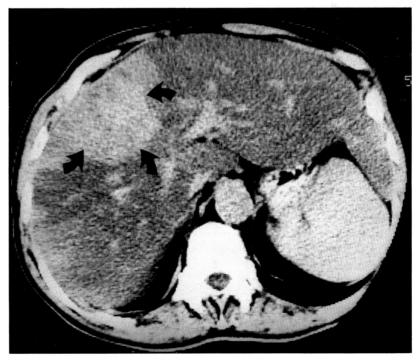

Fig. 3.6 Hepatoma (*arrowed*) in a fatty liver in a patient with cirrhosis.

fatty infiltration the affected liver has a density less than the other solid organs such as the spleen. Mild degrees of fatty infiltration may be subtle and not appreciated unless comparative density measurements are made with the spleen. While values vary widely between individuals, for a given subject the liver is normally 6–12 Hounsfield units denser than the spleen. Where this ratio is altered, fatty infiltration is likely to be present (Piekarski et al., 1980). In more advanced cases the vessels stand out as areas of increased density when compared to the liver parenchyma, which is a reverse of the normal. Focal areas of fatty infiltration tend to be lobar or segmental in distribution and the vessels within the area tend to be undistorted. Irregular fat distribution can resemble neoplastic change, and where doubt exists guided needle biopsies will resolve the dilemma (Fig. 3.6).

When quantitative assessment of infiltration is being measured it must be remembered that the CT numbers will be altered by the scanning techniques. A significant difference in readings will exist on scans performed at 120 kVp from those done at 80 kVP (Haaga & Alfidi, 1983). The importance of identical technique when doing comparative studies is obvious.

Finally, in addition to the quantitative and qualitative information that has been discussed, the information about surrounding changes accompanying liver disease such as ascites, splenomegaly or lymphadenopathy, or changes in surrounding organs, considerably increases the radiologist's potential for accurate diagnosis of disease processes involving the liver.

References

Baert, A.L., Wackenheim, A. & Jeanmart, L. (1980) Abdominal Computer Tomography. Springer-Verlag, New York.

Barnett, P.H., Zerhouni, E.A., White, R.I. Jr. & Siegelman, S.S. (1980) Computed tomography in the diagnosis of cavernous haemangioma of the liver. American Journal of Radiology, 134, 439–447.

Berland, L.L., Lawson, T.L., Foley, W.D. Melrose, B.L., Chintapalli, K.N. & Taylor, A.J. (1982) Comparison of pre- and post-contrast CT scans in hepatic masses. American Journal of Roentgenology, 138, 853–858.

Bernardino, M.E., Erwin, B.C., Steinberg, H.V., Baumgartner B.R., Torres, W.E. & Gedgaudas-McClees, R.K. (1986) Delayed hepatic C.T. scanning: increased confidence and improved detection of hepatic metastases. Radiology, 159, 71–74.

Biello, D.R., Levitt, R.G., Siegel, B.A., Sagel, S.S. & Stanley, R.J. (1978) Computed tomography and radionuclide imaging of the liver: a comparative evaluation. Radiology, 127, 159–163.

Bryan, P.J., Dinn, W.M., Grossman, Z.D., Wistow, B.W., McAfee, J.G. & Kieffer, S.A. (1977) Correlation of computed tomography, gray scale ultrasonography and radionuclide imaging of the liver in detecting space occupying processes. Radiology, 124, 387–393.

Foley, W.D., Berland, L.L., Lawson, T.L., Smith, D.F. & Thorsen, M.K. (1983) Contrast enhancement technique for dynamic hepatic computed tomographic scanning. Radiology, 147, 797–803.

Freeny, P.C. & Marks, W.M. (1983) Computed tomographic arteriography of the liver. Radiology, 148, 193–197.

Haaga, J.R. & Alfidi, R.J. (1983) Computed Tomography of the Whole Body. C.V. Mosby, Toronto.

Itai, Y., Araki, T., Furui, S. & Tasaka, A. (1981) Differential diagnosis of hepatic masses on computed tomography with particular reference to hepatocellular carcinoma. Journal of Computer Assisted Tomography, 5, 834–842.

Lamarque, J.L., Bruel, J.M., Dondelinger, R., Vendrell, B. Pelissier, O., Rouanet, J.P., Michel, J.L. & Boulet, P. (1979) The use of iodolipids in hepatosplenic computed tomography. Journal of Computer Assisted Tomography, 3, 21–24.

Lee, J.K.T., Sagel, S.S. & Stanley, R.J. (1983) Computed Body Tomography. Raven Press, New York.

McCullough, E.C. (1977) Factors affecting the use of quantitative information from a C.T. scanner. Radiology, 124, 99–107.

Marchal, G.J., Baert, A.L. & Wilms, G.E. (1980) CT of non cystic liver lesions: Bolus enhancement. American Journal of Radiology, 135, 57–65.

Moss, A.A., Dean, P.B., Axel, L., Goldberg, H.I., Glazer, G.M. & Friedman, M.A. (1982) Dynamic CT of hepatic masses with intravenous and intra-arterial contrast material. American Journal of Radiology, 138, 847–852.

Moss, A.A., Schrumpt, J., Schnyder, P., Korobkin, M. & Shimshak, R.R. (1979) Computed tomography of focal hepatic lesions: a blind clinical evaluation of the effect of contrast enhancement. Radiology, 131, 427–430.

Petasnick, J.P., Ram, P. Turner, D.A. & Fordham, E.W. (1979) The relationship of computed tomography, gray-scale ultrasonography and radionuclide imaging in the evaluation of hepatic masses. Seminars in Nuclear Medicine, 9, 8–21.

Piekarski, J., Goldberg, H.I., Royal, S.A., Axel, L. & Moss, A.A. (1980). Difference between liver and spleen CT numbers in the normal adult: its usefulness in predicting the presence of diffuse liver disease. Radiology, 137, 727–729.

Snow, J.H., Goldstein, H.M. & Wallace, S. (1979) Comparison of scintigraphy sonography and computed tomography in the evaluation of hepatic neoplasms. American Journal of Roentgenology, 132, 915–918.

Vermess, M., Doppman, J.L., Sugarbaker, P., Fisher, R.I., Chatterji, D.C., Leutzeler, J., Grimes, G., Girton, M. et al. (1980) Clinical trials with a new intravenous liposoluble contrast material for computed tomography of the liver and spleen. Radiology, 137, 217–220.

4: Radionuclide Liver Imaging

D.M. ACKERY AND V.B. BATTY

Introduction

Liver disease can be categorized by a variety of laboratory, imaging and tissue-sampling procedures. Investigations should be selected to follow a logical progression so that a correct diagnosis is made with the least inconvenience to the patient, and for the lowest cost. Imaging investigations used for hepatic disease differ in their capability to answer a particular clinical question. Radionuclide imaging provides a sensitive assessment of regional function and morphology, although it cannot compete with the anatomical resolution of ultrasound and computed tomography. It has the advantages of availability, convenience, and relatively low cost, and its interpretation is not subject to the expertise to the operator. Following intravenous administration of a radiopharmaceutical, uptake by the liver depends both upon hepatic and portal regional blood flow and extraction by liver cells. The time course of uptake and retention by the liver can be quantified to give indices of total or regional hepatic function. Despite the fact that radionuclide techniques rely upon regional function for their success, the diagnostic value often comes from changes in the morphological appearances of the images.

The clinical value of radionuclide imaging needs to be considered independently for focal and diffuse hepatic disease. In general it is sensitive (low false-negative rate) for the detection of focal liver conditions such as metastases, cysts, and abscesses (Clarke et al., 1986), but it has a low diagnostic specificity, i.e. it cannot distinguish between the different causes for a focal defect. Usually radionuclide imaging has little to offer in the differential diagnosis of diffuse hepatic conditions. It is limited in comparison with other imaging procedures which can show the structural relationship of the liver to other abdominal organs. These drawbacks restrict radionuclide imaging for many patients with suspected liver disease, although it continues to have a place when alternative procedures are not available or are overloaded by demand. It also has a supporting role when other investigations give an equivocal result, or fail for technical reasons. Certain special techniques are unique to radionuclide methodology, e.g. measurement of relative hepatic blood flow.

Liver physiology

The concentration of radioactive pharmaceuticals by the liver is a function of both hepatic vascular perfusion and cellular extraction. The product of these factors is termed the *effective hepatic blood flow*.

Of the two afferent vascular supplies to the liver, the hepatic artery supplies approximately 25–30% of total blood flow and 50% of available oxygen. The portal vein, draining from the splanchnic region and spleen, is responsible for the remaining proportion, but is relatively deficient in oxygen content. Both systems mix at the level of the hepatic lobule, and blood passes via the hepatic veins into the inferior vena cava. Variations in vascular structure are common. Pathological conditions such as hepatic fibrosis (cirrhosis) impede the normal flow of blood through the liver giving increased pressure in the portal system, with engorgement of the spleen and development of collateral venous return to the heart, and the development of varices. Thrombosis of the portal vein gives few constitutional symptoms, and ligation or embolization of the hepatic artery, which may be used as a therapeutic measure, does not usually result in hepatic necrosis.

The liver macrophages or reticuloendothelial cells (Kupffer cells) comprise about 2% of the hepatic cellular volume. Their position as endothelial cells, adjacent to the lumen of the vascular sinusoids, permits effective removal of colloid particles from the circulation. Normal extraction

31

efficiency is about 80—90%, and a colloid size of 200—500 nm appears to be optimal for liver imaging. Uptake may be reduced by impairment of either blood flow or Kupffer-cell function. In normal individuals 5—10% of radiocolloid is localized in the spleen, with a small percentage in bone marrow and other sites of reticuloendothelial cell function, but these levels are usually insufficient for diagnostic imaging with a gamma camera. There is a theoretical correlation between size of colloid and uptake at sites of reticuloendothelial function. The largest particles tend to localize in the spleen, smaller particles in the liver and the smallest are taken up in the bone marrow. For a known colloid size, excessive uptake in the spleen or visualization of the bone marrow in an otherwise technically satisfactory liver image, is a pathological finding to be discussed in later chapters.

Hepatocytes (large polygonal cells) comprise 80—90% of the parenchymal volume of the human liver. These are metabolically active, and responsible for the passage of dyes and other chemicals into bile. Function is impaired by inflammation and obstructive jaundice.

Instrumentation

Nowadays a gamma camera is almost always used for radionuclide imaging. This consists of a collimated sodium iodide crystal in which gamma photons interact and are converted into light photons. These in turn are detected by an array of photomultipliers, which convert the information into a set of electronic signals. These signals provide the co-ordinate data for each gamma interaction and the number of interactions at that position in the crystal. As detection events occur in the camera these are recorded on an oscilloscope, and gradually build up an image of the distribution of activity within the patient.

The lead collimator in front of the disc of sodium iodide ensures that only gamma photons perpendicular to the face of the crystal enter and are detected, and the diameter and length of the collimator holes dictate the spatial resolution of the system. Electronic analysis rejects the recording of those gamma photons which are not within a predetermined energy range. This effectively avoids all scattered photons (or reduced energy) which otherwise would lead to impairment of image resolution.

By the very nature of the principle of action of the gamma camera there is reciprocal relationship between spatial resolution and detector sensitivity. The consequence of this is that resolution can be improved only at the expense of reduced count-rate, or if this is unacceptable, with greater administered activities of radionuclide with consequent higher radiation doses to the patient.

Emitted photon energies of between 100 and 300 keV are optimal for the gamma camera, as at this energy range the sensitivity of the scintillation crystal is greatest, and scatter of photons within the patient is not too great. Radionuclides for gamma camera imaging are chosen with photon emission within this range, and preferably with a radioactive half-life measured in hours and with no beta-particle emission, so that patient radiation doses are minimized.

Most images are taken with the gamma camera viewing the anterior, posterior or lateral aspect of the patient — so-called *planar imaging*. This is in most cases adequate for routine imaging of patients with hepatic disease, although lesions lying deep within the liver may be missed. In these circumstances some improvement in diagnostic sensitivity may be gained by the use of *single-photon emission tomography*. For this procedure the gamma camera is set up to rotate around the patient, and digital images are stored for several incremental angles within the 360° rotation. These images are analysed by a back-projection algorithm similar to that used for transmission computerized tomography, but requiring a correction for attenuation of the gamma photon as it traverses the patient's tissues. The final images are viewed as a series of transaxial slices of radionuclide distribution.

Positron emission tomography

This is a specialized technique in which radiopharmaceuticals are labelled with positron-emitting radionuclides. The positron is a positive electron which decays with the emission of two gamma photons each of 510 keV. These are emitted in directly opposite directions to each other. They are detected by a specially designed scintillation detector with precisely opposed and collimated crystals, which record a signal only within the very short time interval of the coincidence of the detection of the pair of gamma photons. The advantage of such a system is that radionuclides of many of the common biological elements — carbon, oxygen and nitrogen — can be used with theoretically a considerably wider choice of radiopharmaceuticals. Also, improved resolution and absolute quantification of uptake is possible. This type of imaging has been valuable in establishing fundamental physiological principles of blood flow, oxygen consumption, and metabolic turnover, but is expensive and not appropriate for routine diagnostic imaging. It has been used little in the investigation of the liver.

Reticuloendothelial imaging

A number of different colloid preparations are commercially available as pharmaceutically approved products. The usual radioactive label is ^{99m}technetium. There are no clinical contraindications to the investigation. No special preparation of the patient is necessary.

In Britain, levels are laid down by the Administration of Radioactive Substances Committee (ARSAC) of the Department of Health for the usual administration for radionuclide clinical studies. For adult hepatic imaging the maximum usual activity per test is 80 MBq, which gives an effective whole-body equivalent absorbed radiation dose of one mSv. The radiocolloid is administered intravenously, and imaging is commenced after 15 min, when maximum clearance by the reticuloendothelial system is achieved. The patient may be imaged standing or lying, and views are taken from the anterior, posterior, and right and left lateral projections, the liver having been centred in the field of the gamma camera for each view, using a storage oscilloscope display for positioning. Usually 500—1000 thousand counts are obtained per image, and each view takes approximately 2 min to acquire.

Anatomical landmarks should be recorded on the final image and should include the lower costal margin in the anterior and right lateral projections, and the bisection of the mid-axillary line with the costal edge should be marked so that a reference co-ordinate can be given for needle biopsy. When a radioactive marker source is used it is preferable to record these landmarks on a second film so that image detail is not obscured by the marker. The abdomen is palpated before the patient is moved from the gamma camera, so that the position of the hepatic edge and of any abdominal masses is recorded. The position of discrete focal masses may be marked on the patient's skin as a guide to biopsy.

If image resolution is impaired due to diaphragmatic movement over the period of acquisition,

re-imaging at repeated breath-hold may be carried out, or if digital recording is available, by respiratory gating of the acquired data using an electronic triggering circuit. Occasionally oblique views may assist in the identification of lesions not shown by conventional views.

Data is acquired onto a digital computer following a bolus injection of radiopharmaceutical to give an activity—time curve of the arrival of tracer in the liver, or when subtraction techniques are used for multiple isotope studies. Digital analysis is usually unnecessary for the interpretation of the routine colloid image, although quantification of the uptake ratio between spleen and liver can be used to follow changes in function in diffuse hepatic disease.

The effective perfusion rate of the liver can be determined from a mathematical model. This shows that the *rate* of uptake is the same at each site of radiocolloid accumulation (whether hepatic or extrahepatic), and that the relative effective perfusion rates can only be given by the equilibrium plateau values at the individual sites (Karran et al., 1974). Rapid data acquisition following bolus injection can also be used to separate the hepatic and portal arrival of activity, and to determine the relative contribution of each to hepatic perfusion (Fleming et al., 1983). The hepatic:portal ratio of flow may be increased in gastrointestinal malignancy before metastases are evident in the liver (Leveson et al., 1983).

Radionuclide techniques have also been used to assess flow in percutanous hepatic arterial catheters implanted for the direct perfusion of hepatic metastases with chemotherapeutic and other agents (Borzutsky & Turbiner, 1985). The hepatic perfusion pattern is shown by the injection of ^{99m}technetium-labelled microspheres or macroaggregated particles which can then be visualized by conventional planar imaging or single-photon emission tomography (Ziessman et al., 1985).

Normal appearances

Based on functional criteria the liver is a bilobed organ, the division between the right and left lobes being based on blood supply and biliary drainage. The radioisotope image often shows a clear division at the attachment of the falciform ligament, but this should not be confused with the true anatomical separation of the lobes. The right lobe is contained by the rib cage and right hemidiaphragm, and variations in these will affect its

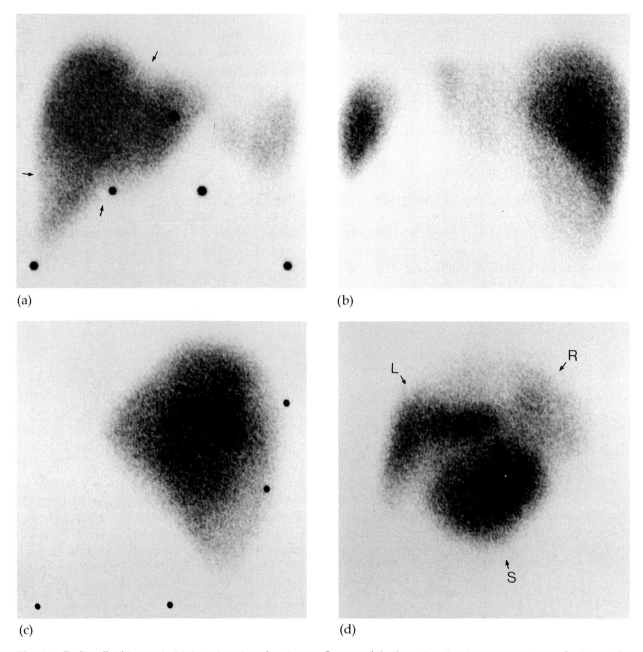

Fig. 4.1 (Radiocolloid images). (a) Anterior view showing confluence of the hepatic veins (*arrow*, superior surface), costal impression (*arrow*, lateral surface), and gall bladder fossa (*arrow*, inferior surface). (b) Posterior view showing on the right the liver with the right renal impression on the inferior surface, and on the left the spleen. (c) Right lateral view of the liver. Markers indicate the costal margin. (d) Left lateral view. R and L indicate right and left lobes of the liver; S is the spleen.

morphological appearance (Fig. 4.1). The lower costal edge can impress the liver so that a linear defect is shown in the right lateral image, and with hepatic enlargement the lower right lobe can often be seen to extend laterally where it is released from the constraint of the thoracic cage. The medial segment of the left lobe is thin, and shows in the left lateral view as a leaf of tissue which projects downwards and anteriorly. Abnormalities of the diaphragm affect the contour of the superior surface of the right lobe. Patients with chronic obstructive airways disease may be referred for radionuclide imaging because the liver is palpable. Often these patients have displacement of the liver from hyperinflation of the lungs, rather than true hepatomegaly.

Several morphological variants of the liver may confuse image interpretation (McAfee *et al.*, 1965).

A palpable mass may be present due to a Reidel's lobe (Fig. 4.2), or the normal hepatic contour may be distorted by compression from adjacent organs. The confluence of the portal vein, bile ducts, and hepatic artery, the *porta hepatis*, may show prominently as a 'cold' region at the junction of the right and left lobes, particularly with extrahepatic biliary obstruction. The gall bladder, especially when enlarged, may indent the inferior surface of the right lobe. Enlargement of the right kidney can impress the posterior surface of the right lobe, causing anterior and caudal displacement, giving a characteristic appearance to the right lateral image. The confluence of the hepatic veins at the cephalic attachment of the falciform ligament can notch the upper hepatic border. Attenuation of counts by breast tissue in female patients may give non-uniformity in the image. (Fig. 4.3). Awareness of such variations minimizes the risk of false-positive interpretation of the images.

Hepatobiliary imaging

Hepatocyte function is utilized when radionuclide investigation of the biliary tract is necessary. [99m]Technetium-labelled chemical derivatives of iminodiacetic acid (IDA) are most suitable for routine clinical use, and give good images of the biliary tract even when bilirubin levels are elevated (Schwarzrock *et al.*, 1986). Radiolabelled rose bengal and bromsulphthalein (BSP) have been used in the past, but these agents must be labelled with radioiodine rather than [99m]technetium and thus give higher absorbed radiation doses to the patient.

Hepatobiliary imaging is used to show intermittent extrahepatic obstruction (when ultrasound may reveal no evidence of duct dilatation), to assess patency of ducts or stents after surgery, and to demonstrate biliary leaks after surgery or trauma. It is both sensitive and specific for the diagnosis of acute cholecystitis, when cystic duct obstruction prevents the flow of activity into the gall bladder (Hall *et al.*, 1981).

IDA agents are available as commercial kits which are readily radiolabelled with [99m]technetium. An intravenous administration of 150 MBq gives an effective whole-body equivalent absorbed radiation dose of 3 mSv. Concentration by hepatocytes is rapid, and with normal function biliary secretion takes place promptly. Images are acquired with the patient supine at 15 min intervals for the first hour. When activity fails to pass into

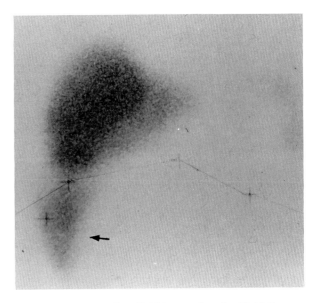

Fig. 4.2 Anterior radiocolloid image showing Reidel's extension of the right lobe of the liver (*arrow*) — a normal variant.

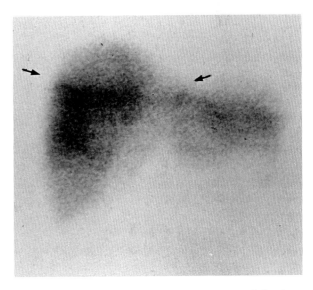

Fig. 4.3 Anterior radiocolloid image. Apparent defect in the upper right hepatic lobe due to attenuation by the overlying breast (*arrows*).

the intestine, or when no concentration is perceived in the gall bladder, biliary flow is encouraged by the administration of milk or other cholegogues and further images obtained at 30 min intervals as necessary. Late examination up to 24 h may be required if bile transit is severely impaired. Overnight fasting is recommended when gall bladder function is being assessed, but is not necessary for the investigation of biliary obstruction.

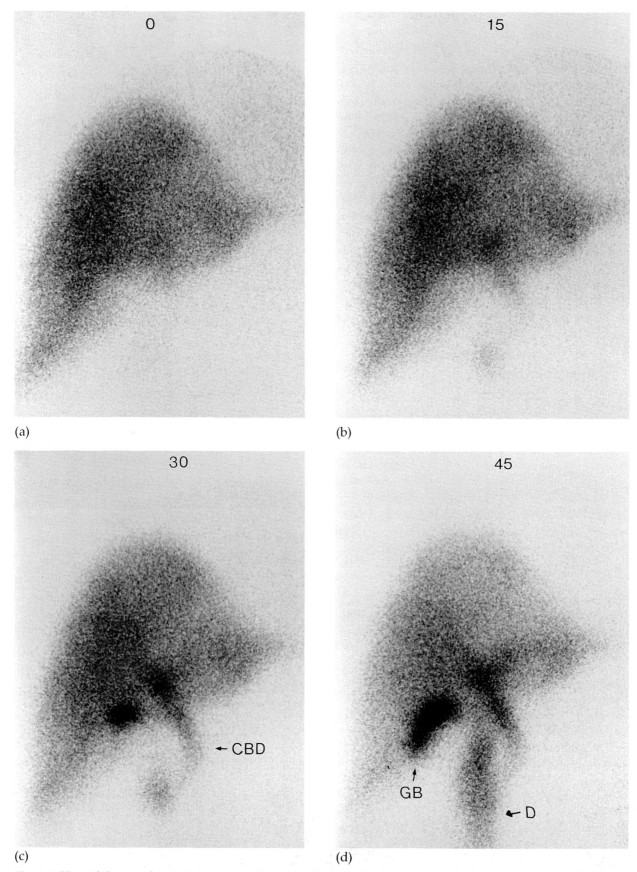

Fig. 4.4 (Hepatobiliary study). Anterior images show normal transit of activity through the liver parenchymal cells into the biliary tree and intestine over 45 min (GB, gall bladder; CBD, common bile duct; D, duodenum).

Normal appearances

The high photon flux available with [99m]technetium ensures perception of the main bile ducts and gall bladder and enables flow of bile into the duodenum to be demonstrated. When function is normal, activity shows in the liver parenchyma 5 min after injection, after which there is progressive clearance from the liver as the radiopharmaceutical is excreted into the biliary tract. The main hepatic ducts, gall bladder, common bile duct and duodenum are usually perceived within 30 min, and the study is complete by 1 h, by which time much of the activity is in the small bowel (Fig. 4.4).

Biliary radiopharmaceuticals are cleared to a small extent from the blood stream by the kidneys and this is greater when the patient is jaundiced. Activity in the renal tract may be misinterpreted as being in the gall bladder or intestine. In some patients, activity in the duodenal loop may overlie the gall bladder. Misinterpretation can be avoided by the use of oblique or lateral views.

Other radionuclide hepatic imaging procedures

The lack of diagnostic specificity of radiocolloid liver imaging has encouraged a search for alternative agents which might concentrate in focal hepatic lesions.

[67]Gallium

This agent has shown its greatest promise in the identification of primary hepatocellular carcinoma. Reports suggest that over 90% of tumours show positive uptake, whereas less than 50% of metastases accumulate gallium. The precise mechanism of uptake is unknown. An adult intravenous dose of 150 MBq is followed by imaging at 48−72 h. Physiological accumulation is shown in normal liver tissue and bone marrow, and frequently large intestinal uptake is also observed. Bowel cleansing with laxatives or enema is usually required for proper interpretation of [67]gallium images.

[75]Selenium selenomethionine

Methionine is taken up by metabolically active cells, and the labelled amino acid has been shown to localize in the liver, pancreas, and in some tumours (Kaplan & Domingo, 1972). Ten MBq [75]selenium activity is administered intravenously, and images commenced 1 h later. A medium energy collimator is essential for the higher-energy photon emission. A complementary hepatic image using substraction of the two images can be used but probably adds little to the accuracy of interpretation.

Abscess localization

Inflammatory tissue may accumulate either [67]gallium citrate (Lavender et al., 1971), or [111]indium-oxide-labelled autologous leukocytes (Segal et al., 1976). Both techniques can show the site of intra- or extrahepatic sepsis. The gallium procedure is identical to that for tumour detection, but imaging at 24 h often successfully localizes the abscess. [111]Indium-oxide-labelled autologous leukocytes separated from whole blood are reinjected, and images obtained at 4 h or later.

Labelled antibody studies

Most of the work done in the field of labelled antibodies has been related to the imaging of malignant tumours. The lack of tissue specificity has up until now limited precise localization of tumour masses. Furthermore, free labelled antibody and antibody complexes result in high uptake of activity by the normal liver, so that hepatic metastases cannot be identified.

Conclusion

Radionuclide hepatic imaging provides a simple, atraumatic and rapid means for the identification of focal liver disease, and for the investigation of biliary function. Its role has declined in recent years with the wider availability of ultrasound and computerized tomography.

References

Borzutzky, C.A. & Turbiner, E.H. (1985) The predictive value of hepatic artery perfusion scintigraphy. *Journal of Nuclear Medicine*, **26**, 1153−1156.

Clarke, D.P., Cosgrove, D.O. & McCready, V.R. (1986) Radionuclide imaging for liver maligancy and its relationship to other hepatic investigation. *Clinics in Oncology*, **5**, 159−181.

Fleming, J.S., Ackery, D.M., Walmsley, B.H. & Karran, S.J. (1983) Scintigraphic estimation of arterial and portal blood supplies to the liver. *Journal of Nuclear Medicine*, **24**, 1108−1113.

Hall, A.W., Wisbey, M.L., Hutchinson, F., Wood, R.A.B. & Cuschieri, A. (1981) The place of hepatobiliary isotope scanning in the diagnosis of gallbladder disease. *British Journal of Surgery*, **68**, 85—90.

Kaplan E. & Domingo M. (1972) 75 Se-selenomethionine in hepatic focal lesions. *Seminars in Nuclear Medicine*, **2**, 139—149.

Karran, S.J., Leach, K.G. & Blumgart, L.H. (1974) Assessment of liver regeneration in the rat using the gamma camera. *Journal of Nuclear Medicine*, **15**, 10—16.

Lavender, J.P., Lowe, J., Barker, J.R., Burn, J.I. & Chaudhri, M.A. (1971) Gallium 67 citrate scanning in neoplastic and inflammatory lesions. *British Journal of Radiology*, **44**, 361—366.

Leveson, S.H., Wiggins, P.A., Nasiru, T.A., Giles, G.R. & Robinson, P.J. (1983) Improving the detection of hepatic metastases by the use of dynamic flow scintigraphy. *British Journal of Cancer*, **47**, 719—721.

McAfee, J.G., Ause, R.G. & Wagner, H.N. (1965) Diagnostic value of scintillation scanning of the liver. *Archives of Internal Medicine*, **116**, 95—110.

Schwarzrock, R., Kotzerke, J., Hundershagen, H., Bocker, K. & Ringe, B. (1986) 99m Tc-diethyl-iodo-HIDA (JODIDA): a new hepatobiliary agent in clinical comparison with 99m Tc-diisopropyl-HIDA (DISIDA) in jaundiced patients. *European Journal of Nuclear Medicine*, **12**, 346—350.

Segal, A.W., Thakur, M.L., Arnot, R.N. & Lavender, J.P. (1976) Indium-111-labelled leukocytes for localisation of abscesses. *Lancet*, **ii**, 1056—1058.

Ziessman, H.A., Wahl R.L., Juni J.E., Gyves, J.E., Ensminger, W.D., Thrall, J.H., Keyes, J.W. *et al.*, (1985) The utility of SPECT for 99m Tc-MAA hepatic arterial perfusion scintigraphy. *American Journal of Roentgenology*, **145**, 747—751.

5: Angiography

H.B. NUNNERLEY

Introduction

The role of angiography in the liver has remained of great importance, though this has changed since it was first described by Bierman *et al.* in 1951, when they used the brachial artery approach. The introduction of the Seldinger technique (Seldinger, 1953) made hepatic angiography a practical procedure. The introduction of ultrasound, particularly Doppler ultrasound, as well as computer tomography scanning and now magnetic resonance imaging has changed the diagnostic role of angiography from being a primary diagnostic tool to that of a technique which has a complementary role, and indeed is used in therapeutic procedures. It must be remembered that in such a complex organ as the liver, many of these diagnostic techniques are complementary. Obviously the management of patients with liver disorders varies from centre to centre, and much depends on the type of treatment being planned, e.g. if partial hepatectomy is a considered option. Angiography is an essential prerequisite for planning surgery and is also needed before such therapeutic procedures as installation of drugs via catheter, including porto-cath infusion pumps, or embolization. In some instances it is the only diagnostic technique that shows pathology such as a small tumour in a cirrhotic liver.

In the transplanted liver, angiography may be the only way of finally deciding the pathological process in certain instances. It can distinguish between acute rejection and narrowing or occlusion of the transplanted hepatic artery at the anastomosis with the recipient's artery, though Doppler ultrasound is now proving to be a helpful and accurate investigation.

Vascular anatomy

The liver has a dual blood supply. It receives its arterial supply in a variety of ways. The conventional hepatic artery arises from the coeliac axis (Fig. 5.1). This classic appearance is seen in only 65% of patients. The coeliac trunk arises from the aorta at the level of T12–L1 and extends caudally for approximately 1–2 cm, then ventrally. Its normal branches are the left gastric artery, the splenic artery and the common hepatic artery. The inferior phrenic arteries may also arise from the coelic artery, as can the dorsal pancreatic artery. The common hepatic artery is slightly smaller than the splenic artery and pursues a course to the right and anteriorly, giving off the gastroduodenal artery and sometimes the dorsal pancreatic artery, before becoming the hepatic artery proper. This enters the porta of the liver and divides into right, left, and middle hepatic arteries.

In only 50% of cases do both the right and left hepatic arteries arise from the common hepatic artery; rarely, in about 10% of patients, the whole of the hepatic artery is supplied from the superior mesenteric artery (Fig. 5.2). More commonly the right hepatic artery can arise from the superior mesenteric artery (Fig. 5.3). The right hepatic artery early gives off the cystic artery before supplying the right lobe of the liver. In 45% of patients the left hepatic artery gives rise to the middle hepatic artery, and in approximately 25% of patients the left hepatic artery arises from the left gastric artery. The origin of the middle hepatic artery is variable. It comes from the common hepatic artery in 10% of patients. Otherwise it is a branch of either the left or right hepatic artery. It supplies the quadrate lobe of the liver and can also sometimes supply the gall bladder. Although the arteries to the liver are end arteries, there are multiple collateral vessels; if one branch is embolized there is a rapid redistribution and supply of that section of the liver by collaterals.

These anatomical variations mean that it is essential to demonstrate both the coeliac axis artery and the superior mesenteric artery to get a full picture of the hepatic arterial anatomy. It is also

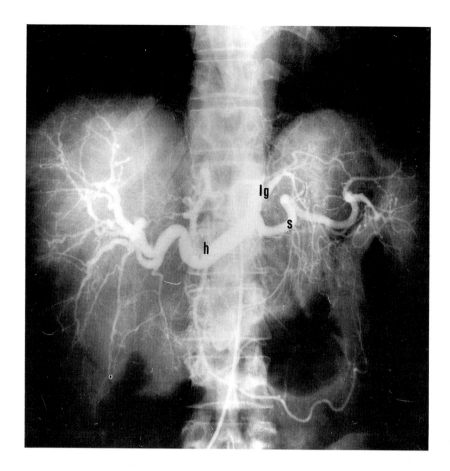

Fig. 5.1 Coeliac axis arteriogram showing the hepatic artery (*h*) arising from this, as well as the splenic(*s*) and left gastric (*lg*) arteries. It divides early into smaller left and larger right branches.

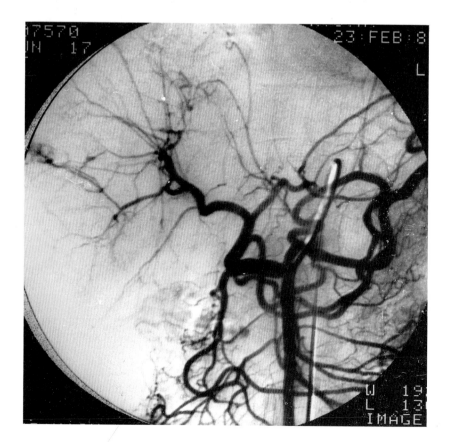

Fig. 5.2 Superior mesenteric artery arteriogram showing the complete hepatic artery arising from it.

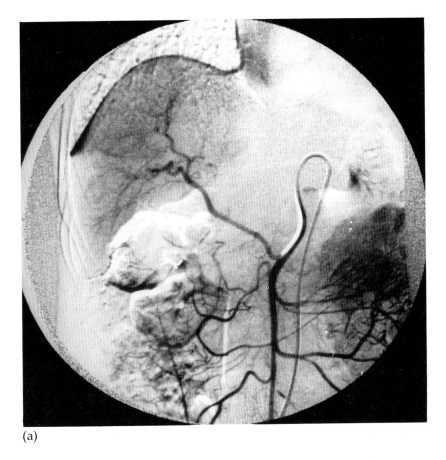

(a)

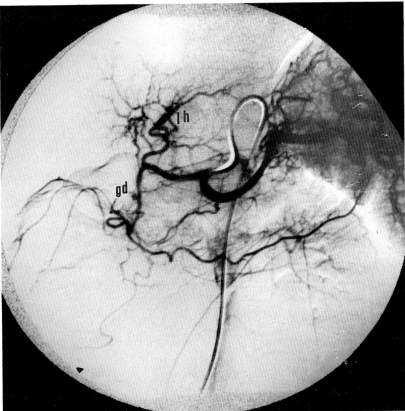

(b)

Fig. 5.3 (a) Superior mesenteric arteriogram showing the right hepatic artery arising from it. (b) Coeliac axis arteriogram shows left hepatic artery (lh) and gastroduodenal artery (gd) arising from it, together with the splenic artery.

worthwhile remembering that occasionally the left hepatic artery can arise directly from the aorta (Fig. 5.4)

The portal vein, which delivers the other blood supply to the liver, is formed behind the neck of the pancreas at the junction of the superior mesenteric vein and the splenic vein. The portal vein ascends to the right in the free edge of the lesser omentum, entering the porta of the liver with the hepatic artery and the common bile duct. It divides into the right and left branches, the right portal vein tends to go somewhat horizontally into the right lobe before dividing into anterior and posterior branches. These are fairly constant and always relatively easy to define (Fig. 5.5). The left portal vein is smaller than the right, but longer and runs upwards and anterior to the caudate lobe before making a fairly abrupt anterior turn to the left, where it gives off medial and lateral branches. One must remember that the remnant of the umbilical vein arises from the anterior margin of the left portal vein.

The hepatic veins are much more difficult to identify angiographically. They lie between the hepatic segments and are useful in describing the anatomy of the liver. The right hepatic vein runs an oblique course in the intersegmental fissure between the anterior and posterior segments of the right lobe; it is the largest hepatic vein and enters the inferior vena cava just below the diaphragm. The middle hepatic vein marks the junction between the right and left lobes of the liver, whilst the left hepatic vein runs in the left intersegmental fissure. All the hepatic veins drain obliquely upwards and medially and enter the inferior vena cava fairly close to its entry to the right atrium. The middle and left hepatic veins may join before they enter the inferior vena cava. There may be other small hepatic veins that enter the inferior vena cava separately; this can cause the surgeon many problems during hepatic surgery.

Technique

Before undertaking any techniques in a patient with liver problems it is essential to check the clotting factors. These patients may well have a low platelet count. If the count is less than 50 000/ml it is important to decide whether the investigation is absolutely essential. If it is, there must be discussion with the clinicians, and probably either the provision of some fresh blood or a platelet transfusion considered. If the prothrombin time is prolonged more than 5 s, it is advisable to have some fresh frozen plasma available; this can be infused slowly during the technique and will cover particularly the end of the procedure. As far as equipment is concerned it is helpful if digital subtraction is available; this is particularly useful in demonstrating the portal venous system. However, if one is using angiography as a final investigation to exclude a possible tumour in a large patient, it may well be necessary to provide cut film angiograms with either a Puck or other form of film changer to obtain full-sized films of the liver.

The usual approach now is via the femoral artery using a Seldinger technique. A torque-controlled catheter is required, and it is useful for the hepatic angiographer to have a variety of catheters available. The most commonly used is the 'Sidewinder II' variety. This catheter is introduced into the aorta, re-shaped at the arch, and brought down the aorta with its curve re-formed into its natural shape, and then hooked into the origin of the coeliac trunk or superior mesenteric artery; with the curve it can then be directed into the common hepatic artery. Some operators prefer to use a 'shepherd's crook' type of catheter, and a 'cobra' catheter can be useful, particularly if the coeliac axis has a very short common trunk. A floppy guide-wire with a small or medium curve can sometimes be used to lead the way along the vessel if it is desired to go superselectively. Entering the hepatic artery can sometimes be very difficult if the anatomy is distorted by previous surgery or a very large tumour. In these cases a helpful technique is to rotate the patient onto the right side; this removes some of the weight of the liver off the origin of the coeliac axis and enables the catheter to pursue a course round to the right and into the hepatic artery. It is important to obtain a stable position of the catheter before injecting contrast.

If conventional angiography is being performed, up to 70 cc of contrast, 350 mg of iodine per cc is injected at a rate of 8–10 ml/s. If looking at the arterial anatomy in the hepatogram phase it is important to film up to 12 s. With a digital subtraction technique, much less contrast is needed, usually about 40 cc, again at 8 cc/s. The strength needed is less, approximately 100 mg of iodine per cc. To obtain an accurate assessment of the blood supply to tumours, and to determine their extent, it is sometimes essential to carry out oblique studies with both the right or left side of the

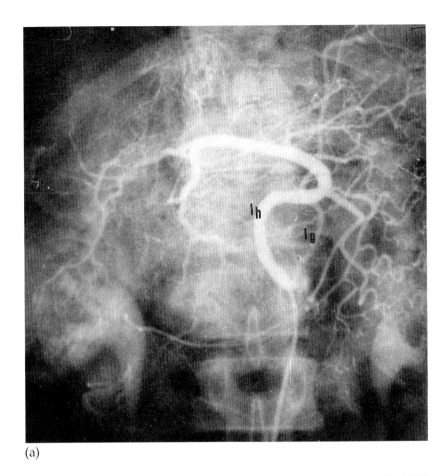

(a)

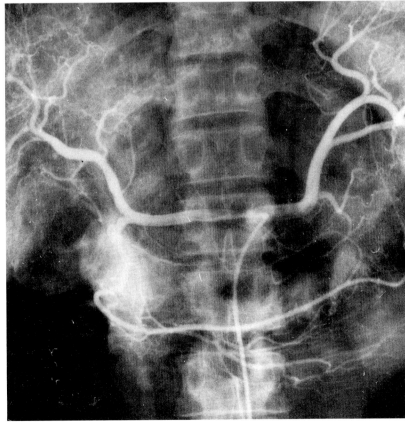

Fig. 5.4 (a) The left hepatic artery (lh) is shown arising separately from the aorta with the left gastric artery (lg). (b) The coeliac axis artery supplies the right and middle hepatic artery as well as the splenic artery.

(b)

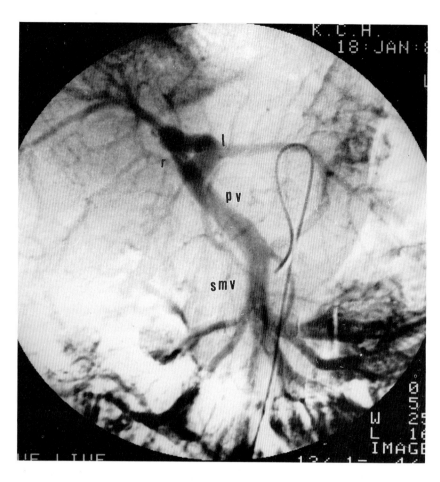

Fig. 5.5 Portal vein (pv) shown with left (l) and right (r) branches filling from a superior mesenteric artery injection via the superior mesenteric vein (smv).

patient raised to approximately 40°. Alternatively, if a C arm is available the axis of this may be swung round. The oblique view chosen depends on the site of the abnormality within the liver, and on any coexisting displacement of structures; it is not always easy to predict which one is needed.

If the hepatic artery arises from the superior mesenteric artery, much patience may be required to enter the vessel; an extra curve may be needed on the catheter to enable it to enter the common hepatic or right hepatic artery. If only the right hepatic artery is being injected, less contrast is needed: 40 cc for a conventional study and approximately 20 cc of dilute contrast for a digital subtraction angiogram. If after reviewing the hepatogram phase of the studies it appears that part of the liver is missing, it is essential to carry out an injection into the aorta itself to see if there is a further hepatic artery arising in some unusual manner, such as directly from the aorta.

Apart from reviewing the anatomy of the vessels and the supply to areas of abnormality such as tumour, it is important to look at the hepatogram phase, as over 90% of tumours receive their blood supply exclusively from the hepatic artery and the majority are hypervascular. These are easier to identify before the hepatoportal venous supply enters the liver.

The portal vein can be demonstrated by a variety of methods. Digital subtraction angiography has made a great contribution to the demonstration of the portal vein. It is best seen on late studies of superior mesenteric artery injections. If conventional cut-film technique is used, a period of 32 s should be covered from the commencement of injection; inject 70 cc of approximately 350 mg iodine strength contrast into the superior mesenteric artery, filming for 32 s after a fairly slow injection at 8 cc. With digital subtraction angiography, 40 cc of 240 mg iodine strength contrast can be used, and a technique again to cover a longer period than the arterial side. The portal vein comes up clearly relatively early on in these studies, and can be seen with its branches through the liver. Obviously, with portal hypertension the portal vein appears later. If there is a reverse flow in the portal vein, the contrast will travel via collaterals either up to the oesophagus, fundus of the stomach or, for example, through a splenorenal shunt into the inferior vena cava. This does not necessarily mean that the portal vein is blocked. Doppler ultrasound is particularly helpful in these situations. To confirm possible controversial findings between ultrasound and angiography it may be necessary to puncture directly a branch of the portal vein within the liver, injecting some contrast to confirm reverse flow in a patent portal vein.

In the past, splenic venograms were often used to demonstrate the portal vein. Here a small cannula was usually introduced into the splenic pulp. Contrast was injected directly into the splenic pulp and followed into the splenic vein and so into the portal vein. Films were taken at 1-s intervals for a period of 12 s. This was an accurate way of showing the splenic and portal veins, and indeed the collateral veins if the portal vein was blocked, but there were complications. It was possible to inject the contrast outside the spleen, and occasionally considerable pain followed the procedure because of a leak of contrast and blood from the spleen into the peritoneal cavity. Using digital subtraction angiography it is possible to put a 23 gauge needle into the spleen and inject contrast by hand, and to follow this with the new technique. Excellent results can be obtained showing the portal vein and collaterals, using only 12−15 cc of 240 mg strength contrast. We have found this of particular use in studying children.

Hepatic veins

The hepatic veins are studied via the inferior vena cava. It is usual to insert a catheter via the femoral vein. A multi-purpose type of catheter is normally used and in a patient with patent hepatic veins it is easy to enter them all. The catheter can be passed down the hepatic vein to a wedge position to carry out pressure studies; these can be of great value to the clinician in determining the vascular state of the liver. If the veins cannot be entered from below, it may be possible to perform a brachial-vein approach, passing through the heart and down into the hepatic veins. The inferior vena cava is normally slightly narrowed as it passes through the liver; however, if the liver, particularly the caudate lobe, is enlarged this can compress the inferior vena cava significantly more. It is often helpful to have studies showing the pressures in the inferior vena cava below and above the liver; one has also to exclude the possibility of a web within the inferior vena cava at the level just above the entrance of the hepatic veins.

The extension of tumour or clot into the inferior vena cava must be confirmed or excluded.

References

Bierman, H.R., Byron, R.L. Jr., Kelly, K.H. & Grady, A. (1951) Studies on the blood supply of tumors in man: vascular patterns of the liver by hepatic arteriography *in vivo*. *Journal of the National Cancer Institute*, **12**, 107.

Seldinger, S.L. (1953) Catheter replacement of needle in percutaneous arteriography; a new technique. *Acta Radiologica*, **39**, 368.

Part 2
Liver Disease

6: Magnetic Resonance Imaging of the Liver

G.M. BYDDER

Introduction

Over 5 years have now elapsed since publication of the first clinical results of magnetic resonance imaging (MRI) in the liver by Smith *et al.* (1981). In this period MRI of the central nervous system has made considerable progress and is now accepted as the imaging technique of first choice for a variety of neurological diseases; however progress in MRI of the liver has been slower. The earliest MRI images produced in 1981–1982 were generally comparable with ultrasound (US) and computerized tomography (CT) in diagnostic content, although at a disadvantage in terms of spatial resolution and susceptibility to motion artefact. This was followed by a relatively static period in which some alternative MRI techniques were applied without notable improvement in results, but over the last year a variety of new techniques have been applied with generally better results. These techniques take into account the difference in magnetic resonance properties of the liver as compared with the brain. In addition several techniques are now available for controlling artefact due to respiratory motion, and over the last year MR contrast agents have become available.

Much of the present work is essentially technical in nature so that some understanding of the basic physics of MRI is necessary to appreciate the differences between the approaches now in use. The first section of this chapter therefore deals with the basic physics of MRI; this is followed by a review of the technical approaches in current use, and finally a review of the clinical results achieved to date.

Basic physics of MRI

Good reviews of the basic physics of MRI exist (Gadian, 1982, Bradley *et al.*, 1984, Petersen *et al.*, 1985) and only aspects of the technique relevant to later sections of this chapter are covered below.

The NMR phenomenon

It is possible to regard the nuclei of hydrogen atoms (i.e. protons) as behaving like tiny spinning magnets. In the presence of a large static magnetic field these tiny magnets are preferentially aligned with the static magnetic field, giving a net nuclear magnetization M_z (Fig. 6.1). When an additional magnetic field rotating at the spin frequency of the protons is applied perpendicular to the main field, the nuclear magnetization M_z can be rotated through any angle such as 90°, as shown in Fig. 6.2. After the magnetization has been rotated and the additional applied magnetic field is turned off, M_z returns to its equilibrium position. This process is called relaxation and is described by two time-constants T_1 and T_2, which refer respectively to relaxation in the longitudinal and transverse axes of the magnet. As the magnetization returns to equilibrium it generates a small voltage in a receiver coil that is placed around the patient. This voltage is the detected signal and it is processed by computer to give the final data in the image.

Obtaining an image

During the process of excitation and relaxation of protons additional magnetic field gradients are applied in order to select a slice and localize the signal from protons within that slice. The spin frequency is proportional to the size of magnetic field at any point. A gradient field produces a systematic change in field, changing the resonant frequency in a regular manner and enabling the location of protons to be determined by their spin frequency.

Pulse sequences

It is possible to represent the recovery and decay of the proton magnetization by exponentials and to represent the signals at each point by a composite graph (Fig. 6.2). During the first phase after

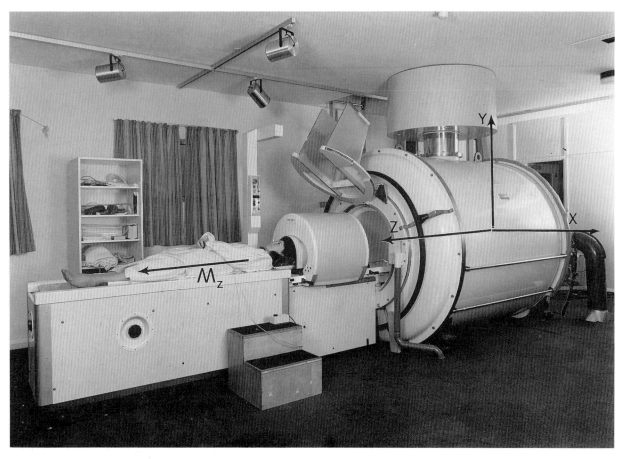

Fig. 6.1 An MRI system. The X, Y, Z axes are shown. The static magnetic field in the Z direction induces the magnetization M_z in the patient.

a 90° pulse the signal recovers with time-constant T_1. The signal is detected after a period TE (the echo time) during which it decays with a time constant T_2. The signal is received during the data collection (DC) and the cycle is repeated after time TR (the repetition time). Figure 6.2 illustrates the simplest pulse sequence available — a partial saturation (PS) sequence. Two other pulse sequences are also in common use, the inversion recovery (IR) sequence (a 180° pulse followed at time TI (the inversion time) later by a 90° pulse and then data collection), and the spin echo (SE) sequence (a 90° pulse followed by a 180° pulse and then data collection with time TE between the 90° pulse and the data collection). The process of data collection can be achieved by a spin echo when the changes caused in the first part of the decay are partially reversed on either side of the 180° pulse, or by a field echo in which the gradient fields are reversed.

The resonant frequencies of protons in water and protons in fat are slightly different, leading to a 'beat' phenomenon between the two. This is analogous to the augmentation and cancellation effect when two musical notes that are slightly out of tune are sounded simultaneously. The type of image that results from this phenomenon is known as a phase-contrast or chemical-shift image (Dixon, 1984).

Determinants of T_1 and T_2

In general terms T_1 and T_2 reflect molecular mobility (Fig. 6.3). Thus, for liquids both T_1 and T_2 are very long but as the liquid becomes more viscous T_1 and T_2 shorten. As this process is continued T_2 shortens but T_1 becomes long again so that solids have long values of T_1 and very short values of T_2. Tissue 'wetness' or viscosity is thus an important factor in determining T_1 and T_2. Another important factor is the presence of proton relaxation enhancement (PRE) agents. These are usually materials that contain unpaired electrons that produce local magnetic fields, which in turn

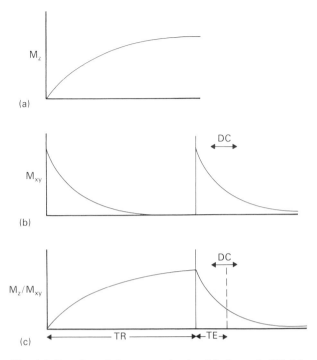

Fig. 6.2 Rotation of the magnetization M_z through 90°. (a) Immediately following the 90° pulse M_z is 0 but recovers exponentially to its original value. (b) With rotation of the magnetization, M_z becomes M_{xy}, following which it decays exponentially with time-constant T_2. (c) Shows M_z followed by M_{xy} with the data collection DC following a second 90° pulse. The height of M_{xy} at the time of the data collection represents the available signal.

accelerate the process of relaxation. Important examples are iron, either as the free iron or in the form of organic complexes such as methaemoglobin or haemosiderin. The liver contains a higher concentration of organic iron than many other organs producing a relatively short T_1 and T_2.

Many pathological processes increase T_1 and T_2. In some cases this may be associated with increased water content due to oedema, but the exact explanation for this phenomenon remains uncertain. In a collation of published data on values of T_1 for the liver, Bottomley *et al.* (1985) point out that values for liver tumours are at least one standard deviation greater than the normal range and that this should provide a useful basis for developing image contrast.

Effects of respiratory motion

Respiratory motion produces a degradation of image quality as a result of blurring during data acquisition. In addition ghost artefacts are produced in the so-called phase-encoded direction

when one particular type of image reconstruction (two-dimensional fourier transformation) is used. Several techniques have been proposed to overcome these problems. One is gating of the pulse sequence to the least active phase of respiratory cycle. Although this can be effective it increases examination time by a factor of 2–3. Another technique is to average data throughout the period of a respiratory cycle — so-called pseudogating. It improves image quality but results in increased imaging time. A third method is respiratory-ordered phase encoding (ROPE) which does not incur a significant time penalty and provides reasonably effective control of respiratory artefact (Bailes *et al.*, 1985).

Approaches to MRI of the liver

The inversion recovery (IR) approach

The initial MRI studies of the liver were performed with IR sequences with medium values of TI (i.e. values of about 200–400 ms). The pulse sequences had short values of TE (typically 10 ms or less), decreasing their T_2 dependence and producing highly T_1-dependent images. The first two studies with this pattern displayed high soft-tissue contrast (Fig. 6.3) with sensitivity about equal to that of ultrasound and CT (Smith *et al.*, 1981, Doyle *et al.*, 1982). Similar results have been obtained since by Henkelman *et al.* (1984). The disadvantage with these early results was that the spatial resolution was low (64 × 64 or 128 × 128) compared with that of X-ray CT which is typically 256 × 256.

The spin-echo (SE) approach

Another early approach to liver imaging was the use of SE sequences. These were used in two forms — T_1-dependent and T_2-dependent. The T_1-dependent form ('short TE, short TR') produced rapid images with good anatomical detail but with much less lesion contrast than with IR sequences (Fig. 6.3C). This early type of T_1-dependent sequence had lower T_1 dependence (because of the not-so-short TE of 28 ms) than IR sequences, and the T_1-dependent contrast opposed the T_2-dependent contrast. The other form of spin-echo, i.e. the highly T_2-dependent form, produced higher lesion contrast but the general signal level was low and the sequence was vulnerable to motion (Fig. 6.3D). In addition, lesions with an increased T_2 tended to show contrast properties

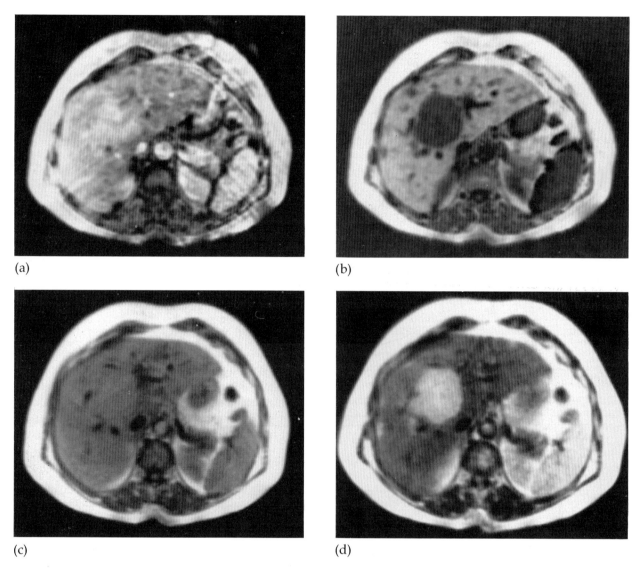

(a)

(b)

(c)

(d)

Fig. 6.3 Liver metastases: $PS_{100/13}$ (a), $IR_{1400/400/13}$ (b), $SE_{540/40}$ (c), and $SE_{1080/80}$ (d) scans. Poor contrast is seen in (a), the lesion is dark in (b), seen poorly in (c), but highlighted in (d).

similar to fat. Results with this approach were either comparable to X-ray CT (Moss *et al.*, 1984) or worse than CT (Heiken *et al.*, 1985b).

THE SHORT TE SPIN-ECHO APPROACH

In order to overcome the problem of the T_2 dependence of the basically T_1-dependent spin-echo, the echo time can be reduced to the range of 10–15 ms as opposed to values of 28 ms used in earlier studies. TR can then be reduced to about the T_1 of the liver to maximize T_1-dependent contrast (e.g. 260 ms). This approach has been used with averaging throughout a respiratory cycle (e.g. 18 averages), producing low-resolution (128 × 128 or 128 × 256) T_1-dependent images. The results with this

approach have compared well with X-ray CT (Stark & Ferrucci, 1986).

THE CHEMICAL SHIFT (PHASE-CONTRAST) APPROACH

This technique was developed by Dixon (1984) as well as by Sepponen *et al.* (1984). It relies on the fact that dephasing or 'beating' occurs between protons in water and those in fat during the period TE. If particular values of TE are chosen, the water and fat signals can be added or opposed. Subtraction or addition of these images gives images of the 'fat' fraction and the 'water' fraction within the liver.

The technique has been used to recognize and

quantify fatty infiltration of the liver (Heiken *et al.*, 1985a). In addition the opposed image is sensitive to the presence of metastases. This is possibly because metastases are frequently accompanied by some degree of fatty infiltration. A metastasis may be highlighted if the signal from adjacent fatty infiltration is reduced by opposing its fat and water components.

THE SHORT TI IR (STIR) APPROACH

When the TI of IR sequences is reduced to about 100–120 ms the signal from fat is reduced to zero. This means that the anterior abdominal wall no longer produces artefacts with respiration. Also the T_1-dependent and the T_2-dependent contrast is additive, giving high sensitivity (Fig. 6.2) (Bydder & Young, 1985). This type of sequence has been used in a limited comparison with CT with favourable results (Bydder *et al.*, 1985b). It also shows high sensitivity to fatty infiltration, periportal changes, and other secondary features accompanying liver disease. Images have been obtained with this sequence at high resolution (256×256 or 256×512), i.e. at higher resolution than with the previous techniques.

THE FAST FIELD-ECHO IMAGING APPROACH

An approach to the problem of respiratory artefact has been the use of rapid images obtained within breath-holding times, using a field-echo data collection (i.e. PS sequences) which gives higher signal than convential spin-echo patterns. This approach was used early in the development of MRI, with typical imaging times of 12.8 s. The value of this approach was limited by the problem of developing adequate T_1 or T_2-dependent contrast. More recently a technique used in MR spectroscopy of reduced pulse angle (i.e. less then 90°) has been used to increase the available signal per unit time, and with short TE values this technique provides rapid images — but with poor lesion contrast. A variant of this approach has been the use of long TE values coupled with a reduced flip angle (e.g. 30°). These images display high T_2-dependent contrast.

Oral contrast agents

Bowel contents have a prolonged T_1 and T_2 relative to liver and may simulate lesions within the liver, depending on their exact position. This type of problem is dealt with in X-ray CT by the use of oral iodinated contrast agents. The first approach in MRI was the use of oral ferric salts, which produced some improvement by shortening T_1 and T_2 of bowel contents to less than the tissue range (Young *et al.*, 1981, Wesbey *et al.*, 1983), but generally the results were inconsistent. Another approach has been the use of oral magnetite (Fe_3O_4) a susceptibility agent that greatly reduces the signal from bowel (Mendonca-Dias *et al.*, 1985, Olsson *et al.*, 1985).

As yet magnetite is only available for animal use, but the material is basically inert. Its formulation for oral use presents problems analogous to those of barium preparations used in radiology.

Intravenous contrast agents

The paramagnetic contrast agent Gadolinium–DTPA (Weinmann *et al.*, 1984) became available for clinical use in 1984 (Carr *et al.*, 1984). After intravenous injection it circulates within the vascular compartment and enters the extravascular fluid. It produces a decrease in T_1 and T_2, and depending on the precise pulse sequence can increase or decrease signal intensity for a lesion.

The normal liver shows moderate enhancement and the results in general terms parallel those seen with contrast-enhanced X-ray CT.

Receiver coils

The use of close-fitting receiver coils — 'corset coils' — has resulted in an improvement in image quality (Bydder *et al.*, 1985a). There is still scope for further coil improvement.

Clinical results

Recent general reviews of MRI of the liver have been published by Smith & Mallard (1984), Haaga (1984) and Stark *et al.* (1986), and there is a fair measure of agreement on the diagnostic potential of MRI, although recent technical developments have meant that much of the work reviewed has become dated.

Normal appearances

The normal appearance of the liver varies strikingly, depending on the pulse sequence used (Fig. 6.3). With IR sequences the parenchyma has a moderately high signal intensity and blood vessels and bile ducts are dark. Fat is highlighted. With spin-echo sequences the liver parenchyma has a lower signal intensity with blood vessels again dark. Phase-contrast images generally appear like spin-echo images. Fast field-echo images generally display low contrast, but in the T_2-dependent form lesions may be highlighted.

Metastases

The diagnosis of metastases is of central importance. The accuracy of US and CT is generally reckoned to be about 60—80%. Where either of these techniques is positive a specific diagnosis may be achieved by fine-needle biopsy and MRI probably has no role. However, if MRI could be established as the most sensitive imaging technique available, it would have a major role in the exclusion of metastases when other imaging techniques were negative. Because of the importance of the liver in staging and operative management of malignancy, this use of MRI would represent a major clinical application. As a result, evaluation of different approaches to the MRI diagnosis of metastases has received considerable attention.

The clinical studies have confirmed the data collated by Bottomley et al. (1985) with metastatic tumours consistently displaying evidence of an increase in T_1 and T_2. This differs from brain for example, where 12% of 278 tumours have shown evidence of a normal or decreased T_1 or T_2 in our experience. Exceptions to the pattern in the liver may be seen where tumours are calcified, and in some areas of necrosis where it is possible that the tumour has undergone haemorrhage, releasing paramagnetic species as breakdown products of blood.

Frequently there are associated changes with metastases. These are probably due to fatty infiltration but may also be due to atrophy, fibrosis, or other pathological processes.

The effect of different sequences is illustrated in Fig. 6.3, which shows a metastases from carcinoma of the breast. The PS sequence (Fig. 6.3a) shows little contrast but the IR sequence displays a low signal intensity. The short TE short TR spin-echo sequence displays little contrast, but as the T_2 dependence of the sequence is increased the tumour is highlighted as a result of its increased T_2 (Fig. 6.3c,d).

The pattern with STIR sequences is demonstrated in Fig. 6.4. The metastases are more obvious in the STIR image and a local dilated bile duct is only seen with the STIR images. A potential difficulty with this type of image is the fact that bile ducts are highlighted, and this puts a limit to the minimum size of a metastasis that may be detected.

A corresponding problem exists with T_1-dependent spin-echo and IR sequences where portal veins (low signal intensity) may simulate metastases.

When fatty infiltration is present this produces a normal or short T_1. With IR sequences this may be of value in determining whether a low-attenuation lesion in the liver on X-ray CT is due to fatty infiltration or a metastasis. With STIR sequences areas of fatty infiltration usually display a moderate increase in T_2 and are seen as higher-intensity lesions, although the intensity is less than metastases. The use of phase-contrast opposed images can lead to cancellation of the signal from the liver adjacent to a metastasis, leaving the metastasis highlighted. This has been the explanation for the high sensitivity of this type of sequence. General considerations help in recognizing metastases, including their multiplicity and the frequent association of a large liver. The tumour boundary is often sharply defined but there may also be a ring-shaped appearance around the lesion.

Comparison with CT shows some general advantages for MRI, particularly in the left lobe, where with CT the liver may be obscured by the presence of linear artefacts from the interface between air and water within the stomach. The same comments apply to areas of 'shadowing' on CT at the surface of the liver immediately beneath ribs. Even outside of these areas the differences between CT and MRI may be striking (Fig. 6.5).

The presence of ascites is usually obvious either with IR sequences or STIR sequences. Ascites may make diagnosis of capsular or subcapsular metastases more difficult.

Following embolization with coils, difficulties may be experienced in obtaining useful images at all because of the presence of metallic artefact. In other cases a decrease in T_1 and T_2 may be seen within the tumour as a result of the embolization.

Gd-DTPA produces a decrease in T_1 and T_2 of the liver. Many metastases also display a marked decrease in T_1 and T_2 with this agent; in fact this decrease may be sufficient to produce an 'isointense' appearance with loss of lesion contrast (Fig. 6.6). The same concentration of Gd-DTPA produces a greater absolute reduction in T_1 and T_2 in metastases than it does for normal liver. In addition,

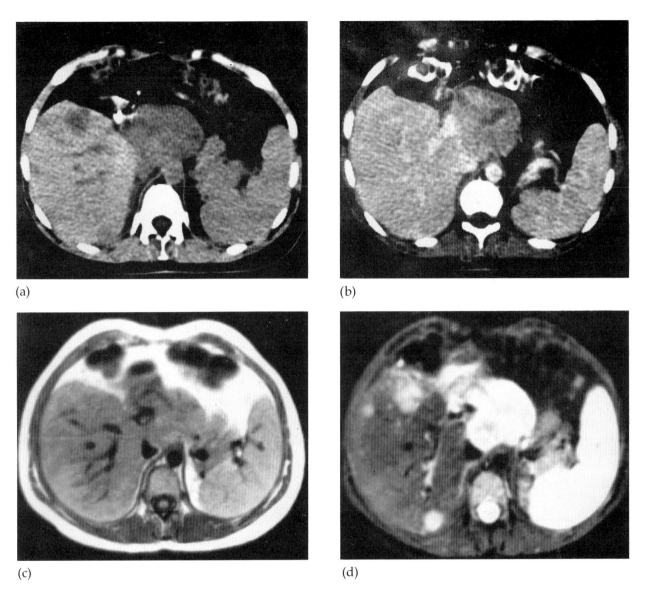

(a)

(b)

(c)

(d)

Fig. 6.4 Metastasis from carcinoma of the colon: CT (a), enhanced CT (b), $SE_{544/44}$ (c), and $STIR_{1500/100/44}$ (d) scans. The recurrent tumour metastases and dilated bile duct are best seen in (d).

abnormal vascular permeability within the blood vessels of tumours results in excessive accumulation of contrast. In some cases less enhancement of tumours may be seen but in general with medium TI IR sequences the additional information provided following the use of Gd-DTPA has been small (Carr *et al.*, 1985).

It is possible to use other strategies with Gd-DTPA and one that has been suggested is the use of fast PS sequences. These show some T_1 dependence and should therefore display enhancement, making metastases more obvious. No clinical results from the use of this technique are yet available.

Non-ferromagnetic biopsy needles are being developed for use in association with MRI and it is possible that biopsies will be performed in a way analogous to X-ray CT.

The presence of long T_1 long T_2 stomach contents adjacent to the left lobe of the liver may make the diagnosis of metastases in this region difficult with both IR and STIR sequences. The use of paramagnetic or susceptibility contrast agents to identify or eliminate this signal is likely to be important.

The studies of metastases performed to date have been mentioned in the techniques section but are summarized again as the IR approach (Smith *et al.*, 1981, Doyle *et al.*, 1982, Henkelman *et al.*, 1984), the SE approach (Heiken *et al.*, 1985b),

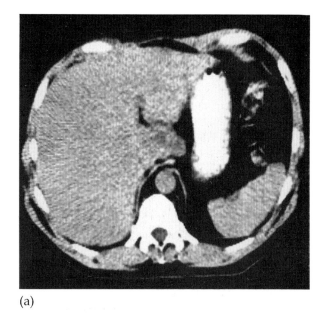

(a)

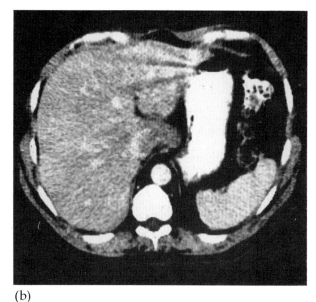

(b)

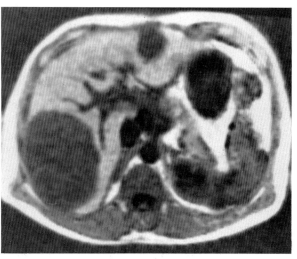

(c)

Fig. 6.5 Metastases from carcinoid tumour: CT (a), enhanced CT (b), and $IR_{1400/400/13}$ (c) scans. The three metastases are better seen in (c).

the short TE SE approach (Stark & Ferrucci, 1986), and the STIR approach (Bydder *et al.*, 1985b).

Primary malignant tumours

As with malignant metastases, an increase in T_1 and T_2 of primary tumours is seen but the situation may be complicated by the fact that hepatomas may occur in livers with cirrhosis, and both these pathological conditions increase T_1 and T_2, leading to a net loss of lesion contrast. In these circumstances an abnormal vascular pattern may be of diagnostic value. Hepatomas may also be multifocal, making differentiation from metastases difficult.

Not infrequently hepatomas are large at the time of diagnosis, but may show only a limited difference in attenuation on CT, so that they may be missed or poorly localized in spite of their size. MRI has an advantage in these circumstances (Vermess *et al.*, 1985).

As with metastases, fatty infiltration is a frequent association (Fig. 6.7).

Patterns of infiltration along portal veins have been identified. Subcapsular changes, even in the absence of biopsy, have been seen and are usually more extensive than on CT. They may represent haemorrhage.

Identification of recurrence can be useful with MRI (Fig. 6.8). Note that the original resection line is highlighted in this case.

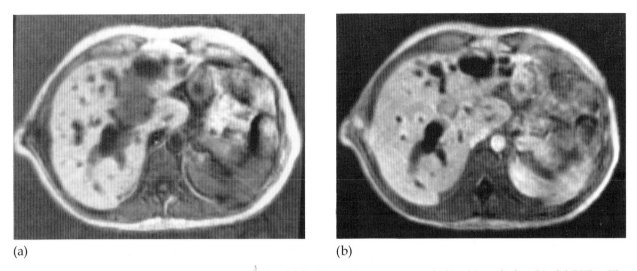

(a) (b)

Fig. 6.6 Adenocarcinoma at the liver hilum with dilated bile ducts: $IR_{1400/400/13}$ scans before (a), and after (b), Gd-DTPA. The tumour becomes isointense. Definition between bile ducts and portal veins is improved in (b).

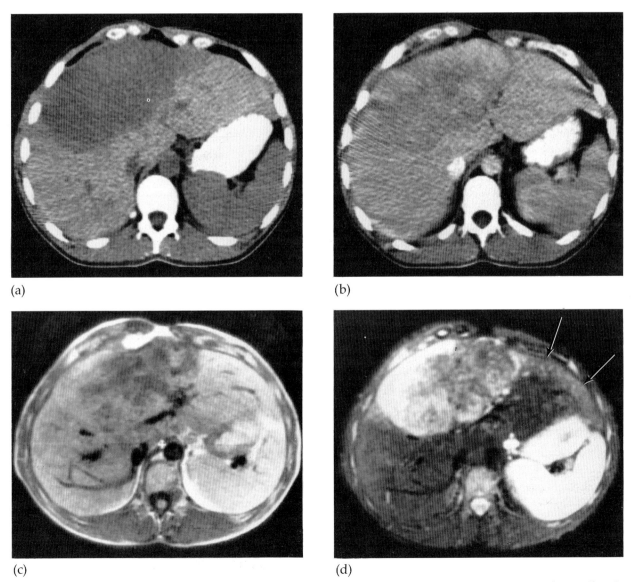

(a) (b)

(c) (d)

Fig. 6.7 Hepatoma: CT (a), enhanced CT (b), $SE_{544/44}$ (c), and $STIR_{1500/100/44}$ (d) scans. The tumour is seen in (d) as well as the secondary changes at the surface of the left lobe (*arrows*).

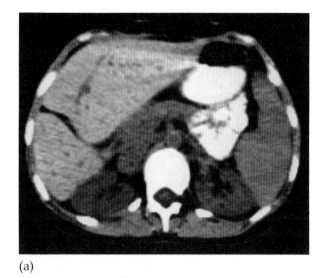

(a)

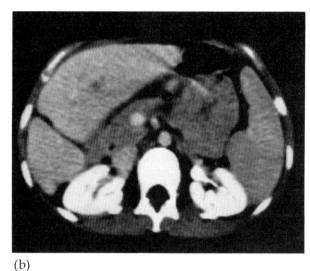

(b)

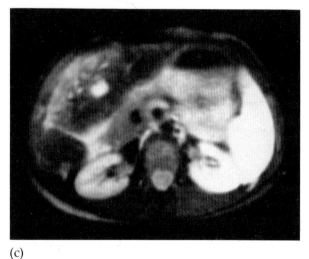

(c)

Fig. 6.8 Recurrent hepatoma: CT (a), enhanced CT (b), and STIR$_{1500/100/44}$ (c) scans. Metastases are better seen in (c), as is the fatty change at the anterolateral surface of the liver.

As with metastases, Gd-DTPA has displayed contrast enhancement but the contribution to diagnosis has been relatively small. The value of MRI to date has principally been in defining the extent of liver involvement prior to surgery.

Cholangiocarcinomas present particular problems in diagnosis when they are small, and the role of MRI is more in defining the extent of larger tumours (Fig. 6.9) and the associated changes, rather than in recognition of small tumours and differentiating these from bile duct strictures.

Hepatic adenoma

Two cases have been identified in our experience. Both have been well defined and presented as multiple lesions. In the case illustrated (Fig. 6.10) the liver displays features of iron overload with a very low signal and the tumour is highlighted. This was in a child with Fanconi's anaemia treated with multiple transfusions and androgenic steroids. The tumour regressed following withdrawal of the steroids.

Haemangioma

Haemangiomas may present difficulties, since the differential diagnosis is usually metastasis, and yet needle biopsy is contraindicated by the possibility of haemorrhage. These lesions are quite common, and are variable in size and histological pattern. In fact, large haemangiomas may show areas of infarction, necrosis, and lamellar changes and thus mimic hepatomas or metastases (Fig. 6.11).

Using the SE approach a long T_2 has been identified in haemangiomas with MRI, and upper limits have been proposed for tumours, giving about a 90% cut-off between metastases and haemangiomas (in small lesions). This cut-off has been

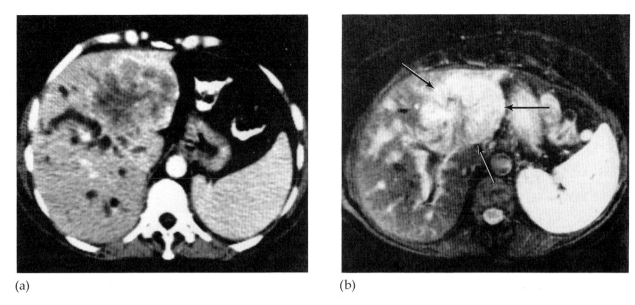

(a)

(b)

Fig. 6.9 Cholangiocarcinoma: enhanced CT (a) and STIR$_{1500/100/44}$ (b) scans. The tumour margins are better defined in (b) (*arrows*).

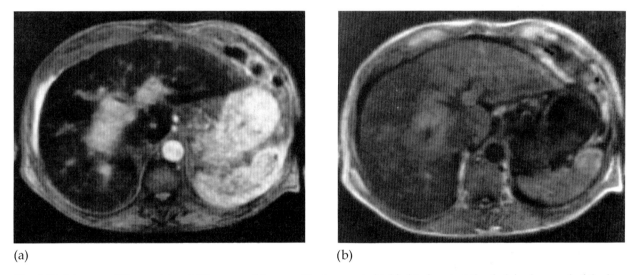

(a)

(b)

Fig. 6.10 Adenoma: PS$_{1000/13}$ (a) and IR$_{1400/400/13}$ (b) scans. The tumour is highlighted against the dark background of the liver parenchyma.

supported by two groups (Stark *et al.*, 1985a, Ohtomo *et al.*, 1985a) but not by a third (Glazer *et al.*, 1985).

The margins of haemangiomas are usually well defined and the smaller examples have not been associated with secondary changes, although changes with larger lesions have been seen.

Gd-DTPA has been used to display peripheral filling in a way analogous to X-ray CT. As yet no flow-specific sequences have been used to identify the slow flow in these lesions, but this might provide additional specificity.

Cysts

These lesions are usually sharply defined with very long values of T$_1$ and T$_2$. The T$_1$ and T$_2$ may shorten, depending on the contents of the cyst, with haemorrhage and protein both decreasing T$_1$ and T$_2$.

Cysts may be difficult to distinguish from haemangiomas and cystic tumours.

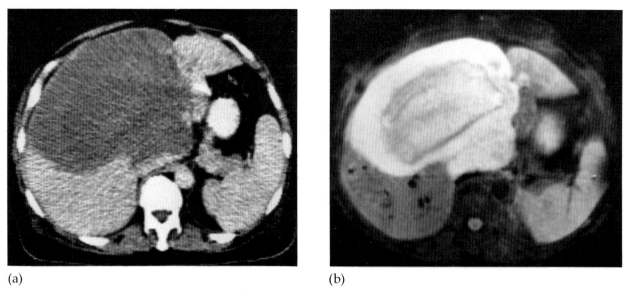

(a)   (b)

Fig. 6.11 Giant haemangioma: enhanced CT (a) and STIR$_{1500/100/44}$ (b) scans. The haemangioma is seen, together with the atrophic left lobe, which is highlighted on (b).

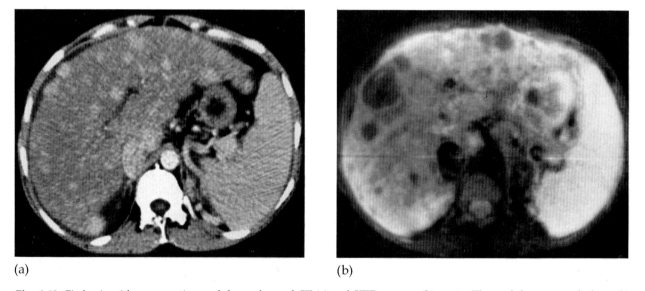

(a)   (b)

Fig. 6.12 Cirrhosis with regenerating nodules: enhanced CT (a) and STIR$_{1500/100/44}$ (b) scans. The nodules appear dark on (b) indicating that they are relatively normal parenchyma.

Dilated bile ducts

These also have an increased T_1 and T_2 but conform to a specific anatomical pattern from centre to periphery in association with portal veins.

There is no difficulty in distinguishing portal veins (dark) from dilated bile ducts (light) using the STIR approach.

Vascular diseases

The normal vascular pattern of the liver as seen with the SE approach has been described by Fisher *et al.* (1985). Patency of a portasystemic shunt has also been accurately diagnosed with MRI. Several patients with the Budd−Chiari syndrome have been imaged. Secondary parenchymal changes

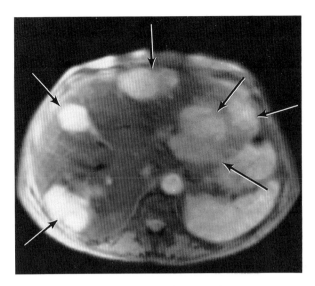

Fig. 6.13 Fatty infiltration of the liver with metastases: PS$_{1000/13}$ scan. The signal from liver is cancelled, leaving the metastases highlighted (*arrows*).

is not an invariable pattern and the appearances of the liver may be heterogenous, with areas of fatty infiltration and fibrosis. Other features such as the liver size, irregular nodules, sparing of the caudate lobe, irregular and disjointed vascular pattern, the presence of ascites, features of portal hypertension, and the increased spleen size may all be of value in diagnosis.

The pattern of regenerating nodules can be quite striking (Fig. 6.12). The nodules have a normal value of T_1 and T_2 and with STIR images give a lower signal intensity than the surrounding parenchyma.

No specific features have been detected in Wilson's disease.

have been more extensive than those displayed by CT in this condition.

Portal-vein thrombosis secondary to hepato-cellular carcinoma has also been described (Ohtomo *et al.*, 1985b).

Abnormal, irregular and small vascular patterns are also seen in cirrhosis, usually associated with some sparing of the caudate lobe.

Cirrhosis of the liver

The initial reports on MRI both referred to an increase in T_1 that may be found in cirrhosis. This

Fatty infiltration of the liver

With IR scans fatty infiltration produces a little change, or only a slight reduction in T_2, resulting in a slightly higher signal intensity than normal parenchyma. With SE sequences fatty infiltration causes an increase in T_2, producing an elevated signal intensity. No particular change is seen with the short TE spin-echo.

With phase-contrast sequences it is possible to image the fat and water fraction separately within the liver (Heiken *et al.*, 1985a). The opposed image of this type leads to cancellation of the signal, which may in turn highlight associated pathology (Fig. 6.13).

With STIR sequences fatty infiltration is high-lighted, although not to the degree that tumours are.

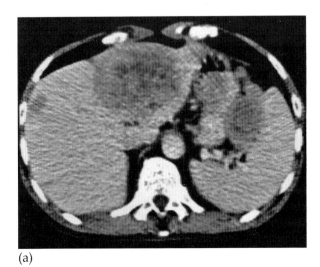

(a)

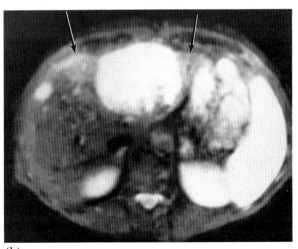

(b)

Fig. 6.14 Metastases with fatty infiltration: enhanced CT (a) and STIR$_{1500/100/44}$ (b) scans. Additional areas of fatty infiltration are highlighted (*arrows*).

The uses of MRI follow from the above considerations. When a low-attenuation lesion is seen on CT with a differential diagnosis between tumour and geographical fatty infiltration, IR images can give a specific diagnosis — fatty infiltration does not show an increase in T_1, liver tumours do so. When STIR images are used it is important to recognize that highlighted areas may represent fatty infiltration as well as tumour (Fig. 6.14).

Quantification of fatty infiltration is possible with the phase-contrast technique.

Fatty infiltration is also seen as part of the pattern of atrophy.

Haemochromatosis

Excessive iron deposition in the liver can produce a radical reduction in T_2, leading to a loss of signal from the liver with all sequences (Leung *et al.*, 1984, Stark *et al.*, 1985b). The liver appears strikingly dark (Fig. 6.15). Less severe degrees of iron overload may result in increased signal intensity as a result of a reduction in T_1.

Trauma

Local changes of increased T_1 and T_2 are seen in contusion. Lacerations are usually associated with more extensive damage. Subcapsular haematoma are frequently seen with an initial long T_1 and long T_2 phase followed by decrease in these parameters. Features of regeneration may be seen later.

Abscess

The general considerations here are whether the abscess is intrahepatic or extrahepatic and what its aetiology is. MRI features include an increase in T_1 and T_2 often with a thick, well-defined capsule, although there are usually abnormal regions outside the capsule (Fig. 6.16). The sagittal and coronal planes may be of value in defining the anatomical relations of the abscess. The presence of gas is well shown although calcification is poorly demonstrated. Daughter cysts are characteristic of hydatid (Fig. 6.17).

The contrast can be monitored with MRI, and drainage of bacterial abscess may soon be possible under MRI control.

Hepatitis

Various forms of hepatitis are usually associated

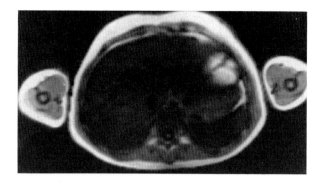

Fig. 6.15 Haemochromatosis: $PS_{1000/13}$ scan. The liver signal is markedly reduced.

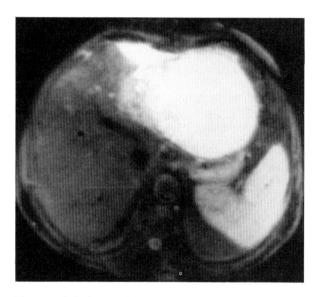

Fig. 6.16 Subphrenic abscess: $STIR_{1500/100/44}$ scan. The abscess is highlighted, as is associated change in the left lobe.

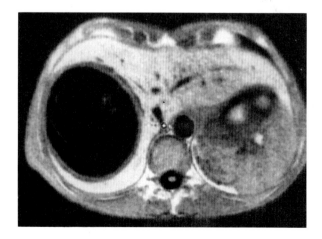

Fig. 6.17 Hydatid cyst: $IR_{1400/400/13}$ scan. The abscess has a thick wall.

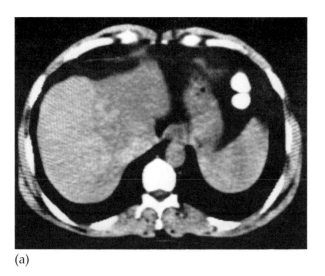

(a)

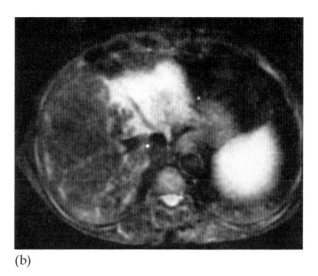

(b)

Fig. 6.18 Liver atrophy: CT (a) and STIR$_{1000/100/44}$ (b) scans. The atrophic left lobe is highlighted.

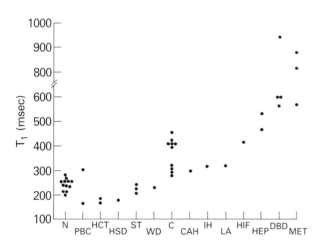

with an increase in T_1 and T_2. The features are generalized. They have been seen in acute viral hepatitis as well as chronic forms of hepatitis and in hepatitis associated with systemic disease. Periportal changes are seen, as well as slight focal areas of fatty change.

Liver atrophy

Atrophy is seen in association with a variety of lesions, but particularly with tumours at the central hilar region. The area of abnormality is highlighted with STIR sequences (Fig. 6.18).

The gall bladder

The gall bladder is well seen, and in the fasting state concentration of bile salts may produce a layering effect. This has been proposed as a test of gall bladder function (Hricak *et al.*, 1983).

Other aspects of MRI

It was hoped that measurements of T_1 and T_2 might provide useful information, allowing some degree of tissue characterization; however, the overlap between different disease states is substantial, and while these parameters are sensitive the specificity is limited (Fig. 6.19).

Fast imaging techniques are now being developed and it is possible to obtain useful contrast with the fast T_2-dependent field-echo sequence (Fig. 6.20). Detailed comparison with other techniques will be necessary to evaluate this approach.

Although magnetite is not available for clinical

	No. of subjects	Range of mean CT attenuation values (H)	Range of mean T_1 values (msec)
Normal volunteers	12		210–270
Normal patients	12	51–65	
Hepatoma	2	41–53	460–530
Metastases	3	28–34	560–810
Dilated bile ducts	4	10–51	550–980
Liver atrophy	2	24	320
Hepatic infarct	1	41	410
Infectious hepatitis	1	57	310
Chronic active hepatitis	1	49	290
Haemochromatosis	2	66–71	170–190
Haemosiderosis	1	81	180
Steatosis	3	3–42	210–240
Cirrhosis	10	41–62	280–450
Primary bilary cirrhosis	2	40–56	160–350
Wilsons disease	1	56	230
Total	33		

N	Normal	CAH	Chronic active hepatitis
PBC	Primary biliary cirrhosis	IH	Infectious hepatitis
HCT	Haemochromatosis	LA	Liver atrophy
HSD	Haemosiderosis	HIF	Hepatic infarct
ST	Steatosis	HEP	Hepatoma
WD	Wilsons disease	DBD	Dilated bile ducts
C	Cirrhosis	MET	Metastases

Fig. 6.19 T_1 values in a range of disease.

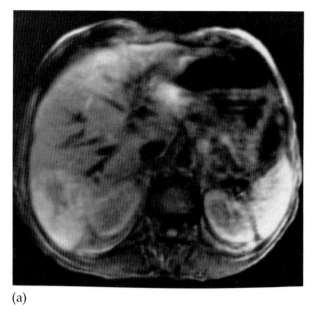

(a)

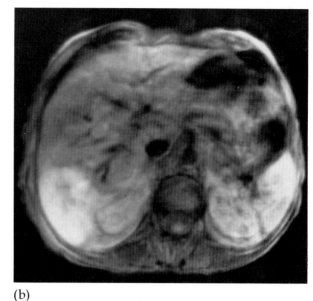

(b)

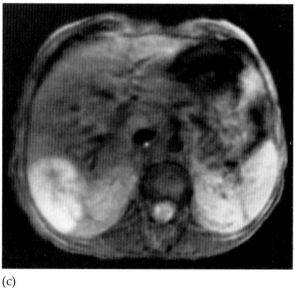

(c)

Fig.6.20 Metastases: $PS_{250/33}$ ($\alpha = 90°$) (a), $PS_{250/33}$ ($\alpha = 60°$) (b), and $PS_{250/33}$ ($\alpha = 30°$) (c) scans. As the rotation angle is reduced the contrast is improved but the images become noisier.

use it is effective in animal studies (Fig. 6.21). It may be of considerable value in clinical practice.

Conclusion

The evolution of MRI in the liver to date has largely been a technical exercise. Problems due to motion, the short T_2 value of liver, and the presence of fat in the abdomen have been recognized and techniques designed to cope with these problems have been developed. This has meant that clinical evaluation in strict terms has lagged behind many other areas of the body, but the general results in common conditions such as liver metastases have continued to improve.

Once artefact is controlled, the sensitivity of MRI to soft-tissue change has provided a high diagnostic yield although the specificity has been much lower.

Magnetic resonance spectroscopy is now available for clinical use and spectra of tumours and various metabolic conditions have already been obtained. This may provide useful biochemical information.

Questions about the cost-effectiveness of MRI in relation to US and CT remain. At the moment MRI is the most expensive technique and may remain so, but work is now in progress aimed at producing cheaper magnets and cheaper imaging systems.

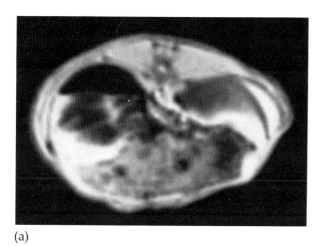 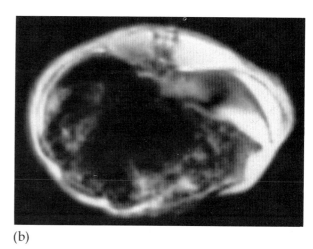

(a)   (b)

Fig. 6.21 Prone normal rabbit: PS$_{1000/13}$ images before (a) and after (b) oral magnetite. The magnetite obliterates much of the signal from the bowel in (b).

Acknowledgements

The help of Dr Ian Young of GEC Hirst Research, Wembley, and Dr H.P. Niendorf of Schering AG, Berlin, is gratefully acknowledged.

References

Bailes, D.R., Gilderdale, D.J., Bydder, G.M., Collins, A.G., Butson, P.R., Gilderdale, D.J. & Young I.R. (1985) Use of closely coupled receiver coils in MRI: Practical aspects. *Journal of Computer Assisted Tomography*, **9(5)**, 987−996.

Bottomley, P.A., Hardy, C.J., Argersinger, R.E. & Allen, G.R. (1985) Relaxation in pathology: are T$_1$'s and T$_2$'s diagnostic? *Abstracts, Society of Magnetic Resonance in Medicine*, 4th Annual Meeting, 1985, The Barbican, London, pp. 28−29. SMRM, Berkeley.

Bradley, W.G. Jnr, Crooks, L.E. & Newton, T.H. (1984) Physical principles of NMR. In: Newton, T.H. & Potts, D.G. (eds) *Modern Neuroradiology Vol. 2, Advanced Imaging Techniques*, pp. 15−61. Clavadel Press, San Francisco.

Bydder, G.M., Curati, W.L., Gadian, D.G., Hall, A.S., Harman, R.R., Butson, P.R., Gilderdale, O.J. & Young, I.R. (1985a) Use of closely coupled receiver coils in MRI: Practical aspects. *Journal of Computer Assisted Tomography*, **9(5)**, 987−996.

Bydder, G.M., Steiner, R.E., Blumgart, L.H., Khenia, S. & Young, I.R. (1985b) MRI of the liver using short TI inversion recovery sequences. *Journal of Computer Assisted Tomography*, **9(6)**, 1084−1089.

Bydder, G.M. & Young, I.R. (1985) MRI: clinical use of the inversion recovery sequence. *Journal of Computer Assisted Tomography*, **9(4)**, 659−675.

Carr, D.H., Brown, J., Bydder, G.M., Steiner, R.E., Weinmann, H.J., Speck, U., Hall, A.S. & Young, I.R. (1984) Gadolinium-DTPA as a contrast agent in MRI: initial clinical experience in 20 patients. *American Journal of Roentgenology*, **143**, 215−224.

Carr D.H., Graif, M., Bydder, G.M., Niendorf, H.P., Brown, J., Steiner, R.E., Blumgart, L.H. & Young, I.R. (1985) Gadolinium-DTPA in the assessment of liver tumours by magnetic resonance imaging. *Abstracts, Society of Magnetic Resonance in Medicine*, 4th Annual Meeting, The Barbican, London, Vol 2, pp. 1135−1136.

Dixon, W.T. (1984) Simple proton spectroscopic imaging. *Radiology*, **153**, 189−194.

Doyle, F.H., Pennock, J.M., Banks, L.M., McDonnell, M.J., Bydder, G.M., Steiner, Steiner, R.E., Young, I.R. et al. (1982) Nuclear magnetic resonance (NMR) imaging of the liver: initial experience. *American Journal of Roentgenology*, **138**, 193−200.

Doyle, F.H., Pennock, J.M., Banks, L.M. et al. (1982) Nuclear magnetic resonance (NMR) imaging of the liver: initial experience. *American Journal of Roentgenology*, **138**, 193−200.

Fisher, MR., Wall, S.D., Hricak, H, McCarthy, S. & Kerler, R.K. (1985) Hepatic vascular anatomy on magnetic resonance imaging. *American Journal of Roentgenology*, **144**, 739−746.

Gadian, D.G. (1982) *NMR and its Application to Living Systems*. Clarendon Press, Oxford.

Glazer, G.M., Aisen A.M., Francis, I.R., Gyres, J.W., Lande, I. & Adler, D.D. (1985) Hepatic cavernous hemangioma: magnetic resonance imaging. *Radiology*, **155**, 417−420.

Haaga, J.R. (1984) Magnetic resonance imaging of the liver. *Radiologic Clinics of North America*, **22**, 879−890.

Heiken, J.P., Lee, J.K.T. & Dixon, W.T. (1985a) Fatty infiltration of the liver: evaluation by proton spectroscopic imaging. *Radiology*, **157**, 707−710.

Heiken, J.P., Lee, J.K.T., Glazer, H.S. & Ling, D. (1985b) Hepatic metastases studied with MR and CT. *Radiology*, **156**, 423−427.

Henkelman, R.M., Poon, P.Y., Broskiel, M.J. & Ege, G.M. (1984) *Optimised MR image contrast for liver metastases*. Presented at the Society of Magnetic Resonance in Medicine, 3rd Annual Meeting, New York City August 16, 1984. SMRM, Berkeley.

Hricak, H., Filly, R., Margulis, A.R., Moon, K.L., Crooks, L.E. & Kaufman, L. (1983) NMR imaging of the gall bladder. *Radiology*, **147**, 481−484.

Leung, A.W-L., Steiner, R.E. & Young, I.R. (1984) NMR imaging of the liver in two cases of iron overload. *Journal of Computer Assisted Tomography*. **8(3)**, 446–449.

Mendonca-Dias, M.H., Bernardo, M.L., Muller, R.N., Acuff, V. & Lauterbur, P.C. (1985) Ferromagnetic particles as contrast agents for magnetic resonance imaging. *Abstracts, Society of Magnetic Resonance in Medicine*, 4th Annual Meeting. The Barbican London, Vol. 2, pp. 887–888. SMRM, Berkeley.

Moss, A.A., Goldberg, N.I., Stark D.D. *et al.*, (1984) Nuclear magnetic resonance imaging of hepatic tumors. *Radiology*, **150**, 141–147.

Ohtomo, K., Itai, Y., Funii, S., Yashiro, N., Yoshikawa, K. & Iio, M. (1985a) Hepatic tumors: differentiation by transverse relaxation time (T$_2$) of magnetic resonance imaging. *Radiology*, **155**, 421–423.

Ohtomo, K., Itai, Y., Furai, S., Yoshikawa, K., Yashiro, N. & Masahino, I. (1985b) MR imaging of portal vein thrombosis in hepatocellular carcinoma. *Journal of Computer Assisted Tomography*, **9**, 328–329.

Olsson, M., Persson, B.R.B., Salford, L.G. & Schroder, U. (1985) Ferromagnetic particles as contrast agent in T$_2$ NMR imaging. *Abstracts, Society of Magnetic Resonance in Medicine*, 4th Annual Meeting, The Barbican, London, Vol. 2, p. 889. SMRM, Berkeley.

Petersen, S.B., Muller, R.N. & Rinck, P.A., (1985) *An Introduction to Biomedical Nuclear Magnetic Resonance*. Georg Thieme Verlag, New York.

Sepponen, R.E., Sipponen, J.T. & Tanttu, J.I. (1984) A method for chemical shift imaging: demonstration of bone marrow involvement with proton chemical shift imaging. *Journal of Computer Assisted Tomography*, **8**, 585–587.

Smith, F.W., & Mallard, J.R. (1984) NMR imaging in liver disease. *British Medical Bulletin*, **40**, 194–196.

Smith, F.W., Mallard, J.R., Reid, A. & Hutchison, J.M.S. (1981) Nuclear magnetic imaging in liver disease. *Lancet*, **i**, 963–966.

Stark, D.D., Felder, R.C., Willenberg, J. *et al.* (1985a) Magnetic resonance imaging of cavernous hemangioma of the liver: tissue specific characterisation. *American Journal of Roentgenology*, **145**, 213–222.

Stark, D.D. & Ferrucci, J.T. (1986) Technical and clinical progress in MRI of the abdomen. *Diagnostic Imaging International*, **2(1)**, 26–35.

Stark, D.D., Moseley, M., Bacon, B.R. *et al.* (1985b) Magnetic resonance imaging and spectroscopy of hepatic iron overload. *Radiology*, **154**, 137–142.

Stark, D.D., Moss A.A. & Goldberg, H.I. (1986) Nuclear magnetic resonance of the liver, spleen and pancreas. *Cardiovascular and Interventional Radiology*, **8**, 329–341.

Vermess, M., Leung, A.W-L., Bydder, G.M., Steiner, R.E., Blumgart, L.H. & Young, I.R. (1985) MR imaging of the liver in primary hepatocellular carcinoma. *Journal of Computer Assisted Tomography*, **9**, 749–754.

Weinmann, H-J., Brasch, R.C., Press, W.R. & Wesbey, G.E. (1984) Characteristics of Gadolinium-DTPA complex: a potential NMR contrast agent. *American Journal of Roentgenology*, **142**, 619–624.

Wesbey, G.E., Brasch, R.C., Engelstad, B.L., Moss, A.A., Crooks, L.E. & Buto, H.C. (1983) Nuclear magnetic resonance contrast enhancement study of the gastrointestinal tract of rats and a human volunteer using non-toxic oral solution. *Radiology*, **149**, 175–180.

Young, I.R., Clarke, G.J., Bailes, D.R., Pennock, J.M., Doyle, F.H. & Bydder, G.M. (1981) Enhancement of relaxation rate with paramagnetic contrast agents in NMR imaging. *Computed Tomography*, **5(6)**, 543–547.

7: Diffuse Liver Disease — Cirrhosis

K.C. DEWBURY AND COLLEAGUES

Pathology and clinical manifestations

Cirrhosis is a pathological term to describe hepatic fibrosis and nodule formation involving the major portion of the liver. This is the common end-response of the liver to many different types of injury or insult. Initially injury produces damage and necrosis of liver cells, leading to a collapse and distortion of the collagen framework of the liver and the formation of fibrous septa. Continuing liver injury leads to the formation of regenerative nodules of liver cells and increasing fibrosis, the hallmarks of cirrhosis. The distribution of fibrous septa varies with the cause of liver necrosis. In biliary cirrhosis fibrosis occurs in the portal tracts around the bile ducts, and extends into the lobules.

Three anatomical types of cirrhosis are recognized, classified according to the size of the nodules. In a micronodular cirrhosis the liver contains small nodules that vary little in size. This is usually associated with a continuing liver injury such as alcohol abuse. In a macronodular cirrhosis the liver contains larger nodules of varying sizes, usually reflecting post-hepatitic injury. A cirrhosis containing both large and small nodules is described as a mixed pattern.

Causes of cirrhosis include the following:
1 Alcohol.
2 Virus hepatitis (Type B and non-A, non-B).
3 Prolonged obstructive jaundice.
4 Drugs (e.g. methotrexate).
5 Primary biliary cirrhosis.
6 Chronic active hepatitis.

The majority of the cirrhosis in the UK is related to alcohol and hepatitis virus infection. There remains, however, a large group in whom no cause is found. These are termed 'cryptogenic', and at present account for up to 40% of all patients diagnosed as having cirrhosis in the UK.

Cirrhosis, irrespective of cause, results in two major events: *hepatocellular failure* due directly to liver-cell damage, and *portal venous hypertension*, which is a mechanical effect of the regenerative liver nodules distorting the hepatic vascular tree, impeding the drainage of blood from the liver, and thus producing back pressure in the portal system. Direct portal vein—hepatic vein communications may also occur, diverting blood past functioning tissue within regenerating nodules. This leads to ischaemia of the cells in the centre of the nodules and further progression of the cirrhosis, even after removal of the primary causative factor. Prognosis and treatment depends in large part on the severity of these two changes. Clinically the cirrhosis may be either latent and well compensated or active and decompensated. Patients with compensated cirrhosis may have the skin stigmata of liver disease such as spider naevi, red palms, white nails, and scanty body hair, as well as gynaecomastia, testicular atrophy, and hepatosplenomegaly, but otherwise be quite well. Vague symptoms of morning indigestion and flatulent dyspepsia may be early signs of alcoholic cirrhosis.

Patients with decompensated cirrhosis usually present with ascites and jaundice. Their general health is poor, with muscle wasting and weight loss. The signs of hepatic encephalopathy, drowsiness, and fetor hepaticus, may be present. In general, the deeper the jaundice the more severe the hepatocellular dysfunction. The development of a primary liver cancer may cause sudden decompensation in a previously well-compensated patient.

Portal venous hypertension is indicated by the presence of splenomegaly and abdominal-wall venous collaterals. Portal venous hypertension leads to the development of oesophageal varices that may rupture, causing torrential haemorrhage. This is not only serious in its own right, but may also precipitate hepatocellular failure. Biochemical liver function tests are usually of little value for making the diagnosis of cirrhosis. A hepatitic or cholestatic pattern may help point to the cause. Reduced protein synthesis by the liver, indicated by a low serum albumin concentration and a prolonged prothrombin time, is an index of hepatic decompensation. A raised gammaglobulin concentration is usual. In decompensated cirrhosis complex electrolyte disturbances may develop, including functional renal failure. Cirrhotic patients are especially susceptible to bacterial infections including bacteraemia, urinary-tract infections, and occult bacterial peritonitis. Unexpected clinical deterioration in a cirrhotic is commonly due to bacterial infection. There are numerous special investigations including tests for type B hepatitis virus markers, the mitochondrial antibody (primary biliary cirrhosis), and smooth muscle antibody (lupoid chronic active hepatitis). A raised serum alphafetoprotein suggests the development of a primary liver cancer.

Chronic active hepatitis

This is a precursor of cirrhosis in most cases. It is characterized by chronic inflammatory changes in the portal areas of the liver extending into the liver parenchyma. There are many causes including lupoid hepatitis, which is a multisystem disease with an autoimmune basis.

Primary biliary cirrhosis

This is an uncommon form of intrahepatic cholestasis occurring mainly in females from 40 to 60 years of age. Histologically, in the early stages, nodular regeneration is inconspicuous and the features are of a chronic non-suppurative granulomatous obliteration of the interlobular and septal bile ducts, with an infiltration of mononuclear inflammatory cells. Pruritus is the most common presenting symptom, followed by jaundice. When this is deep and prolonged, skin xanthomata develop. Prolonged cholestasis produces osteomalacia and osteoporosis. Hypertrophic osteoarthropathy and avascular necrosis are also described, and pulmonary fibrosis may occur. Mitochondrial antibodies are present in over 80% of cases.

The radiology of cirrhosis

Conventional radiology has a relatively small part to play in the specific diagnosis of cirrhosis, which is made definitively by liver biopsy. Certain features may be demonstrated by radiological techniques, particularly in relation to assessing the stage of disease, its progression, and the effects of therapy. Radiology is also of value in the diagnosis of the complications and associated diseases of cirrhosis, including gallstones, peptic ulcer, pancreatitis, hepatoma, portal-vein thrombosis, cardiomyopathy, pulmonary shunting, emphysema, and the various bone changes associated with primary biliary cirrhosis.

Plain films

Chest X-ray

Alcohol may cause a cardiomyopathy, probably mainly due to a direct toxic affect of alcohol on the myocytes. Other contributory factors may be the general nutritional deficiency found in some alcoholics, and a thiamine deficiency causing beriberi. The radiological changes are of cardiac enlargement with signs of left and right heart failure. Enlargement of the azygos vein and widening of the left paravertebral shadow due to dilatation of the hemiazygos vein may be seen.

The pulmonary circulation in cirrhotic patients may be abnormal in a number of ways. About one-third of patients with decompensated cirrhosis have reduced arterial saturation and are sometimes cyanosed. This is probably due to intrapulmonary shunting through microscopic arterial venous fistulae. The chest X-ray may show a nodularity in the lower zones usually attributed to dilatation of normal small pulmonary blood vessels. This is a local manifestation of the general vessel dilatation and increased peripheral blood flow seen in the systemic circulation.

There is a significantly increased incidence of pulmonary oedema in patients with fulminant hepatic failure (decompensated cirrhosis) (Warren *et al.*, 1978), which does not appear to be secondary to heart failure. Many of these patients with pulmonary oedema later develop pulmonary infection.

In chronic liver disease with ascites, ventilation of the lung bases is restricted by mechanical factors. Elevation of the diaphragm and the basal collapse may be seen.

Alpha$_1$-antitrypsin is a glycoprotein whose synthesis in the liver is controlled by a pair of autosomal codominant genes (Cohen, 1975). Decreased serum levels are found in homozygos zz phenotype patients. Up to 10% of this group develop a cirrhosis that typically is rapidly progressive. The cirrhosis may be macronodular, micronodular or biliary in type. The pulmonary manifestations are typically of a progressive panlobular basal emphysema (Hutchinson, 1973).

Plain abdominal X-ray

The lower edge of the liver is usually demonstrated on the plain abdominal film, but what forms this visible boundary is unclear. Because of the complex shape of the liver simple linear measurements of size are at best only guidelines. A length of 15 cm in the mid-clavicular line is used by some as the upper limit of normal. Enlargement of the liver may cause displacement of the hepatic flexure of the colon downwards, the diaphragm up, and the stomach to the left. If the right lobe of the liver is decreased in size, as may occur in severe cirrhosis, the hepatic flexure of the colon may conversely lie in a rather high position. The soft-tissue outline of the spleen is also visible on the plain abdominal film, characteristically lying along the left 10th rib. When the spleen enlarges it indents the greater curvature of the stomach, eventually displacing it. The splenic flexure of the colon may be pushed downwards. Marked splenomegaly is easily recognized.

Ascites occurs in all types of liver cirrhosis. Large amounts may be suggested on the plain abdominal film, characteristically causing a greyness and haziness of the film and medial displacement of the bowel loops. The colon is apparently shortened and appears more vertical than usual.

Calcified gall stones may be shown on the plain film, as may calcification in the pancreas in alcoholic cirrhosis. An example of this is shown in Fig. 7.1. Alcoholic pancreatitis is the commonest cause of pancreatic calcification and may be complicated by portal vein thrombosis.

Bones and joints

The skeletal changes of chronic liver disease include a destructive arthropathy, inflammatory polyarthritis, and osteomalacia. The latter occurs due to malabsorption of vitamin D and calcium, associated with cholestasis. The features of the osteomalacia are not unusual, with osteopenia and Looser zones. Clinical arthritis and joint pains are common in liver disease but radiological changes are found infrequently.

The destructive arthropathy described in patients with primary biliary cirrhosis (Clark *et al.*, 1978) is striking, showing the radiological appearances of an avascular necrosis. The head of

the humerus or femur is most commonly involved; an example of this is shown in Fig. 7.2.

Barium studies

The two main reasons for performing barium studies of the gastrointestinal tract in patients with cirrhosis are to demonstrate the signs of portal hypertension and to investigate the cause of bleeding. Varices present in the oesophagus may be demonstrated in the majority of cases by careful radiological technique. The examination is carried out with the patient recumbent. Multiple films are taken of the relaxed oesophagus with a thin coating of barium. Varices present as nodular filling defects of various sizes in the lower one-third of the oesophagus (Fig. 7.3). When large varices are present the oesophagus is always dilated. Enhanced visualization of varices may be achieved by the use of i.v. Buscopan. Varices in the stomach present as lobulated filling defects in the gastric fundus and along the lesser curve of the stomach. Visualization is often best seen on the erect double-contrast views of the fundus. Gastric varices are almost always associated with oesophageal varices. During the search for suspected varices in a patient who has had a haematemesis from an unknown site, it is most important to search for other causes of upper gastrointestinal tract haemorrhage, even when varices are shown, since there is an increased incidence of peptic ulcer in liver disease.

To some extent barium studies have been replaced by endoscopy, which may not only be more accurate in the demonstration of oesophageal varices in particular, but will also be able to demonstrate the precise cause and site of bleeding.

Vascular studies

Vascular studies have no real place in the specific diagnosis of cirrhosis, but since the prognosis of cirrhosis is determined by the severity of the liver disease and the occurrence of haemorrhage, studies of the portal system become necessary in order to assess the patency of the splenoportal axis and to demonstrate the presence of varices, and the predominant flow patterns in the portal vein and the portal systemic collaterals.

Splenoportography

For many years direct-puncture splenoportography was the primary angiographic method for

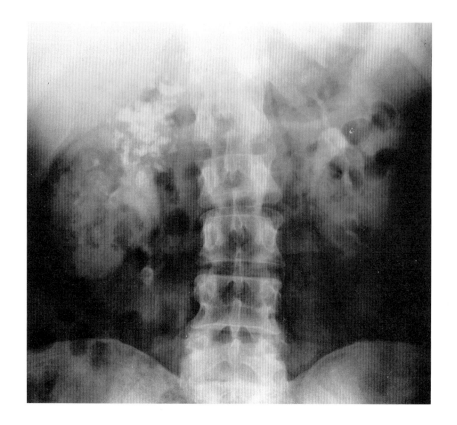

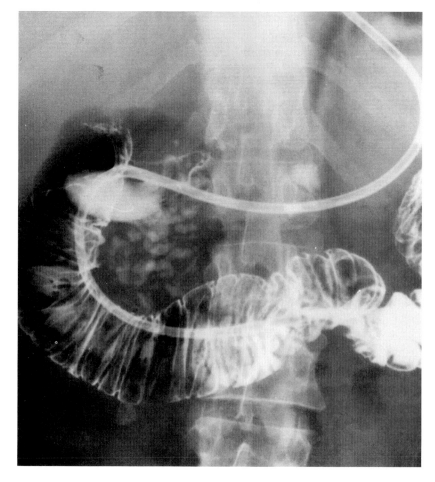

Fig. 7.1 Extensive pancreatic calcification in a patient with cirrhosis.

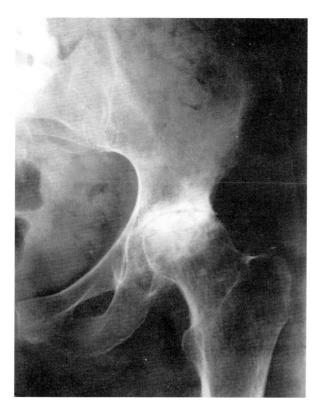

Fig. 7.2 Extensive arthritis and avascular necrosis in the hip of a patient with primary biliary cirrhosis.

evaluating patients with cirrhosis and portal hypertension. The measurement of splenic pressure gives an accurate indication of portal pressure in patients with both post-sinusoidal and pre-sinusoidal blocks. Injection of contrast into the splenic pulp demonstrates the systemic collateral veins that develop in patients with increased intrahepatic resistance of portal blood flow. In patients with splenic-vein or portal-vein thrombosis it demonstrates the site of obstruction and the periportal collateral veins that regularly develop. The splenoportogram gives a good demonstration of the intrahepatic portal radicals and an assessment of the rapidity of wash-out of the vessels in a hepatopetal direction. When portal vein blood flow is reversed the portal vein is not demonstrated. In established cirrhosis there may be distortion of the peripheral portal radicals in the liver and apparent reduction in the number of side branches.

Arterioportography

The portal venous system of the liver may be demonstrated by selective angiography of the coeliac axis, splenic artery, or superior mesenteric artery. Arterioportography has become popular in recent years, replacing direct-puncture splenic portography, particularly in the presence of ascites and coagulation defects. It is essential in the assessment of the portal system after splenectomy. Filming must be extended to at least 25 s, as flow is slowed in patients with portal hypertension. One advantage of this technique is that arterial studies of the liver may be carried out at the same time as arterioportography.

Arterial studies

Coeliac angiography has three main functions in the evaluation of patients with cirrhosis and portal hypertension in addition to demonstration of the portal system and collateral channels. Arteriography may be of help in excluding other causes of massive upper gastrointestinal tract bleeding, particularly when the source has not been shown in gastroscopy. Approximately 20%—30% of patients with cirrhosis and upper gastrointestinal bleeding are actually bleeding from sources other than varices. If varices are demonstrated the figure is only 10%. The most common causes of bleeding are duodenal ulcer, gastric ulcer, gastritis, and Mallory—Weiss tears. The technique may be used to control bleeding by selective embolization.

Arteriography may also be used to study the haemodynamics of the hepatic arterial system during the various stages of cirrhosis. In early cirrhosis there may be intrahepatic artery stretching with hepatomegaly. In more advanced disease the hepatic artery and its branches become more dilated, elongated, and tortuous. Occasionally the peripheral branches have the appearance of being duplicated. Finally in severe disease, when the liver begins to shrink, the combination of tortuosity and retraction of the hepatic artery branches gives the characteristic angiographic appearance of cirrhosis frequently called 'corkscrewing' (Fig. 7.4). Unfortunately the variation in the amount of hypervascularity accompanying cirrhosis is wide and correlation of any angiographic appearance of hepatic arteries with the stage of cirrhosis is difficult. In advanced cirrhosis the hepatic venous resistance to outflow of the portal vein and hepatic artery may become so great that hepatic artery blood drains from the liver through the portal vein.

When a hepatoma develops in a patient with cirrhosis it is often more difficult to identify than in a patient with an otherwise normal liver. The

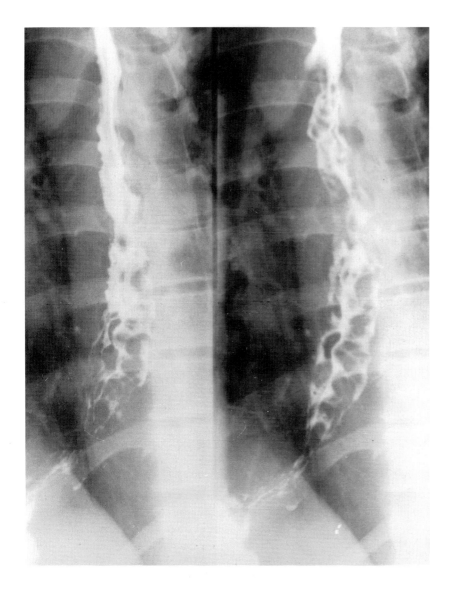

Fig. 7.3 Large oesophageal varices.

diffuse form of hepatoma in particular may be extremely difficult to differentiate from the already diffusely abnormal cirrhotic liver on which it is superimposed. In general a hepatoma stands out as a hypervascular mass with tumour vessels. With hepatoma, the place of angiography is not so much in the diagnosis of the lesion, but in an accurate mapping of the vascular supply when surgery is being considered.

Radioisotope imaging

Radioisotopes have been used for many years to study the function and morphology of the liver. Function may be impaired by focal or diffuse disease. Irregular or patchy hepatic uptake of radiocoloid is seen in many disorders which alter normal hepatic function and architecture. The

mechanisms for these appearances include impairment of normal hepatocyte macrophage function, alterations in blood flow, and replacement of liver parenchyma by fibroid tissue. When hepatic function is impaired, macrophages of spleen, bone marrow, and lung clear a large proportion of radiocoloid from the circulation. The characteristic image appearance is an enlarged liver, usually with irregular distribution of radiocoloid, and splenomegaly with increased radiocoloid uptake and a high proportion of activity in bone marrow (Fig. 7.5). These appearances reflect the functional deficit that occurs in cirrhosis. The appearances are not, however, specific and are also seen in hepatitis, portal fibrosis, and extensive metastatic replacement. Fatty infiltration on its own shows as hepatic enlargement with minimal functional impairment. The non-specific image appearances

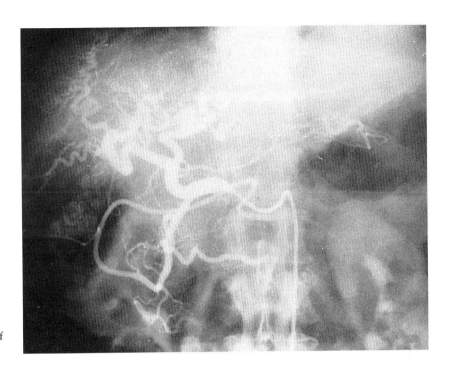

Fig. 7.4 Selective hepatic arteriogram showing duplication and 'corkscrewing' of peripheral vessels in a patient with cirrhosis. There are stones in the gall bladder (courtesy of Dr S.J. Birch).

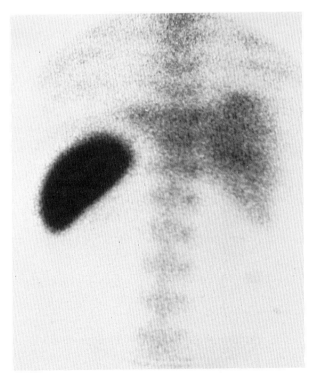

Fig. 7.5 Posterior view of an isotope scan in alcoholic cirrhosis showing poor radiocolloid uptake in the liver and increased uptake in spleen and spine.

shown by many generalized disorders of the liver limit the diagnostic contribution made by radio-isotope imaging. Serial studies may be of value in mapping the changing functional status of the liver.

Ultrasound

The size and texture of the normal liver can usually be clearly demonstrated with ultrasound. The appearances seen in cirrhosis may be divided into those of the liver itself, and the associated findings. The liver may be enlarged in the early stages where there is inflammatory and fatty change, normal in size, or shrunken and scarred in the late stages. The caudate lobe of the liver often appears particularly large relative to the rest of the liver. This may form a useful index of the presence of cirrhosis. The lateral edge of the portal vein in a transverse section of the liver is taken as demarcating the caudate from the right lobe. The lobes are measured from this point to their free edges medially and laterally, respectively (Fig. 7.6). The caudate lobe is usually less than half the width of the right lobe, and never more than two-thirds (Harbin *et al.*, 1980). Though easy to gauge and usually abnormal in cirrhosis, this ratio may also be abnormal in other diffuse disorders and especially in the Budd–Chiari syndrome.

In cirrhosis the liver surface usually appears smooth but the larger regenerative nodules may produce lobulation of the surface. The echoes returned are variable and indeed may be quite normal. Characteristically, however, the cirrhotic liver returns high-level echoes, producing the so called 'bright' liver echo pattern (Saverymuttu *et al.*, 1979, Taylor *et al.*, 1981). The assessment of

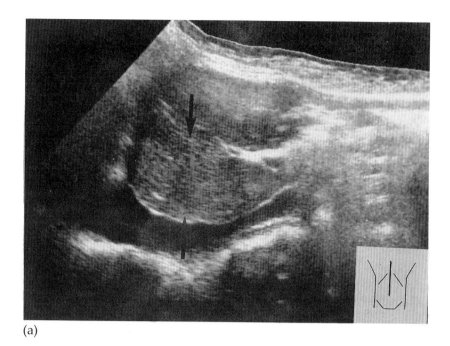

(a)

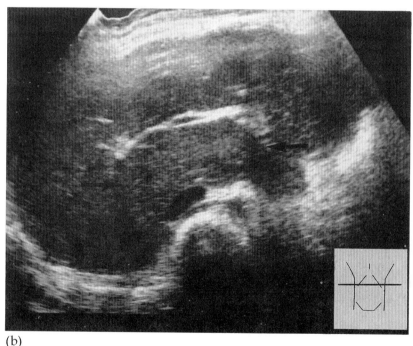

(b)

Fig. 7.6 (a) Longitudinal and
(b) transverse scans showing marked
enlargement of the caudate lobe
(*arrowed*) in a patient with post-
hepatitic cirrhosis.

the amplitude of the parenchymal echoes of the liver is usually of necessity somewhat objective, but two internal features are particularly useful in making this assessment more reliable. In the normal patient the renal cortical echoes are usually only slightly less reflective (or bright) than the hepatic echoes. When the liver is abnormally reflective the kidney appears unduly dark in contrast to the abnormal liver. This exaggerates the hepatorenal contrast. For the same reasons, structures that normally return strong echoes from within the liver lose contrast compared with the liver parenchyma, so that for example the normally echogenic periportal tissues may become inapparent, the portal veins appearing to no longer have walls and showing as simple tubular structures within the liver, rather like the hepatic veins seen in normal patients (Fig. 7.7).

Changes in liver texture are also inconstant and subjective, but in some cases the echoes seem smaller and tightly packed to give a fine texture. Likewise in some cases the attenuation of the liver

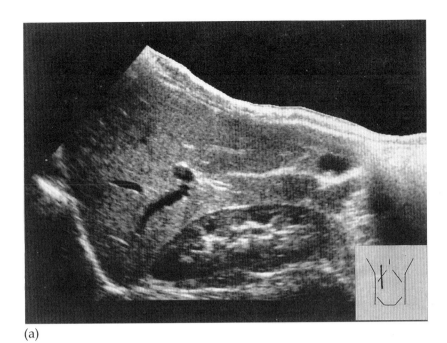

(a)

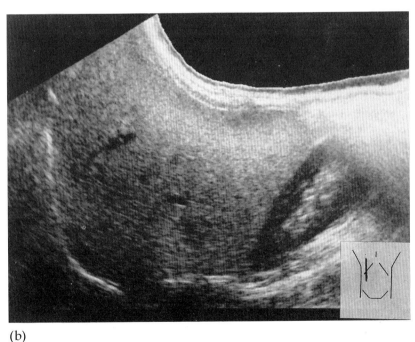

Fig. 7.7 (a) Longitudinal scan of the liver in a normal patient. (b) Comparative section in a patient with cirrhosis showing a high amplitude liver echo pattern.

(b)

seems to be high so that deeper parts cannot be registered without considerable changes in the swept gain characteristics. Whilst these textural features are inconstant and it has been difficult to relate them to the severity of the histological change in cirrhosis, none the less they are commonly encountered and may be a useful diagnostic feature. In micronodular cirrhosis as many as 80% of the patients will show abnormality in the liver echo pattern, although in a macronodular cirrhosis the proportion will not be so high. This difference

may well reflect the amount of fat in the liver in alcoholic cirrhosis, and recent studies suggest that this may be the key to amplitude changes (Joseph & Dewbury, 1985, Unpublished data). Identical features may be seen in cases of fatty infiltration of the liver and in some granulomatous diseases as well as in rare cases of miliary malignancy (Dewbury & Clarke, 1979).

Over many years there has been the hope that more objective measurements may be made in an attempt to be more 'tissue specific' in ultrasound diagnosis. Preliminary results are now available from a prototype system that performs sophisticated computerized measurements of the frequency of echoes returning from within patients. In all biological tissues the higher-frequency component of ultrasound signals is attenuated to a greater degree than the low-frequency components. The normal range of values for frequency-dependent attenuation in the human liver have been established and measurements obtained in patients with a wide range of known liver pathologies. Results available to date indicate that the normal range is wide and there is considerable overlap between normals and abnormals. However, in general the presence of fat deposition within the liver substantially increases the attenuation, whilst active inflammatory disease causes a reduction in frequency-dependent attenuation. This system does not and cannot 'characterize' liver conditions, but does offer additional information over and above that available in the conventional amplitude image (Meire, 1985, Personal communication).

Large regenerating nodules of the liver are occasionally discernible as regions of slight alteration in the texture of the liver. Usually, though, they are best detected as a slight lobulation of the liver surface. This feature is much more apparent in the presence of ascites, where it may be quite a useful diagnostic feature (Fig. 7.8).

The associated findings in cirrhotic patients are both of ascites and of portal hypertension. Ultrasound is sensitive in detecting even small amounts of ascitic fluid.

Unless it is massive, postural shift of the fluid can be demonstrated. Since in cirrhosis the ascites is an exudate, the bowel remains normally mobile and gut containing gas will float into the central part of the abdomen with the patient supine. The presence of peritoneal fluid often allows excellent visualization of abdominal structures, including specifically the surface nodularity of the cirrhotic liver. Ascites is a feature of cirrhosis when there is a critical combination of liver protein synthesis failure producing hypoalbuminaemia, and of portal hypertension. It is not always present in cirrhosis but it is very rarely found in other conditions that may simulate the ultrasonic features of cirrhosis such as fatty change and biliary malignancy.

In portal hypertension the portal vein dilates, the spleen shows congestive enlargement, and the portasystemic anastomotic channels may open up. The normal portal vein is extremely variable in calibre and may measure up to 1.5 cm in diameter, and the splenic vein up to 1 cm. Enlargement much beyond these dimensions is indicative of portal hypertension, but one must be careful that a true diameter has been measured and also note that there is only poor correlation between the portal pressure and the degree of vein distension. It has been noted that in portal hypertension the

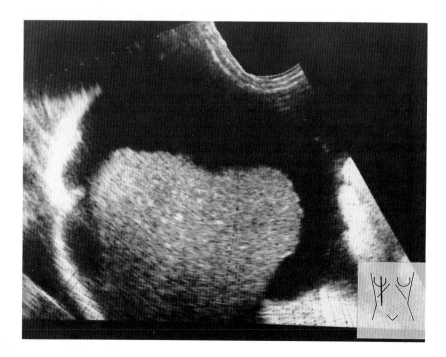

Fig. 7.8 There is marked ascites. The liver texture is uniformly high in amplitude. There is surface nodularity of the liver typical of the regenerative nodules of cirrhosis.

normal calibre change in the portal system occurring with respiration is no longer seen, and this may be a more sensitive indicator of portal hypertension. With pulsed Doppler equipment the flow within the portal venous system may be directly measured. The intrahepatic portal-vein branches do not share in the dilatation that occurs in portal hypertension, presumably because they are splinted by the fibrotic component of cirrhosis. Rarer causes of portal hypertension are venous occlusion of the main portal vein or the splenic vein by mass, or inflammatory lesions. An ultrasonic clue to these conditions may be obtained by an unexpected distribution of venous enlargement.

Of the portasystemic anastomoses that may open up in portal hypertension, those that can be imaged on ultrasound are the gastric, splenic, and umbilical vein sites (Fig. 7.9) (Subramanyan *et al.*, 1983). The gastric and splenic varices appear as tortuous collections of narrow vessels more easily imaged on real time when the typical 'bag of worms' arrangement can be appreciated. The umbilical-vein communication appears as a cannalization of the normal solid ligamentum teres. In cross-section it is seen as a concentric ring, and in longitudinal scan as a central free line within the echogenic round ligament (Glazer *et al.*, 1980). Care must be taken not to confuse this appearance with the normal branches of the left portal vein.

Persistent jaundice in known cirrhosis is a serious sign of liver failure. It is usually accompanied by ascites. It is, however, important to exclude an extrahepatic cause of cholestasis in cirrhosis. Ultrasound is extremely sensitive in the demonstration of biliary-duct dilatation and will often show its cause (Fig. 7.10).

When there is hepatomegaly of a recent onset or an arterial murmur over the liver, hepatoma should be considered. Hepatoma has an extremely variable appearance on ultrasound imaging, appearing echo-poor or echogenic. Tumours may be poorly defined and rather diffuse, and thus are extremely difficult to pick out from the background of the already abnormal liver texture (Fig. 7.11).

CT scanning

As with ultrasound, the value of CT in assessing diffuse parenchymal liver disease is less well established than its role in evaluation of focal hepatic disease. Usually in cirrhosis the density of the liver parenchyma is within the normal range, although in cirrhosis secondary to haemochromatosis there is a generalized increase in liver density.

Fatty infiltration is a common accompaniment of cirrhosis and its presence results in a decrease in hepatic density. Mild degrees of change may be subtle and not appreciated unless liver density is carefully compared to that of other abdominal organs such as the spleen. Although the attenuation values of the normal liver and spleen may

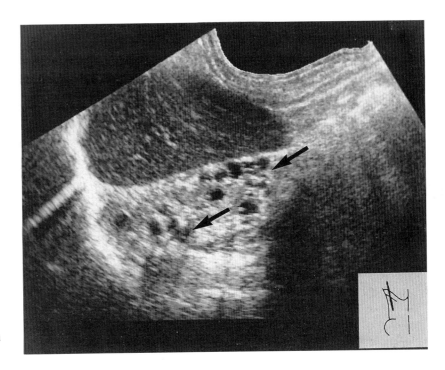

Fig. 7.9 A coronal scan through the spleen showing a mass of collateral veins extending towards the stomach (*arrowed*).

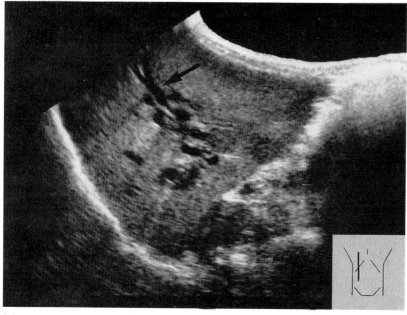

(a)

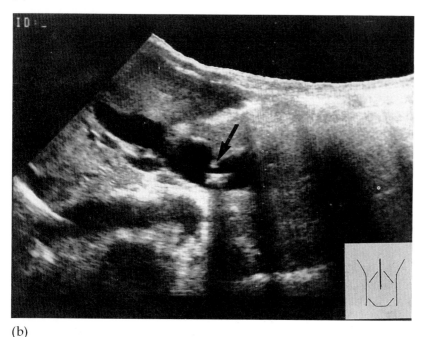

(b)

Fig. 7.10 (a) Dilated intrahepatic biliary ducts in a cirrhotic patient (*arrow*). (b) The dilated common bile duct containing a calculus (*arrow*).

vary widely from person to person, in a given subject the values will be concordant, with the liver by being slightly more dense than the spleen. The reversal of this normal relationship is the earliest CT indication of fatty infiltration. A relatively linear relationship between the amount of fat deposited and the attenuation value appears to exist. The distribution of fat within the liver may be rather patchy (Fig. 7.12) (Halvarsen *et al.*, 1982). In more advanced cirrhosis lobar or segmental atrophy may be seen, with gross nodular irregularity of the surface and overall contour of the liver related to the presence of regenerative nodules and interposed fibrotic bands (Fig. 7.13). As with ultrasound, CT will readily allow recognition of the relative enlargement of the caudate lobe compared with the right lobe. Measurement of ratios is a sensitive and fairly specific sign of cirrhosis (Harbin *et al.*, 1980).

CT will frequently show the complications of

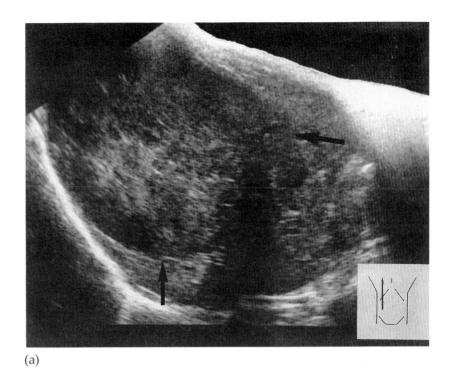

(a)

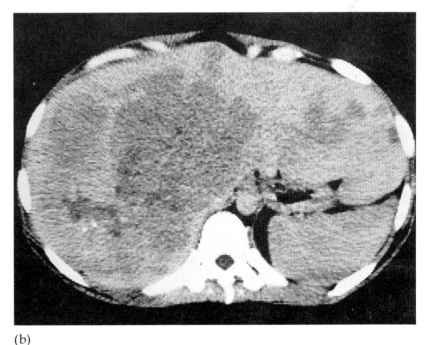

Fig. 7.11 (a) Longitudinal ultrasound scan showing a large hepatoma in the right lobe. (b) CT section through the same lesion as (a) (courtesy of Dr R.M. Blaquiere).

(b)

cirrhosis, ascites, splenomegaly, and dilated collateral veins. Collateral veins appear as a lobulated mass or a cluster of discrete or tubular structures in the typical sites for varices. Pre- and post-contrast scans may be useful for more clear elucidation. Regenerating nodules, which may appear as focal lesions on a radionuclide scan, are most often isodense with the liver. Hepatocellular carcinoma is the most common primary tumour of the liver in adults and has a high association with cirrhosis. Certain CT features favouring the diagnosis of hepatoma rather than metastases include a solitary lesion and attenuation values very close to normal parenchyma, a tendency to alter the contour of the liver by projecting beyond the surface, and dense, diffuse non-uniform enhancement following bolus contrast. Involvement of the portal vein is a recognized complication of this tumour, which may be shown on both ultrasound and CT (Fig. 7.14).

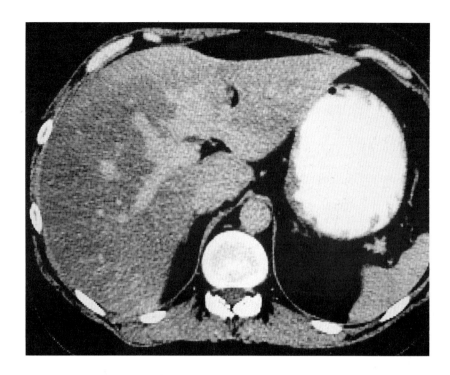

Fig. 7.12 A CT scan showing focal fatty change in the right lobe of the liver. The normal portal vessels contrast with the abnormal areas of low attenuation (courtesy of Dr R.M. Blaquiere).

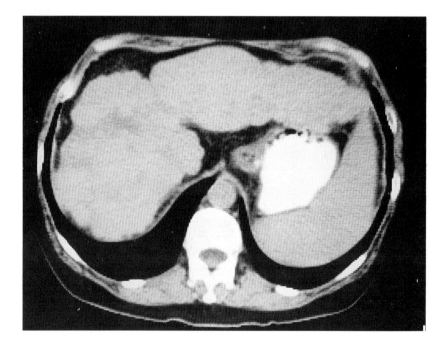

Fig. 7.13 A shrunken cirrhotic liver with an irregular outline due to regenerative nodules. There is splenic enlargement (courtesy of Dr R.M. Blaquiere).

Summary

Radiology is clearly of limited value in making a specific diagnosis of liver cirrhosis; however, it is extremely valuable in assessing the complications of the condition. Whilst barium studies remain useful, the more widespread use of endoscopy has in practice meant that barium studies have to some extent been bypassed. Vascular studies are now much less commonly performed and their main indication is if active surgical intervention is planned. Ultrasound is probably the most commonly performed imaging procedure in patients with suspected or established cirrhosis. It will give a clue as to the presence of cirrhosis by echo-pattern changes in the liver. Spleen size and portal-vein size can be assessed. The status of the gallbladder and biliary system can be evaluated

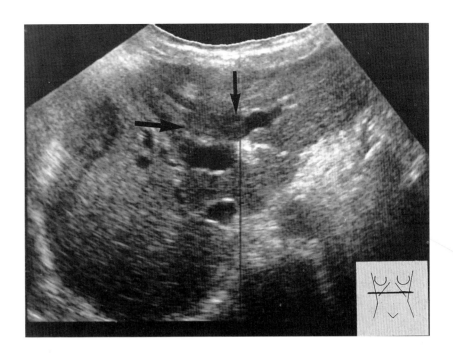

Fig. 7.14 Invasion of the left branch of the portal vein by hepatoma (*arrowed*).

and the presence of focal lesions in the liver detected. Ascites is sensitively shown. The increasing use and value of ultrasound has tended to lessen the use of radioisotope imaging in patients with cirrhosis, although of course the parameters being measured are totally different. The use of CT very much overlaps the use of ultrasound. In clinical practice CT does not tend to be used as a first-line technique in the evaluation of cirrhotic patients, but is reserved for specific problems that have not been resolved with ultrasound examination. The sequenced use of expensive resources is clearly essential to maximize their value.

References

Clark, A.K., Galbraith, R.M., Hamilton, E.B.D. & Williams, R. (1978) Rheumatic disorders in primary biliary cirrhosis. *Annals of Rheumatic Diseases*, **37**, 42—47.

Cohen, C. (1975) Liver pathology in alpha-1-antitrypsin deficiency: A review. *South African Medical Journal*, **49**, 849—852.

Dewbury, K.C. & Clark, B. (1979) The accuracy of ultrasound in detection of cirrhosis of the liver. *British Journal of Radiology*, **52**, 945—948.

Glazer, G.M., Laing, F.C. & Brown, N.W. (1980) Sonographic demonstration of portal hypertension — the patent umbilical vein. *Radiology*, **136**, 161—162.

Halvarsen, R.A. Korobkin, M., Ram, P.C. & Thompson, W.M. (1982) CT appearances of focal fatty infiltration of the liver. *American Journal of Radiology*, **139**, 277—281.

Harbin, W.P., Roberts, N.J. & Ferrucci, J.T. (1980) Diagnosis of cirrhosis based on regional changes in hepatic morphology. *Radiology*, **135**, 273—283.

Hutchinson, D.C.S. (1973) Alpha-1-antitrypsin deficiency and pulmonary emphysema: The role of proteolytic enzymes and their inhibitors. *British Journal of Diseases of the chest*, **67**, 171—196.

Saverymuttu, S.H., Joseph, A.E.A., & Maxwell, J.D. Ultrasound scanning in the detection of hepatic fibrosis and steatosis. *British Medical Journal*, **292**, 13—15.

Subramanyan, B.R., Balthazar, E.S. & Horii, S.C. (1983) Sonography of portosystemic venous collaterals in portal hypertension. *Radiology*, **146**, 161—166.

Taylor, K.J.N., Gorelick, F.S. & Rosenfield, A.T. (1981) Ultrasonography of alcoholic liver disease with histological correlation. *Radiology*, **141**, 157—161.

Warren, R., Trewby, P.N., Lans, J.W. & Williams, R. (1978) Pulmonary complications in fulminant hepatic failure: Analysis of serial radiograph from 100 consecutive patients. *Clinical Radiology*, **29**, 363—369.

8: Diffuse Liver Disease other than Cirrhosis

A.H. CHALMERS

There is a heterogeneous group of diseases affecting the liver diffusely which do not fit into any convenient classification. Jaundice is common in their presentation, and imaging plays a relatively small role in their investigation. Liver biopsy is generally the most valuable diagnostic technique.

In patients with known diffuse liver disease imaging is required for:
1 Exclusion of focal liver lesions.
2 The diagnosis of secondary effects of liver disease such as portal hypertension.
3 The guiding of percutaneous needle biopsy.

Of the non-invasive techniques computerized tomography (CT) is superior to either ultrasound (US) or scintigraphy, as image production and interpretation are less operator dependent and while CT does not produce a tissue diagnosis it produces a shorter differential diagnostic list (Berland, 1984). Tissue characterization using CT attenuation numbers has been disappointing except in haemachromatosis. The role of magnetic resonance imaging (MRI) has still to be assessed but it offers improved prospects compared with CT in some diseases (Doyle *et al.*, 1982).

Ultrasound will show alterations in liver size and shape, enlargement of the caudate lobe relative to the right lobe being an important indicator of cirrhosis. Increased echogenicity of the liver is another sensitive, early, but non-specific sign of cirrhosis and fatty change. The interpretation of ultrasound images is difficult and has so far not contributed greatly in the investigation of diffuse liver disease (Scott *et al.*, 1981).

Scintigraphy of liver and spleen is performed with ^{99m}technetium-sulphur colloid. In diffuse liver disease there is decreased tracer uptake in the liver on the posterior view and increased uptake in the spleen and bone marrow. Focal defects down to 2 cm in diameter can be seen using a gamma camera. Emission tomography, although theoretically more sensitive, has been overtaken by computerized (transmission) tomography,

which affords much better anatomical detail (Fig. 8.1). The secondary effects of cirrhosis may be seen on scintigrams, when portal hypertension causes splenic enlargement and ascites, which displace the liver away from the abdominal wall.

Haemochromatosis

AETIOLOGY AND PATHOLOGY

Haemochromatosis is divided into two main groups:(1) genetic (formerly idiopathic), and (2) acquired.

Genetic haemochromatosis is due to an iron-loading gene on chromosome 6, which is linked to the HLA−A locus. The disease is inherited as an autosomal recessive but the expression of the gene is modified by iron intake and loss from the body. Its mechanism of action is unknown. There is a juvenile form of haemochromatosis that differs in its clinical features from the adult form, but it is not known whether this represents a different genetic defect.

Acquired haemochromatosis is usually seen in sideroblastic anaemias and thalassaemia, and results from increased intestinal absorption in response to anaemia, from release of iron from red-cell destruction, and by blood transfusion.

In both forms of haemochromatosis iron is deposited in the parenchymal cells of the liver, causing cirrhosis, in the pancreas, and in the heart, causing a cardiomyopathy. Deposition also occurs in the pituitary, leading to gonadal failure and in other tissues including the skin. Reticuloendothelial iron stores are raised by iron transfusions but this is less damaging than parenchymal iron overload.

CLINICAL FEATURES

The major presenting symptoms are of weakness, weight loss, increased pigmentation of the skin, loss of libido, abdominal pain and diabetes

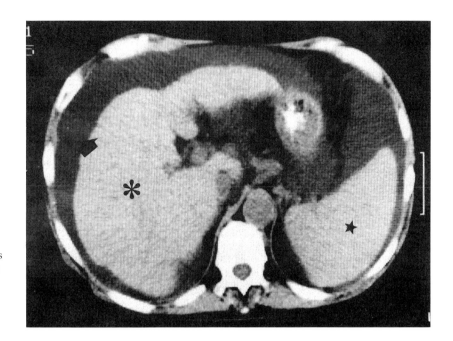

Fig. 8.1 CT of cirrhotic liver. Non-specific features in the liver, which is small with an irregular outline (*large star*). Ascites is present (*arrowhead*). Similar attenuation of liver and spleen (*small star*) (courtesy of Dr R. Dick, London).

mellitus. In advanced disease, symptoms due to jaundice, portal hypertension, gonadal failure, congestive cardiac failure, and arthropathy occur.

Hepatomegaly occurs in at least 95% of symptomatic patients. As the cirrhosis progresses there is splenomegaly, portal hypertension, ascites, jaundice, and abdominal pain. Thirty per cent of patients develop hepatocellular carcinoma, which is the commonest cause of death in treated patients.

Bronzing of the skin is due to melanin and iron deposition and is generalized. Diabetes mellitus is due to pancreatic damage and shows an increased incidence of insulin resistance. Failure of gonadotrophin production leads to loss of libido, testicular atrophy, and loss of body hair. Iron deposition in the heart causes congestive cardiac failure and dysrhythmias. Cardiac and gonadal failure are the commonest manifestations in juvenile haemochromatosis patients.

Arthropathy may antedate other symptoms but ultimately is present in up to 50% of patients. It characteristically affects the second and third metacarpophalangeal joints but other limb joints are also involved.

These manifestations can be prevented by early diagnosis of genetically at-risk individuals who can then have their iron stores kept at normal levels. Hepatocellular carcinoma only occurs in cirrhotic patients. Although pigmentation, diabetes, and cardiac failure are improved in symptomatic patients, cirrhosis, gonadal failure, and arthropathy are irreversible

INVESTIGATIONS

Blood tests

These are the main method of screening suspected individuals for genetic haemochromatosis and for assessing the response to treatment in known cases. Unfortunately these tests lack specificity so the following are usually performed:

Serum ferritin concentration accurately reflects hepatic and total body iron stores. The upper limit of normal is 150–200 ng/ml. Levels over 1000 ng/ml occur in patients with haemochromatosis but normal levels may be found in the important pre-cirrhotic subject.

Transferrin saturation is the earliest and most sensitive indicator of increased iron stores (Gollan, 1983). The normal value is about 30%. Virtually all haemachromatosis patients over 20 years old have levels over 50%. If serum ferritin and transferrin saturation levels are raised, hepatic parenchymal iron stores are probably also raised.

Liver biopsy

This provides an objective measurement of hepatic iron concentration (normal is 7–100 pg/100 mg). Biopsy also allows assessment of the degree of liver damage.

Liver biopsy is invasive and carries some risk in all patients and may be contraindicated in advanced disease. This makes a non-invasive diagnostic technique attractive.

Computerized tomography

It has been recognized since 1975 that CT attenuation figures in the liver are increased by raised tissue iron levels. Normal unenhanced liver attenuation values are 11–36 Hounsfield Units (HU). Attenuation limits are raised in haemochromatosis subjects and correlate directly with serum ferritin levels (Howard *et al.*, 1983). If dual-energy scanning is performed there is 0.993 correlation between hepatic attenuation and tissue iron concentration, which is a better correlation than with serum ferritin (Chapman *et al.*, 1980), and this is a realistic alternative to liver biopsy even in pre-cirrhotic patients. Increased liver attenuation is also seen in glycogen storage disease, parenteral hyperalimentation and long-term amiodarone therapy (Patrick *et al.*, 1984). The images show liver denser than spleen, and within the liver the vascular structures are abnormally prominent (Fig. 8.2). If hepatocellular carcinoma develops, this shows as a circumscribed low-attenuation area (Fig. 8.3). The differential diagnosis includes localized hepatic fibrosis, regeneration nodule, and focal fatty infiltration.

Scintigraphy

Liver/spleen scintigraphy relies on uptake of [99m]technetium-sulphur colloid by the reticuloendothelial cells in these organs, and if their function is impaired, activity is seen in the bone marrow. Using a gamma camera the normal posterior view of the liver and spleen shows more tracer uptake in liver than spleen. In early haemochromatosis, iron accumulates in the hepatic reticuloendothelial cells and damages them. A sulphur colloid scan shows diminished uptake of tracer in the liver with an increase in spleen and bone marrow. Hepatobiliary imaging at this stage with [99m]technetium-DISIDA is normal, as the hepatocytes are still normal. Although this discordance in uptake of the two tracers is of pathophysiological interest it has not found a clinical application.

In advanced haemochromatosis the additional signs of cirrhosis and portal hypertension will be seen on scintigraphy, i.e. splenomegaly and ascites, displacing the liver from the abdominal wall. This is much less common than in Laënnec's cirrhosis.

Ultrasound

Non-specific features of cirrhosis are seen on ultrasound with a 'bright', even pattern to the liver (Fig. 8.4).

Magnetic resonance imaging (MRI)

In haemochromatosis the paramagnetic effect of the excess iron decreases the T_1 and T_2 relaxation times (Doyle *et al.*, 1982, Stark *et al.*, 1983) but the effect on T_1 may be counteracted by hepatic fibrosis, which lengthens it. MRI is most sensitive to changes in hepatocellular hydrogen nuclei, and hepatocytes occupy 78% and reticuloendothelial

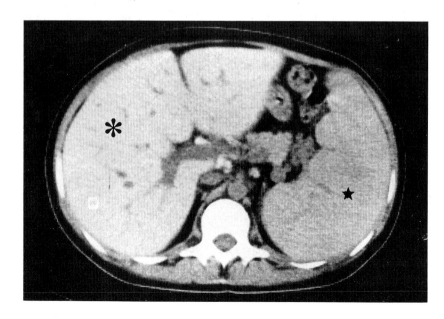

Fig. 8.2 CT of excess iron in the liver following long-term treatment for renal failure. The liver (*large star*) has an attenuation of 88 HU and is denser than the spleen (*small star*). Compare with Fig. 8.1 (courtesy Dr R. Dick, London).

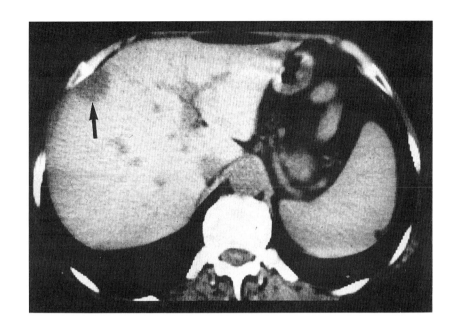

Fig. 8.3 CT of haemochromatotic liver with peripheral hepatocellular carcinoma (*arrow*). Note the dense liver and low attenuation tumour (courtesy Dr R. Dick, London).

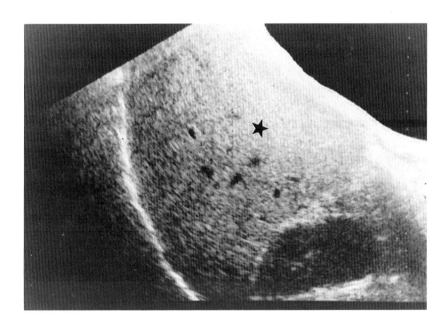

Fig. 8.4 Ultrasound of liver in haemochromatosis (head to left). There is a bright, even echo pattern in the liver (*star*). The appearances are a non-specific indicator of cirrhosis (courtesy Dr K. Dewbury, Southampton).

cells only 20% of liver volume. It is probable that MRI will be able to differentiate iron excess confined to reticuloendothelial cells (which causes little clinical effect, e.g. haemosiderosis and early haemochromatosis) from hepatocellular iron excess (as in haemochromatosis), which is associated with tissue damage. This may be useful in the assessment of patients with iron overload.

Wilson's disease

AETIOLOGY AND PATHOLOGY

Wilson's disease is due to an autosomal recessive gene present with a frequency of 0.53% in the population, giving a disease incidence of about 30 per million. The disease is always manifest in homozygotes, while heterozygotes may show some biochemical but not clinical abnormalities.

The metabolic defects seem to be (i) failure of the normal excretion of copper from the liver into the biliary system, and (ii) deficient production of caeruloplasmin, the protein in the blood to which 95% of copper is usually tightly bound.

The excess copper is stored in hepatocytes but leaks out and damages other tissues such as basal ganglia and renal tubular cells. Initially the liver is grossly functionally and histologically normal despite the raised copper content, but the condition then progresses to chronic active hepatitis and cirrhosis. The brain may show slight generalized atrophy, especially in the basal ganglia, and rarely there may be areas of cavitation. The kidneys show functional rather than structural abnormalities. Copper pigment deposited around the margin of the cornea constitutes the Kayser–Fleischer ring.

CLINICAL FEATURES

Younger patients tend to present with hepatic symptoms such as:
- An acute illness with jaundice, malaise and fever.
- A more insidious onset mimicking chronic active hepatitis.
- Cirrhosis associated with portal hypertension, ascites and coma. Less than 50% of patients present with hepatic symptoms, but in this group neurological symptoms may be absent or minimal.

Patients present with neurological symptoms from childhood through to the fifth decade. Tremor, worse on movement, rigidity, dysarthria, dysphagia, abnormal movements, and psychiatric symptoms all occur and untreated progress to immobility, dementia, and death. All patients with neurological symptoms have the Kayser–Fleischer ring, though a slit lamp may be required to detect it. Rarely a similar ring may occur in biliary cirrhosis or intrahepatic cholestasis.

INVESTIGATIONS

Treatment of asymptomatic patients with the genetic abnormality of Wilson's disease will prevent the disease manifesting itself and symptomatic patients improve, sometimes dramatically, so the most important step towards the diagnosis is to consider it. If cirrhosis has developed the radiological findings are similar to other cases with portal hypertension.

Serum caeruloplasmin

This is low (less than 20 mg/100 ml or 125 μmol/l in 95% of patients. In the remaining 5% it is normal.

Urinary copper excretion

This is raised (> 100 pg/day or 1.6 μmol/day), but excretion is also raised in biliary cirrhosis and other liver disease.

Liver biopsy

Liver biopsy shows histological abnormalities including fat droplets, glycogen deposits, and on electron microscopy mitochondrial abnormalities that appear to be specific.

The *hepatic copper content* is raised (> 200 pg/g dry weight; normal, less than 55 pg/g), but the copper level is also raised in other liver diseases, so in the 5% of patients with normal serum caeruloplasmin and raised liver copper content it is necessary to perform:

Radioactive copper studies

In Wilson's disease incorporation of copper into caeruloplasmin is reduced, there is prolonged turnover of body copper and an alteration in the rate of uptake of copper by the liver (Sternlieb, 1978). These tests enable a firm diagnosis to be made.

Scintigraphy

Multiple areas of increased tracer uptake in the liver have been reported which correspond with regeneration nodules following massive hepatic necrosis.

Computerized tomography

CT of the liver is usually normal or may show slight nodularity due to the cirrhosis. Attenuation values are not altered and cannot be used for diagnosis or assessment of the effect of treatment (Dixon & Walshe, 1984). Ultrasound is also nonspecific with an irregular nodular reflective pattern due to cirrhosis (Fig. 8.5).

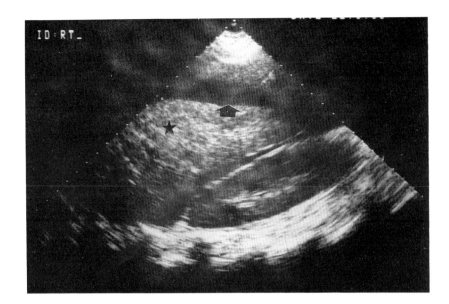

Fig. 8.5 Longitudinal ultrasound scan of liver in Wilson's disease (patient's head to left). Non-specific increased echo pattern in the liver (*star*). Ascites (*arrowhead*) is present (courtesy Dr K. Dewbury, Southampton).

Amyloidosis

AETIOLOGY AND PATHOLOGY

Amyloidosis is a disease of unknown aetiology, characterized by the deposition of abnormal proteins in a wide variety of tissues. The majority of the amyloid protein is structurally similar to some immunoglobulin light-chain fragments and has the form of fibrils on electron microscopy. Other proteins have been found in some forms of amyloidosis, but it seems that all are produced by or related to immunologically active cells, suggesting that the disease is mediated by the immune system.

Amyloid protein is deposited in a perivascular distribution, particularly in the spleen, kidney, and liver though virtually any organ may be involved. In the liver the parenchymal cells are also always affected. Hepatomegaly is present in over 50% of patients but functional impairment is late.

Amyloidosis can be divided pathologically and clinically into the following types:

1 Primary: No known association with other disease.

2 Secondary:

(a) Associated with multiple myeloma. Eight to twelve per cent of myeloma patients develop amyloidosis.

(b) Associated with chronic inflammation, e.g. osteomyelitis, tuberculosis, rheumatoid arthritis, ankylosing spondylitis.

(c) Associated with familial Mediterranean fever and similar syndromes (heredofamilial amyloidosis)

3 Local amyloidosis. Focal and tumour-like deposits develop in organs.

4 Ageing-related amyloidosis.

CLINICAL FEATURES

Symptoms and signs depend on the organs involved but only occur when deposition of amyloid is advanced. Symptoms are due either to loss of function or to a mass effect by amyloid deposits. Hepatic symptoms on presentation include right upper quadrant pain due to hepatomegaly, pruritus and ascites. Non-specific symptoms include malaise and loss of weight. Jaundice can occur due to intrahepatic cholestasis, and portal hypertension occurs, but is uncommon.

Amyloidosis in the kidney causes renal failure and in the heart arrhythmias and congestive failure. In the gastrointestinal tract there may be haemorrhage, malabsorbtion, loss of motility, and mass lesions simulating tumours. Large and small joints are affected. Mass lesions in the upper airways and reduced compliance in the lungs may cause the most serious manifestations of the disease. In the nervous system there may be peripheral neuropathies and plaques in the brain. Plaques also occur commonly in the skin.

INVESTIGATIONS

Biopsy

The unequivocal diagnosis of amyloid can only be achieved by biopsy. Liver, kidney, bone marrow, gingival, or rectal mucosa may all be used. Congored staining of biopsy tissue shows a unique apple-green birefringence on polarizing light microscopy.

Electron microscopy shows the delicate non-branching fibrils of amyloid.

Blood tests

Serum alkaline phosphatase is raised and bromsulphthalein extraction reduced in hepatic amyloidosis.

Scintigraphy

Hepatic scanning with ^{99m}technetium-sulphur colloid may be normal, show generalized reduced hepatic uptake, a non-homogeneuos distribution, or focal defects similar to mass lesions (Waxman, 1982). The liver is usually enlarged.

^{99m}Technetium pyrophosphate, used for bone scintigraphy, is taken up by hepatic amyloid in both primary and secondary amyloidosis. Its use as a screening technique in patients suspected of hepatic involvement but unfit for liver biopsy has been suggested. The specificity of this test is unknown.

Angiography

Amyloid is deposited within blood vessel walls and the appearances in the liver are similar to those in the gastrointestinal tract and kidney. It may show as a hypovascular mass lesion or as luminal irregularity of vessels with abrupt changes in their diameter.

Ultrasound

The findings are non-specific with hepatomegaly and an irregular, dense echo pattern occurs.

Sarcoidosis

AETIOLOGY AND PATHOLOGY

Sarcoidosis is a disorder of unknown aetiology characterized by granulomata in multiple systems. The granulomata are composed of macrophages, epithelioid cells, Langerhan's type giant cells, and lymphocytes. Central necrosis is uncommon, in contrast to tuberculosis. The granulomata are non-specific and are indistinguishable from those due to berylliosis, hypersensitivity reactions, and Crohn's disease.

Hepatic involvement with granulomata is found in about 70% of patients with sarcoidosis but is commoner in people of African origin, in whom the disease is frequently more severe. The liver is enlarged in about 20%. In the vast majority of patients the granulomata resolve with no sequelae. Progression of the disease to cirrhosis and portal hypertension is rare but can occur. Chronic intrahepatic cholestasis with biliary cirrhosis is reported but is uncommon (Bass *et al.*, 1982).

CLINICAL FEATURES

Sarcoidosis is marginally commoner in women (1.36 : 1 female : male ratio) and usually presents in young adults. The manifestations are protean, affecting the respiratory, ocular, cutaneous and nervous systems, and although hepatic involvement is usually present it is clinically silent. Symptomatic hepatic sarcoidosis is rare but presents with upper abdominal pain and fever (Israel *et al.*, 1984). The liver may be enlarged. Respiratory symptoms are usually absent. Symptoms may persist for months but this group of patients do not seem to progress to cirrhosis. If the disease is causing cholestasis it frequently progresses to cirrhosis and there will be jaundice and pruritus or signs of portal hypertension.

INVESTIGATIONS

There are no tests specific for sarcoidosis and the diagnosis is made on the basis of compatible clinical features, the exclusion of other disorders, and the following investigations:

Plain film radiography

Ninety per cent of patients have abnormal chest radiographs. Bilateral hilar lymphadenopathy occurs in 60%, adenopathy and parenchymal shadowing in 25%, and parenchymal shadowing alone in 10%. It should be stressed that the majority of these patients have abnormal liver biopsies but no hepatic symptoms.

Plain films of the abdomen may show hepato-splenomegaly or rarely ascites.

Biopsy

Liver biopsy is the only way of showing hepatic involvement and has long been used to confirm the diagnosis of pulmonary sarcoidosis by demonstrating granulomata and hence the involvement of another organ. Biopsy of other areas (e.g. lymph nodes or skin) or symptomatic areas such as salivary glands of the lower lip (positive in 60%) are used. Transbronchial lung biopsy is positive in 60–85% of pulmonary cases depending on the stage. Mediastinoscopy and biopsy is positive in 85–90% and open lung biopsy in 100%, even in stage I respiratory disease.

Serum angiotensin converting enzyme (ACE)

This enzyme is believed to be produced in the epithelioid cells of granulomata. It is raised in about 75% of patients with active sarcoidosis and in 55% of patients with inactive sarcoidosis. Although serum ACE levels are raised in a variety of other disease (e.g. primary biliary cirrhosis, miliary tuberculosis, fibrosing alveolitis, etc.) it is useful for diagnosis when combined with other tests, especially a gallium scan, and can also be used for assessing disease activity in patients not being treated with steroids.

Scintigraphy

^{99m}Technetium sulphur colloid scans are either normal or show the pattern of diffuse liver disease, i.e. increased uptake in the spleen on the posterior view, and marrow uptake (Fig. 8.6).

Of more use is scintigraphy with ^{67}gallium citrate, which is taken up in areas of active sarcoidosis as well as in inflammatory tissue and some tumours. In the majority of sarcoid patients the liver is normal but uptake is seen in hilar and mediastinal lymph nodes, lung parenchyma, or salivary or lacrimal glands. A positive gallium scan and raised ACE level has a diagnostic specificity for sarcoidosis of 99%. Diffuse hepatic uptake can occur but is uncommon and only differs in degree from the uptake of gallium seen in the normal liver.

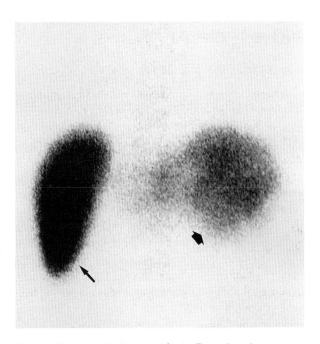

Fig. 8.6 Scintigraphy in sarcoidosis. Posterior view. Diminished uptake in liver (*arrowhead*) with increased uptake in enlarged spleen (*arrow*).

Kveim–Siltzbach test

An intracutaneous injection of 'Kveim antigen', made from human sarcoid spleen or lymph node, will produce a non-caseating granuloma at the injection site after 6 weeks in about 97% of patients with active sarcoidosis. The main disadvantages of this test are the difficulty in obtaining adequate validated antigen, and false-positive reactions due to Crohn's disease, infectious mononucleosis, and chronic lymphatic leukaemia, though these are rare (Sharma, 1983). Steroid treatment suppresses the reaction.

Bronchoalveolar lavage

Lavage is performed by wedging a fibreoptic bronchoscope into the middle or lingular lobes, injecting 200 ml of isotonic saline in 30 ml aliquots, and then aspirating. Cells in normal washings comprise alveolar macrophages (90%), lymphocytes (<10%), and polymorphonuclear leukocytes (<1%). In sarcoidosis there is an increase in T-lymphocytes and their numbers are proportional to the activity of the sarcoid alveolitis. Although this test is relatively invasive it is reliable and repeatable.

Alpha$_1$-antitrypsin deficiency

AETIOLOGY AND PATHOLOGY

Alpha$_1$-antitrypsin is the major plasma protease inhibitor. It is a glycoprotein with a molecular weight of 54 000 and is manufactured in the endoplasmic reticulum of hepatocytes. Its production and plasma level are controlled by multiple codominant alleles. Twenty-six different alleles are known with corresponding phenotypes. Normal people have the Pi MM genotype; the homozygous deficiency state is Pi ZZ, and in adults with liver disease Pi ME is frequent.

People with the Z allele produce an abnormal alpha$_1$-antitrypsin which accumulates as globules in hepatocytes, stains with periodic acid−Schiff, and is resistant to diastase digestion. Failure to release this abnormal substance from the hepatocytes leads to the low level of alpha$_1$-antitrypsin in the blood, levels of 10−15% of normal being found in Pi ZZ homozygotes. The mechanism by which patients develop liver disease is unknown and does not seem to depend solely on the presence of the abnormal alpha$_1$-antitrypsin in hepatocytes, but probably on a number of as yet unknown factors.

CLINICAL FEATURES

Liver disease associated with alpha$_1$-antitrypsin deficiency was first described in 1969 in children (Sharp et al., 1969), and subsequently in adults. In childhood 25−30% of Pi ZZ homozygotes will develop neonatal hepatitis, usually in the first 4 months of life. There is evidence that cirrhosis can develop in utero. Conjugated hyperbilirubinaemia may follow on from normal physiological jaundice. One quarter of these babies with hepatitis will develop cirrhosis during early childhood, one-quarter will die by the second decade, one quarter continue to have abnormal liver function tests and the remaining one-quarter recover (Leader, 1981).

The incidence of hepatic dysfunction in adults and its relation to alpha$_1$-antitrypsin deficiency is less clear than in infancy. There is a significant correlation between Pi MZ with cryptogenic cirrhosis and chronic active hepatitis. Adult liver disease need not follow childhood liver disease, though the same cholestatic pattern is seen in adults. There is also portal fibrosis or cirrhosis, either macro- or micronodular. An increased incidence of hepatoma and cholangiocarcinoma is suspected. Probably only about 10% of adults with Pi ZZ develop liver disease and there is no correlation with lung disease.

INVESTIGATIONS

Blood tests

(a) Serum alpha$_1$-antitrypsin is low (normal 200−400 mg/dl) in the majority of patients. (b) Protease inhibitor (Pi) phenotyping by isoelectric focusing enables the Z allele to be found. It is of value in identifying patients with the Pi Z phenotype as they may have normal serum alpha$_1$-antitrypsin levels. (c) A ratio of serum glutamic oxaloacetic transaminase (SGOT) to serum glutamic pyruvic transaminase (SGPT) of greater than 2:1 in the absence of alcoholic disease has been reported in elderly patients with alpha$_1$-antitrypsin deficiency; which is of interest because in most forms of chronic liver disease the SGOT : SGPT ratio is approximately 1.

Liver biopsy

In the majority of cases this is the definitive test showing cirrhosis with periodic acid−Schiff positive, diastase-resistant globules. In children under 3 months old the globules may not be present despite severe liver damage. Cirrhosis is seen as described above.

Ultrasound

This shows non-specific features of cirrhosis, ascites and splenomegaly.

Scintigraphy

^{99m}Technetium-sulphur colloid scans are also non-specifically abnormal, showing hepatosplenomegaly with increased splenic uptake (Fig. 8.7).

Endoscopic retrograde cholangiopancreatography (ERCP)

Biliary duct narrowing or non-filling and extra-hepatic duct hypoplasia has been reported in infants and adults.

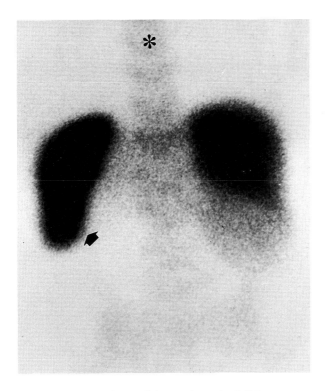

Fig. 8.7 Scintigraphy in alpha₁-antitrypsin deficiency (posterior view). There is increased uptake in spleen (*arrowhead*) and the bone marrow (*star*) (courtesy Dr D. Ackery, Southampton).

Hepatobiliary diseases associated with inflammatory bowel disease

Both hepatic and biliary disease may accompany inflammatory bowel disease and both will be discussed here as they overlap pathologically and clinically. Significant hepatobiliary disease, as defined by persistently abnormal liver function tests, is found in about 5% of patients with inflammatory bowel disease, and incidence seems to be similar in both ulcerative colitis and Crohn's disease. There is no difference histologically in the hepatic changes produced by the two diseases.

AETIOLOGY

The aetiology of the various hepatobiliary disorders is unknown. The favoured hypotheses are:
(i) Chronic portal bacteraemia and toxin absorption through the ulcerated intestinal mucosa damages the liver and portal tracts. One problem of this argument is the lack of protection which colectomy gives to the development of later cholangiocarcinoma.
(ii) A genetic predisposition to an immune disease affecting both the bowel and liver. The occurrence of hepatobiliary disease before the onset of inflammatory bowel disease favours this argument as well as the association of common haplotypes of the human leukocyte antigen system with sclerosing cholangitis, cholangiocarcinoma, and ulcerative colitis.

Hepatic disorders

Fatty infiltration

This occurs in many severely ill patients and is common in both ulcerative colitis and Crohn's disease but is only severe in about 10–15%. It is usually asymptomatic, though the liver may be enlarged. Resolution occurs with improvement of the patients general nutritional state and it usually has no sequelae.

Pericholangitis (portal triaditis)

PATHOLOGY

In pericholangitis there is an inflammatory cell infiltrate around the interlobular bile ducts accompanied by oedema of the bile ductules. This stage is reversible, but may then become irreversible with the development of periductular fibrosis, periportal fibrosis, canalicular plugging, and piecemeal hepatic necrosis. This may progress to cirrhosis and portal hypertension.

CLINICAL FEATURES

Pericholangitis occurs equally in ulcerative colitis and Crohn's disease and is the commonest hepatic disorder associated with inflammatory bowel disease. Its prevalence is unknown as there are no data on liver biopsy findings in patients with asymptomatic inflammatory bowel disease, but it probably occurs in at least 30%.

Most patients are asymptomatic. Symptoms when present are of recurrent acute attacks of jaundice and pruritus. The liver size is normal or only slightly enlarged. In the rare event of progression to cirrhosis the signs of portal hypertension and oesophageal varices develop.

INVESTIGATIONS

Blood tests

Serum alkaline phosphatase is the most useful

test, and is raised, though it has been normal in some patients with biopsy-proven pericholangitis.

Bromsulphthalein retention is increased in both asymptomatic and symptomatic patients.

Liver biopsy

This will confirm the diagnosis, but the distribution of the disease may be patchy. Features of sclerosing cholangitis are also shown in 30–60% of patients.

ERCP

This test is normal in pericholangitis, but may still be necessary to exclude sclerosing cholangitis, which has a much worse prognosis if cholestasis occurs.

Cirrhosis

Post-necrotic cirrhosis occurs in 2–5% of patients, usually young colitics with severe disease requiring surgery. The usual complications of varices and portal hypertension may occur and it accounts for 10% of deaths of patients with inflammatory bowel disease (Kern, 1976).

Chronic active hepatitis

About 1% of patients with inflammatory bowel disease, mainly ulcerative colitics, have chronic active hepatitis, although the number of chronic active hepatitis patients who have inflammatory bowel disease is as high as 30%. Either disease may precede the other and the severity of the liver disease is unrelated to the activity of the bowel disease, though hepatic improvement may follow colectomy.

Amyloidosis

Crohn's disease is rarely associated with secondary amyloidosis affecting the liver as well as kidneys, spleen and other organs.

Granulomatous hepatitis

This is an uncommon complication of Crohn's disease in which there are non-caseating granulomata in the liver similar to those found in the bowel. Most patients are asymptomatic though there may be hepatomegaly, jaundice, fever, and a raised alkaline phosphatase.

Biliary disorders

Primary sclerosing cholangitis

PATHOLOGY

There is progressive sclerosis and obliteration of extra- and intrahepatic bile ducts. This leads to secondary biliary cirrhosis and portal hypertension.

CLINICAL FEATURES

Sclerosing cholangitis occurs in 1–4% of patients with inflammatory bowel disease and is commonest in those with long-standing severe, ulcerative colitis (Shepherd *et al.*, 1983), but is also reported in Crohn's colitis. However, 31% of a series of ulcerative colitis patients with persistently abnormal liver function tests were found to have primary sclerosing cholangitis on biopsy and cholangiography. (Nearly 70% of patients with sclerosing cholangitis have inflammatory bowel disease.) Presenting features are of upper abdominal pain, fever, vomiting, jaundice, and pruritus. Later signs are of cirrhosis and portal hypertension. The prognosis is generally poor with average survival after diagnosis being 7 years, but in some patients the disease may cause no symptoms for years.

INVESTIGATIONS

ERCP (Kolmannskog et al., 1981)

This is essential to exclude other causes of obstructive jaundice, as 75% of cases show multiple strictures and dilatations of bile ducts (Fig. 8.8). Both intra- and extrahepatic ducts are affected in 70%. If cirrhosis is present the intrahepatic ducts are always abnormal. Of all cases, 25% have a localized stricture, in which event differentiation from cholangiocarcinoma may be impossible without biopsy.

Liver biopsy

This will confirm the histological features mentioned above.

Cholangiocarcinoma

Carcinoma of the biliary tract and gall bladder

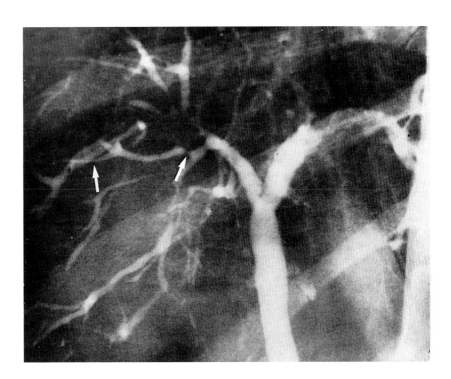

Fig. 8.8 ERCP in sclerosing cholangitis. The intrahepatic ducts show multiple strictures (*arrows*) but the extrahepatic ducts are normal (courtesy Dr R. Dick, London).

occurs about 10 times more frequently in patients with inflammatory bowel disease than in the general population, though it is still uncommon with an incidence of 0.4–1.4%. Most cases are in ulcerative colitis patients though it has been reported in Crohn's disease. It is usually found in patients with severe, chronic colitis, but it may antedate the colitis or occur some years after colectomy, which seems to afford no protection (Christophi & Hughes, 1985).

PATHOLOGY

The tumours are adenocarcinomas, frequently multicentric, affecting extrahepatic and intrahepatic ducts. The gall bladder is involved in 15% of cases. Gall stones are uncommon in comparison to cholangiocarcinoma in non-colitics, in whom cholelithiasis is present in over 50%.

CLINICAL FEATURES

Patients present in their 4th–5th decade with right upper quadrant pain and usually progressive obstructive jaundice. The prognosis is poor with a mean survival of 6 months after diagnosis.

INVESTIGATIONS

Endoscopic retrograde cholangiography or percutaneous transhepatic (fine-needle) cholangiography

(Fig. 8.9) are required in patients with inflammatory bowel disease who become jaundiced. Local expertise should determine which technique is used, and both may required depending on the site and severity of the strictures. As previously mentioned cholangiocarcinoma may be radiologically indistinguishable from sclerosing cholangitis so biopsy, percutaneous or open, is usually required.

Biopsy. Biopsy may be undertaken at laparotomy for relief of the jaundice but may also be performed with less trauma to the patient, using a 22-gauge needle percutaneously with ultrasound or CT guidance.

Congenital non-haemolytic hyperbilirubinaemias

There are four conditions which have raised serum bilirubin levels due to an inherited metabolic abnormality in the hepatocytes; they are described here, as imaging techniques are of some value in their diagnosis.

Gilbert's syndrome

AETIOLOGY AND PATHOLOGY

This syndrome is probably inherited as an autosomal dominant and is due in part to a decrease in glucuronidation in the liver, causing a

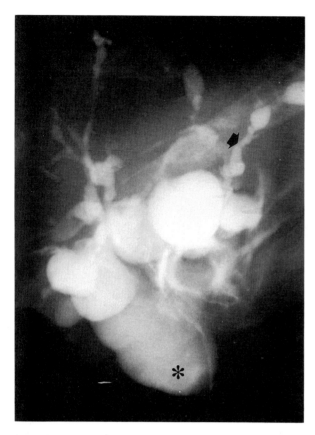

Fig. 8.9 Percutaneous cholangiogram in ulcerative colitis complicated by sclerosing cholangitis (*arrowhead*) and cholangiocarcinoma. The dilated common bile duct (*star*) tapers to an occlusion by a cholangiocarcinoma (biopsy proven).

Liver biopsy is normal, though an increase in lipofuscin in centrilobular hepatocytes may be seen.

Bromsulphthalein clearance is decreased in some patients.

Crigler—Najjar syndrome

AETIOLOGY AND PATHOLOGY

The Crigler—Najjar syndrome is divided into type I, in which there is no bilirubin glucuronidation in the liver, and type II, in which there is some and the enzyme can be induced by phenobarbitone. In type I an autosomal recessive inheritance is probable. Type II is familial and in some patients there seems to be a homozygous state of Gilbert's syndrome.

CLINICAL FEATURES

Type I. Severe unconjugated hyperbilirubinaemia presents in the neonatal period, proceeding to kernicterus; it is unaffected by phenobarbitone. Death usually occurs in the first year, but some patients survive, only to die in the second decade from neurological disease.

Type II. Jaundice presents later, is less severe, and is reduced with phenobarbitone. Kernicterus seldom occurs.

rise in unconjugated bilirubin (Fevery, 1981). Other cellular abnormalities are thought to be present and the 'syndrome' may not consist of a single disorder.

CLINICAL FEATURES

Hyperbilirubinaemia usually not exceeding 3 mg/100 ml may be noted incidentally or the patient may be discovered with mild jaundice after an intercurrent illness, especially if there has been a period of reduced food intake. Males are affected four times as commonly as females. Treatment is with phenobarbitone lowers bilirubin levels by enzyme induction.

INVESTIGATIONS

Blood tests reveal hyperbilirubinaemia with normal alkaline phosphatase and transaminases, and no evidence of haemolysis.

INVESTIGATIONS

Blood tests show unconjugated hyperbilirubinaemia, but normal alkaline phosphatase and transaminases. In type I the bile contains no bilirubin glucuronides, so is colourless, but in type II glucuronides are present and the bile is deeply pigmented. There are no signs of haemolysis.

Liver biopsy is normal.

Bromsulphthalein clearance is normal in both types.

Dubin—Johnson syndrome

AETIOLOGY AND PATHOLOGY

In this syndrome there is a failure of excretion of conjugated bilirubin and other organic anions from the liver into the biliary tree. The reflux of conjugated bilirubin into the blood causes jaundice. There is also accumulation of a black pigment in the hepatocytes, which may be melanin, and which gives a characteristic naked-eye appearance to liver biopsies. Inheritance is probably due to an autosomal recessive trait.

CLINICAL FEATURES

Jaundice due to conjugated hyperbilirubinaemia may be precipitated by pregnancy or oral contraceptives. There are no other definite symptoms or signs ascribable to the syndrome, though malaise, upper abdominal pain, and tiredness are described.

The condition is benign and there is no treatment.

INVESTIGATIONS

Blood tests. There is a raised level of conjugated bilirubin with normal alkaline phosphatase and transaminases.

The bromsulphthalein (BSP) clearance test shows a rise in plasma BSP at 90 min compared with the 45-min level due to release of conjugated BSP from the liver.

Urinary coproporphyrin levels. In normal people the ratio of urinary coproporphyrin I to coproporphyrin III is 1:3, but in homozygous Dubin–Johnson syndrome it is at least 4:1.

Cholangiography. Oral cholecystography and intravenous cholangiography show no excretion of contrast media because of the underlying biochemical defect (Javitt, 1979).

Scintigraphy. Biliary imaging with ^{99m}Tc-HIDA (hepatic iminodiacetic acid) shows rapid clearance of tracer from the blood into the liver, failure of visualization of the biliary tree, but tracer accumulation in the gall bladder in the majority of patients by 90 min (Bar-Meir *et al.*, 1982). Tracer reaches the gut in all patients by 1 h.

This pattern is different from that seen in diffuse hepatocellular disease where there is delayed clearance of tracer from the blood, and from the appearances in biliary obstruction where there is rapid clearance of tracer which then accumulates at the level of the obstruction.

Rotor syndrome

AETIOLOGY AND PATHOLOGY

This is a rare familial disorder manifested by a fluctuating conjugated hyperbilirubinaemia. The defect appears to be one of hepatic uptake and storage (Javitt, 1979), rather than of excretion as in the Dubin–Johnson syndrome. Inheritance is probably as an autosomal recessive trait.

Liver biopsy shows no accumulation of pigment.

CLINICAL FEATURES

Clinically, Rotor syndrome resembles the Dubin–Johnson syndrome.

INVESTIGATIONS

Blood tests. There is a conjugated hyperbilirubinaemia with normal alkaline phosphatase and transaminases.

The bromsulphthalein retention test is normal, without the secondary rise seen in the Dubin–Johnson syndrome.

Urinary coproporphyrin levels. The total excretion is raised as well as the ratio of coproporphyrin I to III.

Cholecystography. The gall bladder opacifies normally.

Scintigraphy. There is a failure to visualize the liver, gall bladder or biliary tree with ^{99m}technetium-HIDA (Bar-Meir *et al.*, 1982). A similar appearance is seen in hepatocellular disease, but the blood tests will differentiate this from the Rotor syndrome.

Gaucher's disease

AETIOLOGY AND PATHOLOGY

Gaucher's disease is due to a deficiency of the lysosomal enzyme glucosylceramide-B-glucosidase. This deficiency leads to accumulation of the enzyme's substrate, glucosylceramide, in the reticuloendothelial cells of the body. The abnormality is inherited as an autosomal recessive and is most common in Ashkenazi Jews with an incidence of 1:2500 births, though it occurs world-wide.

Pathologically, macrophages laden with lipid accumulate in various organs, especially the spleen, liver, bone marrow, and lymph nodes. These 'Gaucher' cells have characteristic light and electron microscopic features, but may also occur in granulocytic leukaemia and myeloma.

CLINICAL FEATURES

There are three varieties of the disease, the commonest of which is the 'Adult', non-neuronopathic type I. Despite its name this may present from childhood through to old age and runs a chronic course. Massive splenomegaly, hepatomegaly, bone pain due to infarctions and fractures, bleeding diathesis, and fever occur. Conjunctival pingueculae and skin pigmentation are seen, but neurological signs do not develop.

The degree of liver involvement correlates with the severity of extrahepatic disease. With extensive replacement of liver by 'Gaucher' cells, cirrhosis and portal hypertension will develop and this occurred in 12% of patients in one series (James *et al.*, 1981).

Type II, acute neuronopathic Gaucher's disease, presents in infancy with both brain-stem and cerebral signs, as well as hepatosplenomegaly, and death occurs by the age of 3 years.

Type III or juvenile subacute neuronopathic disease is intermediate between types I and II, and presents with fits and myoclonus.

INVESTIGATIONS

Blood tests. Serum non-prostatic acid phosphatase and angiotensin-converting enzyme are both raised. Liver function tests are abnormal in some patients but are non-specific.

Bromsulphthalein clearance is reduced, with a raised level at 45 min.

Leukocyte enzyme analysis is a sensitive and non-invasive technique for demonstrating the biochemical abnormality (Lee *et al.*, 1981).

Biopsy. Detection of lipid-laden macrophages in bone marrow or liver biopsy is the main diagnostic technique. The cells have a characteristic appearance of pale cytoplasm with one or more eccentric hyperchromatic nuclei between which run fibrils.

Plain films. Abdominal radiographs show hepatosplenomegaly. Multiple, well-circumscribed hepatic calcifications of varying size have been described (Stone *et al.*, 1982).

Bone changes are frequent, with avascular necrosis of the femoral heads, modelling deformities of the lower femoral shafts and pathological fractures. Vertebral body collapse occurs.

Scintigraphy. Non-specific findings of hepatosplenomegaly and diminished tracer uptake by the liver are present.

References

Bar-Meir, S., Baron, J., Seligson, U., Gottesfeld, F., Levy, R. & Gilat, T. (1982) ^{99m}Tc-HIDA cholescintigraphy in Dubin–Johnson and Rotor syndromes. *Radiology*, **142**, 743–746.

Bass, N.M., Burroughs, A.K., Scheuer, P.J., James, D.G. & Sherlock, S. (1982) Chronic intrahepatic cholestasis due to sarcoidosis. *Gut*, **23**, 417–421.

Berland, L.L. (1984) Screening for diffuse and focal liver disease: The case for hepatic computed tomography. *Journal of Clinical Ultrasound*, **12**, 83–89.

Chapman, R.W.G., Williams, G., Bydder, G., Dick, R., Sherlock, S. & Kreel, L. (1980) Computed tomography for determining liver iron content in primary haemochromatosis. *British Medical Journal*, **280**, 440–442.

Christophi, C. & Hughes, E.R. (1985) Hepatobiliary disorders in inflammatory bowel disease. *Surgery, Gynecology & Obstetrics*, **160**, 187–193.

Dixon, A.K. & Walshe, J.M. (1984) Computed tomography of the liver in Wilson's disease. *Journal of Computer Assisted Tomography*, **8(1)**, 46–49.

Doyle, F.H., Pennock, J.M., Banks, L.M. *et al.* (1982) Nuclear magnetic resonance imaging of the liver: Initial experience. *American Journal of Roentgenology*, **138**, 193–200.

Fevery, J. (1981) Pathogenesis of Gilbert's syndrome. *European Journal of Clinical Investigation*, **11**, 417–418.

Gollan, J.L. (1983) Diagnosis of hemochromatosis. *Gastroenterology*, **84**, 418–421.

Howard, J.M., Ghent, C.N., Carey, L.S., Flanagan, P.R. & Valberg, L.S. (1983) Diagnostic efficacy of hepatic computed tomography in the detection of body iron overload. *Gastroenterology*, **84**, 209–215.

Israel, H.L., Margolis, M.L. & Rose, L.J. (1984) Hepatic granulomatosis and sarcoidosis. Further observations. *Digestive Diseases and Sciences*, **29**, 353–356.

James, S.P., Stromeyer, F.W., Chang, C. & Barranger, J.A. (1981) Liver abnormalities in patients with Gaucher's disease. *Gastroenterology*, **80**, 126–133.

Javitt, N.B. (1979) Hyperbilirubinemia and cholestatic syndromes. *Postgraduate Medicine*, **65**, 120–130.

Kern, F. (1976) Hepatobiliary disorders in inflammatory bowel disease. *Progress in Liver Diseases*, **5**, 575–589.

Kolmannskog, F., Aakhus, T., Fausa, O., Schrumpf, E., Ritland, S., Gjore, E. & Elgjo, K. (1981) Cholangiographic findings in ulcerative colitis. *Acta Radiologica:Diagnosis*, **22**, Facs 2, 151–157.

Leader. (1981) Alpha-1-antitrypsin deficiency and liver disease. *British Medical Journal*, **283**, 807.

Lee, R.E., Robinson, D.B. & Glew, R.H. (1981) Gaucher's disease. Modern enzymatic and anatomic methods of diagnosis. *Archives of Pathology and Laboratory Medicine*, **105**, 102–104.

Patrick, D., White, F.E. & Adams, P.C. (1984) Long-term amiodarone therapy: a cause of increased hepatic attenuation on CT. *British Journal of Radiology*, **57**, 573–576.

Scott, W.W., Donovan, P.J. & Sanders, R.C. (1981) The Sonography of diffuse liver disease. *Seminars in Ultrasound*, II, **3**, 219–225.

Sharma, O.P. (1983) Diagnosis of sarcoidosis. *Archives of Internal Medicine*, **143**, 1418–1419.

Sharp, H.L., Bridges, R.A., Krivit, W. *et al.* (1969) Cirrhosis associated with alpha-1-antitrypsin deficiency: a previously unrecognized inherited disorder. *Journal of Laboratory and Clinical Medicine*, **73**, 934–939.

Shepherd, H.A., Selby, W.S., Chapman, R.W.G., Nolan, D., Barbatis, C., McGee, J.O'D. & Jewell, D.P. (1983) Ulcerative colitis and persistent liver dysfunction. *Quarterley Journal of Medicine*, **208**, 503–513.

Stark, D.D., Bass, N.M., Moss, A.A. *et al.* (1983) Nuclear magnetic resonance imaging of experimentally induced liver disease. *Radiology*, **148**, 745–751.

Sternlieb, I. (1978) Diagnosis of Wilson's disease. *Gastroenterology*, **74**, 787–793.

Stone, R., Benson, J., Tronic, B. & Brennan, T. (1982) Hepatic calcifications in a patient with Gaucher's disease. *American Journal of Gastroenterology*, **77**, 95–98.

Waxman, A.D. (1982) Scintigraphic evaluation of diffuse hepatic disease. *Seminars in Nuclear Medicine*, **12**, 75–88.

9: Circulatory Changes in Liver Disease

J. W. LAWS

Although the main circulatory changes in patients with liver disease occur in the hepatic arterial or portal venous systems, profound changes of clinical importance may take place elsewhere, notably in the systemic and pulmonary circulations.

Systemic circulation

Two of the most obvious manifestations of liver disease are palmar erythema and liver 'spiders.'

Palmar erythema, which is much more common than plantar erythema, is due to vasodilatation of the small vessels of the hand. This is merely one obvious manifestation of a generalized hyperdynamic state in which there is increased cardiac output and decreased peripheral resistance, often associated with an increased blood volume. These circulatory changes may wax and wane quite rapidly, depending on the severity or otherwise of the patient's liver dysfunction. The generalized reduction of the peripheral resistance in patients with liver disease means that systemic hypertension is relatively uncommon and that the blood pressure of patients previously hypertensive may return to normal if they develop cirrhosis (Loyke, 1962). Hypertension is rare in patients with hepatic dysfunction.

There is some evidence to suggest that this generalized cutaneous vasodilatation, with hot hands and liver palms, may allow shunting through cutaneous vessels at the expense of the muscular branches. This is analogous in some ways to the shunting which may occur in the lungs in patients with fulminant hepatic failure which will be discussed later. Liver spiders or spider naevi may occur in crops within the catchment area of the superior vena cava. These also may appear rapidly and disappear in a matter of

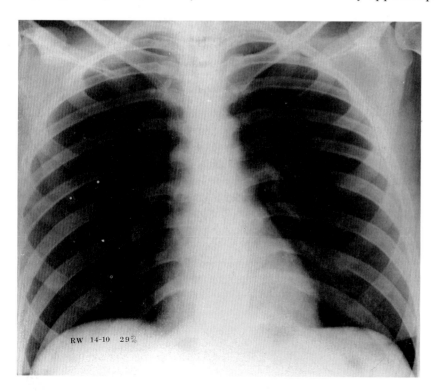

RW 14-10 29

Fig. 9.1 Chest film of a patient in fulminant hepatic failure with 29% intrapulmonary shunt. Note the normal heart size and clear lung fields.

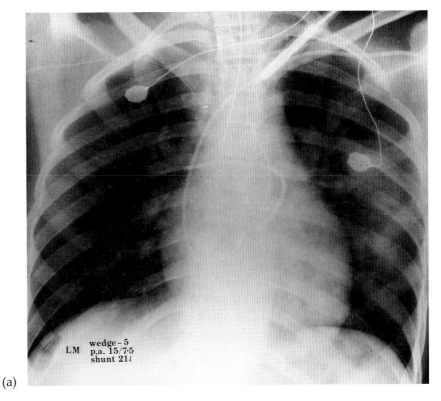

LM wedge – 5
p.a. 15/7·5
shunt 21%

(a)

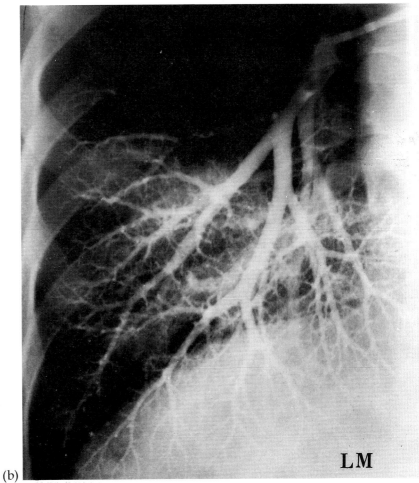

LM

(b)

Fig. 9.2 Fulminant hepatic failure. (a) Chest film showing normal heart size and clear lungs except for a small area of pulmonary oedema in the left mid-zone; 21% intrapulmonary shunt. (b) Wedge pulmonary angiogram showing no evidence of a macroscopic shunt or early venous filling.

days as liver function recovers; for example in a patient recovering from a fatty liver of pregnancy.

Pulmonary circulation

Patients with hepatic failure may develop two main types of circulatory change in their lungs: pulmonary oedema and intrapulmonary shunting.

About one-third of patients with fulminant hepatic failure develop radiological evidence of intra-alveolar pulmonary oedema during the course of their illness. The changes are initially peribronchial and perihilar. They may be unilateral for a time but are commonly bilateral and extensive. The septal lines of interstitial pulmonary oedema are not seen. This oedema occurs with a normal heart size and with a normal pulmonary wedge pressure, indicating that it is probably due to reduced capillary permeability. It is sometimes associated with cerebral oedema (Warren *et al.* 1978).

Rather fewer patients with hepatic cell failure develop intrapulmonary shunting during the course of their illness at a time when the chest radiograph may be entirely normal. Such patients, when assessed by measuring their arterial oxygen saturation after breathing pure oxygen for 15 min, have been shown to have shunts as high as 20–30%, i.e. as though 20–30% of the output of the right ventricle was passing through the lungs without being oxygenated (Fig. 9.1). These shunts may vary in severity, disappearing as the patient comes out of coma and returning when the patient relapses into coma again. Wedge pulmonary angiograms in two such patients were normal with no premature venous filling and no other evidence of shunting on a macroscopic scale (Fig. 9.2). Post-mortem angiograms have also been normal. Precise morphometric techniques have shown dilatation at all levels of the vascular tree (Trewby *et al.* 1978).

The mechanism of this reduction in arterial saturation, which is reversible and may vary from time to time, is uncertain. Pleural spiders occur similar to those that appear on the skin, but are unlikely to be of functional significance. The dilatation of the peripheral branches of the pulmonary artery as shown post-mortem is of a minor degree and should not by itself be the cause. One possibility is the relaxation of a precapillary sphincter mechanism in response to high cardiac output, allowing the blood to short-circuit the alveolar network, similar to the shunting which occurs in the systemic circulation in palmar erythema; 'liver lungs' rather than 'liver palms' (Trewby *et al.* 1976).

The hepatic circulation in health and disease

Normal liver

Normally the liver contains about 15% of the total blood volume of the body. This may be increased many times in heart failure or constrictive pericarditis and may be reduced to half in response to acute haemorrhage. The liver normally receives about a quarter of the cardiac output, say 1500 ml of blood per minute, of which 25% comes from the hepatic artery and 75% from the portal vein (Fig. 9.3). Although the hepatic artery supplies only a quarter of the blood, it has a higher oxygen saturation and is responsible for 50% of the oxygen supply of the liver (Lautt, 1977, Brooks, 1983).

Under normal circumstances, the flow through the hepatic artery is kept fairly constant by autoregulation. If the perfusion pressure rises, the resistance of the liver also increases, so that the flow remains approximately constant (Greenway & Stark, 1971). On the other hand, the flow through the portal vein may vary considerably during the course of the day. Measurement by Doppler ultrasound has shown that the flow through the portal vein may double within an hour of a meal and fall to the resting level within the next 2–3 h. (Fig. 9.4a,b). The volume of the liver may increase at the same time, probably due to the storage of

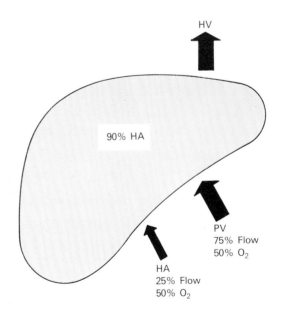

Fig. 9.3 Normal hepatic circulation. Although the hepatic artery supplies only 25% of the blood, it is responsible for over 50% of the oxygenation of the normal liver, and for 90% of the blood supply of most hepatic tumours.

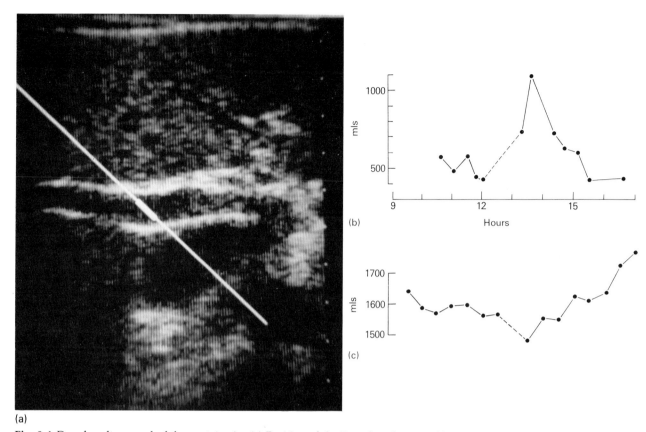

(a)

(b)

(c)

Fig. 9.4 Doppler ultrasound of the portal vein. (a) Position of the Doppler ultrasound beam within the portal vein. (b) Rise and subsequent fall of the portal blood flow following a meal. (c) Variation in the volume of the liver as estimated by ultrasound. There is an increase in volume following the meal. (Courtesy of Dr H.B. Meire.)

glycogen, since the administration of glucagon results in a rapid reduction in the size of the liver and rise of blood sugar due to mobilization of liver glycogen (Fig. 9.4c) (Leung *et al*. 1986).

Moderate cirrhosis

In patients with moderate cirrhosis there is periportal fibrosis with reduction in the sinusoidal volume and distortion of the portal veins. This gives rise to increased resistance to portal blood flow and reduced flow in the portal vein. There is a compensatory increase in blood flow through the hepatic artery, which may rise to double the normal value (Fig. 9.5).

In more severe cirrhosis the central veins are obliterated, and the resistance to portal vein flow increases still further so that eventually the balance of flow in the portal vein is away from, rather than into, the liver. The flow through the hepatic artery is increased still further (Fig. 9.6). This disturbance in portal vein flow gives rise to numerous collateral veins, which for convenience may be grouped

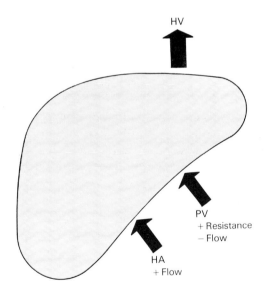

Fig. 9.5 Hepatic circulation in moderate cirrhosis. Portal blood flow is reduced with a compensatory increase in blood flow through the hepatic artery.

into: (1) reverse flow in normal tributaries; (2) watershed collaterals; (3) embryonic veins; and (4) confusing collaterals.

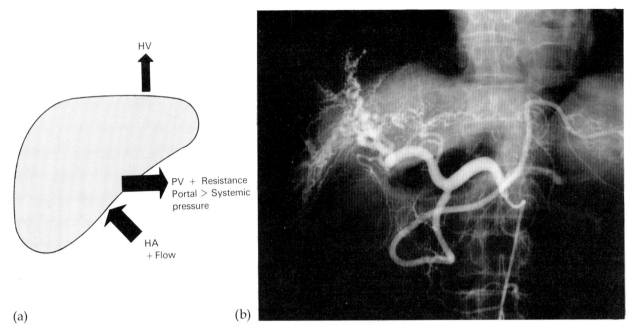

Fig. 9.6 Hepatic circulation in severe cirrhosis. (a) Increased hepatic artery blood flow with centrifugal flow in the portal venous system. (b) Hepatic angiogram showing large hepatic arterial flow in a small, cirrhotic liver.

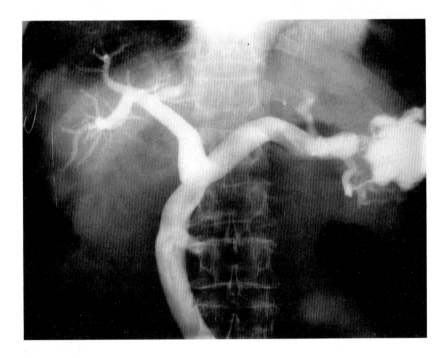

Fig. 9.7 Splenic venogram showing a very large superior mesenteric venous collateral channel. The patient had portasystemic encephalopathy.

1 The most common collaterals are those in which there is reversed flow in veins that are normally tributaries of the portal vein, particularly the gastric and oesophageal veins and the superior and inferior mesenteric veins (Figs 9.7, 9.8).

2 Watershed collaterals refer to those veins, mainly retroperitoneal, in which under normal conditions the blood may flow either towards or away from the liver. The lienorenal, gastrorenal and testicular veins fall into this category.

3 The main embryonic vein is the umbilical vein (Fig. 9.9).

4 Occasionally a collateral vein by its unusual size or position may masquerade as some quite different lesion and give rise to problems in diagnosis. For example, an aneurysm of the portal vein in the

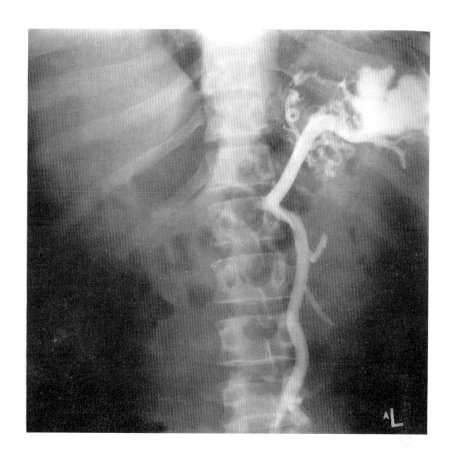

Fig. 9.8 Splenic venogram showing diversion of blood from the splenic vein into the inferior mesenteric vein.

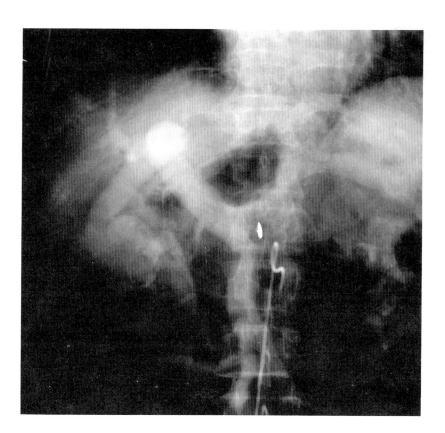

Fig. 9.9 Umbilical vein. Late phase of a superior mesenteric angiogram showing small intrahepatic branches of the portal vein with most of the flow entering a massive umbilical vein in a patient with severe cirrhosis.

porta hepatis, usually in a patient with cirrhosis, may give rise to obstructive jaundice by pressing on the common bile duct, or may present to the surgeon at laparotomy as a large unexpected vascular 'tumour'. Veins in the lienorenal ligament may give rise to filling defects in the substance of the left kidney, demonstrable on intravenous urography. Large varices of the haemorrhoidal and inferior mesenteric veins may give rise to filling defects visible on barium enema examination. These defects may be more evident when the colon is relatively collapsed than when it is fully inflated for a double-contrast examination, when the veins may be compressed. Collaterals passing up through the hemiazygos and azygos venous systems may give rise to a giant azygos vein, simulating a paratracheal 'mass' on the chest film: an appearance for which at least one patient has had a bronchoscopy. Such an appearance may be associated with absence or thrombosis of the inferior vena cava.

Portal hypertension with a normal liver biopsy

By far the most common cause of portal hypertension with a liver biopsy which is normal or

shows only mild periportal fibrosis is extrahepatic portal-vein thrombosis, often following umbilical sepsis in childhood. A much less common cause is hyperkinetic portal hypertension, in which there is a 'steal' of blood from the superior mesenteric and hepatic arteries into the spleen, presumably because of low splenic resistance. In such cases the splenic artery is usually large, sometimes with

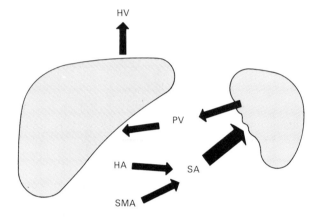

Fig. 9.10 Hyperdynamic portal hypertension. There is a 'steal' of hepatic artery and superior mesenteric blood into the spleen, resulting in a large blood flow through the splenic artery and vein.

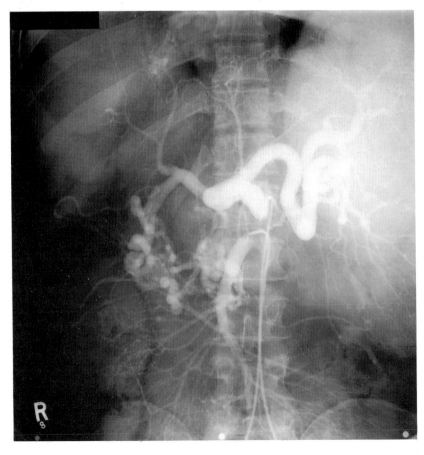

Fig. 9.11 Hyperdynamic portal hypertension. Male, aged 29 years, with haematemesis from oesophageal varices due to portal hypertension but with a normal liver biopsy. Simultaneous injection into the superior mesenteric artery and coeliac axis shows torrential flow through a large splenic artery into a large spleen, splenic artery aneurysms and 'steal' of blood from the superior mesenteric artery through duodenal channels into the spleen. Direct arterial flow into the liver is very small.

numerous aneurysms arising from it (Figs 9.10, 9.11).

Haemangioma of the liver

Haemangiomata vary vastly in their clinical behaviour and the effects they have on the hepatic circulation. Some cause no symptoms, have no haemodynamic effect, and may be chance findings during an ultrasound examination, while others may present with life-threatening heart failure due to massive shunting of blood through the liver.

Cavernous haemangiomata

These occur mainly in adults and are often a chance finding, but may cause symptoms of local pain by bleeding either into the liver or rupturing into the peritoneum. They are usually sited peripherally in the liver and may even be pedunculated. They may calcify. Their peripheral situation in the liver is well demonstrated by ultrasound as a localized, highly reflective lesion, sometimes with a less reflective centre (Fig. 9.12a). Angiographically they cause only a few scattered pools of contrast medium during the arterial phase and may be relatively avascular during the early hepatogram phase, filling with contrast only slowly, and late in the examination, sometimes from the portal vein. (Fig. 9.12b, c). They appear to function as a low-pressure sponge without forming a shunt. They may require treatment because of their size, discomfort or intraperitoneal bleeding.

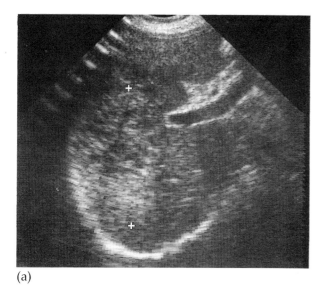

(a)

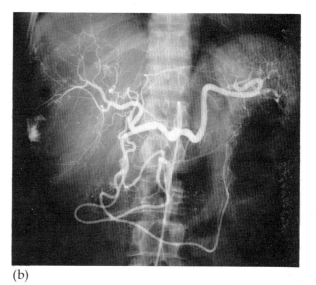

(b)

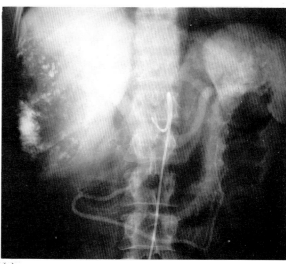

(c)

Fig. 9.12 Cavernous haemangioma. (a) Transverse ultrasound scan through the liver showing a highly reflective lesion with a less reflective centre in the periphery of the right lobe. (b) Coeliac axis angiogram showing pools of contrast scattered throughout the right lobe of the liver with some displacement of branches of the hepatic artery. The plain film showed some calcification in this area. (c) Hepatogram phase showing pools of contrast in some areas of the haemangioma although the bulk of the lesion is avascular relative to the rest of the liver.

Haemangioendothelioses

These occur in neonates and may be associated with haemangioma of the skin, particularly the scalp. The liver is usually diffusely affected. The high blood flow through the liver gives rise to a high-output cardiac failure occurring shortly after birth. Angiographically these demonstrate a variety of appearances. The most striking is torrential flow through the hepatic artery, which may become as large as a normal iliac artery, and effectively steal blood from the lower limbs. (Fig. 9.13a). There is a variable degree of pooling of blood within the liver before filling of large hepatic veins. The flow through the liver varies considerably in different patients. In the most severe cases the hepatic veins and right atrium may be seen to fill almost immediately after the hepatic artery. (Fig. 9.13b). If the flow can be reduced by hepatic-artery embolization or ligation, there is a good chance that the condition will remit, the flow continue to get less, and the liver develop normally, so that the child may recover completely.

Blood supply of hepatic tumours

Over 90% of the blood supply to both primary and metastatic hepatic tumours is derived from the hepatic artery. If an attempt is to be made to reduce the blood supply to a hepatic tumour it may be done either by surgical ligation of the hepatic artery or by selective embolization of the tumour itself by radiological methods.

Surgical ligation of the hepatic artery may reduce the blood supply to the tumour immediately but, since the arterial anatomy of the liver is very variable, the blood supply to normal liver tissue may be reduced also. Moreover, it has been estimated that there are at least 26 arterial collateral pathways by which blood can reach the liver following ligation of the hepatic artery, so that collateral pathways soon form, usually in a matter of days, and the blood supply to the tumour is at least partially restored quite quickly.

Selective embolization on the other hand often results in a permanent reduction in the blood supply that may be confined to the part of the liver involved in tumour. If the tumour is particularly vascular and has been stealing blood from the rest of the liver, the effective blood supply to the normal liver may be actually increased (Chaung & Wallace, 1980).

Although the flow through the hepatic artery may increase and partially compensate for a reduction in portal-vein blood flow, the reverse happens to only a very minor degree. For this reason, hepatic artery ligation is contraindicated in most patients with impaired portal-vein blood flow, for example in cirrhotics. Thus, localized embolization, which may need to be repeated at intervals, is preferable to ligation of the hepatic artery in most instances. Occasionally the sequence of events may be dictated by the arterial anatomy, which may make embolization impossible. Once the hepatic artery has been ligated, embolization of the tumour becomes impossible.

Focal nodular hyperplasia

The lesion of focal nodular hyperplasia is always hypervascular and is usually associated with a large hepatic artery, presumably because the lesion develops slowly over the course of many years. About 20% of them are pedunculated and 20% are multiple. Forty per cent take up sulphur colloid and, if present, this may be a useful diagnostic sign. The CT scan shows a circumscribed lesion, enhancing after injection of contrast, and frequently with a central scar of reduced attenuation (Fig. 9.14a). Angiographically a large hepatic artery divides into numerous branches which supplies the lesion from the periphery (Fig. 9.14b). Later films show extreme generalized vascularity (Fig. 9.14c). The flow may be brisk enough for the hepatic veins to outline clearly on the later films (Fig. 9.15). Embolization of focal nodular hyperplasia results in a dramatic reduction in the vascularity of the lesion, with an increase in the supply to the normal liver.

Contraceptive pill tumour

The hepatic tumours associated with the contraceptive pill vary considerably in their nature, from a single encapsulated benign adenoma to a frankly malignant lesion, which spreads within the liver and metastasizes freely. It is usually hypervascular, but the main hepatic artery is not as large and the outline of the lesion not as regular as in focal nodular hyperplasia (Fig. 9.16). The sulphur colloid scan shows a cold area. There may be areas of 'peliosis', dilated blood spaces, elsewhere in the liver. Embolization of the tumour may result in total necrosis of the tumour, sometimes with the formation of a sterile abscess which may need to be drained. In other patients the tumours may be

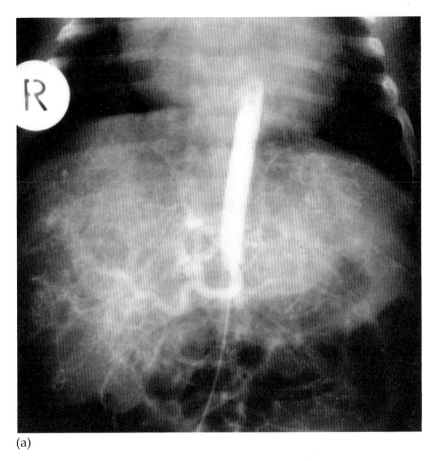

(a)

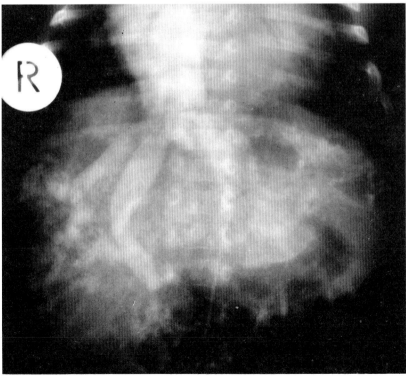

(b)

Fig. 9.13 Haemangioendotheliosis. A male neonate presenting with heart failure during the first week of life. There were haemangiomata on the scalp and right thumb. (a) Arterial phase of aortogram showing large main hepatic artery supplying a very hypervascular liver. (b) Venous phase showing massive veins entering the right atrium.

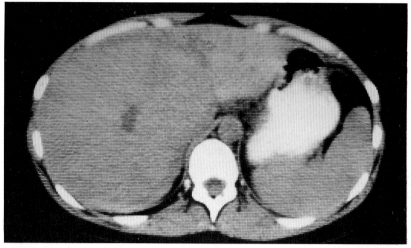

(a)

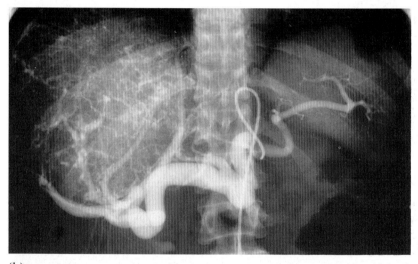

(b)

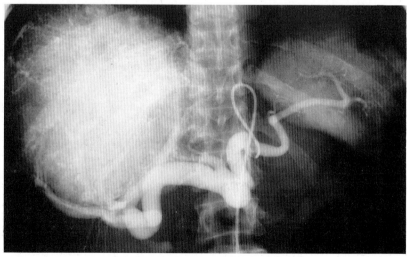

(c)

Fig. 9.14 Focal nodular hyperplasia. Female, aged 33 years, with pain in the right hypochondrium, for 2 years. (a) CT scan showing a large circumscribed lesion in the right lobe of the liver, with reduced attenuation in the centre. (b) Coeliac axis angiogram showing massive right hepatic artery supplying a hypervascular lesion, with the main blood supply entering from the periphery. (c) Later film showing the vascular nature of the lesion.

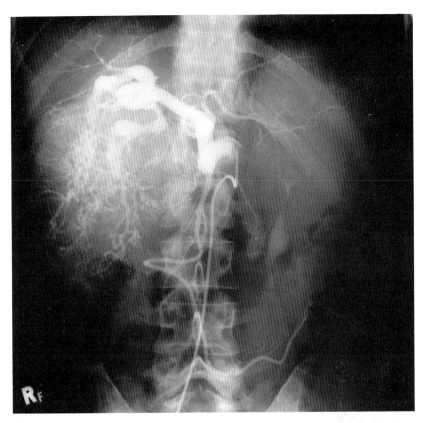

(a)

Fig. 9.15 Focal nodular hyperplasia. Male, aged 29 years, with a history of slowly enlarging liver for 8 years with recent pain. No stigmata of chronic liver disease. A sulphur colloid isotope scan showed increased uptake in the right lobe of the liver. (a) Hepatic arteriogram showing a very large hepatic artery with tortuous branches entering the periphery of the lesion. Note the small size of the hepatic arteries supplying the rest of the liver. (b) Later film showing generalized uptake of contrast into the lesion with filling of the hepatic veins (*arrows*).

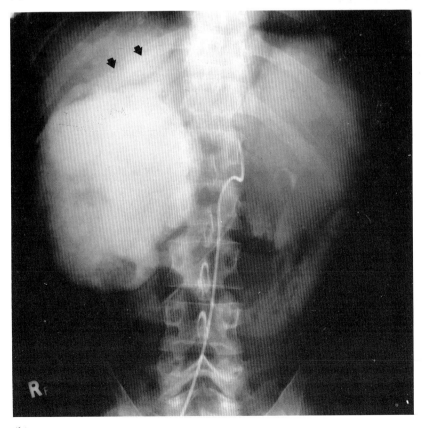

(b)

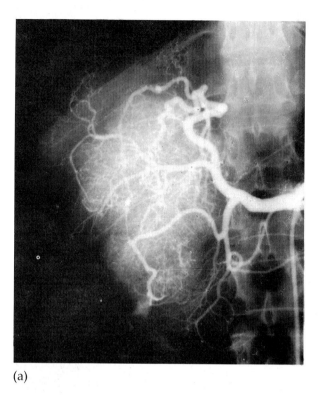

(a)

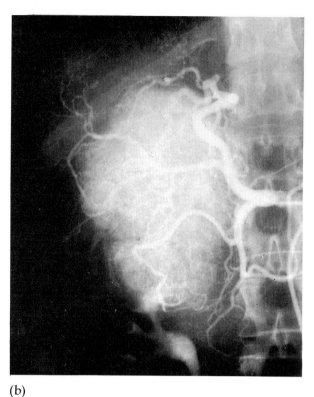

(b)

Fig. 9.16 Contraceptive pill tumour. Female, aged 29 years, on high-oestrogen pill for 6 years. Pain in the right hypochondrium. Cold areas in colloid scan in the right lobe of liver. (a) Hepatic arteriogram showing a localized but irregular area of hypervascularity with vessels of irregular calibre entering the main lesion from the periphery. Elsewhere in the liver there are dilated blood spaces. (b) Later film showing the extreme hypervascularity of the tumour. The tumour was embolized, a sterile abscess developed which required surgical drainage, but there was no recurrence at 3 years.

localized initially, but recur following excision or embolization before metastasizing widely.

Hepatoma

The circulatory changes in hepatoma vary widely. They may be circumscribed or multifocal. They are usually hypervascular, but may be avascular with a hyperaemic rim. Direct communication between the hepatic artery and the hepatic or portal vein may occur within the tumour, usually spontaneously but occasionally as a result of biopsy. Tumour tissue may be demonstrated within the lumen of the portal vein (Fig. 9.17).

Metastatic tumours

Embolization of hepatic metastases may be indicated for a number of reasons. The most common is in an attempt to alleviate pain, and this may be very successful. The embolization may need to be repeated at intervals. The other main group in which embolization may be helpful is the endocrine-secreting tumours, particularly in patients with the carcinoid syndrome associated with massive deposits in the liver. Repeated embolization of carcinoid metastases may well relieve the patient of the distressing symptoms of the carcinoid syndrome and keep the tumour under control for many years (Fig. 9.18). The very slowly growing metastases of medullary carcinoma of the thyroid may give rise to greatly increased circulation through the liver, even causing high-output heart failure, which may be alleviated by repeated embolization (Fig. 9.19).

Budd–Chiari syndrome

Some of the more common causes of the Budd–Chiari syndrome are given in Table 9.1. Underlying thrombotic disease needs to be excluded. A mechanical cause such as direct invasion by a tumour or a web across the inferior vena cava is very uncommon. Veno-occlusive disease, affecting the small veins, may result from a variety of drugs or poisons, including most of the cytotoxic drugs.

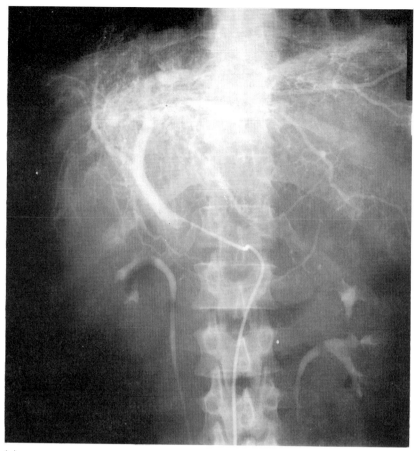

(a)

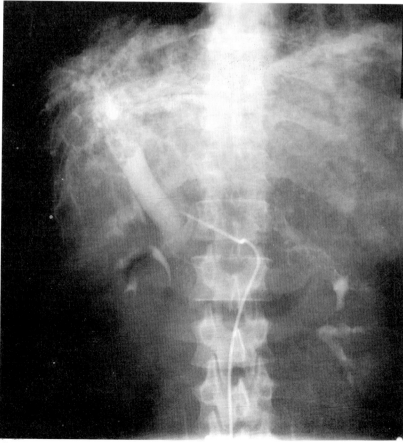

Fig. 9.17 Hepatoma in the portal
vein. Male, aged 64 years, with
cirrhosis and hepatoma. (a) Early
arterial film showing tumour
circulation in the right lobe of the
liver. (b) Film 2 s later showing direct
shunting from the hepatic artery into
the portal vein, with tumour in the
portal vein.

(b)

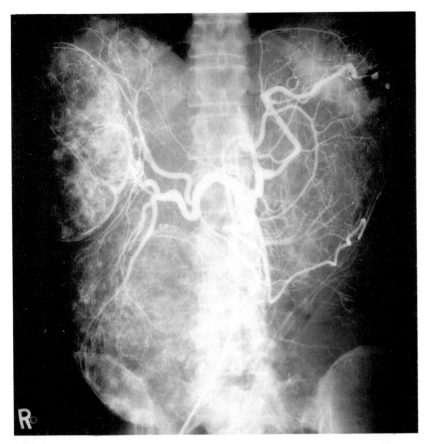

(a)

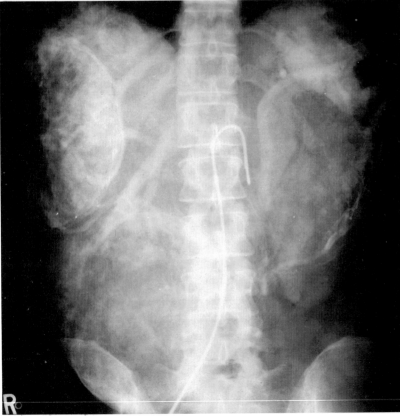

(b)

Fig. 9.18 Carcinoid syndrome. Female, aged 37 years, with increasing oedema of the legs due to a large abdominal mass shown at laparotomy to be a very vascular liver. She developed the carcinoid syndrome with flushing and thickening of the pulmonary and tricuspid valves. 5-Hydroxyindoleacetic acid excretion was greatly increased. (a) Early arterial phase showing massive hypervascular lesions throughout the whole of an enormous liver. (b) Later film showing circumscribed metastases with filling of the hepatic veins. Repeated embolization of the carcinoid metastases reduced the size of the liver and relieved the symptoms of the carcinoid syndrome. The patient later developed retroperitoneal fibrosis, a known complication of the carcinoid syndrome.

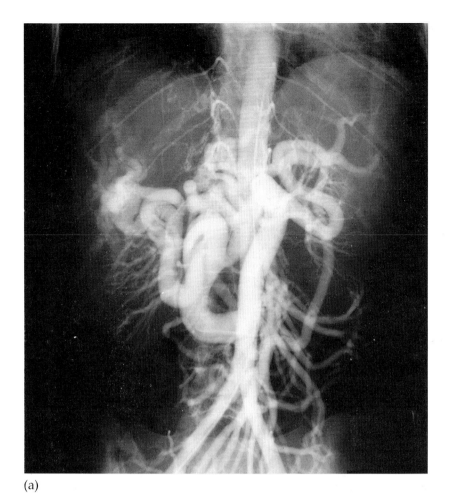

(a)

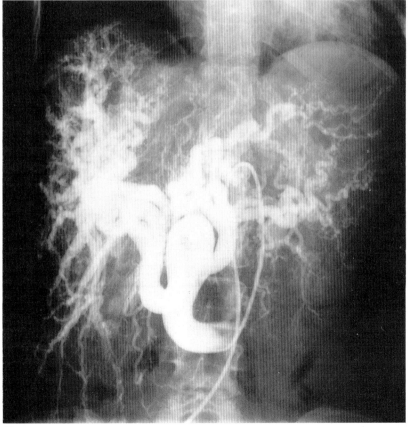

(b)

Fig. 9.19 Medullary carcinoma of the thyroid. Female, aged 37 years, with a history of diarrhoea for 20 years, lassitude for 1 year and increasing shortness of breath for 3 months. Partial thyroidectomy 19 years ago. On examination there was pigmentation, high-output cardiac failure, and nodular thyroid enlargement. (a) Aortogram showing torrential flow through a grossly enlarged hepatic artery. (b) Localized injection into the main hepatic artery demonstrates this torrential flow. Hepatic artery embolization failed to relieve the high-output failure. Laparotomy revealed an enormous liver studded with metastases from a medullary carcinoma of the thyroid. The hepatic artery was ligated, but the patient died of high-output cardiac failure. Review of the histology of the partial thyroidectomy performed 20 years earlier showed that it was the same as had been found in the hepatic metastases.

Table 9.1 Budd–Chiari syndrome

1 Thrombotic disease
  Polycythaemia vera
  Paroxysmal nocturnal haemoglobinuria
  Contraceptive pill
  Renal disease

2 Mechanical
  Hepatic and renal tumours
  Inferior vena-caval web

3 Veno-occlusive disease
  Crotalus or *Senecio* poisoning
  Cytotoxic drug therapy

4 Idiopathic

A knowledge of the anatomy of the hepatic veins is necessary for an understanding of the radiological diagnosis of the Budd–Chiari syndrome. The main part of the liver is drained by three large veins, the right, middle, and left hepatic veins, while the caudate lobe is drained by a number of small veins that enter directly into the inferior vena cava. Commonly in the Budd–Chiari syndrome the large veins are affected and the small veins of the caudate lobe are spared. In such a case, the sulphur colloid scan will show some uptake in an enlarged caudate lobe overlying the spine and some in a large spleen, but none in the rest of the liver.

It should be possible to demonstrate the main right, middle, and left hepatic veins by ultrasound in a normal-sized liver, but failure to demonstrate them in a swollen liver is not conclusive evidence of thrombosis. The ascites, which is nearly always present, should be demonstrable.

Direct catheterization of the hepatic veins may demonstrate their patency or, if they are thrombosed, the characteristic 'spider's web' of collateral veins on the surface of the liver. This is the most direct method of confirming the Budd–Chiari syndrome. There may also be a side-to-side narrowing of the portal vein by the swollen liver and an indentation of its anterior surface by the enlarged caudate lobe, which lies immediately anterior to it. Rarely, a web may be demonstrated in the inferior vena cava between the point of entry of the hepatic veins and the right atrium.

Conclusion

In health, the circulation of the liver is constantly adapting to changing circumstances. In disease, there may be not only severe disturbances of the circulation locally around the liver, but also profound changes elsewhere in the systemic and pulmonary circulations, which may be of considerable importance in the proper management of patients with liver disease.

References

Brooks, F.P. (1983) The physiology of the liver. In Herlinger, H., Lunderquist, A. & Wallace, S. (eds) *Clinical Radiology of the Liver*. Dekker, New York.

Chuang, V.P. & Wallace, S. (1980) Hepatic arterial redistribution for intraarterial infusion of hepatic neoplasms. *Radiology*, **135**, 295–299.

Greenway, C.V. & Stark, R.D. (1971) Hepatic vascular bed. *Physiological Reviews*, **51**, 23.

Lautt, W.W. (1977) Hepatic vasculature; a conceptual view. *Gastroenterology*, **73**, 1163.

Leung, N.W.Y., Farrant P. & Peters, T.J. (1986) Liver volume measurement by ultrasonography in normal subjects and alcoholic patients. *Journal of Hepatology*, **2**, 157–164.

Loyke, H.F. (1962) Reduction of hypertension after liver disease. *Archives of Internal Medicine*, **110**, 45–49.

Michels, N.A. (1953) Collateral arterial pathways of the liver. *Cancer*, **6**, 708–724.

Trewby, P.N., Warren, R., Contini, S., Crosbie, W.A., Wilkinson, S.P., Laws, J.W. & Williams, R. (1978) The incidence and pathophysiology of pulmonary edema in fulminant hepatic failure. *Gastroenterology*, **74**, 859.

Trewby, P.N., Williams, R. & Reid, L. (1976) Intrapulmonary vascular shunts in fulminant hepatic failure. *Digestion*, **14**, (abstract) 466.

Warren, R., Trewby, P.N., Laws, J.W. & Williams, R. (1978) Pulmonary complications in fulminant hepatic failure: analysis of serial radiographs from 100 consecutive patients. *Clinical Radiology*, **29**, 363–369.

Wallace, S. & Chuang, V.P. (1983) Liver tumours; diagnosis and management. In Herlinger, H., Lunderquist, A. & Wallace, S. (eds) *Clinical Radiology of the Liver*. Dekker, New York.

10: Portal Hypertension

R. DICK

Introduction

Portal hypertension is defined as increased hydrostatic pressure within the portal vein and/or its tributaries. In normal man portal venous pressure is about 7 mmHg. A pressure consistently above 11 mmHg indicates the presence of portal hypertension (Sherlock, 1985).

Included in the portal system are all veins which carry blood from the abdominal part of the alimentary tract, the spleen, pancreas and gall bladder. The portal vein enters the liver at the porta hepatis in two main branches, one to each lobe. It is without valves in its larger channels. Branches have a segmental distribution within the liver. Normally the hepatic artery provides the liver with a small volume of blood at a high pressure, whilst the portal vein delivers a large volume at a low pressure. Portal blood flow in man is 1000–1200 ml/min, and the portal vein contributes 72% of the total oxygen supply to the liver. Figure 10.1 shows the normal portal vein, linked via the sinusoids to the hepatic vein and thence the systemic circulation.

Four important factors determine portal pressure: the volume of splanchnic blood flow, the extent of portasystemic shunts, the intra-abdominal pressure (represented by inferior vena caval pressure), and the resistance to flow of blood between the portal and systemic venous circulations. In portal hypertension, the last named is the predominant cause, the site of resistance to venous outflow from the portal system being disease anywhere between the origin of the splenic vein and the heart.

Imaging techniques have a seminal role in the investigation and management of patients with portal hypertension. Gastrointestinal haemorrhage, haematemesis and/or melaena is the most common presentation, though splenomegaly may be the first indication of disease. Radiological imaging, endoscopy, laboratory tests, and liver biopsy are the four major investigations needed to confirm a diagnosis of portal hypertension and to localize the site of causation.

Aetiology

Obstruction to portal flow anywhere along its course usually results in portal hypertension. Intrahepatic obstruction from liver disease or obstruction in the extrahepatic portion of the portal vein are the two commonest causes. The so-called idiopathic portal hypertension marked by splenomegaly and mild changes in liver function tests is rare, as is active (non-cirrhotic) portal hypertension, which is hyperkinetic in type and occurs in patients with myelofibrosis, leukaemia, lymphoma, and Gaucher's disease. Felty's syndrome may fall into this group, and imaging relative to the particular disease is indicated. All in this group have splenomegaly, and the persistently elevated flow may cause increased vascular resistance in the liver, so that 'passive' portal hypertension supervenes. Active portal hypertension may also occur in hereditary haemorrhagic telangiectasia (Osler–Rendu–Weber syndrome) or be

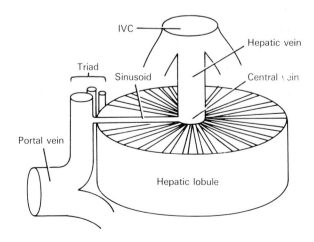

Fig. 10.1 Normal relationship between portal vein, sinusoids, and hepatic vein within the hepatic lobule.

115

acquired from stab wounds etc. involving the hepatic artery, portal vein, or hepatic vein (Fig. 10.2).

For practical purposes, the commonest causes of portal hypertension are illustrated in Fig. 10.3. Obstruction of the main splenic or portal vein by thrombosis or by tumour invasion/compression is shown in Fig. 10.3a. In Fig. 10.3b, obstruction to the portal vein is seen at the presinusoidal level. This may occur in a number of diseases, including early primary biliary cirrhosis, chronic active hepatitis, granulomatous disease such as sarcoidosis, schistosomiasis, congenital hepatic fibrosis, and toxins including vinyl chloride, arsenic, and copper.

Sinusoidal obstruction as shown in Fig. 10.3c is the commonest overall cause of portal hypertension. All late cirrhoses, including alcoholic and post-hepatitic, affect this level, as do a few non-cirrhotic conditions such as acute alcoholic hepatitis and cytotoxic drugs. Hepatic vein obstruction is the final group. Figure 10.3d shows veno-occlusive disease affecting the small hepatic veins,

whereas in Fig. 10.3e the portal pressure will be increased behind webs, tumours, or thrombosis in the main hepatic vein or in the hepatic portion of the inferior vena cava.

Attempts to localize the level of the pathology causing portal hypertension either by imaging or by liver biopsy are of real practical value. For example, in patients with presinusoidal cellular infiltrate or in those with a portal vein thrombosis, a major haemorrhage will rarely be followed by liver failure. In contrast, the intrahepatic types frequently go into liver failure after haemorrhage because of their gross hepatocellular disease.

Pathology

Obstruction to the portal circulation either within the liver or outside it results in an extensive collateral circulation to carry portal blood into the systemic veins (Fig. 10.4). Collateral veins which travel caudally will finally join the inferior vena cava, whilst those travelling cephalad will drain into the superior vena cava.

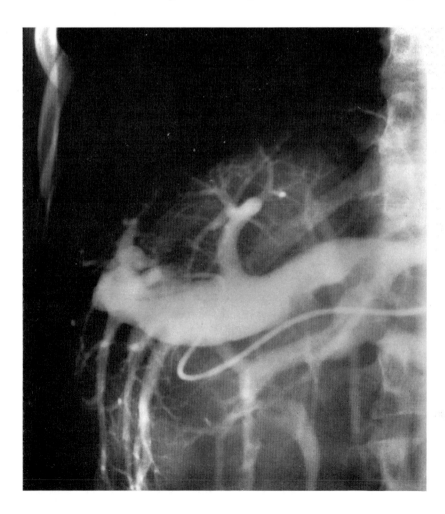

Fig. 10.2 This 16-year-old boy has portal hypertension following a stab wound. Superselective hepatic arteriogram shows fistula carrying blood at arterial pressure into the portal vein (dilated from site of fistula).

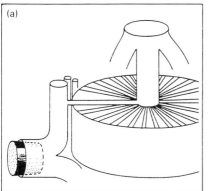
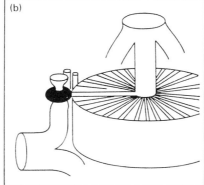
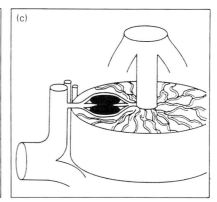
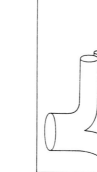
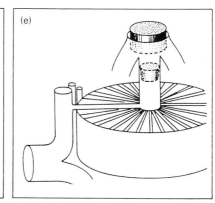

Fig. 10.3 Causes of portal hypertension. (a) Extrahepatic; (b) intrahepatic presinusoidal; (c) sinusoidal; (d) postsinusoidal (some of which may have a sinusoidal component); (e) post-hepatic.

Four main groups exist:

1 Para-umbilical veins in the falciform ligament, which open up and join systemic veins in the anterior abdominal wall (caput medusae).

2 Veins where abdominal organs are in contact with retroperitoneal tissues (veins from liver to diaphragm), or adherent to the abdominal wall (via omentum, or developing in a laparotomy scar).

3 Via the left renal vein, portal blood entering it directly from splenic vein or by pancreatic, left adrenal or gastric veins. This is often a major shunt (Figs 10.5 and 10.16). Mental disturbance (portasystemic encephalopathy) is common with such shunts only if the patient has poor hepatocellular function. Portal blood enters the systemic veins and reaches the brain without first being metabolized by the liver.

4 Where absorptive epithelium lies next to protective epithelium. Two common sites are at the anus, and stomach cardia where the left gastric (coronary) vein and short gastric veins of the portal system anastomose with the azygos vein and thence the superior vena cava (Fig. 10.6). Communications in the submucosa of the oesophagus and upper part of stomach lead to varicosities known as 'varices'. This is the commonest site for bleeding in portal hypertension.

Around the anus, varices may form in connections between the superior haemorrhoidal veins of the portal system and the middle and inferior haemorrhoidal veins of the caval system.

Intrahepatic shunts may also occur between portal and hepatic veins within the liver, and between portal and pulmonary veins (Taguchi *et al.*, 1983). These shunts are small compared with the main four listed above, which may lead to hepatic encephalopathy, septicaemia (due to intestinal organisms), and other circulatory and metabolic effects.

The liver in portal hypertension

Liver size correlates poorly with the height of the portal venous pressure, though high pressures are more often found with the small, contracted fibrotic organ, and correlate well with the degree of nodule formation. When the liver is deprived of portal blood by growth of the collateral circulation it depends more and more upon hepatic blood supply. The splenic artery and portal vein are enlarged, and may be tortuous and aneurysmal. Mural thrombi and calcified plaques may be seen. Splenic enlargement occurs. Extensive collateral

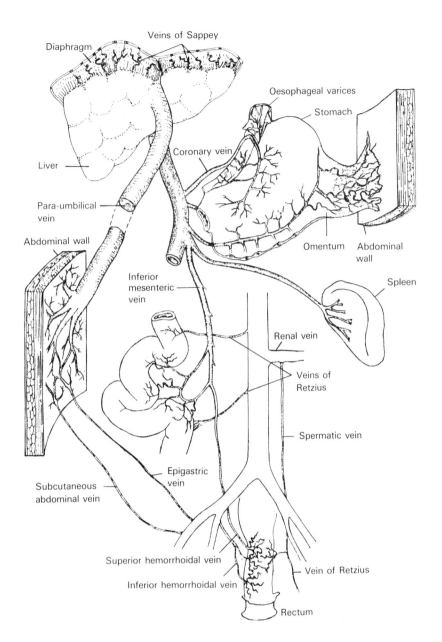

Diaphragm

Veins of Sappey

Oesophageal varices

Stomach

Liver

Coronary vein

Para-umbilical
vein

Abdominal wall

Inferior
mesenteric
vein

Omentum Abdominal
wall

Spleen

Renal vein

Veins of
Retzius

Spermatic vein

Subcutaneous
abdominal vein

Epigastric
vein

Superior hemorrhoidal vein

Inferior hemorrhoidal vein

Vein of Retzius

Rectum

Fig. 10.4 The sites of the portasystemic collateral circulation in cirrhosis of the liver (after McIndoe, 1928).

veins form, but rarely succeed in lowering the portal pressure to normal.

In post-sinusoidal obstruction such as occurs in hepatic-vein occlusion of the Budd—Chiari syndrome, the liver is enlarged, purplish and smooth, though in the chronic case the caudate lobe, which has separate venous drainage into the cava, is enlarged and areas less affected by obstruction may form nodules.

Imaging in portal hypertension

Although endoscopy is of primary importance for establishing the presence of oesophageal and gas-

tric varices and whether they are the source of haemorrhage, and laboratory tests and liver biopsy characterize liver disease, imaging techniques are invaluable at all stages of the patient's clinical course. Imaging ranges from simple studies such as the barium swallow to sophisticated ones including angiograms and dynamic CT. Much of the imaging for portal hypertension is invasive, though the use of non-invasive methods is increasing. Selecting the correct investigation for a particular problem is important and is to be preferred to using multiple imaging techniques. The cost-conscious department must remember this.

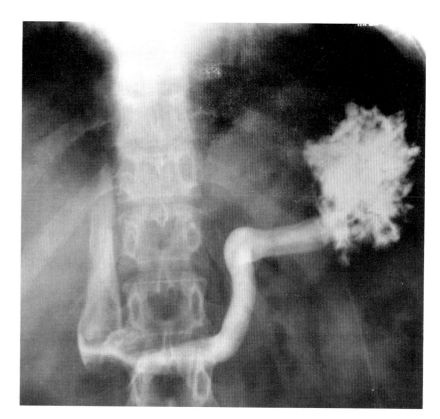

Fig. 10.5 A large shunt from the splenic vein to the left renal vein and thence the inferior cava is shown in this trans-splenic portogram. Such shunts may be spontaneous or follow surgery.

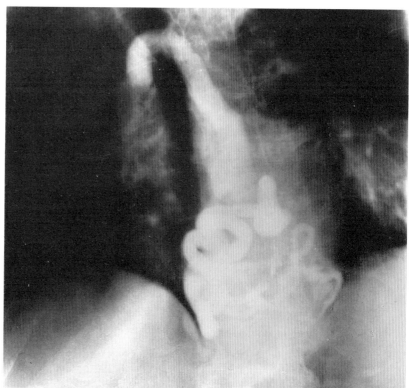

Fig. 10.6 Trans-hepatic portogram. Contrast injected into the left gastric vein fills the azygos vein and thence the superior vena cava.

Simple radiography

In a patient with chronic liver disease, the presence of portal hypertension may first be suspected on a chest film, which may show a dilated azygos vein or a lobulated venous mass in the posterior mediastinum (Fig. 10.7). An abdominal radiograph may reveal a small liver and enlarged spleen, and

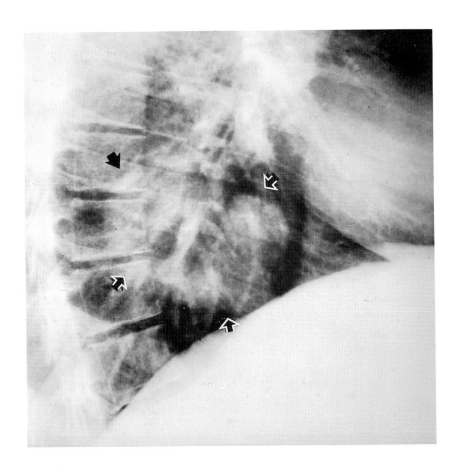

Fig. 10.7 Lateral chest radiography. Arrows indicate a lobulated mass in the posterior venous mediastinum. In this patient with portal hypertension these were venous collaterals.

occasionally calcification in thrombus in the portal or splenic veins or in collaterals (Fig. 10.8).

Barium studies

A barium swallow is contraindicated in the *acute* upper gastrointestinal bleed, and in the non-bleeder the question 'are there varices?' can probably be answered equally well by a competent radiologist or endoscopist (Waldram *et al.*, 1977). A barium swallow is still more widely available than endoscopy and does not require premedication. An excellent technique is required.

For an oesophagogram, small volumes of a standard barium preparation are used, the swallow being performed with the patient supine or prone, and during quiet respiration. The Valsalva or Mueller technique is unnecessary. Worm-like submucosal defects due to varices have a typical appearance. If not seen, repeat films or a video study should be obtained after paralysis of oesophageal motility with intravenous Buscopan (hyosine-N-butylbromide), as described by Ghahremani *et al.*, 1972. Recently, glucagon has proved as effective and lacks the side-effects of the

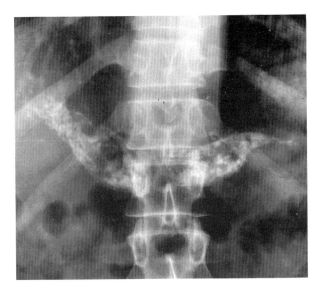

Fig. 10.8 Plain abdomen X-ray. Calcification in portal and splenic veins. This may follow splenectomy, trauma, portal pyaemia, or inflammatory or neoplastic disease of the pancreas.

anticholinergics (Fig. 10.9). Studies without intravenous spasmolytic and using a thick paste miss up to 25% of varices (Khosla *et al.*, 1984). The grading of varices by size is important, since in one study varices smaller than a critical size were shown to be unlikely to bleed, although once patients had bled, variceal size is of limited value in predicting the rate of bleeding (Westaby *et al.*, 1982).

A dilated oesophagus is seen with moderate to large varices, with no obstruction at the cardia. However, occasionally there may be a coexistent reflux oesophagitis or hiatus hernia, though the theory that erosion of mucosa precipitates variceal bleeding is much weakened by a study showing no reduction in bleeding from varices in patients given cimetidine compared with controls (MacDougall & Williams, 1983).

Candidiasis can readily be distinguished from varices. It causes fine ulceration, usually extending down the oesophagus from mouth and pharynx. Should the lower third be spared, the differentiation from varices is simple. The defects are not serpiginous, and there may be intense spasm unrelieved by glucagon. Varices, on the other hand, extend up the oesophagus from the lower third, and may be seen well above the level of the azygos vein arch in the thorax. Occasionally *candida* oesophagitis and varices coexist in debilitated patients (Dick, 1984).

Gastric varices cause polypoid defects in the gastric fundus (Fig. 10.10). They are occasionally found without oesophageal varices, whence splenic vein occlusion or pancreatitis or pancreatic neoplasm should be higher in the differential than liver disease (Hunter, 1983). The position of the gastric fundus should be noted, splenomegaly displacing it medially.

A limitation of the barium swallow is that it cannot determine if a varix is bleeding or indeed has recently bled. Endoscopy will answer this, and varices may be imaged by direct injection into them, usually performed in conjunction with sclerotherapy (Fig. 10.11). Notwithstanding the advantages of direct vision, close agreement occurs between the incidence of varices seen at endoscopy and on barium swallow using spasmolytics when performed in a liver unit. An advantage of endoscopy is that a pressure transducer may be attached to the tip of the endoscope to measure variceal pressure directly.

Occasionally rectal varices dilate and rupture, causing massive bleeding. They are sometimes shown on a double-contrast enema (Fig. 10.12), and have also been described in a family who were non-cirrhotics (Hawkey *et al.*, 1985). Whether barium is introduced orally or rectally, large volumes should be avoided in the patient with chronic liver disease, for if it remains in the large bowel for a long period it may contribute to amine retention and portasystemic encephalopathy.

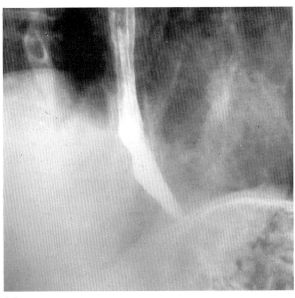

(a)

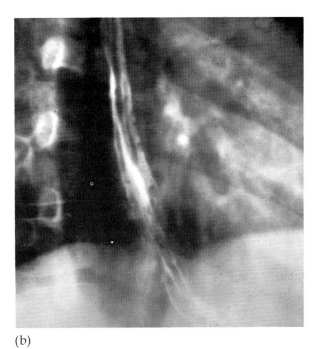

(b)

Fig. 10.9 Barium swallow in cirrhotic patient. (a) Mucosal pattern of lower oesophagus normal; (b) study repeated after i.v. glucagon — definite varices are present.

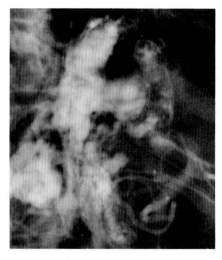

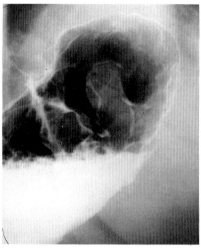

Fig. 10.10 Patient with long-standing splenic vein thrombosis due to sepsis. Barium study shows large submucosal varix in gastric fundus. Portogram on left confirms.

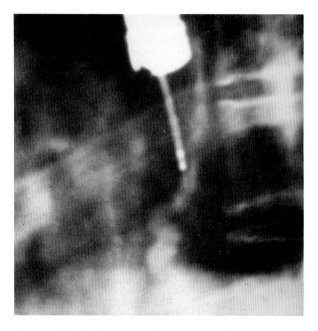

Fig. 10.11 Endoscopic injection of contrast into an oesophageal varix at the time of endoscopic sclerotherapy (courtesy of Drs P.N. Smith and J.D.R. Rose).

Ultrasound (US) and computerized tomography (CT)

Both non-invasive techniques are valuable in the investigation of portal hypertension. Each can demonstrate the patency of the portal and splenic veins and measure their calibres, as well as identifying venous collaterals and portal vein thrombosis. This is important, as in some centres early management of bleeding varices may include transhepatic sclerosis or surgical shunts, both depending upon the patency of the portal vein. Differentiation between cirrhosis and an extrahepatic cause of portal hypertension is also important, as

the natural history of variceal bleeding differs between the two groups.

Normal US appearance has been discussed in Chapter 2. In portal hypertension, scanning in the left lateral decubitus position will cause the portal vein to dilate, whilst the superior mesenteric and splenic veins may be best seen after eating (Bellamy *et al.*, 1984). Gastric and retroperitoneal collateral veins will be best shown in the right lateral decubitus position, using the spleen as a window. A portal vein greater than 15 mm in diameter is virtually pathognomonic of the presence of portal hypertension. In portal vein thrombosis, US is highly accurate (Fig. 10.13). Echogenic thrombus may be seen within the lumen, also small transonic veins in the 'cavernoma' around the block. A diagnosis may be made in 86–95% of patients (Webb *et al.*, 1977; Van Gansbeke *et al.*, 1985). Partial blockage may be seen as a single irregular channel. Both make the diagnosis of portal hypertension certain. The inexperienced ultrasonographer must not diagnose portal vein block without good evidence. Inability to demonstrate the portal vein or reverberation in it may be caused by inexperience or artefact. Ultrasound is less successful at diagnosing splenic vein thrombosis.

Doppler US can be undertaken down the oesophagus through the endoscope and accurate flow patterns established. It has not yet been possible to relate the different patterns to the likelihood of variceal rupture (McCormack *et al.*, 1983).

On CT the portal vein appears as a tubular structure of low attenuation at the hilum of the liver (Chapter 3). Enhancement is mandatory for unequivocal identification, tubular structures due

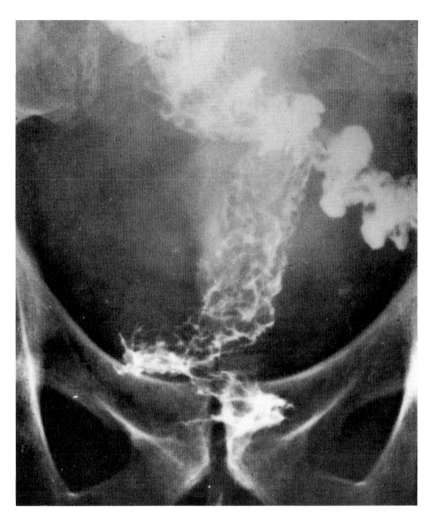

Fig. 10.12 Submucosal rectal varices in a patient with cirrhosis and portal hypertension.

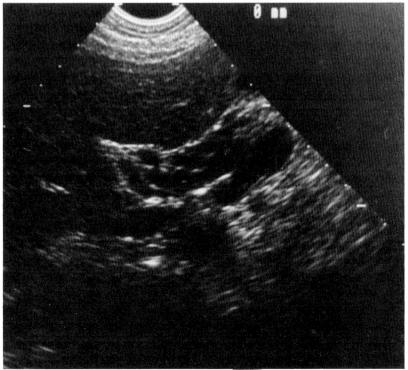

Fig. 10.13 US scan demonstrating multiple irregular veins replacing the single, normal portal vein.

to bile ducts remaining with low attenuation in both studies.

A portal vein diameter greater than 20 mm suggests increased flow and portal hypertension (Fig. 10.14). Contrast-enhanced CT readily diagnoses portal-vein thrombosis, especially using a dynamic mode (Mathieu *et al.*, 1985), whereas the presence of a dilated umbilical vein in the anterior abdominal wall indicates cirrhosis as the cause of portal hypertension (Fig. 10.15). CT portography (scanning after contrast injection into the portal system, either directly or after arterioportography) has also been described (Reinig *et al.*, 1985) and the technique is widely practised.

Enhanced CT is advantageous over US in showing the extent of retroperitoneal and mediastinal collateral shunting veins, but it is both more invasive and less flexible than US. For example, CT may miss thrombus limited to a short segment of portal vein outside the planes scanned (Van Gansbeke *et al.*, 1985), whereas the more flexible US can be used in any number of axes to visualize the vessels. Retroperitoneal 'masses' seen on CT in patients with portal hypertension are likely to be venous collaterals, and biopsy must never be considered before an enhanced study has been performed (Fig. 10.16).

Magnetic resonance imaging (MRI) has limited availability and is rarely used in this group of patients. Nevertheless, flowing blood in veins of the portal system, hepatic veins, and in oeso-phageal varices can be elegantly demonstrated (Fig. 10.17).

Vascular and haemodynamic studies in portal hypertension

Pressure and flow studies provide essential information in patients with portal hypertension. Contrast portography, either direct (trans-splenic, trans-hepatic, trans-umbilical) or direct (arterio-portography) will be needed in the majority of patients and will be discussed in the next section.

Pressure studies

Pressure within the portal system can be measured (i) in the splenic pulp, (ii) in the portal vein, and (iii) at the tip of a catheter 'wedged' in a small hepatic vein. The last-named technique is simple to perform and safe for the patient. It is readily carried out using a balloon-occlusion 'Cobra' or 'Sidewinder' catheter introduced percutaneously via the antecubital, internal jugular, or femoral vein (Fig. 10.18). Unlike puncture of the liver or spleen, haemostatis at the entry site is guaranteed even in the presence of severe clotting defects. Liver biopsy may also be performed should the approach have been transjugular.

A corrected sinusoidal pressure (CSP) is reached by subtracting the pressure in the free hepatic vein close to the inferior vena cava (FHP] from the

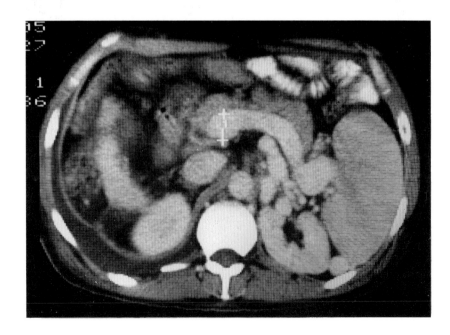

Fig. 10.14 Enhanced CT scan showing a 21 mm diameter portal vein origin. Also dilated splenic vein and splenomegaly.

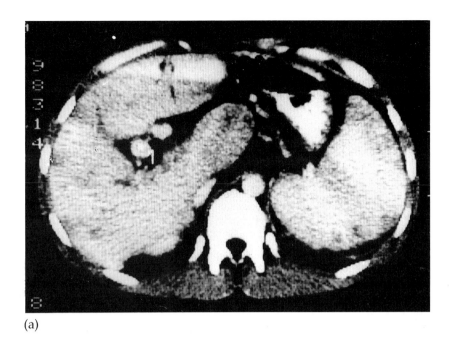

(a)

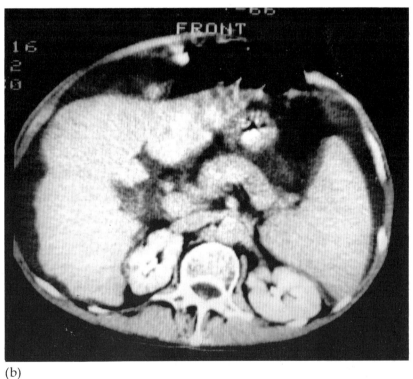

(b)

Fig. 10.15 (a) Enhanced CT in 23-year-old man with long-standing portal vein thrombosis. A cavernous system of veins (two large and several small) replaced the original (non-identified) thrombosed portal vein. (b) Enhanced CT in patient with cirrhosis and ascites. Liver irregular and atrophic. Anterior to the left lobe the umbilical vein can be seen coursing towards the anterior abdominal wall.

wedged ('occlusal balloon') hepatic venous pressure (WHP). This removes from the wedged total the contribution resulting from raised intra-abdominal pressure due to causes such as ascites, obesity, and posture. Normal values are FHP 4–7 mmHg and WHP 4–11 mmHg, the normal upper limit of CSP being 7 mmHg. The degree of portal hypertension is graded by the level of CSP as:

Mild 7–14 mmHg
Moderate 15–30 mmHg
Severe 30 mmHg and above.

The presence of an intrahepatic cause of portal hypertension (commonly cirrhosis) may thus be proved and its severity indicated without contrast studies by the simple means of placing a balloon catheter in one or more hepatic veins, recording

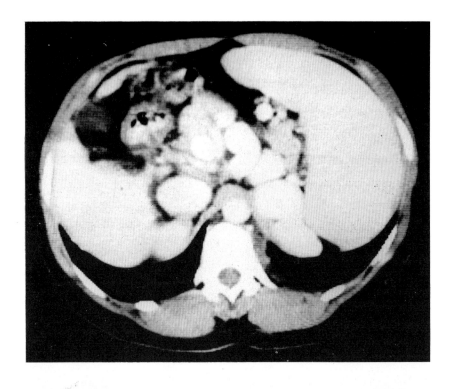

Fig. 10.16 Dynamic enhanced CT. Numerous dilated retroperitoneal collaterals arise from the splenic hilum. They feed to the dilated inferior vena cava. In an enhanced scan, the veins resemble lymphadenopathy.

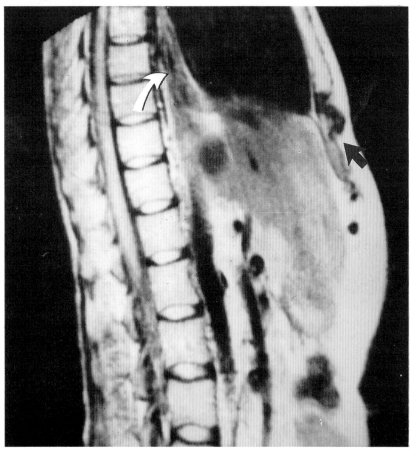

Fig. 10.17 Magnetic resonance imaging in patient with portal hypertension. Oesophageal varices (*curved arrow*), dilated umbilical vein (*short arrow*), and large visceral veins (courtesy Dr A. Leung).

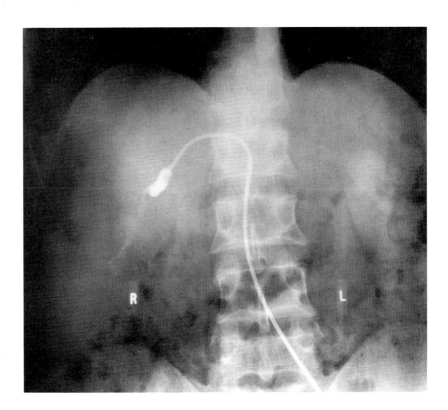

Fig. 10.18 Selective catheterization of a right middle hepatic vein. Balloon occluded with 2 ml dilute contrast. Air may also be used.

pressures both before and after balloon distension, and averaging results from the sets of hepatic veins.

Should the CSP be normal, the patient will require further pressure measurement taken in the prehepatic territory of the portal circulation. Comparison of portal venous pressure (PVP) with the CSP will pinpoint the site of resistance to flow to either presinusoidal hepatic disease or extra-hepatic venous obstruction. Angiography will be needed in some of these patients to delineate the portal tree.

Azygos vein blood-flow studies

At the conclusion of pressure studies, the catheter may conveniently be repositioned to measure the rate of collateral blood flow through the azygos vein (Fig. 10.19). Azygos blood flow is considerably greater in portal hypertension and correlates with the height of the portal pressure. The measurement of azygos venous blood flow by a continuous thermal dilution technique (Bosch & Grossman, 1984) provides an index of blood flow through gastro-oesophageal collaterals, since collateral blood flow from stomach and oesophagus drains largely into the azygos vein (Fig. 10.6). Azygos flow in the normal is 0.08–0.19 l/min, whilst in cirrhotics with portal hypertension it is 0.22–1.61 l/min, a highly significant difference. Changes in portal haemodynamics during drug therapy may be accurately monitored during azygos flow studies.

Contrast studies

Hepatic venography

Rappaport first described this technique in 1951. Today it remains a simple method without contra-indications, and with minimal morbidity and high success rate in excess of 95%. It may be conveniently performed after pressure readings, up to three hepatic veins being studied. A French gauge 7100 cm long, curved occlusion balloon catheter is used. To engage the main right hepatic vein, the catheter and wire are advanced into the high inferior vena cava. When the wire is gradually withdrawn, the catheter curve forms, and is rotated to the right. Gentle manipulation engages the hepatic-vein orifice. A heavy-duty wire may be then needed for further catheter advancement into the hepatic vein.

Iopamidol 300 (30 ml) is injected beyond the inflated balloon at a rate of 5 ml/s using an automatic injector, eight films being obtained at the

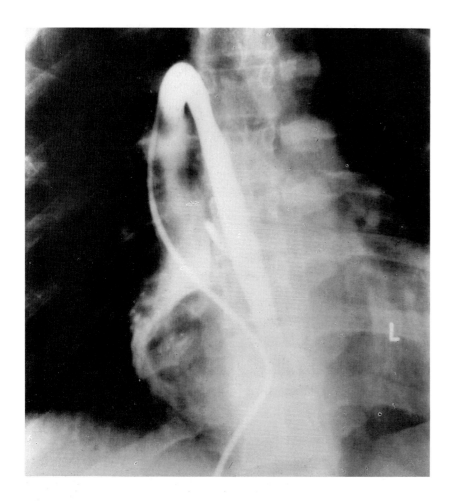

Fig. 10.19 Contrast injected into the (dilated) azygos vein as part of azygos blood flow study in patient with suspected increased portal blood flow.

rate of one per second. The regularity of normal hepatic veins is characteristic (Fig. 10.20). Equally, the distorted patterns in a moderate (Fig. 10.21) and severe (Fig. 10.22) cirrhosis are obvious, the changes correlating with severity of liver disease on biopsy (Bookstein *et al.*, 1975). In a normal patient, adjacent hepatic veins commonly fill, as may portal radicles if injection is too forceful. Rapid filling of portal vein branches, and indeed of the main vein itself, may occur in a patient with a high CSP, indicating reversed ('hepatofugal') flow in the portal system.

Prior to the introduction of balloon catheters, ionic contrast medium was injected once a catheter had been peripherally wedged (Fig. 10.20). This method should be avoided, as haemorrhagic necrosis of liver cells may result, with subsequent pyrexia and elevation in liver enzyme levels.

Occlusive disease of the hepatic veins has been described in the previous chapter. The pathognomonic 'spider's web' is seen on the contrast venogram, whether viewed in the AP or lateral plane (Fig. 10.23). Inferior cavography is also obtained, the cava being typical indented by an enlarged caudate lobe on the lateral projection (Fig. 10.24). Pressure studies in the right atrium and supra and infrahepatic vena cava are even more important in management. Compression of the hepatic cava by the tense, congested liver will elevate the subhepatic vena caval pressure, which may only be a few mmHg less than the portal. This will exclude treatment of portal hypertension using a compressive portacaval or splenorenal shunt, and perhaps indicate a shunt between a superior mesenteric vein and a vein or chamber above the diaphragm. Radiology and pressure measurements are thus vital parts of patient management.

Trans-splenic portography

First described by Abeatici & Campi (1951), this remains a simple diagnostic tool of low morbidity. It is the quickest way of delineating portal venous anatomy in addition to allowing measurement of portal pressure (Fig. 10.25).

Suspected portal hypertension with a bleed is the common indication. Contraindications are a

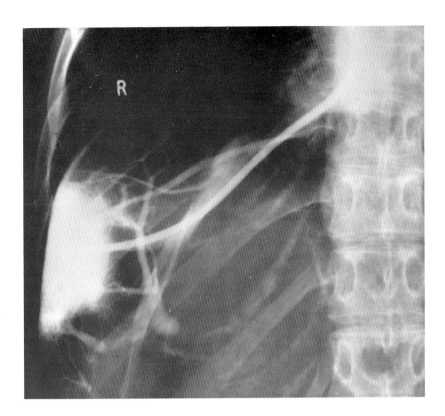

Fig. 10.20 Normal right hepatic venogram. Note homogeneous filling of peripheral sinusoids and reflux to portal vein radicles. Wedge pressure gradient was 1 mmHg. This type of 'wedged' venogram is harmful to liver (see text) and should be replaced by balloon-occlusion method.

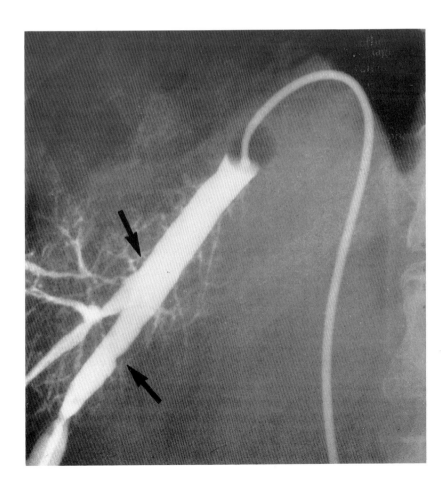

Fig. 10.21 Hepatic occlusion balloon venogram in patient with cirrhosis. Proximal part of hepatic vein is irregular (*arrows*). Peripheral branches show multiple strictures. Wedge pressure gradient 14 mmHg.

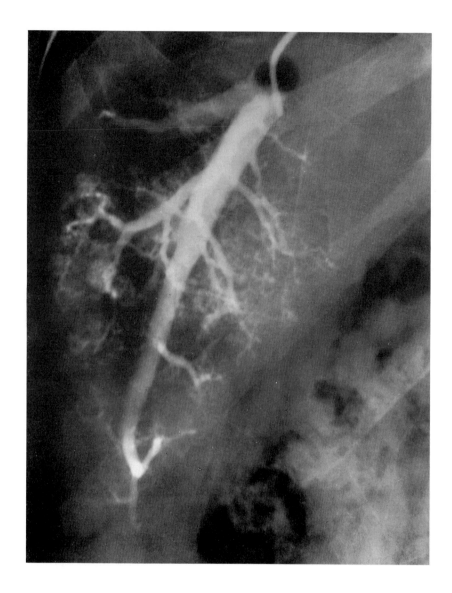

Fig. 10.22 Gross cirrhosis. Hepatic venogram indicates very irregular venous filling and poor parenchymal filling. Wedge gradient 23 mmHg.

prothrombin time prolonged 4 s beyond the control value (despite correction), and a platelet count of less than 75 000 mm³. Deep jaundice and gross ascites make the procedure more risky, whilst the operator must take precautions in patients who are hepatitis b antigen positive.

Technique. After analgesia and skin anaesthesia, the splenic pulp is punctured under fluoroscopy and during apnoea, using a needle cannula (Vygon Intranule; Ecouen, France, FG 6, 90 mm). The assembly is directed from the mid-axillary line 15° cephalad towards the hilum of the spleen to a depth of 4–5 cm. Once the needle is withdrawn, the patient breathes and a steady flow of blood from splenic pulp should immediately leave the cannula. After the position is checked with a test

dose of contrast, the splenic pulp pressure (normally less than 11 mmHg) is measured using a physiological pressure transducer. A cut film or DSA sequence is then obtained over 20 s whilst 50 ml iopamidol 370 is injected at a rate of 8–10 ml/s.

Reversed flow into gastric and oesophageal collateral veins in a patient who has recently bled is usually accepted as clinical evidence of a variceal bleed. A splenic or portal-vein block is a common finding in younger patients with portal hypertension. Collateral veins around the site will confirm this (Fig. 10.26). However, an important limitation of trans-splenic portography is that non-filling of a portal or even splenic vein may occur due to 'steal' by generous collateral veins, or due to hepatofugal blood flow. In this situation, trans-hepatic

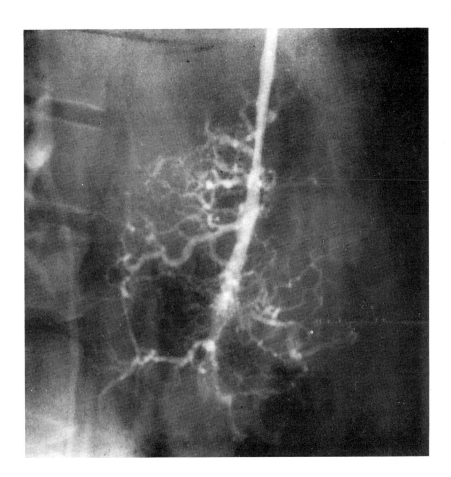

Fig. 10.23 Lateral projection. Wedge hepatic venogram in suspected Budd–Chiari syndrome. 'Spider's web' pattern of collaterals replacing blocked small hepatic veins confirms diagnosis.

portography or superior mesenteric arteriography is required.

As the cannula is withdrawn, Gelfoam suspended in normal saline is injected by syringe to occlude the tract in the spleen. Provided this practice is adhered to, the complications of massive haemorrhage and splenic rupture should be avoided, the reported incidence being less than 1% (Dick, 1983).

Trans-splenic portography is being replaced by angiographic methods discussed below. It remains a reliable means of quickly introducing contrast into the portal system, and in a large series recently reviewed by Zamir *et al.* (1984) a portogram could not be produced after injection into the splenic pulp in only 4%.

Splenomegaly that is persistent and undiagnosed is another indication for trans-splenic portography. Pulp may be aspirated by the radiologist and sent to haematology, microbiology, or cytology if required. In the acute bleeder, however, the method has nothing to offer therapeutically in the patient with portal hypertension, and one of the next two procedures is preferred.

Trans-hepatic portography

Rich opacification of the portal venous tree is provided by this technique (Fig. 10.27). Although markedly superior to trans-splenic portography and arterioportography as regards opacification and details of collaterals (Fig. 10.28) it may occasionally not fill known varices (Smith-Laing *et al.*, 1980). It has long learning curve, and being more a therapeutic than a diagnostic technique, will be described in detail in the section on the acute bleeder.

Arterioportography

Selective coeliac and superior mesenteric arterioportography has a great advantage over direct portography in demonstrating both arterial capillary and venous abnormalities in the portal hypertensive, the venous phase showing the distribution of blood to the liver from all of the gut. Subtraction angiography, either photographic or digital, is preferred if available.

Coeliac and superior mesenteric arterioportography is well tolerated under local anaes-

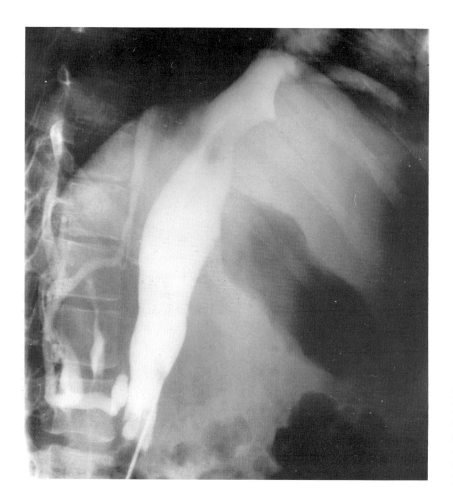

Fig. 10.24 Same patient as Fig. 10.23. Lateral inferior venacavogram. Note smooth identification on anterior surface of cava due to enlarged caudate lobe, also venous return aided by azygos system of veins posteriorly.

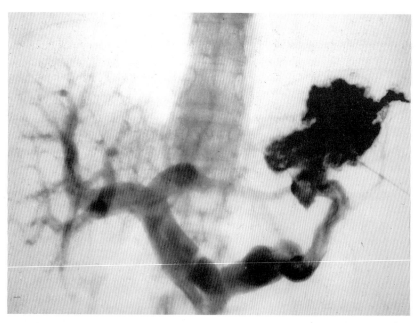

Fig. 10.25 Subtraction study. Normal trans-splenic portogram. All of the flow is hepatopetal. None of the tributaries of the splenic or portal veins should fill with contrast.

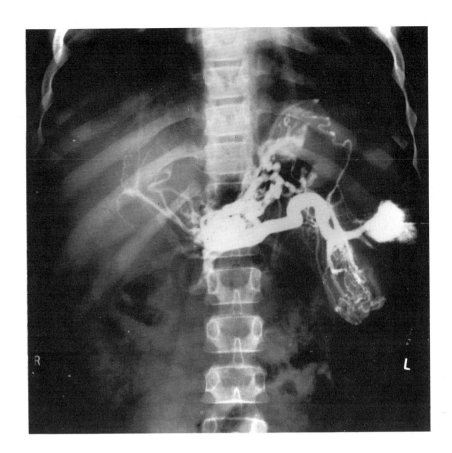

Fig. 10.26 Trans-splenic portogram in patient with previous portal pyemia following septic appendix. Thread-like channels replace the normal portal vein. Gastric varices fill.

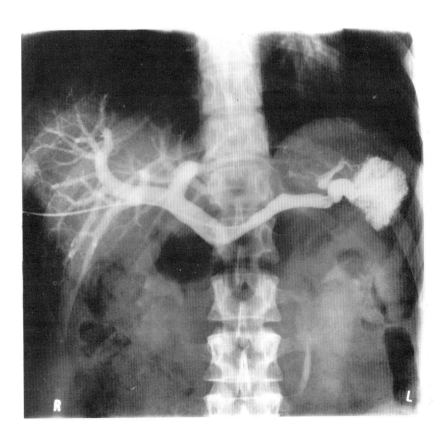

Fig. 10.27 Trans-hepatic portogram. Normal study (performed during sampling for suspected gastrinoma stomach).

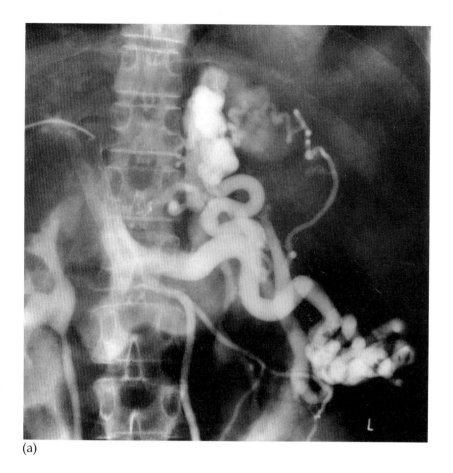

(a)

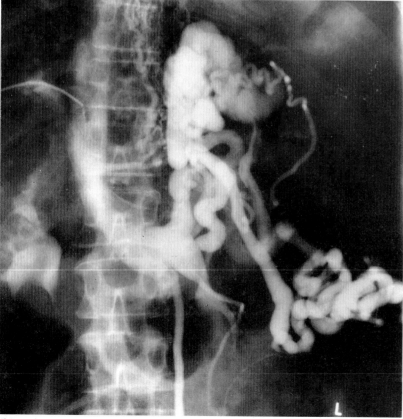

(b)

Fig. 10.28 Trans-hepatic portogram in patient where trans-splenic study failed to show varices. (a) Hepatofugal flow occurs in the portal vein and fills inferior and superior mesenteric veins, gastric and subsplenic collaterals, but no oesophageal varices show. (b) Later film in same study shows huge shunt to left renal vein and thence to inferior vena cava. Oesophageal varices now fill via a connection to the stem of the portal vein.

thesia, and involves placing a Sidewinder-type catheter into each artery and injecting 40–60 ml of contrast at a rate of 8 ml/s. A 30-s sequence is required to ensure full venous filling. Gaseous distention of stomach and duodenum may enhance the study, as may 2 mg sodium nitroprusside given intra-arterially just before the contrast (Fig. 10.29).

In the arterial phase, a corkscrewed pattern of vessels is seen if the liver is contracted from cirrhosis, and in the late phase, a patchy hepatogram and irregular liver contour (Fig. 10.30). Some patients will have a superadded primary liver-cell cancer (hepatoma), which may have invaded the portal vein and caused dramatic portal hypertension (Fig. 10.31). Angiomata anywhere in the gut are not uncommon (Fig. 10.32).

When chronic gastrointestinal bleeding occurs in a portal hypertensive patient and endoscopy has not revealed the source, coeliac and superior mesenteric arterioportography is indicated. Its major limitation is that in the presence of gross splenomegaly, the splenic vein may not fill on the coeliac injection, due to contrast dilution within the spleen. Retroperitoneal shunts are also not as densely filled as with direct portography, though portal vein block may be consistently shown. Gastric and oesophageal varices are sometimes seen only after selective left gastric arterial injection.

Risks of angiography in patients with portal hypertension

Prothrombin times prolonged 3 s or greater beyond the control value, and platelet counts under 75 000/mm^3 are relative contraindications to angiography. Fresh frozen plasma, platelet infusion and vitamin K injections should be given prior to arrival in the angiogram suite, and timed

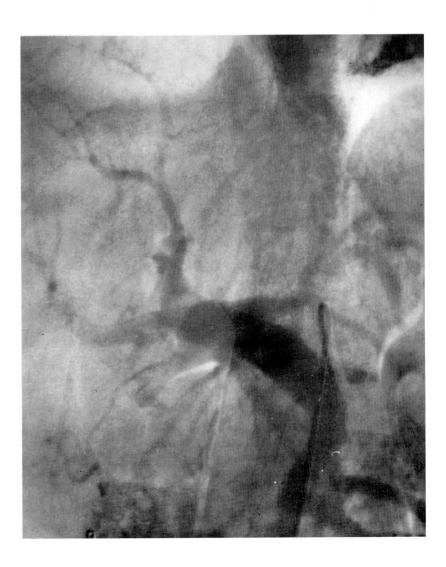

Fig. 10.29 Subtraction study of venous-phase superior mesenteric arteriogram. Widely patent portal vein clearly shown, also left gastric vein filling oesophageal varices.

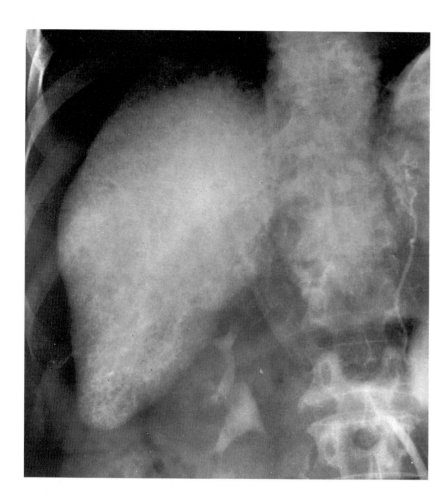

Fig. 10.30 Selective hepatic arteriogram. Parenchymal phase indicates patchy parenchymagram of small, irregular right lobe in this cirrhotic with portal hypertension.

to give maximal haemostasis after the arterial catheter is withdrawn. Haematoma around the femoral artery puncture site is unfortunately not uncommon, though surgical repair of a persistently bleeding artery should never be necessary.

Four factors have emerged in the past 5 years to reduce the risks of angiography in portal hypertension:

1 Improved catheter design now permits the use of smaller-diameter arterial catheters (FG 5 or 6 rather than 7 or 8). This reduces arterial-wall trauma without compromising on flow rate.

2 Digital subtraction angiography allows vital questions about the portal circulation (such as the patency of the portal vein) to be answered by superselective arterial injections of small amounts of dilute contrast, with consequent decrease in insult to liver cells.

3 Contrast media have improved. Low-osmolality agents such as iopamidol (Niopam, E. Merck Ltd) and iohexol (Omnipaque, Nycomed Ltd) are less toxic to body tissues than hyperosmolar ionic agents, produce less hypersensitivity reactions,

and are painless, so that even children find angiograms tolerable under local anaesthesia. Hepato-renal failure after angiography has ceased to be a complication in these patients if newer media are used, and the many clinical advantages to the patient with portal hypertension justify the extra expense of the contrast media.

4 Angiographic catheter exit tracts from either liver or spleen should routinely be plugged in patients with portal hypertension and coagulopathy. Pledgets of Gelfoarm or steel-wire coils must be injected (Fig. 10.33) as the catheter is withdrawn (Dooley & Dick, 1987).

Acute bleeding in portal hypertension: Emergency radiological techniques

Before coming to the angiogram suite the patient must be resuscitated. A tamponade balloon must be ready to inflate should a massive bleed occur. Titrated doses of vasopressin will act as a splanchnic vasocontrictor, the drug being easier to administer intravenously than intra-arterially, and is just

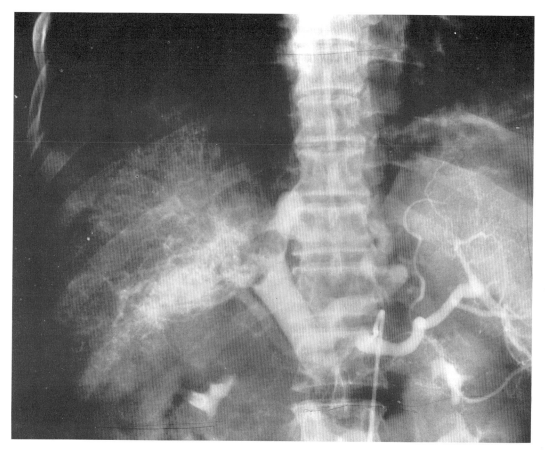

Fig. 10.31 Coeliac arteriography in patient with recurrent variceal bleeding, deteriorating liver function tests, and rising serum alphafetoprotein levels. Arterial phase (note splenic artery) yet immediate filling of portal vein at liver hilum. Tumour circulation liver and filling defect in portal vein is likely to be tumour invasion of it. Early death from a massive bleed may occur in some patients.

as effective. Synthetic vasopressin (Glypressin) 2 mg 6 hourly i.v. is also effective.

Various techniques are available to occlude varices, which may be injected with sclerosant endoscopically or by venous and hepatic access routes.

Direct injection sclerotherapy

This is usually performed under general anaesthesia, using a fibreoptic endoscope within a rigid tube which compresses the varices. If bleeding is torrential the procedure cannot continue, as varices are obscured by blood. Remarkable success may be achieved (Williams & Dawson, 1979), multiple sessions of injections being undertaken over a period of 1–4 weeks, during which all the veins in the lower oesophagus are obliterated. Sclerosants used include ethanolamine oleate and sodium tetradecyl sulphate, 2 ml being injected per varix,

and up to 30 ml per session. There is no consensus as to whether the injection should be intra- or peri-variceal, though the latter may favour oesophageal ulceration and stenosis (Rose *et al.*, 1983). Obliteration is achieved by mural necrosis followed by fibrosis. Control of bleeding is achieved in 80%, and long-term follow-up shows fewer recurrent bleeds compared with controls (Terblanche *et al.*, 1981).

Trans-hepatic portography

This may be extended to selective catheterization of all gastro-oesophageal varices arising from the portal system, and thence their embolization. Lunderquist & Vang described the technique in 1974. Lack of available expertise is its major limitation, the procedure being technically difficult and time consuming (sometimes in excess of 1½ h).

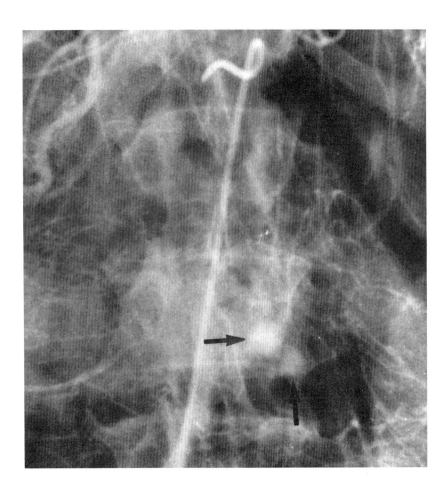

Fig. 10.32 Superior mesenteric arteriogram. Two small bleeding points (*arrowed*) are present in the upper jejunum. Suitable for embolization.

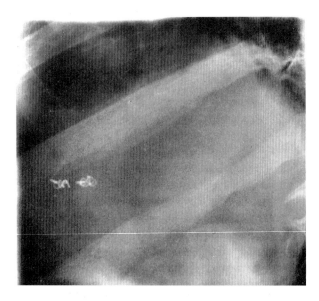

Fig. 10.33 Trans-hepatic portogram. Two steel-wire coils have been injected into the catheter tract in liver during final catheter withdrawal.

Trans-hepatic embolization of varices involves localizing the intrahepatic right branch of the portal vein by angiography or ultrasound, and making this site in the right hypochondrium. Under local anaesthesia, it is approached from the mid-axillary line in the right lower thorax with a long trocar sheathed in a matching length polyethylene catheter (William Cook, Europe). Using a series of guide wires, including moveable core 'J' and rigid stainless steel 'Surgimed' types (Meadox Surgimed Ltd), the catheter is advanced deeply into the portal system. An angiogram is obtained (15 films at 1/s) during injection of 30 ml iopamidol 370 at 10 ml/s. Active bleeding may be shown (Fig. 10.34). Using a tip deflector mechanism, or exchanging the straight catheter for a pre-shaped one, left and short gastric veins are successively entered and embolized with a mixture of 50% dextrose, absolute alcohol, Gelfoam, lyodura, and wire coils (Fig. 10.35). In acute bleeding, a cessation rate of 70% may be achieved, (Smith-Laing *et al.*, 1981); 66% of patients will re-bleed over the following 4 months, therefore additional therapy must be used

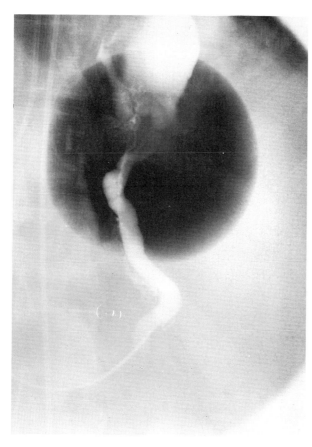

Fig. 10.34 Trans-hepatic portogram. Short gastric vein injection. There is a pool of contrast in the fundus above the inflated gastric balloon, due to active bleeding. Embolized.

in this 'breathing space', including oesophageal injection sclerotheraphy and surgical shunts. Emboli must not be allowed to reflux into the splenic or portal vein or thrombosis may supervene, both exacerbating the degree of portal hypertension and making a future surgical bypass impossible. Injudicious use of guide-wires may also damage the endothelium of a vein and make thrombosis more likely. Surprisingly, symptomatic pulmonary emboli are an uncommon complication of this therapeutic procedure (Pereiras, 1987).

Other methods

Embolization techniques include approaches to varices via the inferior vena cava and a spontaneous splenorenal shunt (Olson *et al.*, 1984), and embolizing both the splenic artery and left gastric vein (Del Guercio *et al.*, 1984). Recently the Japanese have approached varices from the ileocolic vein (Ido & Hiramatsu, 1985). Up to 10% of

patients will have a non-variceal cause for acute bleeding including oesophageal, gastric, and duodenal ulcers, erosions and small angiomata. Arterial embolization should be undertaken with Gelfoam and dura mater fragments, and is an attractive alternative to surgery. Hepatic artery embolization may also be used to cure haemobilia after liver biopsy or to occlude an arteriovenous fistula (either congenital or due to hepatoma) where it is contributing to the level of portal hypertension.

Great care must be taken in performing angiograms during acute bleeding. Many patients are poor risks in Child's grade 3 category, and prone to develop liver or renal failure. They may be restless and impossible to sedate with standard medication, particularly if the liver disease results from alcohol. Where possible it is helpful to have a member of the liver unit or an anaesthetist in attendance. Volumes of contrast medium used must be minimized.

The role of imaging during follow-up of treatment for portal hypertension

Barium studies

Following successful surgical transection or portasystemic shunt, varices disappear, though if the lumen had been previously dilated, or mucosa stretched by large veins, redundant folds may remain (Fig. 10.36).

A barium swallow may also be necessary when a patient develops dysphagia following a course of endoscopic injection sclerotherapy. Approximately 60% of such patients have a disorder of oesophageal motility due to a chemical oesophagitis, and some will develop a stricture disabling enough to merit balloon dilatation. The latter may also be useful after surgical transection. Despite a ring of metallic staples, dilatation achieves an excellent result (Fig. 10.37).

Chest radiography

The chest film plays an important role in the postoperative patient (collapse, effusion, infection), and during a course of endoscopic sclerotherapy. During the latter, pulmonary complications include pleural effusions, aspiration pneumonia, and mediastinitis. Frank oesophageal rupture is rare, but a close scrutiny for mediastinal air must be made in any patient who is febrile

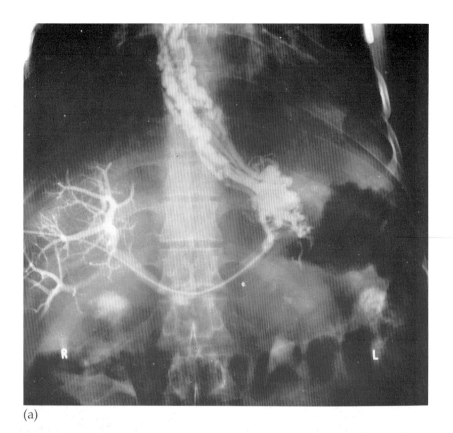

(a)

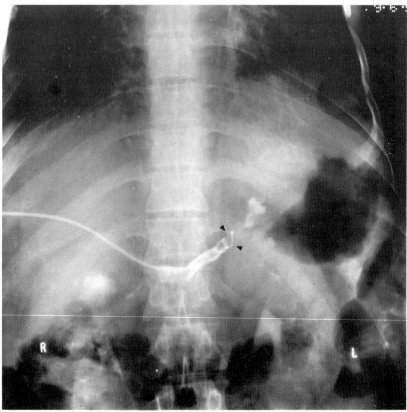

(b)

Fig. 10.35 Alcoholic with acute variceal bleeding. (a) Trans-hepatic portogram. Selective injection of left gastric vein demonstrates gastric and oesophageal varices. (b) After embolization with alcohol, Gelfoam and steel-wire coils.

and complains of searing chest pain after the procedure.

Tests for shunt patency

US, CT and angiography are all useful for showing the patency of a portasystemic shunt, though US may have difficulty with a shunt such as the meso-caval, where bowel intrudes between shunt and transducer. CT with enhancement if performed meticulously will usually demonstrate the site of a shunt, whether contrast is given as a fast intra-venous bolus or via a narrow-gauge needle in the splenic pulp (Fig. 10.38).

Angiography is used to show a long shunt such as a mesoatrial (Fig. 10.39), or when manometry is required. If the spleen remains, a post-shunt pressure measurement may be taken in its pulp with a fine needle. Alternatively, catheters may pass through the shunt from the systemic (caval) side to the portal, embolizing any residual varices (Fig. 10.40). A narrowing shunt may be dilated by balloon catheter (Potts *et al.*, 1984). Finally a shunt may be approached trans-hepatically. Re-bleeding after a shunt usually means closure, and angio-graphy is preferred to US or CT. Certainly bleeding from unusual sites such as ileostomy stomata is best imaged by angiography (Fig. 10.41).

Experimental

In those patients managed medically, progress is gauged by assessing changes in portal pressure (usually by hepatic vein catheter) after treatment with a beta-receptor blocker such as propranolol (Burroughs *et al.*, 1983).

Liver transplantation

Where successful, the operation will remove the

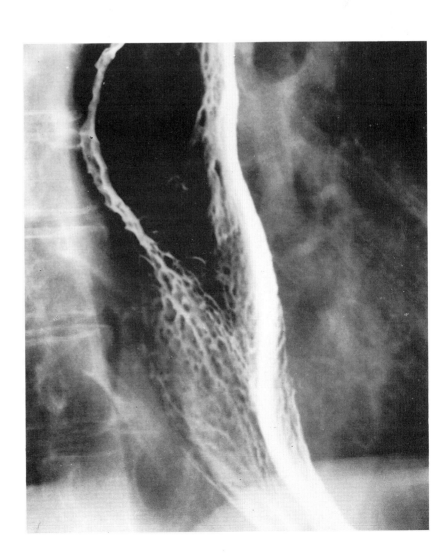

Fig. 10.36 Barium swallow after successful splenorenal surgical shunt. No varices are present (confirmed at endoscopy). Redundant mucosal folds remain over the site of previous large submucosal varices.

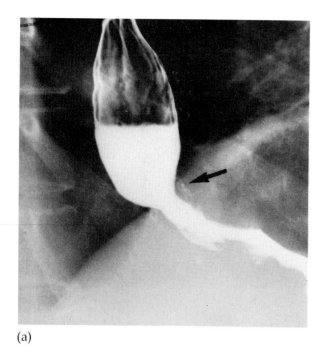

(a)

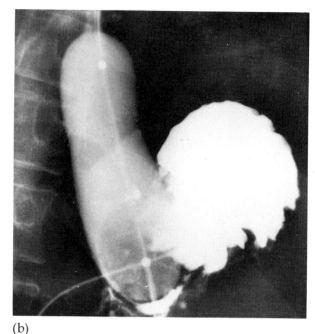

(b)

(c)

Fig. 10.37 Following surgical 'stapling' transection of the cardio-oesophageal junction, this patient's portal hypertension was treated, but a stricture developed after 6 months. (a) Barium swallow. Note fluid level in lower oesophagus above narrowed segment at staples (*arrowed*). (b) Balloon dilatation. (c) Swallow after dilatation. Immediate symptomatic relief.

portal hypertension and its underlying liver disease immediately. The appropriate imaging for patient work-up and for any complications is discussed in Chapter 17.

Summary

Portal hypertension is usually a progressive disease. Whether it is suspected or established, imaging plays a paramount role, and the radiologist is a vital member of the management team.

Non-invasive methods now provide significant information. In those requiring angiography, the investigation must be timed to allow deficient clotting to be remedied as fully at possible, and be performed with the knowledge that the most patients are at risk if underlying hepatocellular failure is present. Figure 10.42 is a flow chart summarizing the role of imaging in portal hypertension and based on the discussion in this chapter.

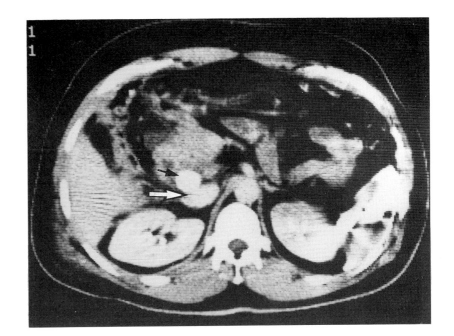

Fig. 10.38 CT during injection of 10 ml dilute contrast into splenic pulp through a French gauge 23 needle. Patent mesocaval shunt demonstrated (*small arrow*, superior mesenteric vein; *large arrow*, inferior vena cava).

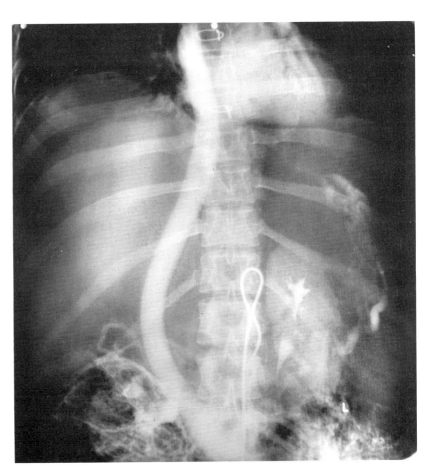

Fig. 10.39 Venous phase of superior mesenteric angiogram. Contrast outlines long prosthetic graft in anterior abdominal wall connecting superior mesenteric vein to right atrium. Female, 24 years old, with Budd–Chiari syndrome. Shunt patent at 3 years.

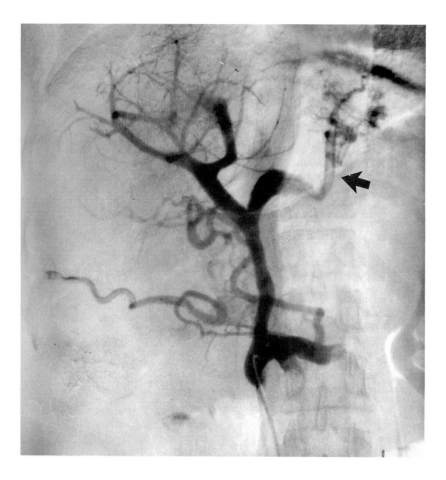

Fig. 10.40 Subtraction venous angiogram. Catheter has passed from the inferior vena cava through a patent portacaval shunt. Filling defects in left gastric vein are due to previous trans-hepatic embolization (*arrow*). Should the surgical shunt stenose, balloon dilatation is an attractive option.

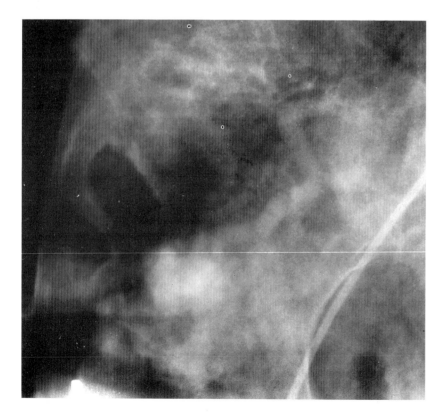

Fig. 10.41 Venous-phase superior mesenteric angiogram in patient with previous colectomy for ulcerative colitis. Portal hypertension resulted from complicating liver disease, and profuse bleeding from ileostomy occurred. Angiogram shows dilated varix above ileostomy and contrast extravasation at soma. Study indicated that a simple surgical procedure to the varix was the best treatment option.

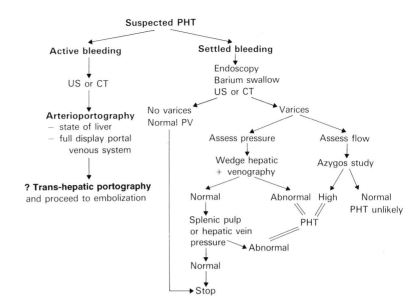

Fig. 10.42 Imaging in suspected portal hypertension (PHT).

References

Abeatici, S. & Campi, L. (1951) La vissualizzaxione radiologica della porta via splenica. *Minerva Medica*, **42**, 593–605.

Bellamy, E.A., Bossi, M.C.C. & Cosgrove, D.O. (1984) Grey-scale ultrasonography of portal vein. *Lancet*, **ii**, 675–677.

Bookstein, J.J., Appleman, H.D., Walter, J.F., Foley, W.D., Turcotte, J.G. & Lambert, M. (1975) Histological venographic correlates in portal hypertension. *Radiology*, **116**, 565–573.

Bosch, J. & Grossman, R.J. (1984) Measurement of azygos venous blood flow by a continuous thermal dilution technique: an index of blood flow through gastro-oesophageal collaterals in cirrhosis. *Hepatology*, **4**, 424–429.

Burroughs, A.K., Jenkins, W.J., Sherlock, S., Dunk, A., Walt, R.P., Osuafor, T.O., Mackie, S. & Dick, R. (1983) Controlled trial of propanolol for the prevention of recurrent variceal hemorrhage in patients with cirrhosis. *New England Journal of Medicine*, **309**, 1539–1542.

Del Guercio, L.R., Hodgson, W.J., Morgan, J.C., Berman, H.L. & Kinkhabwalla, M.N. (1984) Splenic artery and coronary vein occlusion for bleeding esophageal varices. *World Journal of Surgery*, **8**, 680–687.

Dick, R. (1983) The portal and hepatic venous system. In Whitehouse, B.H. & Worthington, G.S. (eds) *Techniques in Diagnostic Radiology*, pp. 165–170. Blackwell Scientific Publications, Oxford.

Dick, R. (1984) Investigation of oesophageal varices. In Watson, R. & Celestin, R.D. (eds) *Disorders of the Oesophagus*, pp. 230–256. Pitman, London.

Dooley, J.S. & Dick, R. (1987) Suspected portal hypertension. In Dooley, J.S., Dick, R., Viamonte, M. Jr. & Sherlock, S. (eds) *Imaging in Hepatobiliary Diseases*, pp. 147–172 Blackwell Scientific Publications, Oxford.

Ghahremani, G.G., Port, R.B., Winans, C.S. & Williams, J.R.

(1972) Esophageal varices. Enhanced radiologic visualisation by anticholingeric drugs. *American Journal of Digestive Diseases*, **17**, 703–712.

Hawkey, C.I., Amar, S.S., Daintith, H.A.M. & Toghill, P.J. (1985) Familial varices of the colon occurring without evidence of portal hypertension. *British Journal of Radiology*, **58**, 677–679.

Hunter, T.B. (1983) Nontraumatic diseases of spleen, pp. 221–229. In Serafini, A.N. & Cutter, M. (eds) *Medical Imaging of the liver and spleen*, pp. 221–229. Appleton Century Crofts, Connecticut.

Ido, K. & Hiramatsu, K. (1985) Transileocolic obliteration of the gastroesophageal varices. *Nichidoku-iho*, **30**, 155–163.

Khosla, S.N., Passi, R.K. & Mishra, D.S. (1984) A comparative study of endoscopic and radiological evaluation of oesophageal varices in portal hypertension. *Journal of the Association of Physicians of India*, **32**, 331–333.

Lunderquist, A. & Vang, J. (1974) Transhepatic catheterisation and obliteration of coronary vein in patients with portal hypertension and esophageal varices. *New England Journal of Medicine*, **29**, 646–649.

MacDougall, B.R.D. & Williams, R. (1983) A controlled clinical trial of cimetidine in the recurrence of variceal hemorrhage: implications about the pathogenesis of hemorrhage. *Hepatology*, **3**, 69–73.

McIndoe, A.H. (1928) *Archives of Pathology*, 5, 23.

McCormack, T., Martin, T., Smallwood, R.H., Robinson, P., Walton, L. & Johnson, A.G. (1983) Doppler ultrasound probe for assessment of blood flow in oesophageal varices. *Lancet*, **1**, 677–678.

Mathieu, D., Vasile, N. & Grenier, P. (1985) Portal thrombosis: dynamic CT features and course. *Radiology*, **154**, 737–741.

Olson, E., Yune, H.Y. & Klatte, E.C. (1984) Transrenal-vein reflux ethanol sclerosis of gastroesophageal varices. *American Journal of Radiology*, **143**, 627–628.

Pereiras, R., (1987) In Dooley, J.S., Dick, R., Viamonte, M.,

Jr. & Sherlock, S. *Imaging in Hepatobiliary Diseases*, pp. 206–229. Blackwell Scientific Publications, Oxford.

Potts, J.R., Henderson, J.M., Millikan, W.J. Jr., Sones, P. & Warren, W.D. (1984) Restoration of portal venous perfusion and reversal of encephalopathy by balloon occlusion of portal systemic shunt. *Gastroenterology*, **87**, 208–212.

Rappaport, A.M. (1951) Hepatic venography. *Acta Radiologica*, **36**, 165–71.

Reinig, J.W., Sanchez, F.W. & Vujic, I. (1985) Hemodynamics of portal blood flow shown by C.T. portography. *Radiology*, **154**, 473–476.

Rose, J.D.R., Crane, M.D. & Smith, P.M. (1983) Factors affecting successful endoscopic sclerotherapy for oesophageal varices. *Gut*, **24**, 946–949.

Sherlock, S. (1985) *Disease of Liver and Biliary System*, pp. 135. Blackwell, Oxford.

Smith-Laing, G., Camilo, M.E., Dick, R. & Sherlock, S. (1980). Percutaneous transhepatic portography in the assessment of portal hypertension. *Gastroenterology*, **78**, 197–205.

Smith-Laing, G., Scott, J., Long, R.G., Dick, R. & Sherlock, S. (1981) Role of percutaneous transhepatic obliteration of varices in the management of haemorrhage from gastroesophageal varices. *Gastroenterology*, **80**, 1031–1036.

Taguchi, H., Horiguchi, Y. & Kitano, T. (1983). The case of intrahepatic portosystemic shunt. *Japanese Journal of Medical Ultrasonics*, **43**, 71–72.

Terblanche, J., Yakoob, H.I., Bornamn, P.C., Stiegmann, G.V., Bane, R., Jonker, M., Wright, J. & Kirsch, R. (1981) Acute bleeding varices: a 5 year prospective evaluation of tamponde and sclerotherapy. *Annals of Surgery*, **194**, 521–530.

Van Gansbeke, D., Avni, E.F., Delcour, C., Engelholm, L. & Struyven, J. (1985) Sonographic features of portal vein thrombosis. *American Journal of Radiology*, **144**, 749–752.

Waldram, R., Nunnerley, H., Davis, M., Laws, J.W. & Williams, J.R. (1977) Detection and grading of oesophageal varices by fibreoptic endoscopy and barium swallow with and without Buscopan. *Clinical Radiology*, **28**, 137–141.

Webb, L.J., Berger, L.A. & Sherlock, S. (1977) Grey-scale ultrasonography of portal vein. Lancet, **ii**, 675–677.

Westaby, D., Macdougall, B.R.D., Saunders, J.B. & Williams, R. (1982) A study of risk factors in patients with cirrhosis and variceal bleeding. In Westaby, D., Macdougall, B.R.D. & Williams, R. (eds) *Variceal Bleeding*, pp. 36–41. Pitman, London.

Williams, K.G.D. & Dawson, J.L. (1979) Fibreoptic injection of oesophageal varices. *British Medical Journal*, **2**, 766–767.

Zamir, O., Mogle, P., Lernau, O. & Nissan, S. (1984) Splenoportography — a reappraisal. *American Journal of Gastroenterology*, **79**, 283–286.

11: Cystic and Infective Disease of the Liver

L.A. BERGER

Introduction

Before the advent of ultrasound, computerized tomography, and more recently magnetic resonance imaging, radiology played a minor role in the diagnosis and management of infective and cystic disease of the liver. The demonstration of calcium or gas on a plain X-ray, of a filling defect on an isotope scan, or of a mass by invasive procedures such as angiography and to a lesser extent percutaneous cholangiography were the major means of preoperative diagnosis in combination with various immunological tests. At that time clinical history and the physical examination were of paramount importance in interpreting the results of these examinations. Despite the ease and elegance with which modern imaging techniques can detect and display disease, this remains as true today as it did then.

In many instances images obtained at scanning are non-specific and can only be interpreted in the light of the clinical situation. Furthermore, unless the radiologist is aware of the diagnostic possibilities he may not look hard enough for the subtle changes that may clarify the nature of a particular lesion, nor look for evidence of disease in other organs when relevant. It is this knowledge of clinical medicine that distinguishes a radiologist from a good radiographer or other technician. There is no substitute for the combination of skillful scanning and interpretation of the images produced, in combination with clinical acumen. The practice of reviewing a series of images produced by a technician cannot be recommended. No apology is therefore necessary for the rather detailed introduction to each section. A thorough understanding of the way in which a disease develops is essential for the correct evaluation of the various tests used to image it.

Throughout the chapter the appearances on ultrasound and CT scanning have been emphasized, as these are now the major means by which infective and cystic disease is demonstrated. Little attention has been paid to the more invasive methods, as these have largely been abandoned. The plain film changes have been described in some detail as a plain film is frequently ordered early on in the patient's management. Although a plain film is frequently normal, on occasions it may provide the diagnosis.

Because ultrasound can resolve small tissue differences better than CT, there are more features to look for and describe. The larger sections devoted to ultrasound compared to CT should not be taken as reflection of personal bias. Both techniques give excellent results in experienced hands. Ultrasound should be the first means by which a patient is examined, as it is more frequently available and cheaper, but it is often helpful to follow it with a CT scan, which may give complementary information.

Although it is not the purpose of this chapter to describe in detail the proper conduct of an ultrasound or CT examination, several points need to be emphasized. When examining an ill patient with a tender liver it is frequently helpful to scan in the left lateral decubitus position. Subcostal and intercostal approaches should be tried and on occasions an erect scan may show areas not visible by other means. It is important to adjust the gain so that the features of any lesion are seen well. Insufficient attenuation is a common cause of loss of vital detail. Once a lesion has been identified it should be scanned in many planes to assess it fully. The flexibility of ultrasound is a great advantage in this respect.

A CT examination is best carried out under the supervision of a radiologist. Injection of contrast is important, as small lesions may be seen that were not visible on the unenhanced scan. The use of the left lateral decubitus position will occasionally clarify difficult areas.

At the Royal Free Hospital, 8 mm slices are used and we inject between 50 and 100 ml of contrast, depending on the circumstances.

Liver cysts

Liver cysts are developmental in origin. They occur twice as frequently in the right lobe as in the left and are unilocular in 95% of cases. They affect women five times as frequently as men and present in middle-age. They may be quite large: a cyst of over 500 ml is not infrequent. Although liver cysts have been found in 0.5% of people at autopsy, their incidence is probably greater and incidental asymptomatic cysts are not uncommonly detected during an ultrasound or CT examination (Taylor & Viscomi, 1980).

Liver cysts are irregularly ovoid in shape and have clearly defined, thin walls. They contain clear, colourless fluid and are therefore completely transonic. There is strong acoustic enhancement posteriorly (Fig. 11.1). Uncommonly, a cyst may exhibit internal septa and raise the suspicion of hydatid disease (Fig. 11.2). In a small number of cysts the contents will be mucoid, purulent, bile-stained, or bloody. The cyst will then appear speckled due to the presence of many fine linear echoes. Posterior enhancement will be less marked (Figs 11.3, 11.4). Approximately 98% of liver cysts greater than 1.5 cm in diameter will be detected by ultrasound or CT. Cysts smaller than this are also frequently shown.

The characteristics of a liver cyst on a CT scan are similar to those seen on ultrasound. A mass of water density (0 ± 15 HU) is seen with well-defined walls that do not enhance. Should haemorrhage or infection occur then a fluid/fluid level may be seen within the cyst.

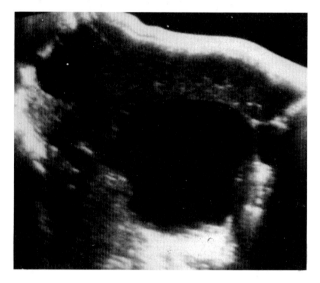

Fig. 11.1 A longitudinal scan showing two cysts in the right lobe. The typical irregularly ovoid shape, absence of internal echoes, and posterior enhancement are well seen.

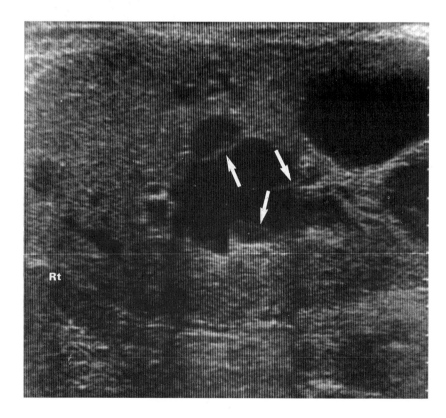

Fig. 11.2 A transverse scan showing two cysts. Septa (*arrowed*) are occasionally seen in simple cysts. Although this is not the typical appearance of a hydatid cyst, hydatid disease should be excluded before attempting aspiration.

Most cysts are silent. They may cause discomfort when large and become painful when internal haemorrhage or secondary infection has developed (Fig. 11.5). Obstructive jaundice due to compression of the biliary tree by a cyst near the porta

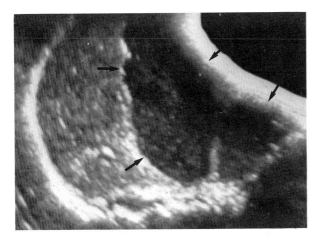

Fig. 11.3 A longitudinal scan. A large cyst occupies the lower half of the liver. It contains clear mucus and appears speckled. Posterior enhancement is not marked.

hepatis is another rare complication, as is rupture into the peritoneal cavity.

A cyst will appear as a filling defect on a radio-nuclide scan, but may not be detected if it lies peripherally. As this may be the first investigation in a patient in whom a mass is suspected in the liver, determination of its exact nature will require an ultrasound or a CT scan. On occasion an incidental cyst will be detected by arteriography. In such cases it will appear as an avascular mass which displaces and stretches vessels locally.

An intrahepatic gall bladder can mimic a liver cyst, but scans in different planes will make this diagnosis obvious. Differentiation of a simple cyst from a hydatid cyst is important, especially when aspiration is being contemplated. At times this distinction cannot be made on ultrasound or CT appearances alone. A solitary uncomplicated hydatid cyst may be indistinguishable from a simple cyst, though in the author's experience this is not common in patients seen in the UK. A hydatid complement-fixation test or one of the immuno-serological tests for hydatid disease should there-

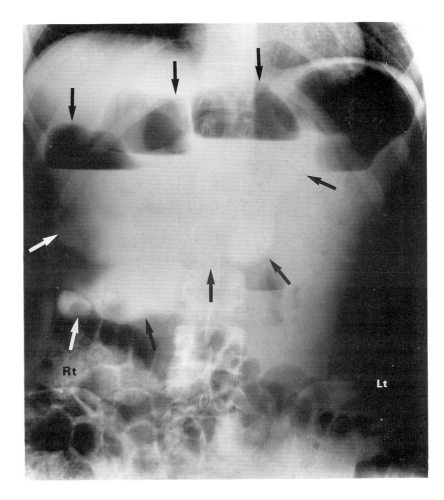

Fig. 11.4 Same patient as in Fig. 11.3. After a diagnostic aspiration, contrast and air were injected into one of the locules. The extent of the multilocular cyst is well shown on this erect abdominal X-ray (*arrows*).

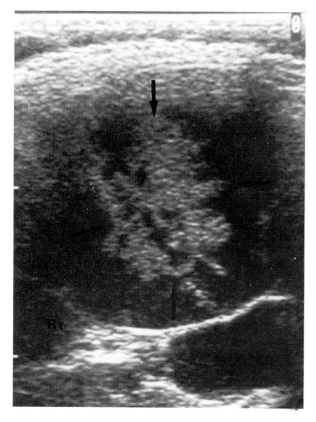

Fig. 11.5 Haemorrhage into a cyst. The irregular echogenic mass (*arrows*) is clotted blood.

fore be performed in a patient from an area where hydatid disease is endemic, though these may be negative in an asymptomatic patient.

Less than 5% of liver metastases are truly cystic, as a result of necrosis or the secretion of mucus, and they may appear identical to a simple cyst at first glance. However, a careful examination may detect localized wall thickening, mural nodules, or septa in many of these 'cysts' and suggest their true nature. In these patients it is important to examine the rest of the liver thoroughly. Space-occupying lesions that are not cystic may be seen, as the appearance of metastases may vary quite considerably in the same patient. The site of origin of cystic metastases is very variable though secondary sarcomas appear to have a greater propensity to become cystic than secondary carcinomas. Although a CT scan is unlikely to provide more detail, as ultrasound is usually more sensitive in the detection of septa, mural nodules and wall thickening, CT may clarify the diagnosis by showing secondaries not seen by ultrasound. The opposite is also the case, and it is unwise to rely only on a CT diagnosis of a solitary simple cyst in a

patient with suspected malignancy. In the end a final diagnosis may depend upon aspiration and cytological examination of the cyst fluid, and this should always be performed in cases of doubt.

Three primary tumours, the biliary cystadenoma, the biliary cystadenocarcinoma and the mesenchymal hamartoma of childhood may present as solitary large cysts, though a mass of small cysts with internal echoes due to trabecula and septa is more common. Wall thickening and mural nodules may also be present. All three are rare (Federle *et al.*, 1981).

There have been reports that primary liver cell cancer may manifest as a solitary cystic lesion. The author has never encountered this in a large experience of this tumour.

Mature liver abscesses containing very thin pus can mimic a cyst, though their walls are usually thicker and irregular and they are less sonolucent than a cyst of comparable size. Moreover, the patient is usually febrile and ill and the liver is tender. Whenever an abscess is suspected, aspiration and bacteriological examination of the contents should be performed. When this is not possible a positive gallium scan is diagnostic of a liver abscess. A CT scan may be helpful in showing small abscesses that have been overlooked at ultrasound.

Haematomas of the liver share some of the characteristics of a liver cyst but the history of antecedent trauma, most commonly liver biopsy, the irregularity of outline, and the relatively poor wall definition and sound transmission makes it easy to differentiate them from simple cysts (Fig. 11.6).

Most liver cysts cause no symptoms and require no treatment. In any case most cysts reaccumulate within weeks or months after aspiration. When the diagnosis is in doubt, for example in a patient with known or suspected cancer or when an abscess is a possibility, aspiration under local anaesthetic is mandatory, as a misdiagnosis could have profound therapeutic consequences (Fig. 11.7).

On the rare occasion when a cyst is painful as a result of internal haemorrhage, needle aspiration will give relief. The technique of needle aspiration is described later in this chapter in the section on liver abscesses.

Polycystic liver disease

This rare condition affects females four times as often as males and is a member of the family of

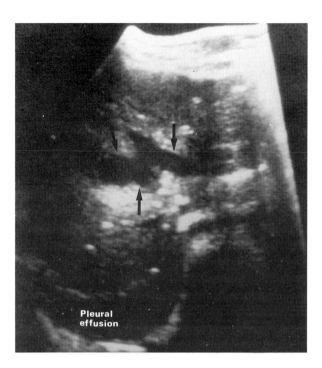

Fig. 11.6 A transverse scan of an anechoic mass with posterior enhancement in the right lobe (*arrows*). Its shape suggests a haematoma secondary to a tear in the liver. Note the pleural effusion. The patient had jumped from a third-floor window.

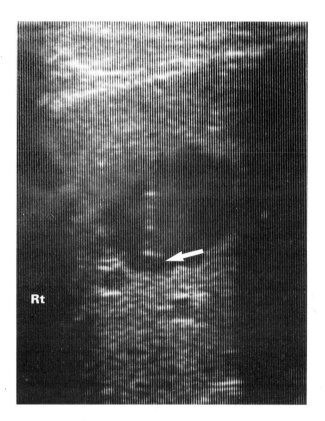

Fig. 11.7 Needle aspiration of a cyst. The needle tip (*arrow*) lies just short of the distal wall. The cyst was emptied, and proved to be simple.

hepatobiliary fibropolycystic diseases. Other members, commonly congenital hepatic fibrosis or Caroli's disease, may be present in patients with polycystic liver disease (Summerfield *et al.*, 1986). The disease is hereditary, but the mode of inheritance is uncertain. The liver is usually enlarged and cysts varying from less than 1 mm to over 12 cm in diameter are present throughout (Fig. 11.8). They contain clear brown fluid unless there has been internal haemorrhage. In 50% of cases the kidneys are involved, and the pancreas, spleen, and lungs may infrequently be similarly affected. Intracranial aneurysms occur with increased frequency. As liver function is not compromised by the cysts the long-term prognosis depends on the degree of renal involvement. Patients rarely present before the fourth decade. Pain and abdominal distension are the usual complaints and this can be relieved by aspirating the largest of the cysts. Unfortunately a symptomatic cyst may refill and cause pain, necessitating further aspiration (Fig. 11.9). At present there is no safe and reliable sclerosing agent available, though absolute alcohol may be effective in some cysts.

On ultrasound the larger cysts exhibit the typical

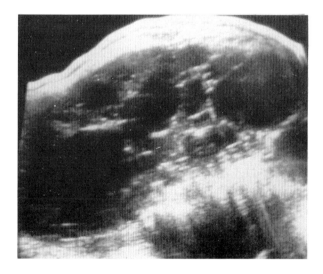

Fig. 11.8 A transverse scan of a liver full of cysts.

features associated with a cyst, but acoustic enhancement may not be present behind smaller cysts. Furthermore, because of the large number of cysts in close proximity to one another, many are compressed into various geometric shapes.

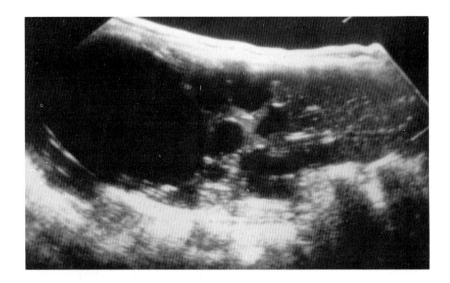

Fig. 11.9 A longitudinal scan of the right lobe. The largest cyst was painful. Aspiration gave relief, but the cyst recurred and required further aspiration.

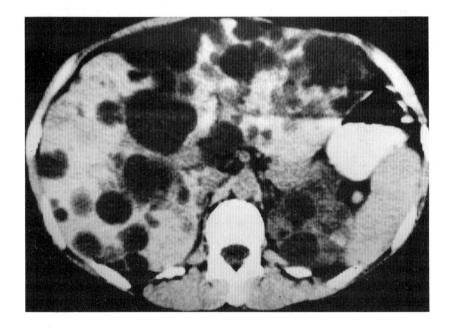

Fig. 11.10 A CT scan of the abdomen showing many liver cysts. Note the cysts in the left kidney.

A CT scan will demonstrate this disease well. The cysts have smooth contours and discrete interfaces (Fig. 11.10). The attenuation value of the cyst fluid lies between −5 to + 20 HU. Although the cysts do not enhance they are easier to see after contrast because of opacification of the surrounding parenchyma and blood vessels (Levine *et al.*, 1985).

A cholangiocarcinoma or a squamous cell carcinoma may very rarely develop in such cysts. The author has seen the latter once. The presence of irregular, solid elements between the cysts suggested the diagnosis. Rupture, haemorrhage, portal hypertension with varices, and jaundice are other rare complications.

Traumatic cysts

These are very rare. They are false cysts and are lined by fibrous tissue rather than by epithelial tissue. They appear identical to developmental cysts in all other ways.

Hydatid cysts

World-wide, the most frequent liver cyst is the hydatid cyst. It occurs predominantly in sheep-raising countries when sheep-dogs are used. Greece, the Middle-East, North America and the Antipodes have a high incidence of the disease, but because of freedom of travel and migration, the disease can present anywhere in the world. Two species of the parasitic tapeworm Echinococcus cause the vast majority of cases. *Echinococcus granulosus* is the more widespread and the dog is the definitive host. The 5-mm long worm lives in the host's small intestine without harming it. There it grows and produces eggs which pass into the dog's faeces. The eggs are then ingested as a contaminant by the intermediate host — cattle, pigs, sheep, camels and humans, usually children. The outer shells of the eggs are digested by the gastric juices and the embryos penetrate the duodenal wall to enter the portal circulation. There they lodge in small capillaries where they either die or develop into hydatid cysts. The liver traps 60%, and 20% of the remainder are trapped by the lungs. The brain is another common extrahepatic site, but almost any organ can be involved.

The wall of the growing cyst consists of an inner germinal layer (the active layer that forms daughter cysts and brood capsules) surrounded by an inert, laminated membrane. The host walls the cyst off by forming a fibrous adventitial capsule, the ectocyst. With time this may become quite thick, and calcify. The laminated membrane, as a result of infection or mechanical shearing forces, can fragment, detach itself from the adventitia and collapse into the cyst fluid.

Eighty to eighty-five per cent of hepatic hydatid cysts are found in the right lobe, and are single in 70% of patients. The cysts grow very slowly (approximately 1 cm in diameter per year) and symptoms rarely occur before a cyst is 10 cm in diameter. Many patients remain asymptomatic even though a cyst is over 20 cm in diameter and clinically palpable. The average age at the time of presentation is 35 years and the symptoms are usually vague abdominal pain. More severe symptoms are usually due to complications, of which the most common is rupture secondary to the high pressure within the cyst. Rupture is usually into the biliary tree, causing jaundice and biliary colic; the peritoneal cavity, causing severe pain and anaphylactoid shock; or the pleural cavity, lung or bronchi. Rupture into the pericardium, duodenum, colon, right renal pelvis and inferior vena cava have been reported. Seven per cent of hydatid cysts develop near the porta hepatis and compress the biliary tree, resulting in jaundice. Secondary infection from a surrounding area of cholangitis or septicaemia will result in abscess formation and death of the parasite.

Diagnosis

Although ultrasound and CT are the best investigations to diagnose hepatic hydatid disease, a plain abdominal radiograph is useful as calcification is present in over 10% of symptomatic cysts. Early on this is semicircular and confined to the periphery (see Fig. 11.29) and is indistinguishable from the calcification that rarely develops in a pyogenic or amoebic abscess or a developmental cyst.

Later the calcification becomes dense and circumferential, with foci of amorphous calcification within the cyst itself (Fig. 11.11). Calcified daughter cysts when present are diagnostic as is the presence of the 'water-lily' sign. This sign develops on the rare occasions in which gas forms in a cyst and strips the laminated membrane off the adventia so that it floats on the cyst fluid.

The variety of appearances seen on an ultrasound scan depend on the stage of evolution of the disease and the presence of the complications described. An uncomplicated cyst has a rounded outline with clear-cut walls and may be undistinguishable from a simple cyst. They may even reach a large size. In some countries this is said to be the commonest appearance of a hydatid cyst. In the author's own experience of patients from the UK, Greece, and the Middle East, tell-tale signs such as localized wall thickening, subtle sagging of the laminated membrane and mural nodules are usually present and suggest the true nature of the cyst (Fig. 11.12). The mural nodules are 2−3 mm in diameter and are the brood capsules, local invaginations of the germinal layer that enlarge to form daughter cysts (Itzchak *et al.*, 1980).

A heavily infested patient may develop multiple 'simple' cysts. As multiple developmental cysts are uncommon these should be considered hydatid in origin until proved otherwise . Occasionally multiple cystic metastases can give a similar appearance. Any patient who comes from an area where hydatid disease is endemic, with one or more 'simple' cysts should have a hydatid complement-fixation test, or one of the other hydatid immunodiagnostic tests. These have an accuracy of over 90%.

In a small number of patients the brood capsules will detach themselves from the wall and form a layer of hydatid 'sand' at the bottom of the cyst. This will manifest on ultrasound as a layer of fine echoes posteriorly.

More often daughter cysts appear as the cyst

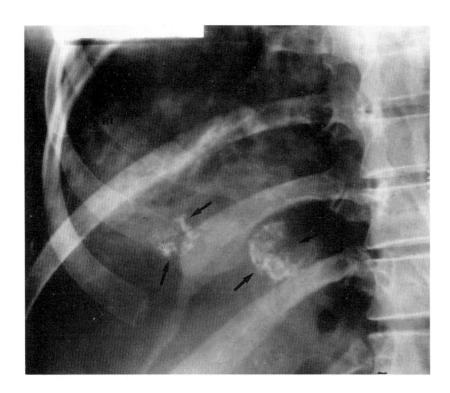

Fig. 11.11 A plain X-ray of two calcified hydatid cysts. Calcification is present in the cyst wall and amorphous calcification is seen within the cyst. The rib abnormality indicates previous hydatid surgery.

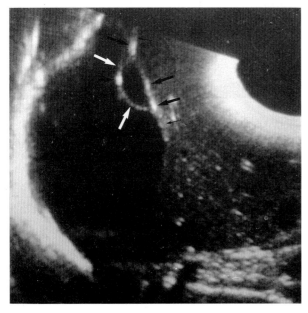

Fig. 11.12 A longitudinal scan of the right lobe showing a large cyst. Localized wall thickening (*thin arrows*) mural nodules (*thick arrows*) and sagging of the laminated membrane (*white arrows*) were apparent on only a few sections. The features are diagnostic of hydatid disease.

continues to develop. They are pathognomonic of the disease and are seen as small round cysts within the mother cyst. As they continue to grow they will only retain their rounded shape when the parent cyst enlarges to accommodate them. Such a

cyst will appear multiloculated or 'honeycomb' in appearance. If on the other hand the surrounding liver parenchyma restrains the further growth of the parent cyst, then the daughter cysts compress and distort each other and the parent cyst appears septated. This appearance can be confused with the appearance of a biliary cystadenoma or a secondary deposit from an ovarian cystadenocarcinoma.

Another pathognomonic sign is infolding of the detached laminated membrane, forming bizarre polycyclic septations in the mother cyst (Figs 11.13, 11.14) or even complete detachment of the membrane giving rise to an ultrasonic 'water-lily' sign. As the daughter cysts continue to grow they will eventually compress the detached membrane into the centre of the cyst and surround it — the 'rosette' pattern (Fig. 11.15).

Calcification may be seen in the wall of a hydatid cyst as fine curvilinear areas of high echogenicity (Fig. 11.16). Cysts that are heavily calcified appear as an echogenic arc with strong acoustic shadowing and are difficult to image by ultrasound. However a plain X-ray or a CT scan will establish the diagnosis in such cases.

The appearance of a hydatid cyst on CT are similar to those seen on ultrasound (Kalovidouris *et al.*, 1986, Pandolfo *et al.*, 1984). Rounded or ovoid cysts of water density are seen which, when less than 3 cm in diameter are indistinguishable

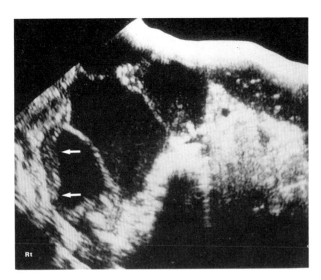

Fig. 11.13 A transverse scan of the liver. Many large cysts compress and distort each other, causing a septate appearance. Infolding of the laminated membrane (*arrows*) is a tell-tale sign of hydatid disease.

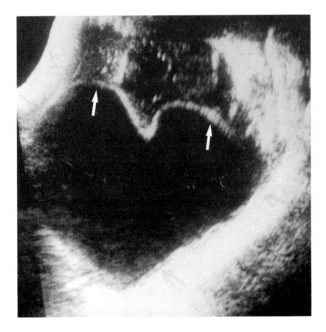

Fig. 11.14 A longitudinal scan of a cyst in the right lobe. The laminated membrane has detached itself from the superior wall (*arrows*). Daughter cysts and debris are present.

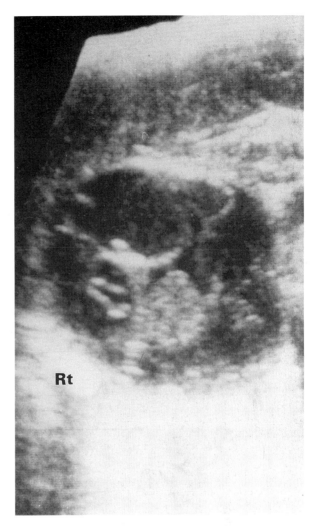

Fig. 11.15 A hydatid cyst exhibiting the rosette pattern. In the centre the infolded laminated membrane appears as a polycyclic septum. It is surrounded by daughter cysts and debris.

from simple cysts, secondaries, or abscesses (Fig. 11.17). Most patients, however, exhibit one or more of the specific signs of hydatid disease.

Calcification of the ectocyst, laminated membrane or daughter cysts is diagnostic and suggests death of the parasite (Fig. 11.18). CT is much more sensitive than plain X-rays at detecting small amounts of calcification, provided that thin contiguous slices are obtained.

The presence of uncalcified daughter cysts is pathognomonic and implies a living cyst. Early on these daughter cysts are small and confined to the periphery of the mother cyst (Fig. 11.19). As they enlarge they occupy the bulk of the cyst and compress each other, appearing irregular or polygonal in outline (Fig. 11.20). They may remain attached to the wall by means of a broad base or by a stalk, or lie free in the cyst fluid. As the cyst becomes more complex the density of the mother and daughter cysts increases.

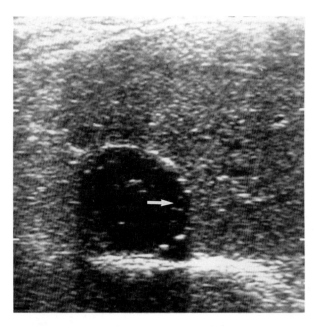

Fig. 11.16 A hydatid cyst with curvilinear calcification in the wall. A small daughter cyst is seen (*arrow*).

Detachment of the laminated membrane is another pathognomonic sign and occurs when the cyst dies (Figs 11.21, 11.22).

Because of the partial volume effect CT is not as sensitive as ultrasound at detecting subtle degrees of detachment.

Complications

Infection

Acute secondary infection should be suspected when a hydatid cyst becomes tender and the patient becomes febrile. On the other hand, a chronically infected cyst may be asymptomatic and appear as a solid mass with a heterogenous internal echo pattern on ultrasound. In the absence of a history, such an abscess may be treated by percutaneous aspiration. A limited experience suggests that this is not harmful because the parasite has usually been killed by the secondary infection. Recent reports suggest that this appearance may occasionally be seen in uninfected cysts also. When hydatid disease is a possibility it should be excluded by laboratory methods before needle aspiration.

When an infected hydatid cyst is suspected a CT scan will frequently confirm the diagnosis. The density of the hydatid fluid will be higher than usual because of the presence of pus; gas may also be present and there will be oedema of the surrounding parenchyma. Contrast will enhance the cyst wall.

Rupture of a cyst

Rupture into the biliary tree causes painful jaundice. Several case reports of ultrasound scans in

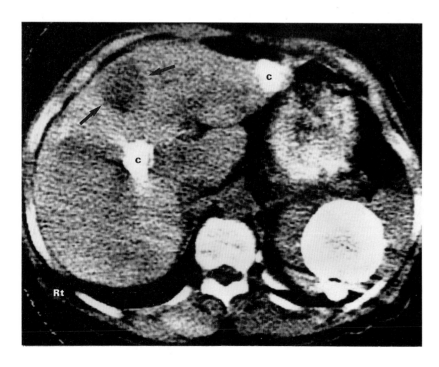

Fig. 11.17 CT scan of the liver showing a 'simple' cyst in the right lobe. Two densely calcified cysts (c) in the liver and a large calcified cyst in the spleen indicate the true diagnosis.

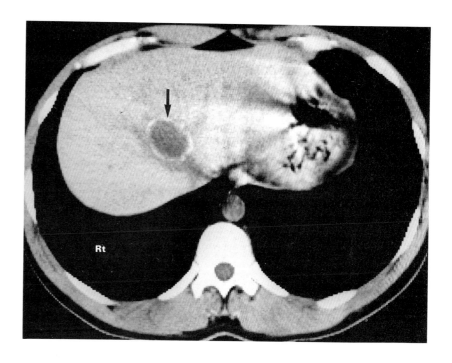

Fig. 11.18 CT scan showing calcification of the ectocyst.

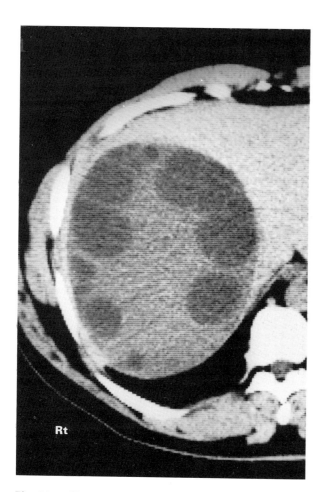

Fig. 11.19 CT scan of a hydatid cyst. The daughter cysts lie in the periphery.

such patients have been published. Dilated intrahepatic and extrahepatic ducts were found communicating directly with the cyst. Filling defects due to scolices (the heads of the tapeworms) were seen in the bile ducts as irregular fine echoes, and daughter cysts were apparent in one patient.

The diagnosis can also be made by CT; five cases were reported by Choliz *et al.* (1982). They found dilated ducts adjacent to a hydatid cyst.

These findings can be confirmed best by a PTC or an ERCP examination (Ertan *et al.*, 1983).

Intraperitoneal dissemination is diagnosed when multiple cysts are present in the peritoneal cavity and the parent cyst is seen on the liver surface, and rupture into the pleural cavity when a cyst is seen in close apposition to the diaphragm and the diaphragm exhibits local irregularity of thickness and outline. A pleural effusion will frequently be present.

Appearances during treatment

The treatment of most hydatid cysts is surgical because the risk of complications is high, and at times fatal. There are, however, a group of patients who are not amenable to surgery. Patients with recurrent disease or polycystic disease are often treated by mebendazole or albendazole, and ultrasound scanning is a useful way to monitor progress. Bezzi *et al.* (1987) followed 141 abdominal

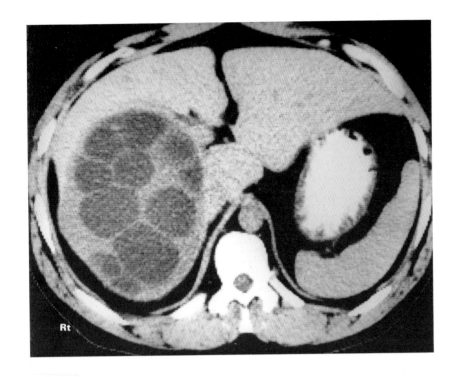

Fig. 11.20 CT scan. The daughter cysts occupy most of the mother cyst. Those in the centre appear polypoid in outline.

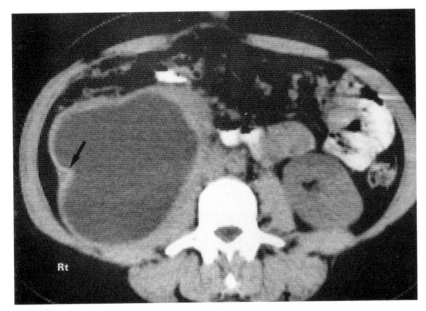

Fig. 11.21 CT scan of a hydatid cyst showing early detachment of the laminated membrane.

hydatid cysts (108 in the liver) in 63 patients treated by these drugs. Forty per cent remained unaltered. Where change occurred there were three patterns.

1 Thirty per cent of cysts shrank and became less rounded, indicating a decrease of intracyst pressure. Ten per cent disappeared completely. This pattern was seen more often in cysts that did not have daughter cysts.

2 In 25% the laminated membrane became detached (Fig. 11.23a). This varied from a split-wall appearance to a true ultrasound 'water-lily' sign. A few became partially calcified.

3 In 30% the cyst became filled by uniform, amorphous, echogenic material (Fig. 11.23b), and some eventually appeared solid (Fig. 11.24). This pattern was mostly seen in cysts that had daughter cysts.

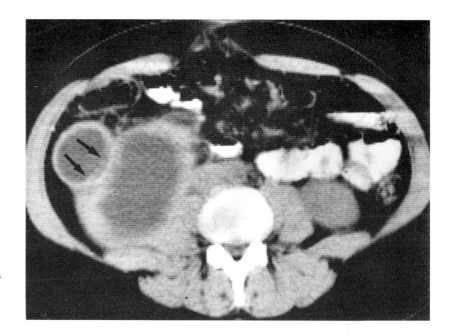

Fig. 11.22 CT scan of two hydatid cysts. The laminated membrane is seen separated from the wall (*arrows*). The wall of the larger cyst is unsharp, suggesting impending detachment of the laminated membrane.

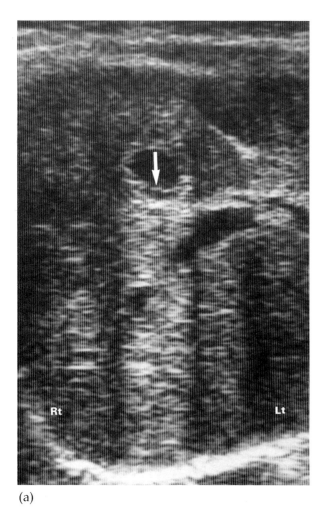

(a)

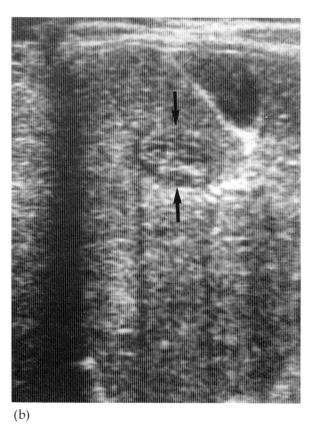

(b)

Fig. 11.23 (a) A transverse scan. The laminated membrane has detached itself from the wall. This cyst appeared simple before treatment was instituted some 2 months before. (b) A transverse scan 4 months later. The cyst is filled by amorphous echogenic material.

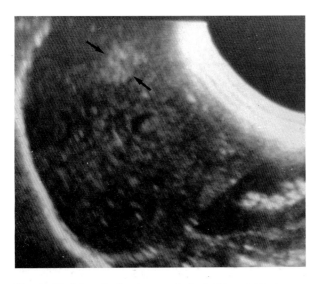

Fig. 11.24 A longitudinal scan of a hydatid cyst. It appears solid, though mild acoustic enhancement is still present.

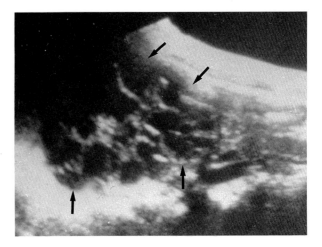

Fig. 11.25 A longitudinal scan of the left lobe. A large cyst filled by many small cysts is seen, typical of *E. multilocularis*. The patient came from Iran.

Echinococcus multilocularis (E. alveolaris)

Echinococcus multilocularis is rarely seen in Great Britain. It occurs in the arctic regions, Russia and southern Germany. The cyst appears macroscopically as a spongy, grey mass of irregular spaces like a Swiss cheese. The ultrasound appearance is that of a cyst filled with many small cysts (Fig. 11.25). Treatment is by lobectomy.

Amoebic abscess

Amoebic abscesses are caused by infection with the protozoan parasite *Entamoeba histolytica*. In the UK it is seen in the main in patients who have returned from a holiday abroad in the past year, though cases do arise in residents who have not been overseas.

The disease is world-wide in distribution, but is particularly prevalent in tropical and subtropical areas and is especially common in South Africa. It is relatively infrequent in temperate regions. Overcrowding and poor sanitation favour the transmission and development of the disease. The organism can remain in the gastrointestinal tract as a non-pathogenic symbiont and it is estimated that 2–4% of the population of the USA are carriers. Thus the demonstration of trophozoites or cysts in the stool does not prove that a patient has clinical amoebiasis. The factors that convert the parasite into its invasive haematophagous form are not known.

Ninety per cent of patients are males and usually in their twenties, the disease being uncommon in the very young or old. The illness develops over a period of 2–3 weeks with right upper quadrant pain, a dry cough, fever and tender hepatomegaly. Only 10–20% will have a history of colonic disease or have cysts in their stools at presentation. In 75% the abscess is solitary and in over 80% the disease involves the right lobe, frequently extending to involve the liver capsule. Although abscesses as small as 5 mm may be seen, most are large at the time of presentation and abscesses of 30 cm in diameter are not unknown. In 10% of patients complications develop. Extension or rupture into the chest is by far the most common of these, but extension into the peritoneal cavity or pericardium is more sinister, with a mortality rate of 20–30%. In uncomplicated cases the mortality rate is less than 1%.

Diagnosis

The diagnosis of an amoebic abscess rests on the demonstration of a liver abscess by scanning in combination with a positive serological test for amoebiasis. Abnormal findings on a chest X-ray are common but non-specific. Elevation of the right dome of the diaphragm, atelectasis, and a modest pleural effusion are common. The right hemithorax may become totally opaque following rupture of an abscess into the pleural cavity. Gas within the abscess cavity is seen only when secondary bacterial infection has developed or after aspiration. A radionuclide scan will show over 80% of amoebic abscesses as a filling defect in the liver. There have been reports that gallium citrate will selectively concentrate in the rim of an amoebic abscess and appear as a halo. However, this is not reliable enough to differentiate it from a pyogenic abscess.

The appearances on ultrasound depend on the maturity of the abscess and the precise nature of its contents. Many variations occur. Most abscesses are irregularly round or ovoid but a lobulated appearance is not uncommon. The wall is moderately well-defined and irregular but it becomes smoother as the abscess matures. No wall may be seen at all or there may be an echo-poor rim, or halo, possibly due to surrounding oedema (Fig. 11.26).

Most amoebic abscesses are echolucent though in some the contents are isoechoic because the infected liver has not yet undergone autolysis. A hyperechoic abscess is the least common and could be mistaken for a primary or secondary tumour. Both isoechoic and hyperechoic abscesses progress to a hypoechoic mass within 1–2 weeks and all abscesses eventually become anechoic as their contents become thinner in consistency (Fig. 11.27), (Boultbee *et al.*, 1979). In mature abscesses necrotic material may sink to the bottom and form an echo level (*see* Fig. 11.31). Distal acoustic enhancement is a very constant and important feature irrespective of the echogenicity of the abscess. Although generally less than that seen behind a cyst of similar size it can, nevertheless, be quite striking.

In the majority of patients the history, the findings at ultrasound, and the serology make the diagnosis. Aspiration is usually unrewarding as the trophozoites are only present in the wall of the abscess and not in its contents even when typical 'anchovy paste' is recovered. Aspiration is helpful when a pyogenic abscess cannot be excluded or to relieve severe pain. It may also be useful when a cystic metastasis or a solitary cyst with internal haemorrhage cannot be excluded, though the clinical setting will usually aid in the differentiation. It is probably important to aspirate all abscesses in the left lobe as in theory they are more likely to rupture into the pericardium or peritoneal cavity than are abscesses in the right lobe (Van Sonnenberg *et al.*, 1985).

Most patients, even those with very large abscesses, respond quickly to appropriate chemotherapy (usually metronidazole) so that aspiration is infrequently performed. In less than 5% delayed resolution will necessitate aspiration because of

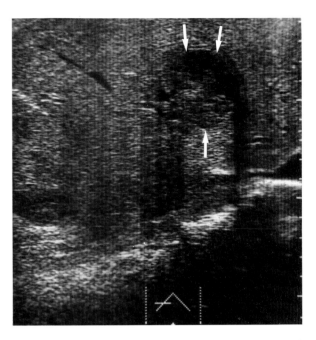

Fig. 11.26 A transverse scan showing an abscess in the left lobe. The walls are poorly defined, the contents hypoechoic compared to the liver and a halo (*arrows*) is seen in places. A moderate degree of acoustic enhancement is present.

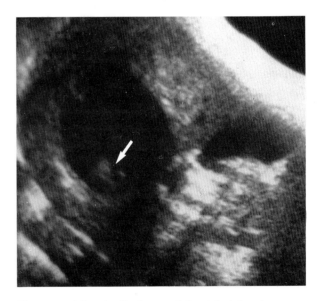

Fig. 11.27 A longitudinal scan of the right lobe. A mature anechoic abscess is seen with well-defined walls. It contains necrotic material (*arrow*). Note the very weak posterior enhancement.

the risk of rupture of the abscess. This is mostly due to failure of the liver to reabsorb the abscess contents. For this reason it is prudent to monitor an abscess under treatment. The rate of resolution depends on the size of the abscess at the time of diagnosis, but even the largest have healed by 4–6 months. The CT appearances are indistinguishable from those of a pyogenic abscess and are described in that section.

Pyogenic liver abscess

An untreated pyogenic liver abscess is fatal. Because of the insidious onset and non-specific nature of the patient's symptoms, and the absence of localizing signs, diagnosis and treatment are often delayed. Fever, malaise and upper abdominal pain are the most common symptoms and tender hepatomegaly the most common sign. Jaundice is unusual in patients with a solitary abscess but relatively common in patients with multiple abscesses. Most patients are middle-aged or elderly. In the past, acute appendicitis was the major source of liver abscesses. In recent years ascending cholangitis, portal bacteraemia, cholecystitis, and secondary infection of necrotic liver metastases or traumatized liver have become the major sources of infection in patients with multiple abscesses, but most patients who have a solitary abscess do not have an obvious primary site. Over half of all abscesses are cryptogenic. Fifteen per cent of patients have diabetes mellitus.

Many enteric bacteria can cause a pyogenic liver abscess and frequently there is a mixed growth of synergistic organisms, 60% of which are anaerobes (Perera *et al.*, 1980).

Diagnosis

An abnormal chest X-ray is present in 50% of cases. An elevated dome, a pleural effusion, atelectasis, or an area of basal consolidation may all be found. An air/fluid level, multiple air/fluid levels, or multiple small collections of gas·in the right upper quadrant, though uncommon, are virtually diagnostic (Figs 11.28, 11.29).

A radionuclide scan will show an abscess as a cold spot in 80% of cases but is non-specific and will miss small abscesses.

Multiple abscesses appear as irregular contrast-filled cavities arising from the biliary tree on PTC or ERCP in a patient undergoing investigation for biliary obstruction and cholangitis.

In most patients the diagnosis will be made by ultrasound or CT scanning. On ultrasound appearances alone it is frequently impossible to differentiate a pyogenic abscess from an amoebic

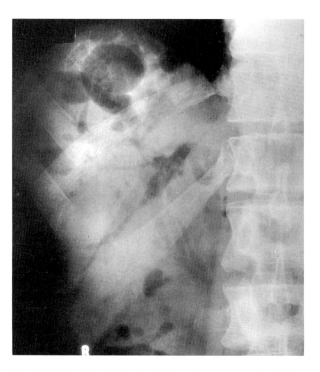

Fig. 11.28 A plain abdominal X-ray in a patient who had undergone biliary tract surgery. Irregular gas-filled abscesses are seen in the right lobe. Note the gas in the biliary tree.

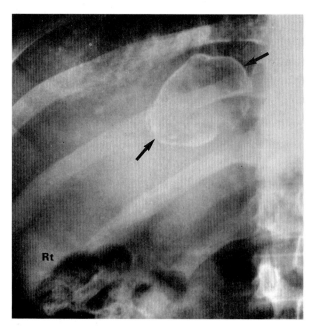

Fig. 11.29 A plain X-ray showing calcification in a healed abscess. This appearance is indistinguishable from calcification in a hydatid cyst.

one, although echogenic abscesses are uncommonly amoebic and suggest a pyogenic abscess (Figs 11.30, 11.31). An abscess will appear very

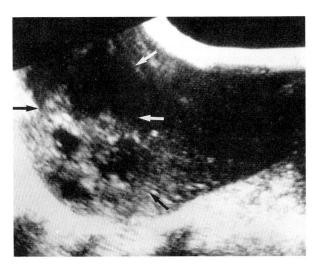

Fig. 11.30 A longitudinal scan showing a large abscess in the right lobe. It contains much echogenic debris. The aspirate was foul-smelling due to the gas within it.

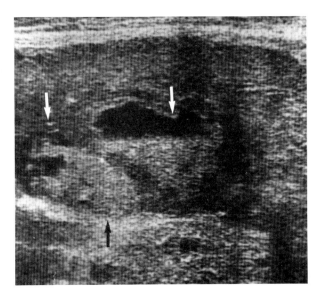

Fig. 11.31 An irregular ovoid, ill-defined, chronic pyogenic abscess. Echogenic debris is seen with a fluid–fluid level posterioly.

echogenic if it contains free gas or microbubbles of gas. The resulting acoustic shadowing will prevent a clear delineation of the abscess, but an erect or left lateral decubitus X-ray of the right upper quadrant, or a CT scan, will reveal the true extent of the abscess cavity. Mature abscesses may appear cystic, and as a pyogenic liver is often unsuspected clinically, the finding of one or more liver 'cysts' in an ill patient should be regarded with great suspicion. Once hydatid disease has been excluded diagnostic aspiration should be performed.

CT scanning is very sensitive at detecting liver abscesses. In a patient with a solitary abscess it has little advantage over ultrasound, but it will demonstrate multiple abscesses in a more easily assimilated format. In a patient with a cluster of small abscesses, CT will show them as discrete lesions when ultrasound may only show an area of ill-defined hypoechogenicity.

Most commonly a single, not completely homogeneous, non-loculated area of low density (2–30 HU) is seen. The walls may be smooth or irregular. A smooth-walled abscess is indistinguishable from a simple cyst or necrotic tumour. Twenty per cent of abscesses are loculated, and 20% contain gas. Multiple small bubbles or a large gas collection with a fluid level may be present, and either is pathognomonic of an abscess. After injection of contrast many abscesses are seen more clearly, and small satellite abscesses may be detected which were not apparent before contrast (Halvorsen et al., 1984) (Figs 11.32, 11.33a). In one-third of patients the liver around the abscess will enhance as two rings — an inner ring that enhances poorly or intensely, and a poorly defined outer hyperdense ring — the 'double target' sign. This is said to be diagnostic of an abscess (Mathieu et al., 1985).

Needle aspiration of pyogenic liver abscesses in combination with modern antibiotic therapy has reduced patient mortality to virtually nil (Berger & Osborne, 1982). In the past surgical drainage had a mortality rate of 20% for solitary abscesses and 77% for multiple abscesses. Although some patients have been successfully treated by antibiotics alone (Herbert et al., 1982) aspiration is advisable in order to obtain pus to determine the nature of the microbes and their antibiotic sensitivities. Blood cultures are unreliable. They are positive in less than 50% of patients and may not grow all the organisms in a mixed growth. Patient recovery time is shortened by aspiration, often dramatically so.

Liver abscesses are particularly well-suited to closed drainage. A safe route to the abscess can usually be found without difficulty, most are unilocular with a well-defined wall and there is usually no significant septation. Furthermore, the pus is usually thin and aspirates easily (Fig. 11.33). Two methods are used, continuous catheter drainage or needle aspiration. The former is favoured by most workers in the United States. Both the trocar and cannula method and the Seldinger technique for insertion of an 8–12F pigtail or straight-

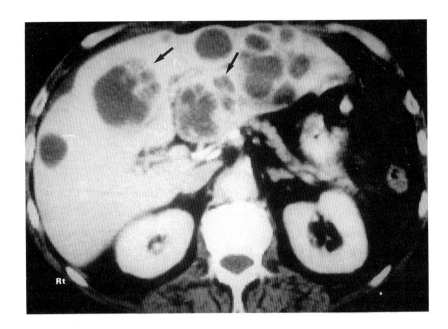

Fig. 11.32 A CT scan showing multiple abscesses in both lobes. Most are smooth-walled, many are not homogeneous and several are very irregular with satellite abscesses (*arrows*).

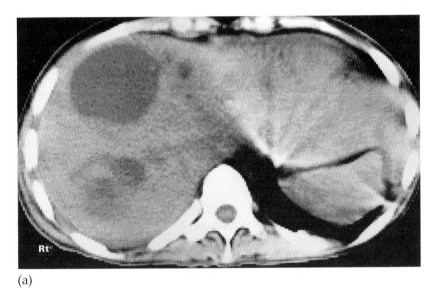

(a)

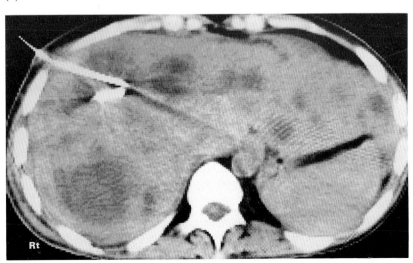

(b)

Fig. 11.33 (a) A CT scan showing a smooth-walled unilocular abscess anteriorly and a more complex abscess posteriorly. (b) A needle has been inserted through the seventh intercostal space and the abscess is being drained. Note the small abscess in the left lobe.

tipped catheter have been used, and the cavity is aspirated as completely as possible. Gentle saline irrigation is recommended by some, but others only irrigate when the pus is too thick to aspirate easily (Gerzof *et al.*, 1985); this is because irrigation increases the risk of bacteraemia and catheter back-bleeding. The catheter is removed once the clinical signs indicate improvement, the aspirate has become clear and is scanty, and a demonstrably reduced cavity as determined by an ultrasound or CT scan or a sinogram is seen. This takes on average 2–3 weeks.

Needle aspiration is a far less traumatic and a quicker procedure. Any bleeding tendency or clotting deficiency should be corrected, though these rarely occur. Local anaesthesia should be generous so that the procedure is pain free. An intradermal weal affords good skin anaesthesia so that the skin can be incised with a scalpel blade in order to facilitate the passage of the needle. Anaesthetic is then infiltrated down to the liver capsule. In most patients a 20 gauge needle is adequate and the relatively thin pus aspirates easily. If the pus is too thick for adequate drainage a larger needle can be inserted. In general a needle consisting of a soft plastic cannula and stylet is the safest, as the cannula causes little trauma to the abscess wall. The use of an extension tube minimizes the risk of trauma to the liver as the needle swings with the patient's respiration. The shortest path to the abscess should be chosen. As most abscesses lie in the right lobe the author has found that turning the patient into the left lateral decubitus position and using an intercostal approach is the easiest way to drain them. When CT is used for guidance a posterolateral approach is best in order to minimize the risk of transpleural passage of the needle.

The distance to the posterior wall of the abscess is measured and a needle of adequate length is selected. It is passed through the centre of the abscess until its tip lies *just short of the distal wall* (see Fig. 11.7). This will prevent the abscess from retracting off the needle as it shrinks. The progressive shrinkage of the cavity is monitored by ultrasound or CT. Near the end of the aspiration, flow will often cease because of occlusion of the cannula by the back wall of the abscess. However, slight withdrawal of the cannula will re-establish flow.

In the author's experience most abscesses can be completely drained through a needle and subsequent recovery is uneventful provided that the appropriate antibiotic therapy has been instituted. A second aspiration is usually unnecessary unless pus reaccumulates and causes symptoms. It is prudent to perform this second aspiration on an X-ray table, and to inject contrast at the end of the procedure in order to exclude an unsuspected fistula to the bowel (Fig. 11.34). This uncommon cause of a liver abscess requires surgery. Communication with the biliary tree may be shown but this is rarely of consequence in the absence of biliary obstruction (Fig. 11.35).

Initial experience of injecting contrast into multilocular abscesses showed that most were successfully drained by a single needle puncture because the locules communicated with each other (Fig. 11.36).

In a 12-year experience of needle drainage of liver abscesses the author has found that the occasional need to reaspirate an abscess is far outweighed by the complications and trauma of catheter drainage. The procedure is well tolerated by even the most ill patient, and apart from pain when the anaesthetic has worn off, no complications have ensued. The insertion of a catheter is more painful, more liable to cause bacteraemia, spill contents into the sub-capsular space or peritoneal cavity, and allow a portal of entry for superadded infection. Furthermore, patients are more uncomfortable after catheter drainage and hospital stay is prolonged. Because of the efficacy of modern antibiotics it is not necessary to drain every last drop of pus in order to achieve complete healing.

In a review of the literature, Gerzof *et al.*, (1985) found a mortality rate of 2.5% after closed aspiration with a needle and 4% after catheter drainage. Fifteen per cent of the catheter group, however, required surgery, whereas surgical drainage has not been necessary in patients treated at the Royal Free Hospital with needle aspiration.

There are those who advocate ultrasound and those who advocate CT as the better method of guidance. CT undoubtedly allows one to plan the route more scientifically, but in most cases this precision is of little importance and is offset by the flexibility of ultrasound and its ability to visualize the liver throughout the procedure. It is also less cumbersome and faster. Gerzof *et al.* (1981) in a large experience of draining abdominal abscesses used CT for planning, and ultrasound for guidance at the time of puncture.

Schistosomiasis (bilharziasis)

Schistosomiasis is an important disease in tropical areas. Over 200 million people are infected, of

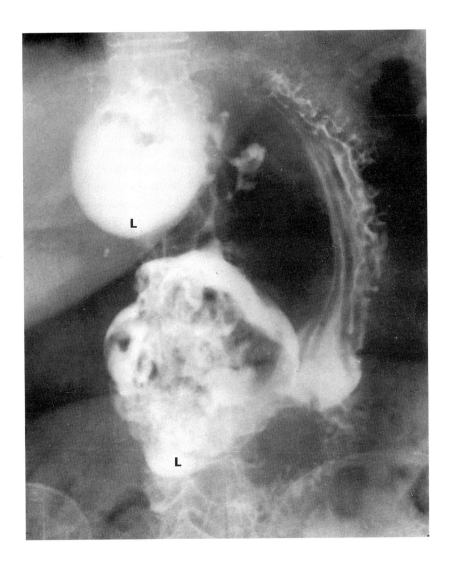

Fig. 11.34 A plain X-ray after puncturing a recurrent liver abscess and injecting contrast. Two communicating locules (L) are shown and contrast is seen in the stomach (and bowel). At surgery a small perforation of the stomach was found in association with an abscess in the lesser sac that had burrowed into the liver.

whom only a small proportion will develop clinically significant chronic disease as a result of years of intensive exposure. Both *Schistosoma mansoni* and *S. japonicum* cause liver disease, whilst *S. haematobium* predominantly affects the urinary tract. Humans are infected by skin contact with water containing the larvae (cercariae) excreted by infected snails. The larvae penetrate the unbroken skin, enter cutaneous venules and travel via the heart and lungs to the systemic circulation. Those that enter the mesenteric arteries pass on to the portal venous system where they stay until mature. The adult worms then migrate against the flow to the intestinal venules where they lodge and lay their eggs. The eggs are excreted into the gastrointestinal tract, but many of them are swept back into the portal system and are trapped by portal venules of 50 μm in diameter — the diameter of the eggs. The eggs produce an inflammatory response

in the host with the formation of granulomas. This manifests as an acute self-limiting febrile illness with tender hepatomegaly.

It should be appreciated that schistosomes do not multiply in the human host, so that light infections remain light. Thus chronic schistosomiasis only occurs in a small percentage of affected persons, and then only after many years of repeated exposure and re-infection. The intensity of infection may be gauged roughly by the egg count in the stools. The HLA alleles A1 and B5 may also be associated with a susceptibility to the chronic form of the disease.

Chronic schistosomiasis is characterized at histology by wide bands of fibrosis around the portal veins, whose cut surface resembles the cross-section of a clay pipe. The parenchyma between fibrotic areas is *not* affected and liver function is therefore well preserved. The fibrosis also occludes

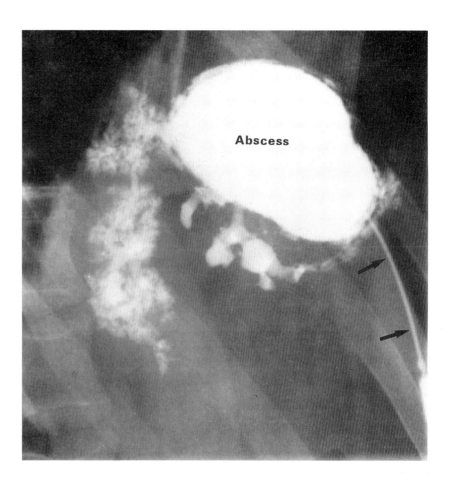

Abscess

Fig. 11.35 A lateral radiograph. An abscess in the right lobe has been punctured by a cannula (*arrows*) through the eighth intercostal space. Contrast has filled the abscess and entered the biliary tree and many small satellite abscesses. The abscess was drained completely and the patient made an uneventful recovery.

many portal radicles, causing presinusoidal portal hypertension, with congestive splenomegaly, oesophageal varices and dilated portasystemic collateral veins. There is always a significant degree of splenomegaly but it may on occasion be massive, in which case a splenic follicular lymphoma may have developed. This rare tumour is found in 1% of spleens removed at splenectomy for chronic schistosomiasis. Schistosomiasis does not cause cirrhosis or hepatoma but portal vein or less often splenic vein thrombosis occasionally develops, especially following splenectomy. Glomerulonephritis and inflammatory intestinal polyps are other complications.

Bleeding from oesophageal varices is the main threat to life in a patient with chronic schistosomiasis. It may on occasion be fatal, but multiple episodes over many years is the usual course of events. Encephalopathy is rare except after shunt surgery. In view of the pathogenesis of chronic schistosomiasis one would not expect the development of liver failure with jaundice, ascites and encephalopathy, yet this does occur in a small

number of patients and is thought to be due to coexisting chronic hepatitis B infection.

A definitive diagnosis can be made only when ova are found in the faeces. When they are absent, serological tests may be helpful. Current drug therapy (oxamniquine, praziquantel) is highly effective if the infection is active. They have no effect on established fibrosis or its sequelae.

Diagnosis

The plain film has little to offer in the diagnosis. A single case of generalized liver calcification in *S. japonicum* has been reported.

The appearances of chronic schistosomiasis on ultrasound reflect the degree of fibrosis present. Characteristically periportal fibrosis results in dense echogenic bands that encase central portal venous branches (Fig. 11.37). Peripherally, the portal veins are not seen, as they are thrombosed. At points where the portal veins divide, two to four radiating bands cause a bird's-claw appearance (Fig. 11.38). The porta hepatis is markedly

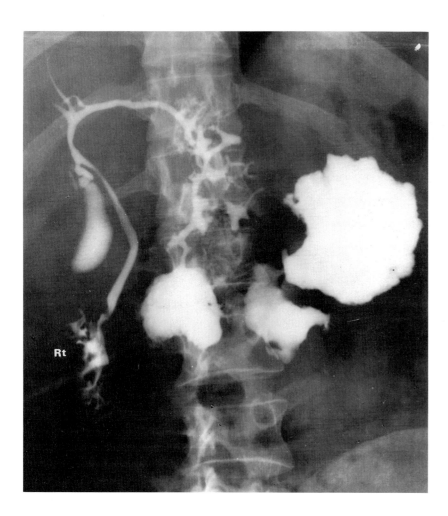

Fig. 11.36 A plain X-ray of a multilocular abscess in the left lobe. The most lateral loculus has been punctured and contrast has filled two other loculi. Contrast then entered the biliary tree and several small abscesses before passing through the main bile ducts and gall bladder to enter the duodenum. After several aspirations the patient recovered completely.

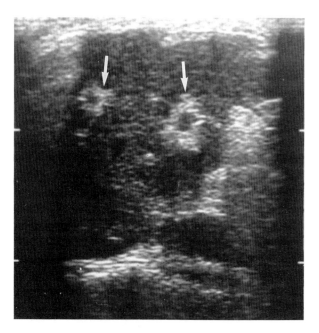

Fig. 11.37 A longitudinal scan of the right lobe. Two central portal vein branches surrounded by dense echogenic bands of fibrosis (*arrows*) are present.

enlarged and 1–2 cm thick echogenic bands radiate from it to the periphery (Fataar *et al.*, 1984). In addition Cerri *et al.*, (1984) noted atrophy of the right lobe of the liver and hypertrophy of the left lobe in 80% of cases. They further observed a thickened gall bladder wall in 60% and echogenic nodules in the spleen in 7% of patients.

By the time portal hypertension has developed, dilatation of the main portal vein and its major tributaries, the superior mesenteric vein and splenic vein, is apparent. The spleen is enlarged, and gastric and retroperitoneal collateral veins are seen (Fig. 11.39). These are most easily demonstrated by scanning the patient in the right lateral decubitus position and angling the transducer towards the gastric bed. Occasionally a spontaneous splenorenal shunt may be demonstrated.

The CT appearances of five patients with hepatic schistosomiasis mansoni have been reported by Fataar *et al.*, (1985). They found low-density periportal zones of fibrosis extending throughout both lobes. Intravenous contrast enhanced these zones

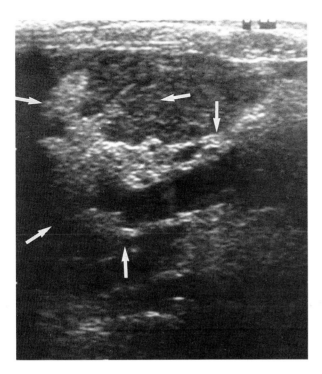

Fig. 11.38 A longitudinal scan. Radiating bands of fibrosis present the 'bird's-claw' appearance.

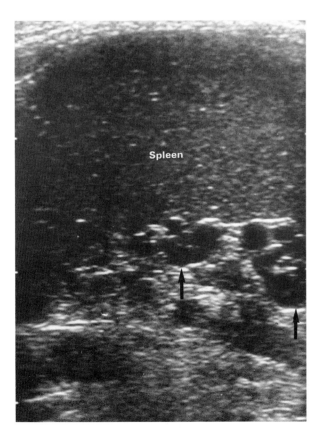

Fig. 11.39 A longitudinal scan through the spleen. There are large varicose collateral veins (*arrowed*).

so that by 60 s they were denser than the surrounding liver. These zones of periportal fibrosis appeared rounded when scanned in cross-section, and as linear bands with occasional branching when scanned longitudinally. In many of the peripheral foci the portal vein branch was thrombosed and could not be identified.

Araki *et al.*, (1985) reporting on the CT scan appearances of 17 patients with chronic schistosomiasis japonica found a characteristic pattern of calcification of the liver capsule and septa, resembling a turtle back. In six patients they found small hepatomas. (A female *S. japonicum* produces 10 times more eggs than a female *S. mansoni* and so this form of schistosomiasis produces much more severe liver impairment. Liver-cell cancer is not an uncommon complication.)

Tuberculosis

Symptomatic tuberculosis of the liver is uncommon in the western world. Although the liver may be frequently involved in a patient with widespread miliary infection, unless it is actively looked for it usually passes undetected. Schuit (1979) in North Carolina found hepatosplenomegaly in 40% and abnormal liver function tests in 25% of 19 children with miliary tuberculosis over a 22-year period. Terry & Gunnar (1975) treated 12 patients with primary miliary tuberculosis of the liver over a 4-year period. Half of their patients were alcoholics.

Alvarez & Carpio (1983) treated 130 patients in the Philippines with hepatobiliary tuberculosis over a 20-year period. Abdominal pain, fever, and a tender, hard, nodular liver simulating malignancy were commonly present in their patients, and the liver function tests were normal except in jaundiced patients. The changes of pulmonary tuberculosis were seen on a chest X-ray in 65% and the plain abdominal X-ray demonstrated hepatic calcification in 50%.

The calcifications in hepatic TB are typically numerous, small (1–3 mm) and rounded. They have ill-defined borders. Similar calcification may also be seen in patients with hepatic histoplasmosis. Calcified miliary nodules are also found on occasion in the spleen.

Although the diagnosis of hepatic tuberculosis rests on the demonstration of caseating granulomata in the liver and the culture of *Mycobacterium tuberculosis* from the liver or other organs, imaging may suggest the diagnosis. In uncomplicated hepatic tuberculosis the appearances at ultrasound are of a 'bright liver' indistinguishable from cirrhosis (Andrew *et al.*, 1982). On the other hand 35% of patients become jaundiced (Alvarez & Carpio, 1983) due to obstruction by enlarged lymph nodes at the porta hepatis or, less commonly, by nodes around the distal common bile duct. In these patients the dilated bile ducts and the large nodes may be demonstrated by ultrasound or CT scanning. At CT the nodes are typically of low density (28–40 HU) and their rims enhance with contrast (Mathieu *et al.*, 1986). Other enlarged abdominal nodes, thickened mesentery, and thickened bowel may be seen and the total picture may suggest the diagnosis (Epstein & Mann, 1982). It is important to define the site of obstruction in these patients as those who do not respond to chemotherapy may benefit from surgical decompression. Glands compressing the distal common bile duct are amenable to surgery, but the removal of obstructing nodes at the porta hepatis is generally not possible as they form a firm mass that makes surgical dissection impossible.

Alvares & Carpio also found tuberculous abscesses on scintigraphy in 50% of their patients.

Brucellosis

Brucellosis is a generalized infection that affects people in the meat-packing industry. Almost 50% of those infected work or have worked in an abattoir. Brucellosis involves the liver in less than 10% of patients. The diagnosis is made by growing the organisms from blood cultures or from a liver biopsy where a non-specific reactive hepatitis is found. In patients who have been infected for less than 3 months granulomas are present. The reported findings on ultrasound and isotope scans are non-specific and of little help in diagnosis.

Occasionally splenic calcifications may suggest chronic brucellosis. Typically these calcifications are small and multiple though they can be as large as 2 cm in diameter (Fig. 11.40).

Syphilis

Syphilis of the liver is rare. Hahn (1943) reported 66 cases of late syphilis in whom 33% had gummas. Symmers & Spain (1946) reported 19 gummas in 102 patients. In neither series did any of the gummas exhibit calcification. There have been reports of large circumscribed calcified masses oc-

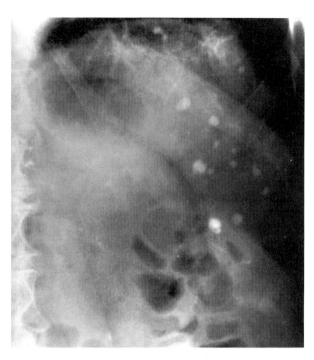

Fig. 11.40 A plain X-ray of the left upper quadrant. Multiple calcifications, some laminated, are seen. These are typical of granulomata but splenic phleboliths can give a similar appearance.

curring in gummata, but this is so rare that in a patient with a positive Wassermann reaction and a large liver with calcification other pathology should be considered more likely than a gumma (Haddow & Kemp-Harper, 1967). To date there have been no reports of the ultrasound or CT findings in hepatic gummata.

Acknowledgements

I wish to thank Sheila O'Riordan for her patience in typing the many drafts of the manuscript, Dr R. Dick for Figs 11.10, 11.17, 11.18, 11.29, 11.33a, b, Mrs Penny Thacker for Figs 11.19–11.22, and Dr S. Edwards for Fig. 11.32.

References

Alvarez, S.Z. & Carpio, R. (1983) Hepatobiliary tuberculosis. *Digestive Diseases and Sciences*, **28**, 193–200.

Andrew, W.K., Glyn Thomas, R. & Gollach, B.L. (1982) Miliary tuberculosis of the liver — another cause of 'Bright Liver' on ultrasound examination. *South African Medical Journal*, **62**, 808–809.

Araki, T., Hayakawa, K., Okada, J., Hayashi, S., Uchiyama, G. & Yamada, K. (1985) Hepatic Schistosomiasis japonica identified by CT. *Radiology*, **157**, 757–760.

Berger, L.A. & Osborne, D.R. (1982) Treatment of pyogenic liver abscesses by percutaneous needle aspiration. *Lancet*, i, 132–134.

Bezzi, M., Teggi, A., De Rosa, F., Capozzi, A., Tusa, G. Bonifacino, A. & Angelini, L. (1987) Abdominal hydatid disease: US findings during medical treatment, *Radiology*, **162**, 91–95.

Boultbee, J.E., Simjee, A.E., Rooknoodeen, F. & Engelbrecht, H.E. (1979) Experiences with grey-scale ultrasonography in hepatic amoebiasis. *Clinical Radiology*, **30**, 683–689.

Cerri, G.G., Alves, V.A.F. & Magalhaes, A. (1984) Hepato-splenic Schistosomiasis mansoni: ultrasound manifestations. *Radiology*, **153**, 777–780.

Choliz, J.D., Olaverri, F.J.L., Casas, T.F. & Zabieta, S.O. (1982) Computed tomography in hepatic echinococcus. *American Journal of Roentgenology*, **139**, 699–702.

Epstein, B.M. & Mann, J.H. (1982) CT of abdominal tuberculosis. *American Journal of Roentgenology*, **139**, 861–864.

Ertan, A., Sahin, B., Kandilci, U., Acikalin, T., Cumhur, T. & Danisoglu, V. (1983) The mechanism of cholestasis from hepatic hydatid cysts. *Journal of Clinical Gastroenterology*, **5**, 437–440.

Fataar, S., Bassiony, H., Satyanath, S. *et al.*, (1985) CT of hepatic Schistosomiasis mansoni. *American Journal of Roentgenology*, **145**, 63–66.

Fataar, S., Bassiony, H., Satyanath, S., Vassileva, J. & Hanna, R.M. (1984) Characteristic sonographic features of schistosomal periportal fibrosis. *American Journal of Roentgenology*, **143**, 69–71.

Federle, M.P., Filly, R.A. & Moss, A.A. (1981) Cystic hepatic neoplasms: Complementary roles of CT and sonography. *American Journal of Roentgenology*, **136**, 345–348.

Gerzof, S.G., Johnson, W.C., Robbins, A.H. & Nabseth, D.C. (1985) Intrahepatic pyogenic abscesses: treatment by percutaneous drainage. *American Journal of Surgery*, **149**, 487–494.

Gerzof, S.G., Robbins, A.H., Johnson, W.C., Birkett, D.H. & Nabseth, D.C. (1981) Percutaneous catheter drainage of abdominal abscesses. *New England Journal of Medicine*, **305**, 653–657.

Haddow, R.A. & Kemp-Harper, R.A. (1967) Calcification in the liver and portal system. *Clinical Radiology*, **18**, 225–236.

Hahn, R.D. (1943) Syphilis of the liver. American Journal of Syphilis, **27**, 529–562.

Halvorsen, E.A., Korobkin, M., Foster, W.L., Silverman, P.M. & Thompson, W.M. (1984) The variable CT appearance of hepatic abscesses. *American Journal of Roentgenology*, **142**, 941–946.

Herbert, D.A., Fogel, D.A., Rothman, J., Wilson, S., Simmons, F. & Ruskin, J. (1982) Pyogenic liver abscesses. Successful non-surgical therapy. *Lancet*, i, 134–136.

Itzchak, Y., Rubinstein, Z., Heyman, Z. & Gerzof, S. (1980) Role of ultrasound in the diagnosis of abdominal hydatid disease. *Journal of Clinical Ultrasound*, **8**, 341–345.

Kalovidouris, A., Pissiotis, C., Pontifex, G., Gouliamos, A., Pentea, S. & Papavassiliou, C. (1986) CT characterization of multivesicular hydatid cysts. *Journal of Computer Assisted Tomography*, **10**, 428–431.

Levine, E., Cook, L.T. & Grantham, J.J. (1985) Liver cysts in autosomal–dominant polycystic kidney disease: clinical and computed tomographic study. *American Journal of Roentgenology*, **145**, 229–233.

Mathieu, D., Ladeb. M.F., Guigui, B., Rousseau, M. & Vasile, N. (1985) Periportal tuberculous adenitis: CT features. *Radiology*, **161**, 713–715.

Mathieu, D., Vasile, N., Fagniez, P.L., Segui, S., Grably, D. & Larde, D. (1985) Dynamic CT features of hepatic abscesses. *Radiology*, **154**, 749–752.

Pandolfo, I., Blandino, G., Scriband, E., Longo, M., Certo, A. & Chirico, G. (1984) CT findings in hepatic involvement by *Echinococcus granulosus*. *Journal of Computer Assisted Tomography*, **8**, 839–845.

Perera, M.R., Kirk, A. & Noone, P. (1980) Presentation, diagnosis and management of liver abscess. *Lancet*, ii, 629–632.

Schuit, K.E. (1979) Miliary tuberculosis in children. *American Journal of Diseases of Children*, **133**, 583–585.

Summerfield, J.A., Nagafuchi, Y., Sherlock, S., Cadafalch, J. & Scheuer, P.J. (1986) Hepatobiliary fibropolycystic diseases: a clinical and histological review of 51 patients. *Journal of Hepatology*, **2**, 141–156.

Symmers, D. & Spain, D.M. (1946) Hepar lobatum. Clinical significance of anatomic change. *Archives of Pathology*, **42**, 64–68.

Taylor, J.K.W. & Viscomi, G.N. (1980) Ultrasound diagnosis of cystic disease of the liver. *Journal of Clinical Gastroenterology*, **2**, 197–204.

Terry, R.B. & Gunnar, R.M. (1975) Primary miliary tuberculosis of the liver. *Journal of the American Medical Association*, **164**, 150–157.

Van Sonnenberg, E., Mueller, P.R., Schiffman, H.R. *et al.* (1985) Intrahepatic amoebic abscesses: indications for and results of percutaneous catheter drainage. *Radiology*, **156**, 631–635.

12: Tumours: Benign, Primary Malignant

J. KARANI

The diagnosis of primary liver tumours

The technological revolution in the last 10 years has produced extensive data on the appearances of primary liver tumours. Consequently there has been a change in emphasis on the role of the radiologist. Diagnosing the presence of a focal lesion is now only the preliminary step in a line which must be followed by an indication of the type of tumour, whether benign or malignant, and accurate tumour mapping. Once the diagnosis is established, the role then switches to therapy with trans-catheter techniques and documenting treatment response with non-invasive imaging. In diagnosis, no imaging technique stands alone and correlation of all modalities may be necessary if all these objectives are to be achieved.

Primary liver tumours are classified histologically as being of hepatocellular, cholangiocellular or mesenchymal origin (Table 12.1). Of these, hepatocellular carcinoma is the most common representing over 80% of all primary hepatic malignancies. However, it should be emphasized that in Western practice metastatic disease involving the liver outnumbers primary tumours by about 50:1 (Pickren et al., 1982). The liver is the most common site of metastases, post-mortem evidence indicates that 40% of adults with primary extrahepatic malignancy will have metastatic involvement. In tumours drained by the portal venous system, such as colon and pancreas, this prevalence may be as high as 70% (Willis, 1973). These statistics highlight the fact that it requires good clinicopathological evidence for diagnosing a primary tumour rather than a metastasis when a focal lesion is demonstrated. An equally important fact is that whereas the prognosis is poor for a patient with colonic hepatic metastases, with a median survival of 150 days (Jaffe et al., 1968), the patient with a primary hepatic tumour may be curable either by surgical resection or orthotopic liver transplantation.

Primary malignant tumours

Hepatocellular carcinoma (hepatoma, HCC)

Although the most common primary malignant tumour involving the liver, hepatocellular carcinoma, is relatively uncommon in Europe and the United States, constituting 1–2.5% of all cancers. This reflects the relatively low prevalence in the West of the aetiological factors associated with their development. Of these, chronic HbV

Table 12.1 Liver tumours

	Malignant	Benign
Hepatocellular	Hepatoblastoma Hepatoma Hepatic mixed tumours	Focal nodular hyperplasia Adenoma
Cholangiocellular	Cholangiocarcinoma	Adenoma Cystadenoma
Mesenchymal	Leiomyosarcoma Rabdomyosarcoma Fibrosarcoma Angiosarcoma Epithelioid haemangioendothelioma	Haemangioma

(Australia antigen, hepatitis B) is the most significant. Prospective population studies have shown that chronic carrier status confirms a relative risk of greater than 200 times of developing this tumour (Beasley et al., 1981). Consequently, in areas of high HBV infection such as the Far East and sub-saharan Africa, the incidence of this tumour is greater than 5 per 100 000, constituting 17% of all cancers. Aflatoxin (Bulatao-Jayne et al., 1982), alcohol (Yu et al., 1983), and the high-dose oral contraceptive pill if taken for greater than 8 years (Forman et al., 1986) are other recognized aetiological factors, and all may act synergistically. Certain metabolic disorders predispose to the development of hepatocellular carcinoma. Tyrosinaemia, porphyria cutanea tarda, and haemochromatosis provide the best examples. A close association exists between cirrhosis and hepatocellular carcinoma Kew & Popper (1984); studies have demonstrated a prevalence of 60–90% in patients developing the tumour.

Throughout the world, hepatocellular carcinoma occurs more frequently in men (Nagasue et al., 1984). If cirrhosis is present, presentation is usually in the 6th decade. In the absence of cirrhosis, there is an equal sex distribution with an earlier mean age of presentation at 35 years (Johnson et al., 1978, Melia et al., 1984).

Clinical features are variable. Right upper-quadrant pain, weight loss, and fever are the most common symptoms. They may be accompanied by hepatic decompensation as indicated by the development of ascites, variceal bleeding, jaundice or encephalopathy. Haemoperitoneum from spontaneous rupture of the tumour may occur, but is far more common in the Far East where it is the presenting feature in 14% of patients (Ong & Taw, 1922).

The tumour marker alphafetoprotein is elevated in 50% of the non-cirrhotic patients and in 85% of those with cirrhosis (Johnson et al., 1978). The level rises exponentially in the absence of effective treatment. The presence of a large tumour, ascites, hypoalbuminaemia and hyperbilirubinaemia are recognized as poor prognostic factors. If all are present, the mean survival is 1 month. This is a relatively common presentation but does not reflect the natural evolution of these tumours, for it has been shown that the 1-year survival of patients with tumours of less than 3 cm is as high as 90% (Ebara et al., 1986). Treatment options are limited. The best chance of a curative approach rests between hepatic resection and orthotopic liver transplantation. The former is limited by the common presence of cirrhosis. Only about 25% of tumours are considered resectable and the operative mortality is as high as 33% with a 5-year survival of less than 5% in patients with coexistent cirrhosis (Huguet & Mouiel, 1983). The rarer fibro-lamellar variant that generally arises in a non-cirrhotic liver carries better surgical results, with a 5-year survival of over 50% (Soreide et al., 1986). Sensitive imaging surveillance of high-risk patients coupled with serial alphafetoprotein estimations may improve survival by detecting small tumours, for although liver transplantation is limited by a high tumour recurrence rate of 60%, in patients where the tumour is an incidental finding the recurrence rate may be reduced by a factor of 10.

Radiological findings

Conventional radiography has been replaced by more accurate imaging techniques. Calcification is seen in 10–25% of hepatocellular carcinomata and results from tumour necrosis, unlike the case in children where the incidence is higher and reflects the osteoid component of the tumour.

Ultrasound

Ultrasound provides an invaluable screening technique for detection or exclusion of a focal liver mass (Fig. 12.1) with a reported sensitivity of 90% (Cottone et al., 1983). The ultrasound appearances of hepatocellular carcinoma are variable, ranging from hypoechoic (47%) to echogenic (23%) (Dubbins et al., 1981). Local invasion of peripheral portal vein radicles (30–60%) and peripheral bile ducts with resultant segmental biliary dilatation or local extrahepatic spread, may be recognized. As stated, the presence or absence of cirrhosis is the most important criterion in judging treatment options. By demonstrating features of cirrhosis and portal hypertension such as ascites and splenomegaly, ultrasound provides important diagnostic information.

There are, however, two problems referrable to the diagnosis of hepatocellular cancer. Firstly, ultrasound does not differentiate benign from malignant focal tumours. Coupled with guided biopsy techniques this may be overcome in most cases. Mengnini and Trucut biopsy techniques have a high diagnostic yield but a significant complication rate with hypotension, haemorrhage, or

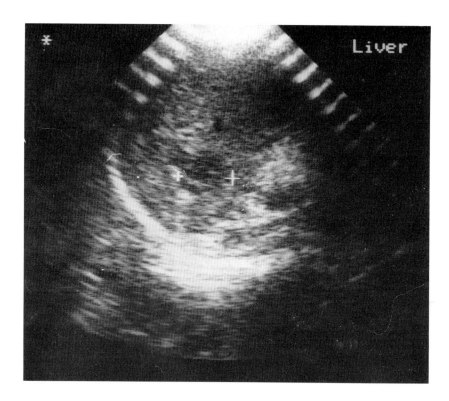

Fig. 12.1 Hepatocellular carcinoma. Ultrasound scan demonstrating development of a small tumour within a cirrhotic liver.

biliary peritonitis occurring in up to 17% of patients (Zamcheck & Klausenstock, 1953). The alternative of fine-needle biopsy with its lower morbidity may result in a sensitivity of 75% (Lees *et al.*, 1985), but the specimen may be insufficient to establish histological differentiation. The second and most significant problem is that although hepatomata may be focal in the majority of cases, in about 15% there is a diffuse pattern of tumour infiltration that may be difficult to differentiate from the heterogeneous and nodular parenchyma of advanced cirrhosis.

Of the newer developments, Doppler ultrasound and intraoperative assessment of hepatic tumours have made the greatest contributions. The latter allows the surgeon to plan the plane of dissection to preserve as much normal liver as possible. Once localized intraoperatively, enucleation of tumours is technically possible.

Computerized tomography

CT is accurate in demonstrating hepatocellular carcinomata and their lobar distribution. As with ultrasound, there is a wide spectrum of appearances reflecting the differentiation, extent, vascularity, and necrosis of these tumours. Individual tumour deposits within the same patient may demonstrate differing appearances. The tumours are generally of low density and appear either as small or large solitary masses or as multicentric nodules. Calcification is recognized in up to 25% of cases (Wallace, 1977). Sensitivity may be increased with dynamic scanning with rapid sequential imaging of the liver over 2–3 min following a bolus injection of contrast. During this period, contrast is present in the intravascular space and results in enhanced differentiation between the normal liver and the reduced density of the tumour. This technique also results potentially in imaging of the portal and hepatic venous anatomy and the relationship of the tumour to these structures. Alternatively a delayed scanning technique may be used where scans are carried out 4–6 h after contrast injection. Approximately 2% of the iodine injected will be excreted into the biliary system. Tumours do not secrete iodine and will appear as lesions of reduced attenuation within normal liver, which will exhibit an attenuation value of about 20–25 Hounsfield units above normal unenhanced hepatic tissue. An increased detection rate in 26% of patients has been reported (Bernardino *et al.*, 1986). As with ultrasound, the presence of features of portal hypertension may be documented. At presentation there may be already evidence of metastatic disease to the lungs (8.3%), portal nodes (3.4%), or central nervous system (1.5%) (Margolis & Homcy, 1972). CT provides high-quality imaging information on these areas for accurate tumour staging.

There are limitations to CT assessment. Firstly, hepatomata may be isodense or become isodense following contrast. Secondly, as with ultrasound, demonstration of diffuse tumour infiltration within a nodular cirrhotic liver may be difficult.

There is now an extensive literature mainly from the Far East, on the role of lipiodol image enhancement in CT diagnosis (Yumoto *et al.*, 1985). The aim of this technique is to opacify the liver on a cellular, rather than a vascular basis. Lipiodol is injected into the hepatic artery at the time of conventional angiography, and sequential CT imaging is carried out, generally over a 2–3-week period. Lipiodol is cleared from normal hepatic tissue over this period (Fig. 12.2) but is said to accumulate in malignant tumours because of the 'leaky' character of neovascular tissue, coupled with the lack of lymphatic clearance of lipiodol from tumour tissue. Histologically, lipiodol is found in necrotic tissue and peritumoural hepatic sinusoids. In our experience, the main role of this technique in the future will probably not be as a diagnostic tool but more as a therapeutic measure using chemotherapy targeting with agents bound to lipiodol. Significant complications are uncommon and appear to be related to the microembolic effects of lipiodol.

Angiography

Angiography plays a major part in both the diagnosis and treatment of hepatocellular carcinoma. Although regarded as an invasive technique, its relative morbidity should not be overstated. It allows detection of tumours as small as 5 mm if vascular and 2 cm when avascular (Wallace & Chuang, 1983). The angiographic characteristic of liver tumours, both benign and malignant, coupled with ultrasound and CT data may be diagnostic and lessen the necessity for histological confirmation. There are no absolute angiographic criteria for malignancy. However, the vast majority of hepatocellular carcinomata are vascular and are characterized by new vessel formation, arteriovenous shunting, and an increased capillary blush in the hepatogram (late venous) phase of the hepatic artery injection (Fig. 12.3). Intravenous extension into the portal vein with arterioportal venous fistulae and hepatic veins are a characteristic feature, particularly in patients with diffuse hepatocellular tumour infiltration. Recent studies suggest that although the predominant vascular supply to these tumours is from the hepatic artery recruitment from portal venous radicles may occur. This is the converse of normal liver tissue, which derives 75% of its blood supply from the portal venous system. In accordance with other imaging, the tumours may be unifocal, multicentric or diffuse. It is in this last category of patients, where as

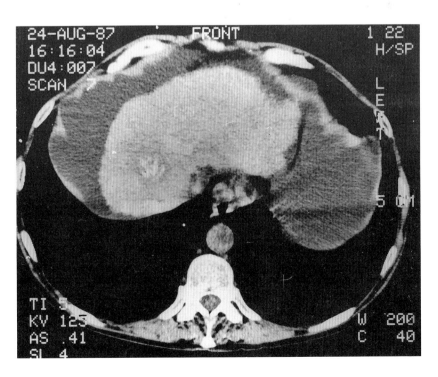

Fig. 12.2 Hepatocellular carcinoma. CT to demonstrate lipiodol retained within a small tumour following selective intrahepatic arterial injection.

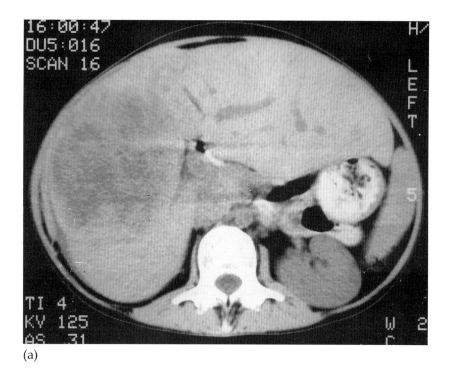

(a)

(b)

Fig. 12.3 Hepatocellular carcinoma. (a) Well-encapsulated tumour within the right lobe, confirmed as malignant by the conclusive pattern of neovascularity demonstrated at arteriography. (b) On selective catheterization of an aberrant right hepatic artery.

previously stated ultrasound and CT may be inconclusive, that angiography may provide a diagnosis. It is our experience that angiography may give a more accurate estimation of the number of tumour nodules or degree of infiltration over these other modalities. Angiographic assessment where the tumours are hypovascular, particularly in the presence of macronodular cirrhosis with regenerating nodules, is generally unrewarding. Accurate mapping of the portal venous system with digital subtraction aorto-portography is necessary if resection or transplantation are being considered as thrombosis is a relative contraindication to both these surgical options. It is important to be aware that non-demonstration of the portal vein by this technique does not necessarily imply occlusion, for in patients with hepatofugal flow from portal hypertension, a preferential flow into portomesenteric or splenoportal collaterals, rather than the intrahepatic portal vein, will occur (Fig. 12.4). This is an area where Doppler ultrasound solves a diagnostic problem.

Trans-catheter techniques with embolization and intra-arterial chemotherapy remains a palliative therapeutic option in a small group of patients. Poor synthetic liver function will be present in those patients with hepatocellular carcinoma and co-existent cirrhosis, so precluding embolization in the vast majority of patients.

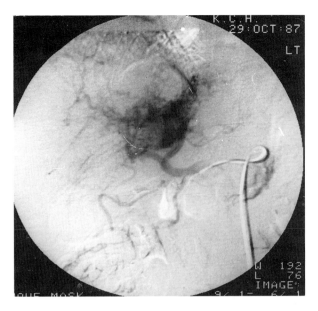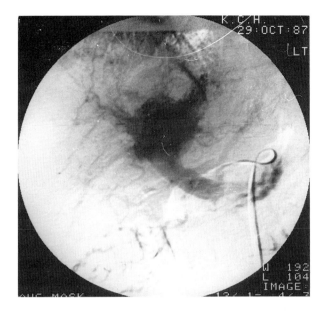

Fig. 12.4 Hepatocellular carcinoma. Invasive tumour at the hilum with tumour propagation into the portal vein, with resultant hepatofugal flow demonstrated at arteriography.

Cholangiocarcinoma

This tumour was first described by Klatskin in 1965, and is characterized histologically by a marked scirrhous reaction with clumps of carcinoma cells surrounded by fibrous tissue, resulting in a malignant stricture. Sclerosing cholangitis and choledochal cysts are recognized predisposing conditions. It develops in association with inflammatory bowel disease even in the absence of pre-existing cholangitis or pericholangitis.

Cholangiocarcinomata are relatively slow growing, spreading into adjacent liver parenchyma with local invasion of the hepatic arteries and portal vein. It is this factor which limits surgical resectability. Its pattern is distinct from the peripheral cholangiocarcinoma which is characterized by diffuse parenchymal infiltration, where jaundice is a late complication. Distant lymphatic and haematogenous metastatic spread is not a major feature, occurring in only 12% of patients at presentation (Wheeler *et al.*, 1981).

Clinical presentation is at a relatively young age with one-third of patients presenting under the age of 50 (Wheeler *et al.*, 1981). Obstructive jaundice that may be intermittent, weight loss, and anorexia are predominant clinical manifestations. Features of portal hypertension may be present if there is pre-existing liver disease or with neoplastic involvement of the portal venous system.

Radiological findings

Ultrasound will confirm the presence of dilatation of the intrahepatic biliary system and delineate the level of obstruction. The site of the tumour may be demonstrable as an area of high reflectivity, its echo characteristics reflecting the fibrous nature of the tumour. Computerized tomography may, similarly, map the extent of local parenchymal involvement and its relation to the portal vein, and assess the presence of lobar atrophy — an important feature if radical surgery is planned. The tumour is avascular and the only signs angiographically demonstrable are encasement or occlusion of the hepatic arteries or portal vein at the site of the tumour (Fig. 12.5).

Unlike the other primary liver tumours, direct cholangiography is the principal diagnostic technique (Fig. 12.6). Both endoscopic and percutaneous cholangiography may be necessary in fully mapping the biliary system proximal and distal to the stricture. Separate puncture of the ducts within the left and right lobes may be necessary in order to fill all the occluded biliary segments.

Differentiation from inflammatory strictures, particularly in the presence of sclerosing cholangitis, may be difficult and highlights the requirement for a histological diagnosis before treatment is instituted. Gall bladder carcinoma and metastatic hilar lymph nodes are alternative malignant

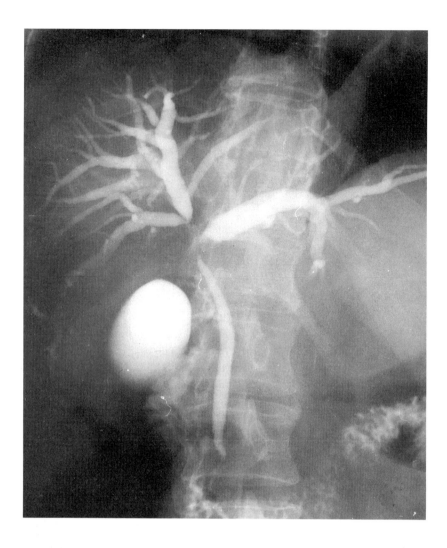

Fig. 12.5 Cholangiocarcinoma. Characteristic appearance of a neoplastic stricture at the confluence of the left and right hepatic ducts.

differentials which carry differing therapeutic implications and prognoses. Fine-needle biopsy may yield representative tissue in over 50% of patients (Blumgart *et al.*, 1984).

Despite the low biological activity of this tumour the success of treatment is disappointing. Preoperative assessment will confirm clinical and radiological criteria precluding curative surgery in up to 80% of patients (Akwari & Kelly, 1979, Blumgart *et al.*, 1984). Even with an aggressive surgical approach, only 10% of patients will have curative surgery and a significant number will have relatively early tumour recurrence. Adequate palliation to relieve biliary obstruction, either surgical or radiological, is the mainstay of treatment, and this may be coupled with local internal irradiation (Karani *et al.*, 1985).

Hepatic sarcomata

These represent relatively uncommon primary malignant liver tumours and fall into three categories: angiosarcoma, epithelioid haemangioendothelioma, and the undifferentiated sarcomata. Differentiation of these tumours from the more common hepatic malignancies is made from clinical and histological data. Predisposing factors such as exposure to arsenic, thorotrast, or vinyl chloride are strong indicators in favour of a diagnosis of angiosarcoma. Patients with epithelioid haemangioendothelioma, which is now recognized more frequently with new histochemical techniques, may survive for several years, even with evidence of metastatic spread to bones and lung, without any specific treatment. The other sarcomata carry a universally poor prognosis (Ishak *et al.*, 1984).

There are no specific radiological parameters by which these tumours may be reliably differentiated. The pattern of multifocal vascular tumour by which they are recognized on ultrasound, CT, and angiography is non-specific, and on statistical grounds metastatic disease or hepatocellular

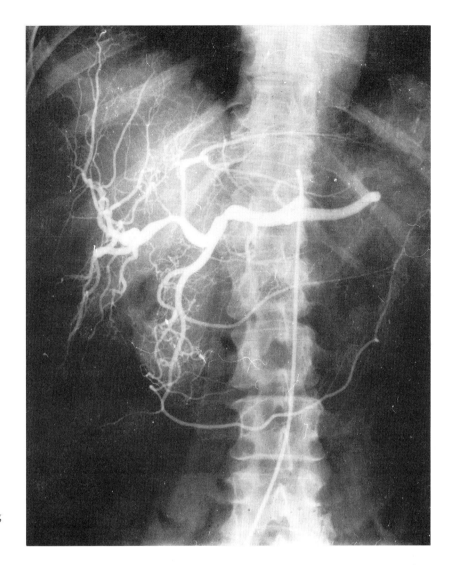

Fig. 12.6 Cholangiocarcinoma. Hepatic arteriography demonstrating encasement of the common hepatic left and right hepatic arteries.

carcinoma are more appropriate interpretations. Biopsy and histological assessment remains the specific diagnostic procedure.

Benign tumours

Haemangioma

This is the most common benign tumour of the liver, observed in 7% of post-mortem series. Over 70% occur in women and though all ages are affected it is uncommon for this tumour to be diagnosed in childhood (Ishak *et al.*, 1975; Freeny *et al.*, 1979). Histologically a haemangioma is characterized by multiple endothelium-lined, cystic, blood-filled spaces, separated by fibrous septae of variable thickness. Calcification occurs with formation of phleboliths in a small group of patients

(Itai *et al.*, 1980). Haemangiomata vary greatly in size but the majority are less than 3 cm in diameter. These small lesions are generally asymptomatic and an incidental finding. Large haemangiomata may be symptomatic with episodic abdominal pain and hepatomegaly. Anorexia and fever may be present and these symptoms may be referrable to central necrosis. Haemoperitoneum is a recognized but uncommon complication. The literature is probably biased towards these large symptomatic haemangiomata which it should be emphasized, are relatively uncommon in the overall prevalence.

Radiological findings

A spectrum of ultrasound appearances have been described. The most common pattern is of a well-circumscribed lesion, of increased echogenicity with posterior acoustic enhancement, sited peripherally in the liver (Fig. 12.7). The larger the haemangioma, the more atypical it will seem, appearing less well-defined and with a hypoechoic or heterogeneous echo pattern. If the ultrasound appearances conform to the typical pattern as described in an asymptomatic patient with normal liver function and a negative alphafetaprotein, further investigation is not warranted. Only if these lesions are large or have an atypical pattern will further imaging with CT and angiography be necessary. In our experience the risk of haemorrhagic complications following guided biopsy is very low and the technique should not be discounted when the diagnosis remains in doubt following imaging.

Differentiation of cavernous haemangiomata from other focal hepatic tumours is possible in up to 90% of cases with computerized tomography (Freeny *et al.*, 1979, Itai *et al.*, 1980, Barnett *et al.*, 1980, Johnson *et al.*, 1981). On the pre-enhancement scan, they usually appear as well-circumscribed homogeneous lesions of low attenuation, sometimes with a central low density cleft. Isodense haemangiomata do occur. Following contrast, immediate enhancement of the rim of the lesion occurs with an attenuation level greater than normal liver. Delayed scans demonstrate a creeping pattern with progressive enhancement of the more central parts of the haemangioma. This pattern is due to accumulation of contrast within the dilated vascular spaces, the slow wash-out reflecting the lack of intratumoral shunting (Fig. 12.8). Transit time through the lesion is slow, and although most haemangiomata will fill in 4–5 min, delay of up to 15 min may occur. Angiography is generally reserved for those patients where the result of CT scanning is equivocal or in those where surgical treatment is planned. The angiographic features of haemangioma are diagnostic. The main hepatic artery and segmental arteries are normal. There is a fine vascular network with small pools of contrast developing on the periphery of the lesion during the early phase of the injection. These form ring-like collections of contrast and persist throughout the venous phase of the injection with delayed clearing of contrast, paralleling the creeping enhancement pattern on CT. Arteriovenous shunting is rare. Displacement of the hepatic arteries and the portal venous radicles around these vascular spaces will be visualized.

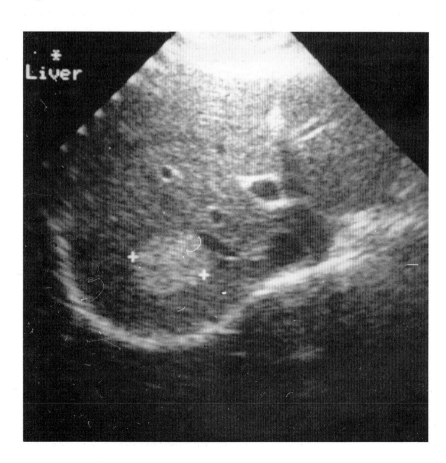

Fig. 12.7 Haemangioma. Characteristic ultrasound appearance.

Focal nodular hyperplasia

Focal nodular hyperplasia is a well-circumscribed, benign, non-encapsulated hamartoma of the liver. It is generally subcapsular but is pedunculated in 20% of cases (Casarella *et al.*, 1978). Multiple lesions are present in 20% of patients and coexistent haemangiomata is a relatively common feature. Pathologically the tumour displays a stellate configuration with radiating septae and a central fibrous scar. The latter feature may be demonstrated on CT. By definition, as a hamartoma, hepatocytes, Kupffer cells, and bile ducts are present in a disrupted pattern.

The tumour has been described in von Gierke's disease (Goldstein *et al.*, 1974) and in association with phaeochromocytoma. The tumours lacks malignant potential. It is generally an incidental finding and has been described in both children and adults. Haemorrhagic complications are rare, with only two reported cases.

It is probable that with the large number of ultrasound scans now performed there will an increasing recognition of these tumours. Therapeutic options vary from the conservative approach to hepatic artery embolization and major hepatic resection. The merits of these varying treatments has not been established in a long-term controlled study to date.

Radiological findings

The ultrasound features of focal nodular hyperplasia are non-specific with a spectrum of appearances varying from hypoechoic to echogenic. They may also appear of the same echogenicity as normal liver and only be recognized by their mass effect displacing local venous structures. The tumour is characteristically supplied by a large segmental hepatic artery that may be demonstrable, particularly with the aid of Doppler scanning. Radionuclide scanning may be valuable as sulphur colloid uptake occurs in 40% of cases because of the presence of Kupffer cells (Casarella *et al.*, 1978), a feature which differentiates this tumour from adenomata, metastases, and hepatocellular carcinoma. On CT, the tumours are generally of lower attenuation than normal liver, with an enhancement pattern reflecting their high vascularity. The central stellate scar, which is recognized histologically, may be demonstrated on CT. However, as with ultrasound, the appearances are non-specific. Even the histological appearances from guided

biopsies may fail to give a conclusive diagnosis. This is because, as the tumour is a hamartoma, sections from it may resemble compressed or minimally distorted normal liver, a pattern that is also seen histologically close to other tumours such as a metastasis.

The angiographic appearances may be diagnostic. Characteristically there is a large segmental artery that supplies the tumour from the periphery of the mass or centrally with a radial distribution of vessels within the tumour (Wallace & Chuang, 1983) (Fig. 12.9). Homogeneous opacification is seen in the hepatogram phase. Arterioportal shunting is not present. The lesions appear as a negative defect in the portal hepatogram phase of the SMA injection, reflecting their lack of portal venous recruitment. Angiographic features of portal hypertension will not be present unless there is coexistent parenchymal liver disease.

Liver cell adenoma

Liver cell adenomata are usually solitary, smooth, encapsulated tumours (Casarella *et al.*, 1978). The majority are 8—15 cm in diameter. Histologically they are characterized by vacuolated, atypical hepatocytes. Unlike focal nodular hyperplasia there are no Kupffer cells or bile ducts. Haemorrhage, necrosis, and biliary stasis are frequently present. Unlike the other benign tumours the lack of malignant potential is not clear-cut (Casarella *et al.*, 1978). The previously reported high recurrence rate of 21% may reflect the difficulty in differentiating this tumour from well-differentiated hepatocellular carcinoma on histological criteria.

A causal relationship with the oral contraceptive pill has been described and this will be supported by the fact that this tumour occurs almost without exception in women of childbearing age, although men taking androgens or anabolic steroids represent a high-risk group (Mays *et al.*, 1976, Ishak *et al.*, 1975). Glycogenosis Type lA is a recognized predisposing condition. It is a very rare post-mortem finding.

Patients generally present because of intra-abdominal bleeding with a subcapsular haemorrhage or haemoperitoneum. An abdominal mass may be palpated. The low malignant potential coupled with the risk of catastrophic haemorrhage are indications for an aggressive therapeutic approach to this tumour, and contrasts sharply with focal nodular hyperplasia and haemangioma. Hepatic resection and hepatic artery embolization

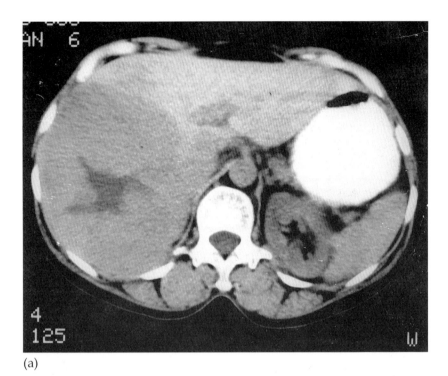

(a)

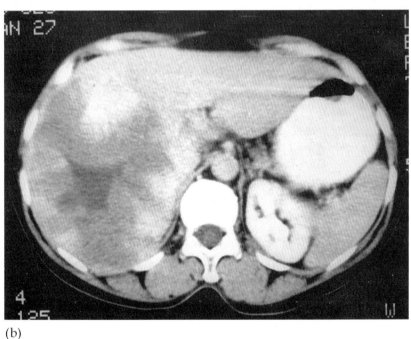

(b)

Fig. 12.8 Cavernous haemangioma. (a) Large low-attenuation tumour with central cleft demonstrating (b) the creeping enhancement pattern of a haemangioma with filling in of the tumour.

are the two primary therapeutic options. Spontaneous regression following withdrawal of the oral contraceptive pill has been documented.

The difference in presentation and treatment of liver cell adenoma makes radiological and pathological differentiation from less significant tumours important.

Radiological findings

There are no specific ultrasound characteristics that differentiate liver cell adenoma from other causes of focal tumour, although the presence of a subcapsular haemorrhage or haemoperitoneum coupled with the clinical and biochemical data

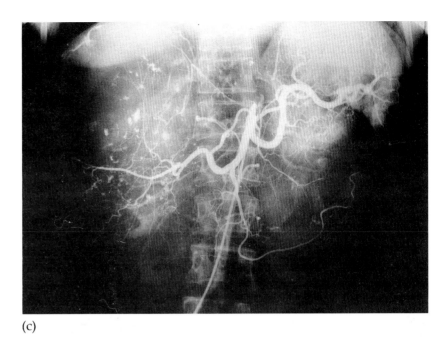

(c)

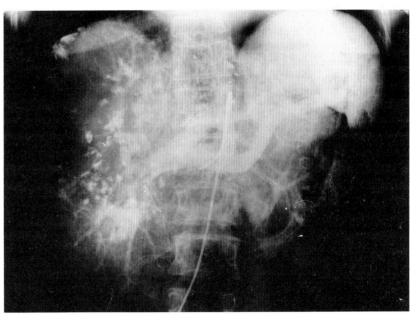

Fig. 12.8 (c), (d) Arteriography of same lesion demonstrating normal sized supplying arteries but with pools of contrast developing and remaining throughout the hepatogram phase of the insertion. This reflects the absence of intratumoral shunting.

(d)

should alert the radiologist to the diagnosis. Areas of central necrosis may be demonstrable. Sulphur colloid scintigraphy will demonstrate a photon-deficient area and this factor may differentiate the tumour from focal nodular hyperplasia but not from other causes (Casarella *et al.*, 1978). No conclusive differentiating features are present on CT. Adenomata are generally of low attenuation on the precontrast scans, although isodense tumours have been described which can only be recognized by their distortion of the surface contour of the liver.

A low-density peripheral ring around the tumour has been described as a characteristic (Angres *et al.*, 1980). This has been attributed to the excess of lipid-laden hepatocytes contained in the tumour capsule. The enhancement pattern varies according to the vascularity of the tumour. Up to 50% of adenomata are avascular and this is reflected in their CT pattern. As with ultrasound, areas of central necrosis and haemorrhage may be visible.

Angiography will generally demonstrate the vascular supply entering from the periphery of the

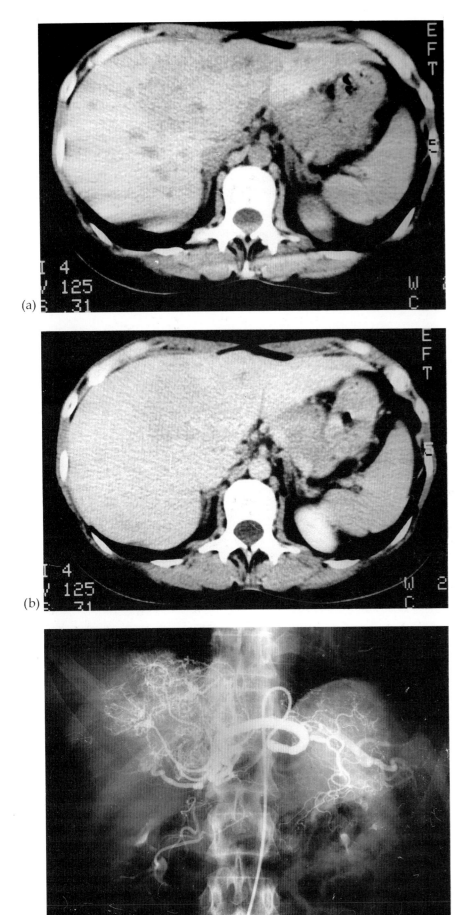

Fig. 12.9 Focal nodular hyperplasia. Non-specific CT characteristics of a low-attenuation tumour which becomes isodense following intravenous contrast (a,b,). Arteriography (c) demonstrates a large left hepatic artery supplying the tumour with a vascular tumour supplied from the periphery of the lesion.

tumour. The vessels may have a bizarre anarchic pattern in the arterial phase but generally exhibit a well-circumscribed homogeneous blush in the hepatogram phase. Irregular attenuated vessels with pools of contrast in the hepatogram phase may be present at other sites in the liver (Wallace & Chuang, 1983). This pattern of peliosis hepatis, which is thought to represent dilated hepatic sinusoid, is a helpful diagnostic feature. The arterial pattern may be indistinguishable from focal nodular hyperplasia and well-differentiated hepatocellular carcinoma. Thus, as with all liver tumours, the diagnosis is made following correlation of all clinical radiological, and histological data. As previously stated, a significant proportion of adenomas will be avascular and may only be demonstrable because of the mass effect they exert with displacement of adjacent arteries and portal vein radicles.

Future trends

The newer techniques, rather than replacing, have tended to complement the pre-existing imaging modalities in the diagnosis of liver tumours. This same development pattern will probably be followed by MRI. Now that improved images are obtained with respiratory and cardiac gating techniques, its role will be fully explored. Its detection of vascular anatomy without contrast allows investigation of the relationship of the hepatic vasculature to focal tumours. Multiplanar imaging will aid tumour mapping and resection evaluation. Focal lesions are well demonstrated (Doyle *et al.*, 1982, Moss *et al.*, 1984). A characteristic pattern has been described for cavernous haemangioma (Itai *et al.*, 1985, Stark *et al.*, 1985). The role of intravenous gandolinium has not been fully evaluated. Long scan times for acquisition of data, and limited resource, will probably result in the reservation of MRI for patients where curative surgery is planned and there remains doubt as to the extent of the tumour.

Intrahepatic arterial antitumour therapy is an area with rapid developments (which are too extensive to review); this will undoubtedly continue to provide a role for the interventional arm of radiology.

References

Akwari, O.E. & Kelly, K.A. (1979) Surgical treatment of adenocarcinoma. *Archives of Surgery*, **114**, 22.

Angres, G., Carter, J.B. & Velasco, J.M. (1980) An unusual ring in liver cell adenoma. *American Journal of Roentgenology*, **135**, 172

Barnett, P.H., Zerhouni, E.A., White, R.I. & Siegelman, S.S. (1980) C.T. in the diagnosis of cavernous hemangioma of the liver. *American Journal of Roentgenology*, **134**, 439.

Beasley, R.P., Lin, C.C., Hwang, Ly & Chien, C.S. (1981) Hepatocellular carcinoma and hepatitis B virus: A prospective study of 22707 men in Taiwan. *Lancet*, **ii**, 1129–1132.

Bernardino, M.E., Erwin, B.C., Steinberg, H.N. *et al.* (1986) Delayed hepatic C.T. scanning. Increased confidence and improved detection of hepatic metastases. *Radiology*, **159**, 71–74.

Blumgart, L.H., Benjamin, I.S., Hadsis, N.S. & Beasley R. (1984) Surgical approaches to cholangiocarcinoma at the confluence of the hepatic ducts. *Lancet*, **ii**, 66–70.

Bulatao-Jayne, J., Almero, E.M, Castro, C.A., Jardeleza, T.H. & Samalat, L.A. (1982) A case control study of primary liver cancer risk from aflatoxin exposure. *International Journal of Epidemiology*, **11**, 112–119.

Casarella, W., Knowles, D., Wolfe, M. & Johnson, P. (1978) Focal nodular hyperplasia and liver cell adenoma: radiologic and pathologic differentiation. *American Journal of Roentgenology*, **131**, 393–402.

Cottone, M., Marcelo, M.P., Maringhini, A. *et al.* (1983) Ultrasound in the diagnosis of hepatocellular carcinoma associated with cirrhosis. *Radiology*, **147**, 517–519.

Doyle, F.H., Pennock, J.M. & Banks, L.M. (1982) Nuclear magnetic resonance imaging of the liver: initial experience. *American Journal of Roentgenology*, **138**, 193–200.

Dubbins, P.A., O'Riordan, D., Melia, W.M. (1981) Ultrasound in hepatoma: Can a specific diagnosis be made? *British Journal of Radiology*, **54**, 307–311.

Ebara, M., Ohto, M., Shinagawa, T. *et al.* (1986) Natural history of hepatocellular carcinoma smaller than three centimeters complicating cirrhosis. *Gastroenterology*, **90**, 289–298.

Forman, D., Vincent, T.J. & Doll, R. (1986) Cancer of the liver and the use of oral contraceptives. *British Medical Journal*, **292**, 1357–1361.

Freeny, P.C., Nimont, T.R. & Barnett, D.C. (1979) Cavernous hemangioma of the liver: ultrasonography, arteriorgraphy and computed tomography. *Radiology*, **132**, 143.

Goldstein, H.M., Neiman, J.L., Mena E., Bookstein, J.J. & Appelman, H.D. (1974) Angiographic findings in benign liver cell tumors. *Radiology*, **110**, 339.

Huguet, C.I. & Mouiel, C. (1983). *Les Tumeurs Primitives du Foie chez L'adulte*. Masson Paris.

Ishak, K.G. & Rabin L.N: (1975) Benign tumors of the liver.*Medical Clinics of North America*, **59**, 995.

Ishak, K.G. Sesterhenn, I.A., Goodman Z.D. *et al.* (1984) Epithelioid hemangioendothelioma of the liver. A clinical, pathologic and follow-up study of 32 cases. *Human Pathology*, **15**, 839–852.

Itai, Y., Furni, S., Araki, T., Yashiro, N. & Tasaka, A. (1980) Computed tomography of cavernous hemangioma of the liver. *Radiology*, **137**, 149.

Itai, Y., Ohtomo, K., Furui, S. *et al.* (1985) Non-invasive diagnosis of small cavernous hemangioma: Advantage of M.R.I. *American Journal of Roentgenology*, **145**, 1195–1199.

Jaffe, B.M., Donegan, W.L., Watson, F. & Spratt, J.S. Jr. (1968) Factors influencing survival in patients with untreated hepatic metastases. *Surgery Gynecology and Obstetrics*, **127**, 1.

Johnson, C.M., Sheedy, P.F II, Stanson, A.W., Stephens, D.H., Hattery, R.R. & Adson, M.A. (1981) C.T. and angiograph of cavernous hemangioma of the liver. *Radiology*, **138**, 115.

Johnson, P.J., Krasner, N., Portmann, B., Eddleston, A. & Williams, R. (1978) Hepatocellular carcinoma in Great Britain: influence of age, sex, HbsAg status and aetiology of underlying cirrhosis. *Gut*, **19**, 1022–1026.

Johnson, P.J., Portmann, B. & Williams, R. (1978) Alpha-feto-protein concentration measured by radio-immunoassay in the diagnosing and excluding of hepatocellular carcinoma. *British Medical Journal*, **2**, 661–663.

Karani, J., Fletcher, D., Brinkley, D., Dawson J., Williams, R. & Nunnerley, H. (1985) Internal biliary drainage and local radiotherapy with iridium-192 wire in treatment of hilar cholangiocarcinoma. *Clinical Radiology*, **36**, 603–606.

Kew, M.C. & Popper, H. (1984) Relationship between hepatocellular carcinoma and cirrhosis. *Seminars in Liver Disease*, **4**, 136–146.

Klatskin, G. (1965) Adenocarcinoma of the hepatic duct at its bifurcation within the porta hepatis. An unusual tumor with distinctive clinical and pathological features. *American Journal of Medicine*, **38**, 241–256.

Lees, W.R., Hall-Craggs, M.A. & Manhire, A. (1985) Five years experience of fine needle aspiration: biopsy of 454 consecutive cases. *Clinical Radiology*, **36**, 517–520.

Margolis, M., Homcy, C. (1972) Systemic manifestations of hepatoma. *Medicine (Baltimore)*, **51**, 381.

Mays, E.T., Christopherson, W.W. Mahr, M.M. & Williams, H.C. (1976) Hepatic changes in young women ingesting contraceptive steroids. Hepatic hemorrhage and primary hepatic tumours. *Journal of the American Medical Association*, **235**, 730.

Melia, W.M., Wilkinson, M.L., Portmann, B.C. *et al.* (1984) Hepatocellular carcinoma in the non-cirrhotic liver: a comparison with that complicating cirrhosis. *Quarterly Journal of Medicine*, **211**, 391–400.

Moss, A.A., Goldberg, H.I., Stark, D.B. *et al.* (1984) Hepatic tumours: magnetic resonance and C.T. appearance. *Radiology*, **150**, 141–147.

Nagasue, N., Yukaya, H., Hamada, T. *et al.* (1984) The natural history of hepatocellular carcinoma. *Cancer*, **54**, 1461–1465.

Ong, G.B. & Taw, S.L. (1922) Spontaneous rupture of hepatocellular carcinoma. *British Medical Journal*, **4**, 146–149.

Pickren, J.W. Tsukada, Y. & Lane W.W. (1982) Liver metastasis: analysis of autopsy data. In Weiss, I. & Gilbert, H.A. (eds) *Liver Metastasis*: pp. 12–18. G.K. Hall, Boston.

Soreide, O., Czerniak, A., Bradpiece, H., Bloom, S. & Blumgart, L (1986) Characteristics of fibrolamellar hepatocellular carcinoma: a study of nine cases and review of the literature. *American Journal of Surgery*, **151**, 518–523.

Stark, D.D., Felder, R.C., Wittenberg, J. *et al.* (1985) Magnetic resonance imaging of cavernous hemangioma of the liver tissue specific characterisation. *American Journal of Roentgenology*, **145**, 213–222.

Wallace, S. (1977) Primary liver tumours. In Parker, B.R. & Castellino, R.A. (eds) *Pediatric Oncologic Radiology*, p. 301. C.V. Mosby, St Louis.

Wallace, S. & Chuang, V. (1983) Liver tumours: diagnosis and management. In Herlinger, H., Lunderquist, A. & Wallace S. (eds) *Clinical Radiology of the Liver*, pp. 715–864. Marcel Dekker Inc., New York.

Wheeler, P.G., Dawson, J.L., Nunnerley, H., Brinkley, D. & Laws, J. (1981) Newer techniques in the diagnosis and treatment of proximal bile duct carcinoma — an analysis of 41 consecutive patients. *Quarterly Journal of Medicine*, **50**, 247–259.

Willis, R.A. (1973) Secondary tumours of the liver. In *The Spread of Tumours in the Human Body*, Butterworths, London.

Yu, M.C. Mack T., Hanisch R. *et al.* (1983) Hepatitis, alcohol consumption, cigarette smoking and hepatocellular carcinoma in Los Angeles. *Cancer Research*, **43**, 6077–6079.

Yumoto, Y., Jinno, K., Tokuyama, K. *et al.* (1985) Intrahepatic arterial administration of Lipiodol for detection of minute hepatocellular carcinoma. *Radiology*, **154**, 19–24.

Zamcheck, N. & Klausenstock, O. (1953) Liver biopsy II: the risk of needle biopsy. *New England Journal of Medicine*, **249**, 1062.

13: Tumours in Children

A.D. JOYCE AND E.R. HOWARD

Introduction

Primary hepatic tumours are the third most common solid abdominal tumour in children. Two-thirds are malignant and the effective management of these tumours relies upon a logical protocol of investigation. In the past it has often been difficult to determine the status of these tumours, but recent advances in diagnostic techniques may now be used to establish accurately the size, location, and anatomy prior to surgery, when the safe resection of up to 85% of the liver substance can safely be performed. The prognosis for benign lesions is excellent, but for those with malignant tumours the cure rate is poor with only 30% of hepatoblastomas being surgically resectable.

Pathology

Hepatic tumours

The common primary tumours are derived either from the hepatocyte or surrounding mesenchymal supporting structures (Fig. 13.1). Benign lesions have a lower incidence than malignant tumours. It is often difficult to determine the diagnosis prior to histological examination.

BENIGN

Haemangioma

Vascular neoplasms are the commonest benign hepatic tumour of childhood, and 90% are discovered before the age of 6 months. Dehner & Ishak (1971) described two histological subtypes; haemangioendothelioma and cavernous haemangioma, but many haemangiomata show features of both types. The tumours, like cutaneous haemangiomata, may enlarge during the first few months of life and undergo subsequent regression. Enlarge-ment of haemangioendotheliomata is associated with arteriovenous shunting (Fig. 13.2) that may precipitate cardiac failure or even spontaneous rupture of the tumour (Rocchini et al., 1976). In contrast, cavernous haemangiomata usually have normal-sized feeding vessels and arteriovenous shunting is rare (Dachman et al., 1983). There is little correlation between tumour size and the degree of cardiac failure, but the high-output failure tends to be unresponsive to medical treatment, with a 50% mortality in young infants not treated by surgery (Braun et al., 1975).

Mesenchymal hamartoma

First described by Maresch in 1903, this is a benign cystic developmental anomaly thought to arise from the connective tissue of the portal tracts. It is characteristically seen in infants and young children, where ultrasonography reveals a collection of fluid-filled cysts. CT examination shows a multilocular cystic mass with septations and variable

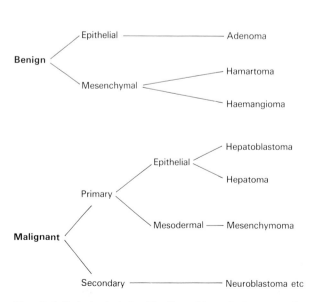

Fig. 13.1 Pathological classification of hepatic tumours of childhood.

187

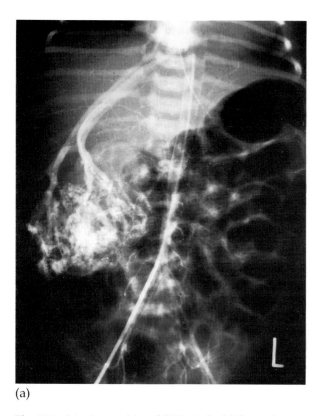

(a)

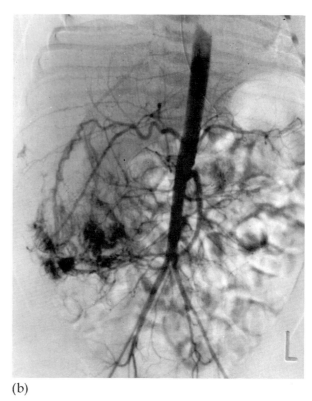

(b)

Fig. 13.2 Arteriogram (a) and DSA study (b) illustrating a cavernous haemangioma and early filling of the hepatic vein due to arteriovenous shunting. The lesion presented as a mass in the right hypochondrium and cardiac failure.

solid components. Typically the tumour is confined to one lobe, often attached to the lower edge via a pedicle, and surgery is indicated if these enlarge and compress adjacent viscera.

Other benign tumours

Adenomata, focal nodular hyperplasia, lymph-angiomata, teratomata and simple cysts may present in childhood, but these are extremely uncommon, comprising 2% of hepatic tumours in the American Academy of Pediatric Surgical Section Survey (Exelby *et al.*, 1974). Adenomata are associated with glycogen storage disease type I (von Gierke's disease) but can be difficult to distinguish histologically from a well-differentiated hepatocellular carcinoma, thus resection is recommended by most authors (Ishak, 1976). Focal nodular hyperplasia has no malignant potential and resection is only necessary if there is histological doubt or the patient is symptomatic (Whelan *et al.*, 1973).

MALIGNANT

Primary hepatic malignancy accounts for approximately 5% of all paediatric neoplasms (Wallace, 1977), whilst metastatic involvement of the liver is even more frequent. Liver tumours have been associated with certain congenital hepatic disorders, extrahepatic anomalies, and metabolic disorders (Table 13.1).

Hepatoblastoma

This is the third most commonly encountered intra-abdominal malignant neoplasm after neuroblastoma, with a peak incidence in infancy. Hepatoblastoma is a malignant tumour arising from primitive epithelial cells characteristic of the fetal liver. In addition to a rapid growth rate the tumour is highly invasive, capable of spreading within the liver and metastasizing to extrahepatic sites, commonly the lungs and abdominal lymph nodes. Bone metastases are rare.

Table 13.1 Reported associations with childhood hepatic tumours (Clatworthy *et al.*, 1974, Weinberg *et al.*, 1976, deLorimier, 1977, Filler & Hagen, 1981, Altman & Schwartz, 1983, Kingston *et al.*, 1983)

Anomalies	Congenital hepatic disorders	Other associations
Hemihypertrophy Haemangioma	Biliary atresia Neonatal hepatitis von Gierke's disease Lipid storage disease Hereditary tyrosinaemia	Osteoporosis Polyposis coli Androgen therapy de Toni–Fanconi syndrome

Hepatocellular carcinoma

Hepatoma is unusual in the very young age group, having a peak incidence in adolescence and accounting for 20% of all primary hepatic tumours (Lack *et al.*, 1983).

Hepatomata have been reported to follow neonatal hepatitis, biliary atresia, and several metabolic disorders (Altman & Schwartz, 1983). Various childhood diseases predispose to cirrhosis, but these do not appear to place the child at risk for hepatoma. A notable exception is hereditary tyrosinaemia, in which it is estimated that 30% of the children will develop hepatoma. Overall the prognosis for this tumour is grim, but the variant fibrolamellar carcinoma has a higher rate of resectability and a longer duration of survival.

Mesenchymoma

Macroscopically these appear as a necrotic cystic tumour mass and microscopically the cells appear anaplastic with frequent mitoses. Smithson *et al.*, (1982) reported a survival rate, at best, of 33% after surgery. One case received postoperative radiation and chemotherapy to survive 6 years.

Metastatic disease

The liver is a common site for metastases from tumours in other organs. This spread may occur by direct extension or from haematogenous spread in patients with neuroblastoma, nephroblastoma, or rhabdomyosarcoma, whilst focal involvement may occur in children with leukaemia or lymphoma. A particular subgroup of disseminated neuroblastoma has been associated with a good prognosis. Classified as stage IV S by Evans these children present with a rapidly growing liver, elevated catecholamines, positive bone-marrow aspirate, and 30% have metastatic skin lesions (Evans *et al.*, 1971). The majority are infants less than 12 months of age and the primary lesions may not be easily identifiable. In 1980 Evans reviewed 17 patients with IV S disease; 55% were found to have spontaneous regression of all or part of their disease and death only occurred as a complication of the local disease.

Bile duct neoplasm

Benign

These are usually inflammatory tumours of the extrahepatic bile ducts and present with obstructive jaundice. The aetiology is unknown but thought to be secondary to a local irritant. The tumour appears yellow-brown with a mixed inflammatory cell infiltrate in a dense fibrous tissue matrix. Excision and reconstruction is usually curative (Stamatakis *et al.*, 1979).

Malignant

The commonest primary tumour of the extrahepatic biliary tract is the rhabdomyosarcoma (Lack *et al.*, 1981). The tumour is an important differential in the diagnosis of obstructive jaundice in childhood. The average survival time is 4.3 months with metastases in 40% of patients, for unlike rhabdomyosarcoma in other sites, radical resection is technically difficult and adjuvant therapy is indicated.

Diagnosis

Clinical findings

Most children present with asymptomatic hepatomegaly which can be of a severe degree, extending to below the level of the umbilicus. The presence of abdominal pain and weight loss is indicative of advanced malignant disease (Ishak & Glunz, 1967), and due to ischaemic infarction or haemorrhage within the tumour. Cutaneous lesions are seen in 45% of haemangiomata, and the diagnosis is reinforced if associated with a high-output cardiac state.

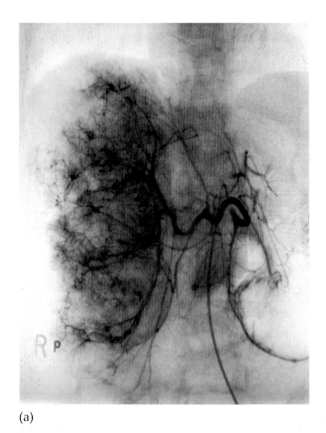

(a)

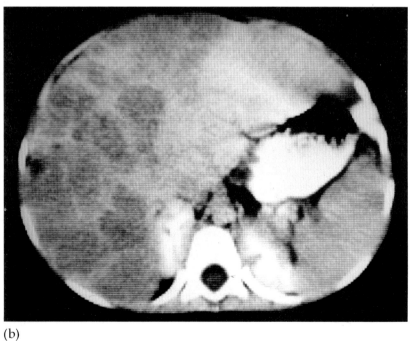

(b)

Fig. 13.3 Angiogram (a) and CT (b) scan illustrating a malignant hepatoblastoma occupying the right lobe of the liver in a 1-year-old child. The tumour was resected completely.

Laboratory investigations are often unremarkable except for a corresponding anaemia or thrombocytopenia if haemorrhage has occurred. Abnormal liver function is only seen in those with pre-existing liver disease or end-stage disease. Serum alphaprotein levels have been more re-warding as a diagnostic tool (Miller *et al.*, 1977). An elevated alphafetoprotein is seen in two-thirds of hepatic malignancies, but notably it is not elevated in fibrolamellar carcinoma and mesenchymoma. In some benign lesions, mesenchymal hamartoma, a mildly elevated alphafetoprotein

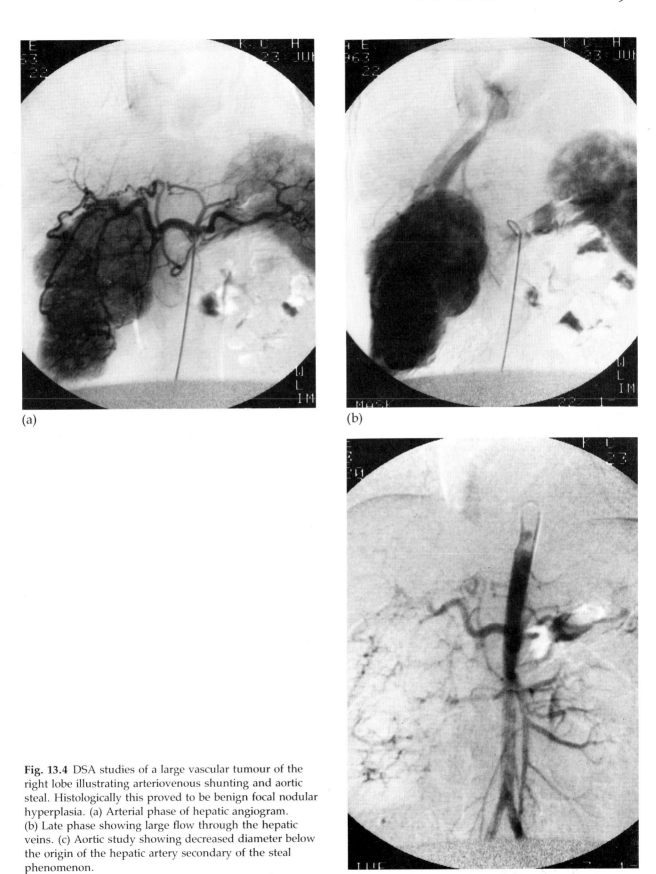

Fig. 13.4 DSA studies of a large vascular tumour of the right lobe illustrating arteriovenous shunting and aortic steal. Histologically this proved to be benign focal nodular hyperplasia. (a) Arterial phase of hepatic angiogram. (b) Late phase showing large flow through the hepatic veins. (c) Aortic study showing decreased diameter below the origin of the hepatic artery secondary of the steal phenomenon.

level can be detected. When positive, alphafeto-protein is a useful tumour marker to assess the efficacy of treatment and the presence of recurrent disease (McIntyre *et al.*, 1976). Malignant liver tumours have also been associated with the abnormal endocrine production of HCG resulting in signs of precocious puberty.

Radiology

Ultrasound is recommended as the screening procedure in children with hepatomegaly (Kaude *et al.*, 1980), as it is inexpensive, non-invasive, and does not involve ionizing radiation. In most cases benign lesions can be identified. However, there are limitations in defining the anatomic location and extent of the tumour (Kirks *et al.*, 1981). Most units use computerized tomography as a screening procedure after ultrasound, so that only children with potentially resectable neoplasms undergo angiography; this is invasive, sometimes technically difficult, and requires a general anaesthetic. Although CT is not totally reliable in assessing tumour extent, it is claimed that the risk of false positive diagnoses is rare so that the disease will not be overestimated (Amendola *et al.*, 1984). Most neoplasms have a characteristic CT appearance and visualization of isodense hepatic tumours may be improved by intravenous administration of urographic contrast media as a bolus or infusion. CT is of unquestionable value in the diagnosis of cavernous haemangiomata and Itai *et al.*, in 1983

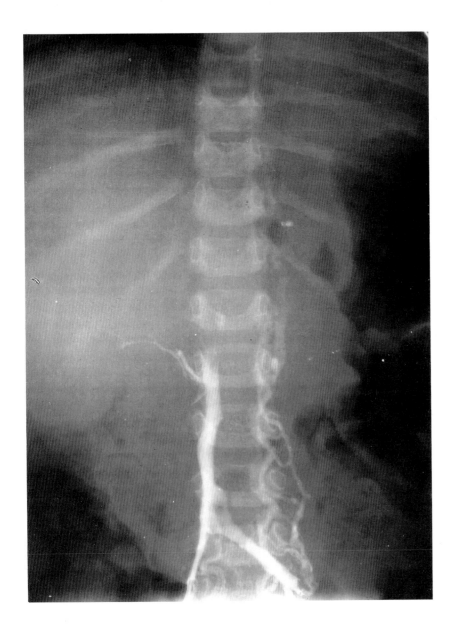

Fig. 13.5 Cavogram performed in a child with a malignant hepatoblastoma, illustrating the difficulty in assessing invasion from extrinsic compression. The inferior vena cava was not invaded by tumour and the tumour was resected.

described four diagnostic CT criteria for a liver haemangioma. However, the uptake of contrast material is not constant, especially if any thrombosis has occurred or there are anomalies of the vascular tree. Computerized tomography has been especially recommended in the determination of malignant neoplasms using contrast enhancement. Hepatoblastomata have a lower attenuation than normal liver and this is accentuated after injection of contrast media. Calcification is highly suggestive of haemangioendothelioma in infants younger than 1 year, though it is non-specific (Dachman *et al.*, 1983) and is seen occasionally in both hepatoblastoma and hepatoma.

Opinions vary on the role of angiography but we consider that selective coeliac arteriography gives important information on tumour pathology, resectability, and the surgical anatomy of the hepatic vasculature, especially as hepatic neoplasms derive their blood supply almost exclusively from the arterial rather than the portal venous system (Figs 13.3, 13.4). The recent introduction of intra-arterial digital subtraction angiography gives excellent imaging of the portal venous system using low-dose selective arterial injections of contrast media and consequent reduction of the examination time (Foley *et al.*, 1983). At present we have relied on the venous phase of the arteriogram to detect the portal vein. Inferior venocavography to assess tumour invasion tends to be misleading, as it is difficult to distinguish occlusion from extrinsic compression (Fig. 13.5). Indeed, the final decision on resectability may be possible only at laparotomy. From our comparison of the merits of ultrasound, computerized tomography, and angiography we suggest an integrated approach to the diagnosis of a child with hepatomegaly (Fig. 13.6). Of the radiological investigations, CT and hepatic angiography have become the most valuable in defining the extent and resectability of the disease, whilst ultrasound is invaluable in the early screening of hepatic masses. Isotope liver scans have a limited value as they lack specificity and often fail to illustrate the full extent of the disease.

Percutaneous liver biopsy may not be totally reliable, and hepatic haemangiomata have been regarded as a contraindication to needle biopsy (Kato *et al.*, 1975). Fine-needle aspiration biopsy has been performed in some centres (Van Sonnenberg *et al.*, 1981) without complications, but it is advised that this technique is performed under CT guidance. Sampling errors can occur, leading to false diagnoses and we have encoun-

tered two cases of tumour seeding onto the abdominal wall after needle biopsy of malignant tumour.

Tumours of the extrahepatic biliary tree are extremely rare and usually present with obstructive jaundice. Diagnosis depends on a combination of ultrasound and cholangiography.

Treatment

Hepatic tumours

It is generally accepted that surgery is necessary for the cure of primary malignant neoplasms of the liver, and resection is necessary for the majority of benign neoplasms.

Haemangiomata less than 3 cm can be managed conservatively with regular ultrasonography, as spontaneous resolution usually starts within 6–8 months. Surgery can thus be reserved for those children with expanding tumours causing symptoms or the development of complications such as high-output failure or haemorrhage. The treatment regimens for these haemangiomata have included steroids (Goldberg & Fonkalsrud, 1969),

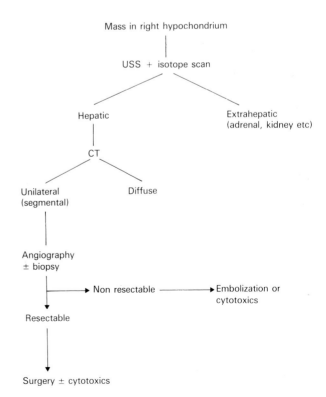

Fig. 13.6 Integrated algorithmic approach to the investigation of a child presenting with a mass in the right hypochondrium.

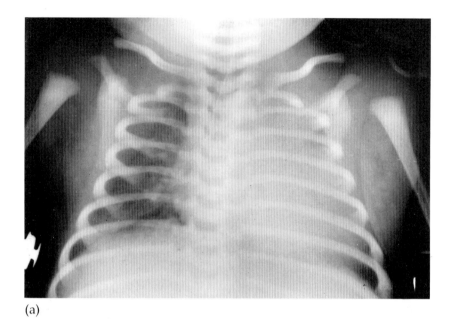

(a)

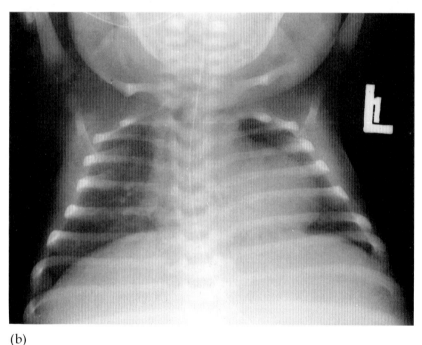

(b)

Fig. 13.7 Chest X-ray, before (a) and after (b) hepatic artery ligation in an infant with congestive cardiac failure secondary to a cavernous haemangioma. The examinations were separated by an interval of 4 weeks.

radiotherapy (Rotman *et al.*, 1980), and hepatic-artery ligation and resection (Larcher *et al.*, 1981). It is now clear that hepatic-artery ligation is very effective in a majority of cases with cardiac failure (Fig. 13.7) and we suggest the following course of management (Larcher *et al.*, 1981):

1 In the absence of complications, infants are simply monitored until regression occurs.

2 Infants under 6 weeks of age in cardiac failure undergo hepatic-artery ligation because of the high mortality in this age group.

3 Infants over 6 weeks of age receive medical management of the cardiac failure, and failure to respond within 2 weeks is an indication for hepatic-artery ligation.

In the absence of liver disease, sepsis, or shock hepatic artery ligation can be performed with the minimum of morbidity even in a sick infant (Moazam *et al.*, 1983). Surgical resection may be necessary for the rare cases complicated by spontaneous haemorrhage (Trastek *et al.*, 1983).

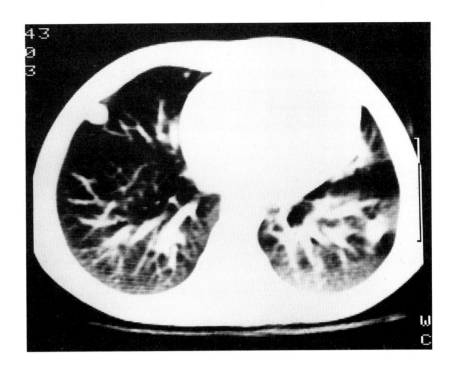

Fig. 13.8 CT scan illustrating a solitary metastasis in the periphery of the right lung.

RESECTION

Eighty-five per cent of the liver may be safely resected and a significant portion will have regenerated by 1 month; full regeneration is seen in 3–6 months. Tumours extending beyond the falciform ligament or around the porta hepatis are deemed inoperable. An attempt at tumour reduction may be obtained by embolization of the relevant hepatic artery or by a course of chemotherapy which may then allow tumour resection. Transcatheter hepatic artery embolization using gelfoam has become an established treatment method for hepatic tumours (Chaung & Wallace 1981, Nakamura *et al.*, 1983). It helps to decrease the vascularity and tumour size preoperatively and may be a palliative treatment option for patients with inoperable tumours. Post-embolization vomiting, pain, and fever may occur but usually resolve with symptomatic treatment. Inadvertent embolization of the gastroduodenal artery may result in peptic ulceration and pancreatitis, and the procedure makes subsequent surgery more demanding due to the increased inflammatory response around the porta hepatis.

We use the standard resection technique described by Starzl & Putnam (1977). We do not employ haemodilution, hypothermia-anaesthesia, or biliary intubation, although supra- and infrahepatic clamping of the inferior vena cava is a valuable method of reducing blood loss with very large tumours. Postoperatively our long-term follow-up of patients includes ^{99m}technetium isotope liver scans to assess regeneration. Serial estimations of alphafetoprotein are used in conjunction with chest radiology and ultrasound to detect tumour recurrence. Any sequential rise in the alphafetoprotein levels merits CT of the lungs (Fig. 13.8) and abdomen to detect any local or distant recurrence. Clinical evidence of local recurrence merits a 'second look' laparotomy with a view to further tumour resection. Other centres are describing similar successes (Andrassy *et al.*, 1980, Weinblatt *et al.*, 1982). Our longest survivor has now completed 4 years after removal of recurrent tumour.

CHEMOTHERAPY

Cure after surgical excision in children with hepatoblastoma and hepatoma is reported as 60% and 33% respectively, but 50% have unresectable disease at diagnosis. Recent studies have assessed the role of cytotoxics in the management of malignant lesions, and Adriamycin and cis-platinum have proved to be the most effective agents (Weinblatt *et al.*, 1982).

Bile duct tumours

The benign tumours are best managed by excision and Roux-en-Y reconstruction, with resection being curative. Rhabdomyosarcomata of the bile duct are curious in that they appear in a site normally devoid of voluntary muscle. In contrast to the treatment successes of tumour in other sites, the biliary tumours have a dismal prognosis with local invasion of the hepatic artery or portal vein rending curative surgery impossible (Longmire *et al.*, 1973). The best results are obtained with a combination of surgery, chemotherapy, and radiotherapy.

References

Altman, R.P. & Schwartz, A.D. (1983) Malignant disease of infance, childhood and adolescence, 2nd ed p.254. W.B. Saunders, Philadelphia.

Amendola, M.A., Blane, C.E., Amendola, B.E. & Glazer, G.M. (1984) CT in hepatoblastoma. *Journal of Computer Assisted Tomography*, **8**, 1105–1109.

Andrassy, R.J., Brennan, L.P. & Siegele M.M. (1980) Pre-operative chemotherapy for hepatoblastoma in children: report of six cases. *Journal of Pediatric Surgery*, **15**, 517–522.

Braun, P., Ducharme, J.C., Riopelle, J.L. & Davignon, A. (1975) Hemangiomata of the liver in infants. *Journal of Pediatric Surgery*, **10**, 121–126.

Chaung V.P. & Wallace, S. (1981) Hepatic artery embolisation in the treatment of hepatic neoplasms. *Radiology*, **140**, 51–58.

Clatworthy, W. Jr., Schiller, M. & Grosfeld, J.L. (1974) Primary liver tumors in infancy and childhood. *Archives of Surgery*, **109**, 143–147.

Dachman, A.H., Lichtenstein, J.E., Friedman, A.C. & Hartman, D.S. (1983) Infantile hemangioendothelioma of the liver: a radiologic–pathologic–clinical correlation. *American Journal of Roentgenology*, **140**, 1091–1096.

Dehner, L.P. & Ishak, K.S. (1971) Vascular tumors of the liver in infants and children. *Archives of Pathology*, **92**, 101–111.

deLorimier, A.A. (1977). Hepatic tumors of infancy and childhood. *Surgical Clinics of North America*, **57**, 443–448.

Evans, A.E. D'Angio, G.J. & Randolph, J. (1971) A proposed staging for children with neuroblastoma. *Cancer*, **27**, 374–378.

Evans, A.E., Chatter, Y., D'Angio, G.J., Gerson, J.M., Robson, J. & Schnaufer, L. (1980) Review of 17 IV S neuroblastoma patients at the Children's Hospital of Philadelphia. *Cancer*, **45**, 833–839.

Exelby, P.R. Filler, R.M. & Grosfeld, J.L. (1974) Liver tumours in children in particular reference to hepatoblastoma and hepatocellular carcinoma. (American academy of Pediatric Surgical Section Survey.) *Journal of Pediatric Surgery*, **19**, 329–337.

Filler, R.M. & Hagen, J. (1981) Liver tumours. *Surgical Clinics of North America*, **61**(5), 1209–1217.

Foley, D.W., Stewart, E.T., Milbrath, J.A., San Dretto, M. & Milde, M. (1983) Digital subtraction angiography of the portal venous system. *American Journal of Roentgenology*, **140**, 497–499.

Goldberg, S.J. & Fonkalsrud, E. (1969) Successful treatment of hepatic hemangioma with corticosteroids. *Journal of the American Medical Association*, **208**, 2473–2474.

Ishak, K.G. (1976) Primary hepatic tumors in childhood. *Progress in Liver Diseases*, **5**, 636–667.

Ishak, K.G. & Glunz, P.R. (1967) Hepatoblastoma and hepatocarcinoma in infancy and childhood. *Cancer*, **20**, 396–422.

Itai, Y., Ohmtama, K., Araki, T., Furui, S., Iis, M. & Atomi, Y. (1983) Computer tomography and sonography of cavernous hemangioma of the liver *American Journal of Roentgenology*, **141**, 315–320.

Kato, M., Sugawara, I. & Okuda, A. (1975) Hemangioma of the liver, diagnosis with combined use of laparoscopy and hepatic arteriography. *American Journal of Surgery*, **129**, 698–704.

Kaude, J.V., Felman, J.H. & Hawkins, I.F. Jr. (1980) Ultrasonography in primary hepatic tumors in childhood. *Radiology*, **124**, 451–458.

Kingston, J.E., Herbert, A, Draper, G.J. & Mann, J.R. (1983) Association between hepatoblastoma and polyposis coli. *Archives of Disease in Childhood*, **58**, 959–962.

Kirks, D.R., Merton, D.F., Grossman, H. & Bowie, J.D. (1981) Diagnostic imaging of pediatric abdominal masses: an overview. *Radiologic Clinics of North America*, **19**, 527–545.

Lack, E.E., Neave, C. & Vawter, G.F. (1983) Hepatocellular carcinoma *Cancer*, **52**, 1510–1515.

Lack, E.E., Perez-Atayde, A.R. & Shuster, S.R. (1981) Botryoid rhabdomyosarcoma of the biliary tract, report of 5 cases with ultrastructural observations and literature review. *American Journal of Surgical Pathology*, **5**, 643–652.

Larcher, V.F., Howard, E.R. & Mowat, A.P. (1981) Hepatic haemangiomata: diagnosis and management. *Archives of Disease in Childhood*, **56**, 7–14.

Longmire, W.P., McArthur M.S., Bastouris, E.A. & Hiatt, J. (1973) Carcinoma of the extrahepatic biliary tract. *Annals of Surgery*, **184**, 68–73.

McIntyre, K.R., Vogel, C.L. & Primack, A. (1976) Effect of survival and chemotherapeutic treatment on alphafetoprotein levels in patients with hepatocellular carcinoma. *Cancer*, **37**, 677.

Maresch, R. (1903) Über ein Lymphangiom der Leber. *Zeitschrift für Kinderheilkunde*, **24**, 39–50.

Miller, J.H., Gates G.F. & Stanley, P. (1977) The radiologic investigations of hepatic tumors in childhood. *Radiology*, **124**, 451–458.

Moazam, F., Rodgers, B.M. & Talbert, J.L. (1983) Hepatic artery ligation for hepatic hemangiomatosis of infancy. *Journal of Pediatric Surgery*, **18**, 120–123.

Nakamura, H., Tanaka, T. & Hori, S. (1983) Transcatheter embolization of hepatocellular carcinoma: assessment of efficacy in cases of resection following embolization. *Radiology*, **147**, 401–405.

Rocchini, A.P., Rosenthal, A., Issenbert, H.J. & Nadas, A.S. (1976) Hepatic hemangioendotheliomatosis: hemodynamic observations and treatment. *Pediatrics*, **57**, 131–135.

Rotman, M., John, M., Stowe, S. & Inamdar, S. (1980) Radiation treatment of pediatric hepatic hemangiomatosis and coexisting cardiac failure. *New England Journal of Medicine*, **302**, 852.

Smithson, W.A., Telander, R.L. & Carney, J.A. (1982) Mesenchymomas of the liver in childhood: 5 year survival. *Journal of Pediatric Surgery*, **17**, 70−72.

Stamatakis, J.D., Howard, E.R., & Williams, R. (1979) Benign inflammatory tumour of the common bile duct. *British Journal of Surgery*, **66**, 257−258.

Starzl, T.E. & Putnam, C.W. (1977) Partial resections of the liver In Robb, C. & Smith, R. (eds) *Operative Surgery*, 3rd edn. Butterworths, London.

Trastek, V.F., Van Heerden J.A., Sheedy, P.F. & Anson, M.A. (1983) Cavernous haemangioma of the liver: resect or observe? *American Journal of Surgery*, **145**, 49−52.

Van Sonnenberg, E., Wittenberg, J., Ferruci, J.T., Mueller, P.R. & Simeone, J.F. (1981) Triangulation method for percutaneous needle biopsy: The angled approach to upper abdominal masses. *American Journal of Roentgenology*, **137**, 757−761.

Wallace, S. (1977) Primary liver tumours. In Parker, B.R. & Castellina, R.A. (eds) *Pediatric Oncologic Radiology*, Ch 13. Mosby, St. Louis.

Weinberg, A.G., Mize, C.E. & Worthen, H.G. (1976) The occurrence of hepatoma in the chronic form of hereditary tyrosiraemia. *Journal of Paediatric Surgery*, **88**, 434−438.

Weinblatt, M.E., Siegel, S.E., Siegel, M.E., Stanley, P. & Weitzmann, J.J. (1982) Preoperative chemotherapy for unresectable primary hepatic malignancies in children. *Cancer*, **50**, 1061−1064.

Whelan, T.J., Baugh, J.H. & Chandor, S. (1973) Focal nodular hyperplasia of the liver. *Annals of Surgery*, **177**, 150−158.

14: The Radiology of Secondary Malignant Neoplasms of the Liver

S.J. GOLDING AND E.W.L. FLETCHER

Introduction

Malignant neoplasms that metastasize to the liver are an important subject for the radiologist. Many malignant tumours involve the liver at some time during their course and in the majority of patients radiology is an essential component of management.

Many patients with hepatic metastases do not have symptoms referrable to the liver until a late stage of the disease, and the radiologist may be the first to detect metastases when carrying out examinations for other purposes. When symptoms do occur, they may consist of discomfort or pain in the upper abdomen, or jaundice due to compression of the intrahepatic bile ducts. Less commonly patients may present with abdominal pain and pyrexia, symptoms which may suggest a hepatic abscess. Metastases may also be detected in patients showing systemic effects of malignancy such as anorexia and weight loss. The demonstration by the radiologist of disease in the liver may not infrequently be the first indication that a patient has a malignant neoplasm.

New imaging techniques have given the radiologist an important place in the management of these patients. Examination of the liver is now an essential part of the initial investigation of many types of neoplasm prior to treatment and these 'staging' examinations are steadily increasing in frequency. Now that effective treatment is available for some neoplasms, examinations may be needed to monitor the response to treatment and detect relapse. Interventional techniques such as guided biopsy and angiographic embolization are also becoming common.

In this chapter we describe the demonstration of hepatic metastases by current radiological techniques and the role of the radiologist in the management of these patients.

Imaging techniques

The abdominal radiograph

Radiographs of the abdomen are usually normal in patients with hepatic metastases, but may occasionally show evidence of hepatic enlargement or calcification.

Hepatic enlargement may be revealed by elevation of the right hemidiaphragm and extension of the inferior liver margin towards or into the right iliac fossa. More commonly an enlarged liver produces a general increase in density over the upper abdomen, often with displacement of the normal gas patterns, particularly that of the transverse colon (Fig. 14.1). Only gross degrees of enlargement are evident on plain radiographs and the finding is a non-specific sign, occurring in many disorders of the liver.

Calcification is seen in a minority of metastases. When demonstrated on plain radiographs, it is frequently poorly defined and may be difficult to detect (Fig. 14.1). It is more readily demonstrated by ultrasound (US) and computerized tomography (CT), which may show calcification not revealed by conventional radiography. Most of the hepatic metastases which calcify originate from the gastro-intestinal tract, but calcification is seen sometimes in carcinoma of the breast or ovary, medullary carcinoma of the thyroid and carcinoid tumours. It is also seen in benign lesions such as cavernous haemangioma and is not therefore diagnostic of malignancy.

For obvious reasons the plain radiograph is an insensitive method of detecting hepatic disease and does not usually have a significant role in practice. It is, however, important for the radiologist to recognize these signs when they are present on abdominal radiographs.

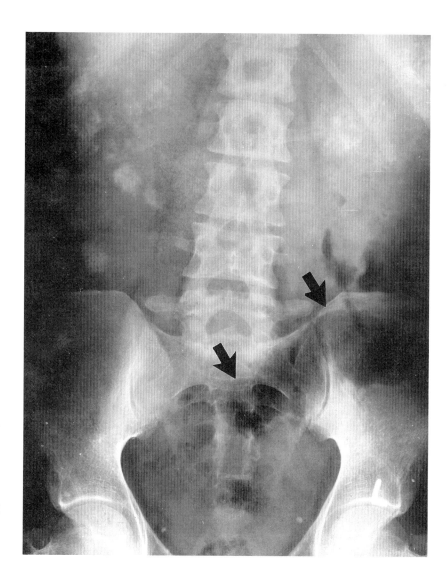

Fig. 14.1 Medullary carcinoma of thyroid. Abdominal radiography showing enlargement of the liver and numerous foci of calcification. The transverse colon (*arrows*) is displaced towards the left iliac fossa.

Ultrasound

Real-time ultrasound machines are so easy to use that it is tempting to think that anyone can be an instant expert. However, poor results are obtained unless technique is meticulous and this is nowhere more true than in the examination of the liver. The liver must be examined in both the sagittal and coronal planes and all the margins of the organ must be identified when metastases are suspected. Technique is considered in detail in Chapter 2.

Abnormal appearances

Metastases may be seen as distortion of the liver outline without any change in echo pattern. However normal bulges in the liver outline must be identified before pathology can be inferred. Normal bulges that can be seen are anteriorly where the liver edge extends below the ribs in the epigastrium, the caudate lobe, a bulge of the left lobe of the liver anterior to the aorta, and a posterior bulge where the liver overlaps the lower pole of the right kidney. Localized humps in the diaphragmatic surface of the liver are common and are usually normal. Any other focal bulge should be considered as a possible lesion. The most common sign to look for is rounding of the normal sharp inferior edge of the liver in the absence of generalized or non-specific hepatomegaly (Fig. 14.2). Less common are individual or multiple humps (Weill, 1978).

Changes in echo pattern are common in metastatic disease of the liver, with or without change in the liver outline. Many distinct patterns have been described and there is considerable overlap between the types. One of the most common is the discrete hypoechoic mass (Fig. 14.3), but echogenic

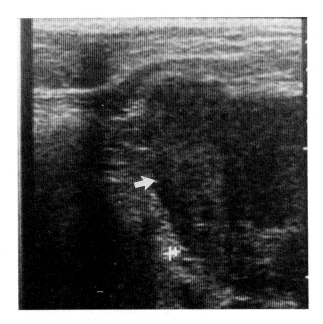

Fig. 14.2 Carcinoma of the bronchus. Sagittal ultrasound image showing rounding of the inferior border of the liver (*arrow*).

(Fig. 14.4), 'bulls eye' (Fig. 14.5) or mixed lesions (Fig. 14.6) are also common (Green *et al.* 1977, Scheible *et al.*, 1977). All these patterns may be seen in multiple or single lesions, with the so-called hail-storm pattern of multiple echo-dense metastases (Fig. 14.7) and 'sieve' pattern of multiple hypoechoic metastases (Fig. 14.8) being particularly striking.

Diffuse infiltration of the liver by secondary neoplasms is common and may produce generalized inhomogeneity of the echo pattern (Fig. 14.9). Discrete anechoic masses are rare and usually indicate necrotic metastases, but unlike benign hepatic cysts they do not have perfectly smooth margins, and an echogenic rim can often be identified (Fig. 14.10). Necrotic debris within these areas may mimic an abscess but the clinical findings usually distinguish these lesions. Large metastases at the liver margin should be examined carefully to ensure that there is no interface between the mass and the hepatic parenchyma, as other upper abdominal tumours, especially of the kidney and adrenal gland, may appear to arise from the liver (Weill, 1978).

Lymphoma, like metastases, may show a generalized alteration in the echo pattern (Fig. 14.11). Focal masses may also occur in the minority of patients. More commonly hepatomegaly is the only finding, and the diagnosis can only be inferred from associated signs such as splenomegaly, retroperitoneal lymphadenopathy and pleural effusions (Ginaldi *et al.*, 1980).

Correlation between the echo pattern and histology of metastases is poor although echogenic metastases are commonly seen in carcinoma of the colon. Infiltration of the portal system occurs in 40% of patients with hepatocellular carcinoma and may distinguish this from other neoplasms (Wong *et al.*, 1985). However, speculation as to the site of

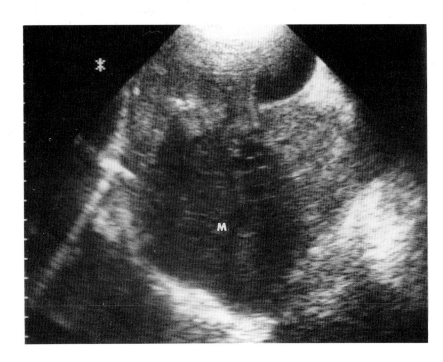

Fig. 14.3 Carcinoma of the colon. Sagittal ultrasound image showing a hypoechoic metastasis (M) in the right lobe.

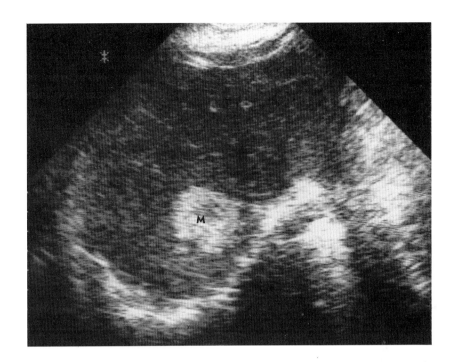

Fig. 14.4 Carcinoma of the colon. Coronal ultrasound image showing an echogenic metastasis (M) in the right lobe.

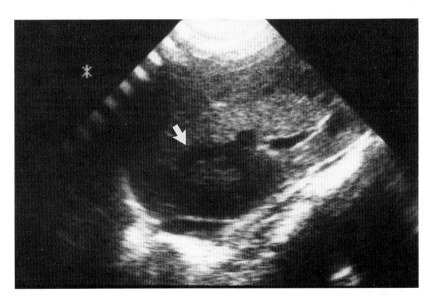

Fig. 14.5 Melanoma of the eye. Coronal ultrasound image showing a 'bull's-eye' metastasis (*arrow*) in the right lobe.

the primary tumour may confuse rather than help the clinician.

Accuracy and limitations

Ultrasound may detect lesions as small as 5 mm in diameter and a diagnostic sensitivity of up to 96% in the detection of hepatic neoplasms has been reported (Wong *et al.*, 1985). A good ultrasound unit should be able to detect over 90% of metastases. Ultrasound has the advantage that it is simple to perform, inexpensive and acceptable to the patient. Furthermore, if metastases are detected, fine-needle biopsy under ultrasound control may be carried out at the first attendance as this is relatively painless and safe (see below).

Difficulties may arise when bowel is interposed between the liver and anterior abdominal wall, particularly on the left side. It may also be difficult to see lesions high under the diaphragm when these are obscured by ribs.

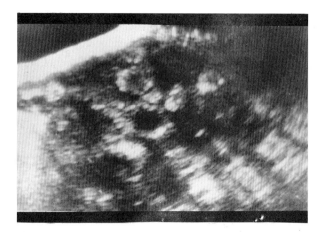

Fig. 14.6 Carcinoma of the colon. Coronal ultrasound image showing a mixed pattern of metastases in the left lobe.

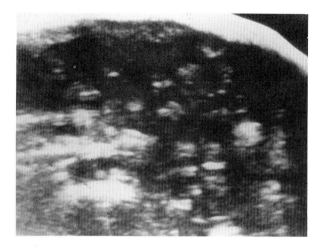

Fig. 14.7 Carcinoma of the colon. Coronal ultrasound image showing the 'hailstorm' pattern of multiple metastases.

Scintigraphy

Like ultrasound, scintigraphy is a convenient and inexpensive method of examining the liver. ⁹⁹ᵐTechnetium sulphur or tin colloid is the radionuclide of choice but more specialized tracers may be used in selected circumstances. No special preparation is required and the standard technique (Chapter 14) is used.

Abnormal appearances

⁹⁹ᵐTechnetium sulphur or tin colloid is taken up in the reticuloendothelial (Kupffer) cells of the hepatic sinusoids. These, like other normal tissues, are displaced by neoplastic tissue, and metastases therefore appear as focal areas of decreased or absent radionuclide accumulation (Fig. 14.12).

A wide range of appearances is possible, depending on the size of the metastases and whether they are well circumscribed or infiltrative. Lesions several centimetres in diameter are readily detected, irrespective of definition. The evaluation of uptake intensity is a subjective process and smaller lesions may be difficult to identify, particularly if they are poorly defined (Figs 14.13, 14.14). Diffuse infiltration of the liver may produce generalized inhomogeneity of uptake and this is easily over-

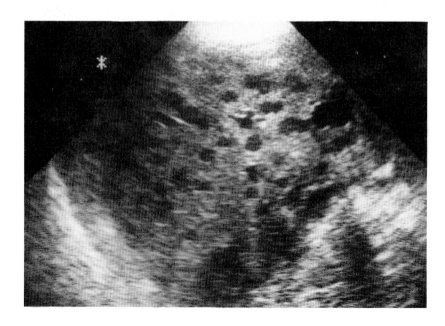

Fig. 14.8 Carcinoma of the bronchus. Coronal ultrasound image showing the 'sieve' pattern of multiple hypoechoic metastases.

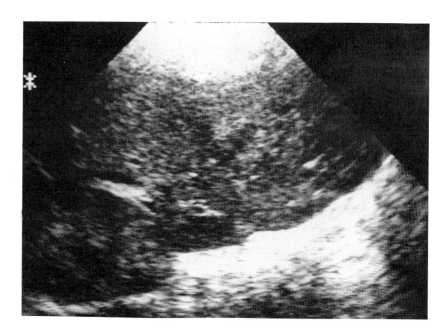

Fig. 14.9 Carcinoma of the bronchus. Diffuse metastatic involvement of the liver is revealed by generalized inhomogeneity of the echo pattern on ultrasound.

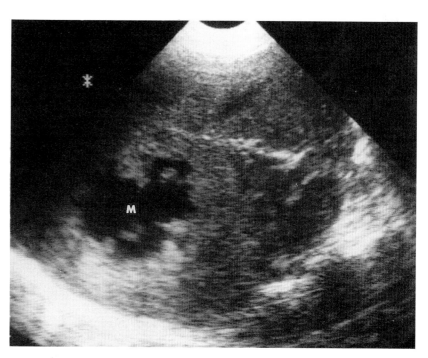

Fig. 14.10 Carcinoma of the rectum. Sagittal ultrasound image showing a necrotic metastasis (M) in the right lobe.

looked. The liver may be enlarged, as may the spleen and there may be greater uptake in the spleen than in the liver (reversed liver—spleen uptake ratio) (Fig. 14.15). Nuclide accumulation in the bone marrow is uncommon in metastic disease and, if present, suggests other causes of hepatosplenomegaly.

Many lesions displace the reticuloendothelial cells and produce focal scintigraphic defects. A specific diagnosis of metastases cannot therefore be made from the scintigraphic appearances alone,

although it may be inferred if there are clinical signs to indicate tumour dissemination. Some correlation has been observed between histology and the scintigraphic findings; there is a tendency for deposits from gastrointestinal neoplasms (Fig. 14.12) to be few and well defined, whereas those from carcinoma of the breast (Fig. 14.14) are often diffuse (Drum & Beard, 1976). This fact is of importance when evaluating examinations carried out for possible spread of known neoplasms: greater care should be used when the disease is

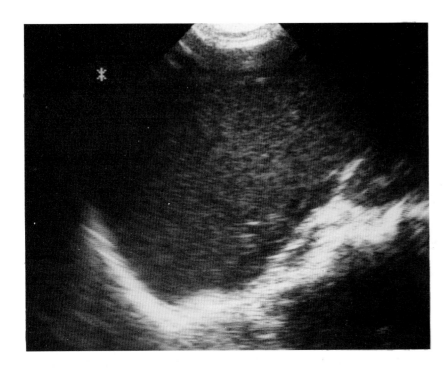

Fig. 14.11 Lymphoma. Sagittal ultrasound image showing generalized alteration in the echo pattern.

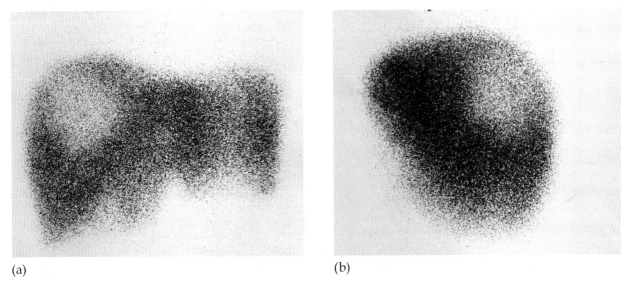

(a)   (b)

Fig. 14.12 Adenocarcinoma of the colon. Frontal (a) and right lateral (b) scintigram showing a large, solitary and well-defined area of reduced uptake due to a metastasis.

known to be difficult to detect scintigraphically.

Scintigraphy may detect lymphoma in the 10% of patients who have large nodules in the liver, but the more common form of diffuse infiltration is not detected and the scintigram may be normal or show only hepatosplenomegaly (Fig. 14.15) (Milder *et al.*, 1973).

In selected circumstances other nuclides may be used to detect metastases.[67] Gallium is taken up by several neoplasms, notably lymphoma, carcinoma of the breast and bronchus, and melanoma

(Bekerman *et al.*, 1984). However, assessment of the liver is difficult because the normal hepatocytes also accumulate the nuclide. This may be overcome by double-tracer scintigraphy and subtraction techniques (Deland & Wagner, 1983) but in practice this is cumbersome and other imaging techniques are more likely to be used.[131] Iodine may be used to detect metastases in carcinoma of the thyroid gland if the tumour takes up the tracer and the primary tumour has been resected. Metastases may be revealed as areas of abnormal nuclide accumu-

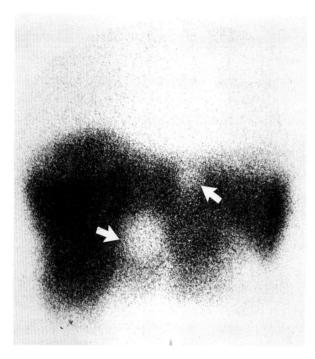

Fig. 14.13 Adenocarcinoma of the kidney. Scintigram showing two well-defined metastases (*arrows*).

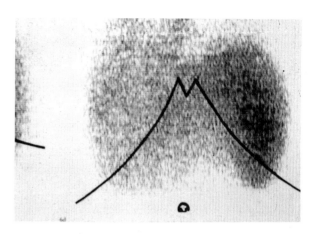

Fig. 14.15 Hodgkin's lymphoma. Scintilligram showing hepatosplenomegaly and reversed liver–spleen uptake ratio.

lation in the liver or elsewhere. Dynamic scintigraphy using ^{99m}technetium-labelled erythrocytes may be used to distinguish cavernous haemangioma from other lesions (Deland & Wagner, 1983); the findings are not completely specific, as a small number of metastases may also show hypervascularity and an increased blood pool (Zeman *et al.*, 1985).

There has been much interest in the possibilities of radiolabelled antibodies directed at specific neoplastic cell antigens. This subject is at an early stage of evaluation and is beyond the scope of the present text but is reviewed by Deland & Goldenberg (1985).

Accuracy and limitations

The accuracy of scintigraphy in detecting metastases using modern techniques appears to be between 74% and 86% (Knopf *et al.*, 1982, Alderson *et al.*, 1983). As discussed above, small lesions are difficult to resolve and in practice it is unusual to identify those less than 2 cm in diameter (Mansfield & Park, 1985). The resolution tends to be best at the liver surface and larger lesions deep in the liver may not be detected (Zeman *et al.*, 1985). The resolution is also affected by organ motion due to respiration. For these reasons the sensitivity is greatest in those tumours which tend to produce large, well-defined metastases, such as carcinoma of the colon (Drum & Beard, 1976, Knopf *et al.*, 1982).

The principal drawback of scintigraphy, apart from the limiting resolution, is the non-specificity

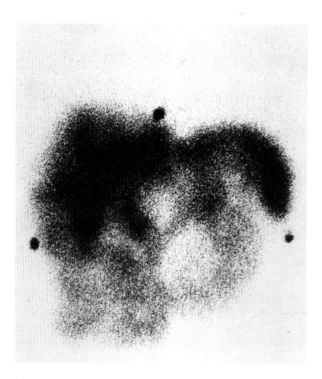

Fig. 14.14 Adenocarcinoma of the breast. Scintigram showing multiple, poorly defined metastases. Two large lesions are evident but elsewhere there is inhomogeneity of uptake due to diffuse infiltration by small, irregular metastases.

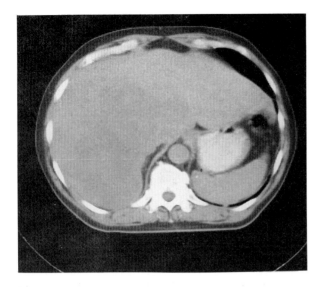

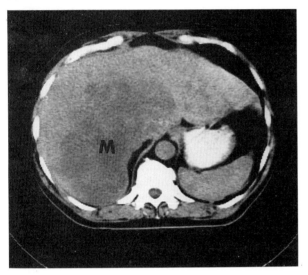

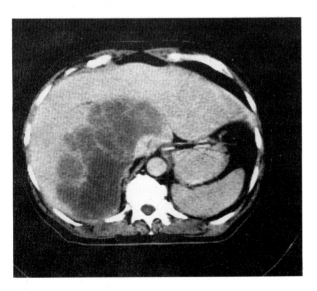

Fig. 14.16 Adenocarcinoma of colon. (a) CT image using routine viewing monitor settings shows no appreciable abnormality (W = 500, L = O). (b) The same image viewed at W = 150 and L = 32 shows a large, solitary metastasis (M). (c) Following enhancement the metastasis is seen more clearly and appears better defined (W = 150, L = 45).

of the findings. Many lesions of the liver produce focal failure of nuclide accumulation and cannot be distinguished by scintigraphy. False-positive results may be produced by pathology in surrounding organs, or by variations in the normal. In practice, awareness of these possibilities should prevent an incorrect diagnosis and suggest another confirmatory investigation, if indicated. The scintigraphic findings should, of course, always be interpreted with information about the patient's clinical state, and further investigation obtained if the findings appear to be at variance.

The sensitivity of scintigraphy may be increased by computer-assisted tomographic techniques (Carrasquillo *et al.*, 1983); an increase in sensitivity of 10% has been claimed for single-photon emission techniques (Ell & Khan, 1981). Cross-sectional display is particularly valuable for detecting deep lesions, and where available this technique may be used to elucidate equivocal findings on conventional scintigraphy (Zeman *et al.*, 1985).

Computerized tomography (CT)

CT of the liver has come of age with the development of machines which have short scan times and excellent contrast resolution. This has overcome many of the difficulties experienced previously and an unsatisfactory examination is now uncommon.

Technique

No specific preparation is required if the liver only is to be examined. Frequently, however, the liver is included in a more extensive examination, and in this case the small bowel should be opacified with a suitable oral contrast medium. It is also advisable to give an antiperistaltic agent intravenously or intramuscularly. The technique is covered in detail in Chapter 3.

Sections 8–10 mm thick are taken from the dome of the diaphragm to the inferior limit of the liver, usually at 1.5 cm intervals unless small lesions are suspected, in which case contiguous sections should be used. Some lesions may be difficult to detect and it is advisable to use the best exposure factors available. Sections should be obtained during suspended respiration.

The sections may be repeated following enhancement with intravenous contrast medium. This is commonly performed using an intravenous bolus injection (e.g. 100 ml Meglumine diatrizoate

65%-Urografin 310 M). More complicated enhancement techniques are available; a continuous intravenous infusion may be used or the injection may be given manually in increments and exposures timed to coincide with the phase of maximal parenchymal enhancement ('dynamic enhancement'). Intra-arterial injection of contrast medium (CT arteriography) has also been recommended (Prando *et al.*, 1979).

Some experimental and early clinical work has been carried out using emulsions of iodized oils which are taken up in the reticuloendothelial cells in the liver and spleen (Vermess *et al.*, 1982). These substances are not generally available and are still under assessment.

Some metastases may have attenuation values similar to those of normal tissue and may be difficult to detect. It is therefore important when viewing images of the liver to use a narrow window width (e.g. 150 Hounsfield units [HU]) and to set the window level close to the attenuation values of normal liver (approximately 50–60 HU) (Fig. 14.16a,b).

Abnormal appearances

Metastases usually produce focal alteration in the attenuation values of the liver. They are usually of lower density than normal tissue, may be multiple or solitary and well or poorly defined (Figs 14.17, 14.18). There is very poor correlation between the appearances and the histological diagnosis. A wide range of attenuation values may be obtained from metastases, even in the same patient, and some lesions have very low attenuation values (Fig. 14.18). This suggests necrosis, but not all lesions with this appearance are in fact necrotic (Scherer *et al.*, 1979). Some metastases may be cystic; the most common example is carcinoma of the ovary, which may produce lentiform subcapsular cysts (Fig. 14.19) indistinguishable from other fluid-containing cavities such as simple cysts or some abscesses.

Patients with diffuse neoplastic infiltration may have a generalized alteration in the attenuation values of the liver, depending on the size of the deposits (Fig. 14.20). Frequently, however, the appearances are normal and this type of hepatic involvement cannot be excluded by CT.

Calcification may be seen in metastases from some primary sites (Fig. 14.21), notably the gastrointestinal tract and pancreas. It is also seen — although much less commonly — in tumours of the breast, kidney, and thyroid gland. Calcification is not an indication of malignancy as it may also be seen in primary malignant or benign lesions (Scatarige *et al.*, 1983).

The majority of metastases are less vascular than normal tissue and appear more obvious and better defined after enhancement (Fig. 14.16c) (Moss *et al.*, 1979). In the early days of CT, contrast enhancement often identified lesions that were not

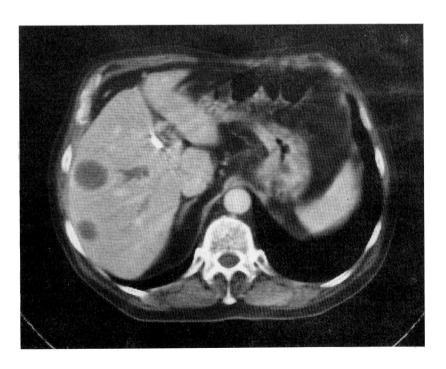

Fig. 14.17 Cholangiocarcinoma. CT image showing two well-defined metastases laterally in the right lobe (W = 500, L = 24).

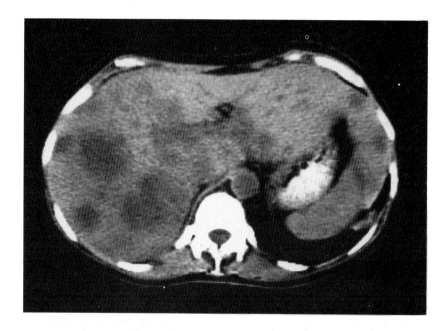

Fig. 14.18 Adenocarcinoma of the pancreas. CT image showing multiple, poorly defined metastases throughout the liver. Some of the lesions have very low attenuation values that may represent necrosis (W = 150, L = 38).

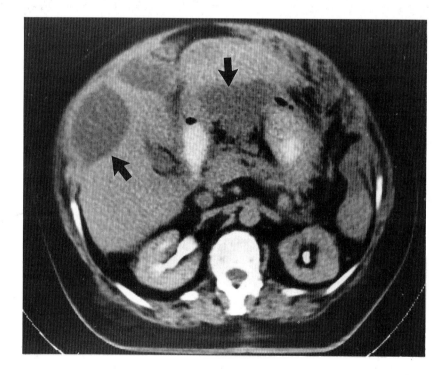

Fig. 14.19 Cystadenocarcinoma of the ovary. CT image showing multiple, well-defined subcapsular cysts (*arrows*). Aspiration revealed fluid containing changed blood and active adenocarcinoma cells (W = 300, L = 28).

seen on initial sections. However, the contrast resolution of modern machines is so good that it is now unusual to find lesions after enhancement if the initial sections have been completely normal (Berland *et al.*, 1982). Enhancement is now most commonly used to confirm an area of suspicion on the initial sections. Berland *et al.* (1982) have suggested that examinations for suspected metastases should be carried out after enhancement

only, but we have seen metastases which enhanced more than the surrounding parenchyma and were poorly visualized after enhancement (Fig. 14.22). It therefore seems sensible practice to start the examination without enhancement and use this only if it should prove necessary.

The enhancement pattern of liver lesions is a complex phenomenon, depending upon the vascularity of the lesion and the dual blood supply of

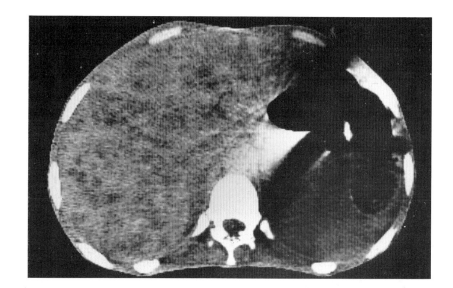

Fig. 14.20 Medullary carcinoma of the thyroid. CT image showing a generalized inhomogeneous parenchymal pattern due to small metastases and diffuse infiltration (W = 150, L = 50).

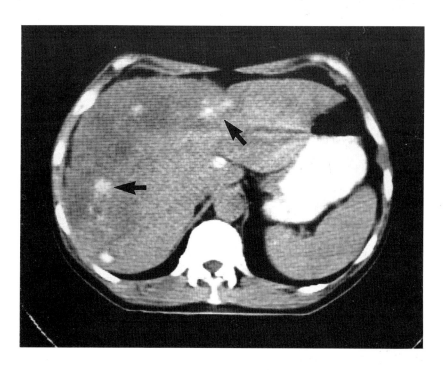

Fig. 14.21 Adenocarcinoma of colon. CT image showing multiple areas of reduced attenuation with foci of calcification (*arrows*) (W = 250, L = 46).

the liver from the hepatic artery and portal vein. Not surprisingly, techniques which produce particularly dense enhancement of the hepatic parenchyma, such as the bolus incremental technique or CT arteriography, tend to produce the greatest difference between normal and abnormal tissues and may be slightly more sensitive (Burgener & Hamlin, 1983, Prando *et al.*, 1979). The different enhancement techniques have been reviewed by Clark & Matsui (1983).

Like other techniques, CT may detect hepatic lymphoma when this is predominantly nodular in type, the appearances being similar to other metastases (Fig. 14.23). However, this type occurs in only 10% of patients, the remainder having diffuse hepatic infiltration, usually microscopic (Zornoza & Dodd, 1980). CT in these patients is usually normal, but just occasionally a generalized inhomogeneity of the parenchymal pattern is seen. It has been suggested that enhancement techniques using emulsified oils may improve the sensitivity of CT for hepatic lymphoma, but these are not yet generally available (Thomas *et al.*, 1982).

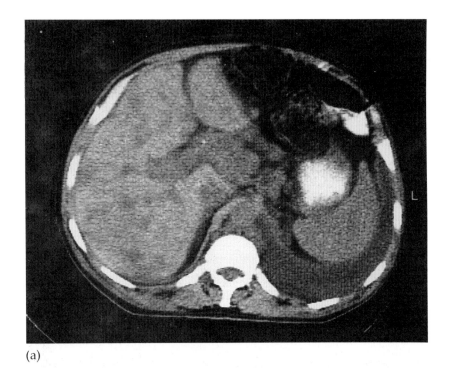

(a)

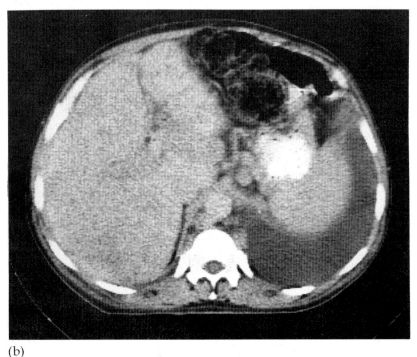

(b)

Fig. 14.22 Malignant insulinoma.
(a) CT image before enhancement
showing small, poorly defined
metastases (W = 250, L = 39).
(b) After enhancement the
metastases are more difficult to detect
(W = 250, L = 20).

Accuracy and limitations

Like ultrasound and scintigraphy, CT is a sensitive
method of detecting focal abnormalities in the
liver. The technique may reveal lesions in up to
98% of patients, marginally more than either
ultrasound or scintigraphy (Finlay *et al.*, 1982,
Knopf *et al.*, 1982, Alderson *et al.*, 1983).

The detection of lesions by CT depends on their
size and the difference in density between normal
and abnormal tissues. Most metastases are clearly
visualized, but those with attenuation values close
to those of their surroundings may be difficult to
detect, even when large, unless there are secondary
signs such as local bile-duct obstruction (Fig.
14.24). Small lesions tend to undergo partial volume averaging with normal tissue, and for this

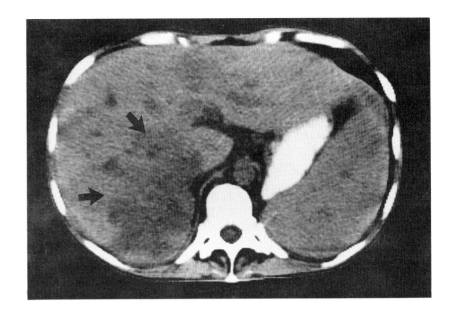

Fig. 14.23 Non-Hodgkin's lymphoma. CT image without enhancement showing a poorly defined area of infiltration in the right lobe of the liver (*arrow*) (W = 150, L = 55).

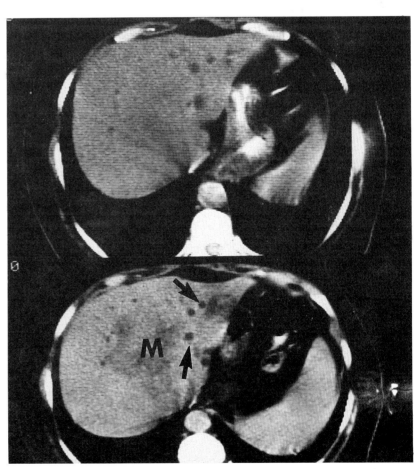

Fig. 14.24 Adenocarcinoma of unknown origin. CT images before (*upper*) and after (*lower*) enhancement. Even after enhancement the metastasis (M) is difficult to define, but there is dilatation of hepatic ducts (*arrows*) due to pressure from the mass (W = 250, L = 42).

reason it is unusual to demonstrate metastases less than 1 cm in diameter. However, when the lesions contain very high or low attenuation values — for example in an area of calcification — those several millimetres in diameter may be detected.

As indicated above, the sensitivity of CT on modern machines is unlikely to be altered radically by enhancement. However, there is no doubt that techniques which produce the most intense enhancement of normal tissue have a slightly greater sensitivity in the detection of focal lesions (Prando *et al.*, 1979, Marchal *et al.*, 1980, Burgener & Hamlin, 1983, Clark & Matsui, 1983). These techniques are more time-consuming in practice, but should be considered when the examination needs to be as accurate as possible, for example when CT is carried out to exclude further lesions in a patient undergoing resection of an apparently solitary metastasis.

CT has the disadvantage of a radiation dose to the patient and it is time-consuming. It is also of limited availability, at least in the UK, and in many centres its use is reserved for clinical problems which cannot be solved by the other available techniques.

Angiography

Ultrasound, scintigraphy and CT have superseded angiography in the diagnosis of hepatic metastases. However, the radiologist still needs to be familiar with the findings, as the technique has an important role in management (Freeny, 1983).

Technique

Both coeliac and superior mesenteric angiography are required to provide a plan of the hepatic arterial and portal venous systems. In coeliac angiography 40–50 ml of contrast medium is injected at 10 ml/s, with radiographs being taken at 1/s for 7 s and then at 1 every 3 s for 12 s. Selective superior mesenteric angiography may be required if an anomalous hepatic artery arises from the superior mesenteric artery; 30 ml of contrast medium is injected at 8 ml/s. The radiographic sequence is similar to coeliac angiography. Superselective hepatic angiography is performed by injecting contrast at 5 ml/s for 8 s, with a similar radiographic sequence as for coeliac angiography.

Abnormal appearances

Hepatic metastases are almost completely supplied by the hepatic artery (Healy & Sheena, 1963). As a result, the coeliac or superior mesenteric angiogram may show hypervascular tumour circulation in metastases, while the same lesions appear hypovascular during the venous phase, as portal blood containing contrast perfuses the surrounding normal tissue. Hypervascular metastases are probably best demonstrated by selective hepatic angiography, as they remain opacified while the

contrast medium is 'washed out' of the normal surrounding tissue by the non-opacified portal venous blood (Chuang, 1983). Improvements in angiographic technique may result in angiography being performed to exclude very small metastases, or to monitor the change in vascularity during treatment.

As in other techniques, metastases may show a variety of appearances on angiography and while there is some correlation with histology, the appearance are not sufficiently specific to make a definite diagnosis. Metastases from carcinoma of the kidney, functioning endocrine tumours, and carcinoid tend to be hypervascular, whereas those from the upper gastrointestinal tract and bronchus are usually hypovascular. Not surprisingly, those that show a characteristic tumour circulation are easier to detect than those that are hypovascular and are seen as space-occupying lesions in the parenchymal phase of the examination. Other metastases from common primary tumours such as carcinoma of the breast may have a similar opacification pattern to normal tissue and may be extremely difficult to detect (Freeny, 1983).

Angiography usually shows characteristic findings in cavernous haemangioma and has been used to confirm the diagnosis when this pathology is suspected on ultrasound or scintigraphy. However, CT with dynamic enhancement appears to be as reliable and is less invasive (Zeman *et al.*, 1985) Angiography also shows characteristic findings in focal nodular hyperplasia of the liver but this diagnosis is also likely to be made by other techniques.

The disadvantages of angiography are that it is an invasive procedure, and carries a relatively high radiation dose and increased risk to the patient from vascular damage or embolization. In our practice it is now common to perform an angiogram only as a prelude to a therapeutic interventional or surgical procedure (see below).

Digital subtraction angiography of the liver may be helpful, in view of the versatility of image processing, allowing arterial and venous phases to be superimposed or subtracted. The technique has the advantage that less contrast medium is required and real-time images are available. However, spatial resolution is poorer than conventional angiography, although this may improve enough to make digital vascular imaging the method of choice in the future (Rossi *et al.*, 1985). Clearly, further evaluation of the role of this technique is required.

Magnetic resonance imaging

This is still a young technique and remains under evaluation. However, it is now well-established that hepatic tumours are relatively easily distinguished from normal tissue because they have increased T_1 and T_2 relaxation times (Fig. 14.25) (Steiner, 1986). As the technique is based on biochemical information from the tissues, the difference between normal and abnormal areas may be more striking than in metastases demonstrated by other techniques. Further, MRI may give additional information compared to other techniques (Moss *et al.*, 1984).

Although the MR image reflects biochemical information, current experience suggests that a specific diagnosis may not be possible with this method, as there is significant overlap between the relaxation times of different hepatic lesions (Ohtomo *et al.*, 1986). It has, however, been suggested that the distinction between cavernous haemangioma and other lesions may be very reliably made by MRI (Stark *et al.*, 1985).

MRI has the disadvantage that the equipment is expensive and of limited availability. The examinations are time-consuming and images of the upper abdomen in particular are subject to movement artefact. It is not yet clear how MRI will compare in practice with other imaging techniques, or how important MR spectroscopy of liver lesions will prove to be, and the technique requires further evaluation.

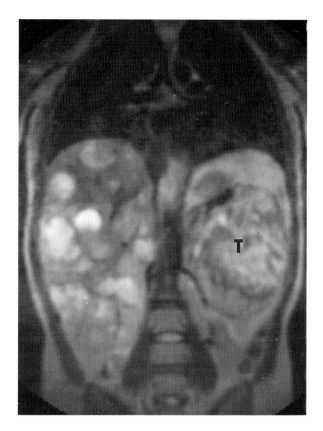

Fig. 14.25 Adenocarcinoma of the kidney. Coronal magnetic resonance image (spin-echo sequence) showing on the left a tumour (T) arising from the kidney. On the right side the liver is enlarged and contains multiple focal lesions of varying signal intensity (TR = 2000, TE = 60). (Reproduced by kind permission of Dr J.P.R. Jenkins, University of Manchester.)

The role of the radiologist in the management of hepatic metastases

Diagnosis

It is good practice in the diagnostic investigation of any patient to use simple, inexpensive and non-invasive methods first, proceeding to more complex techniques as necessary. We recommend that ultrasound should be used first in patients with symptoms referable to the liver. The differential diagnosis is wide and includes pathology of the biliary system and other upper-abdominal organs; ultrasound should distinguish these in the majority of patients, and if disease is not hepatic in origin, will probably indicate what further investigation is appropriate. Confident demonstration by ultrasound of multifocal soft-tissue masses in the liver is virtually diagnostic of metastases; percutaneous biopsy may be carried out for confirmation, depending on the clinical circumstances. It is certainly required if a solitary lesion is identified, because benign lesions may give similar appearances.

Further investigation is required if the ultrasound examination is equivocal, or if no abnormality is seen and there is strong clinical suspicion of disease. Scintigraphy is probably best used where it is thought that the ultrasound findings are due to a normal variant, as normal nuclide uptake in the area of suspicion excludes a space-occupying lesion. In other circumstances CT should be performed as the findings are likely to be more specific. These recommendations are of course influenced by the availability of techniques and local workloads. Serum enzymes such as alkaline phosphatase or gamma-glutamyl transpeptidase may be present in abnormally high levels when there are liver metastases, but these tests are considerably less sensitive than the three main imaging techniques (Schreve *et al.*, 1984).

Alternatively, scintigraphy may be used as the initial investigation, particularly if the clinical picture strongly suggests a hepatic mass. However, in view of the low specificity of the technique a confirmatory investigation, usually ultrasound should be obtained of any abnormalities (Zeman *et al.*, 1985). Indeed, scintigraphy can be used as an initial screen to direct the ultrasonologist to areas of suspicion. Our ideal is for ultrasound to be available at the same attendance, as the nature of a focal scintigraphic abnormality can often be established quickly and effectively by a short ultrasound examination. Combining techniques in this way increases the detection rate (Schreve *et al.*, 1984).

Cavernous haemangioma represents an important diagnostic pitfall. This tumour does not usually give rise to symptoms and is often an incidental finding, but may produce confusion on examinations carried out for suspected metastases. Biopsy of haemangioma should, of course, be avoided and the diagnosis confirmed radiologically if possible. Characteristic patterns may be seen with dynamic scintigraphy, dynamically enhanced CT or CT arteriography, and angiography (Bernardino *et al.*, 1982, Moinuddin *et al.*, 1985). CT with dynamic enhancement is probably the most convenient and gives the most specific appearances, provided that strict diagnostic criteria are used (Barnett *et al.*, 1980, Zeman *et al.*, 1985). Occasionally metastases may show an intense enhancement pattern similar to that of haemangioma (Fig. 14.26). Early experience with MRI suggests that this may ultimately become the technique of choice (Stark *et al.*, 1985).

Focal deposition of fat may also cause difficulty on both ultrasound and CT (Fig. 14.27). This is often more irregular than metastases and may extend to the liver surface. The diagnosis may be obvious if vessels are seen coursing through the lesion, but areas of fatty infiltration frequently have sufficiently normal function to appear normal on scintigraphy and this technique can be used in cases of difficulty (Halvorsen *et al.*, 1982).

Radiologists are often faced with requests to search for an occult primary neoplasm when disseminated disease has been found radiologically. This is rarely rewarding and such requests should be resisted. In our view, percutaneous biopsy of the metastases should be performed instead because this may indicate the primary site of disease. More importantly, the possibility of treatment depends on the histological diagnosis. With the agreement of the referring clinician, fine-needle biopsy may be carried out at the same attendance.

All imaging techniques may fail to diagnose diffuse or microscopic metastases, especially lymphoma. In these circumstances diagnosis is usually made by unguided liver biopsy or laparotomy. However, in our view there is no justification for the practice of carrying out an unguided biopsy when multifocal disease has been demonstrated radiologically, unless it is clear that disease is very extensive. A negative 'blind' biopsy does not exclude disease, is invasive and may be non-contributory, and is illogical where pathology is essentially focal in nature.

Staging

The introduction of modern imaging techniques has given radiology an important role in the pretreatment assessment of malignant disease, a process that until recently was largely clinical. As the liver is a relatively common site of metastases, it is now included in the staging protocols for many malignant tumours.

The extent to which the liver should be investigated depends upon the likelihood of spread to that organ when the patient presents for treatment. Unfortunately the precise incidence of metastases can only be found from histological examination of the liver. Gilbert & Kagan (1976) have pointed out that the post-mortem incidence of liver metastases in tumours with a relatively short natural history (for example, carcinoma of the pancreas) is likely to represent closely the incidence at presentation, whereas in tumours with a protracted course (for example, carcinoma of the kidney) hepatic involvement may represent a late development in the disease. In practice, our assessment of the probability of hepatic involvement depends almost entirely upon imaging studies and constantly changes as these are refined and improved.

It is important to realize that the philosophy of tumour staging is radically different from that of diagnosis. In diagnosis the aim is to demonstrate an abnormality which will explain the patient's symptoms and signs and the diagnostic work-up from simple to complex investigations is sensible. However, in staging, the aim is usually to exclude tumour spread before initiating treatment to the primary neoplasm. Where disseminated disease is found, systemic treatment is necessary and local treatment precluded. This therefore requires the

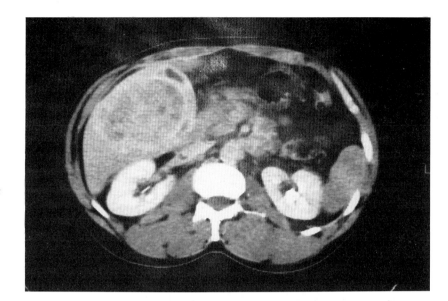

Fig. 14.26 Adenocarcinoma of caecum. CT image after enhancement showing a metastasis in the right lobe of the liver. There is intense uptake of contrast medium in the periphery of the tumour, with some central pooling, appearances which might be produced by a cavernous haemangioma (W = 250, L = 63).

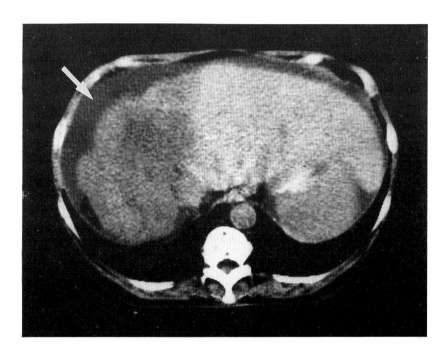

Fig. 14.27 Adenocarcinoma of unknown origin. CT image showing an irregular and contracted right lobe and compensatory enlargement of the left lobe. The variable reduction of density in the right lobe was thought to be due to chronic scarring and deposition of fat, but guided biopsy revealed unsuspected malignant tissue. Note that there is ascites (*arrow*) (W = 250, L = 51).

technique most likely to exclude disease, i.e. the most sensitive. This implies CT, but the technique is of limited availability and ultrasound and scintigraphy are almost comparable. In practice, therefore, the liver is included when patients undergo CT for other staging purposes — usually assessment of the primary tumour — and experience suggests a significant incidence of metastases at presentation. Our current recommendations are given in Table 14.1. Patients who would not ordinarily be referred for CT for other staging purposes may have ultrasound or scintigraphy. In practice this usually means gastric and colonic carcinoma as other tumours are unlikely to have spread to the liver at presentation. We should emphasize that this is a personal view, based on current experience.

No imaging technique can exclude hepatic lymphoma, and radiology has not therefore replaced 'blind' needle biopsy or staging laparotomy in these patients. In practice these tend to be carried out only if there is clinical suspicion of hepatic involvement. Early experience with MRI suggests that it will be no better in the detection of lymphoma (Weinreb *et al.*, 1984).

Table 14.1 Neoplasms in which the liver is included in computerized tomography carried out for tumour staging

Carcinoma:
  Bronchus
  Oesophagus
  Pancreas
  Rectum
  Kidney
  Ovary
Malignant lymphoma
Testicular teratoma and seminoma
Malignant melanoma
Soft-tissue sarcoma
Wilms' tumour
Neuroblastoma

Resection of metastases

The most accurate staging techniques are required when disease appears to be confined to one lobe or segment of the liver, and surgical resection is considered. Such localization of disease is uncommon, occurring in less than 10% of patients with metastases. CT is now used for these purposes and it is logical to use those techniques which have been claimed to be the most sensitive, such as dynamically enhanced CT (Prando *et al.*, 1979, Marchal *et al.*, 1980). In many patients, however, angiography will also be obtained to demonstrate the vascular anatomy and assist the surgeon in planning the procedure (Williamson *et al.*, 1980). Selective hepatic angiography provides only part of the information and it is important to obtain a good portal venogram, either by coeliac or splenic angiography (Roche *et al.*, 1982). It has been claimed that the most sensitive technique of all is to carry out CT during the arteriographic opacification of the liver (Matsui *et al.*, 1983).

Monitoring treatment

In the majority of patients with hepatic metastases follow-up examinations are unnecessary because in disseminated disease treatment is usually directed at symptoms. An accurate assessment of tumour response may, however, be required where alternative therapy is available if the tumour fails to respond, or where aggressive treatment regimes are being used which would be abandoned if failure of response were to be demonstrated.

In general, ultrasound is the most convenient technique provided that there is sufficient difference between the echo pattern of the tumour and that of the normal tissue. Alternatively, CT may be used when precise measurements are required in a reproducible plane.

Interventional techniques

Percutaneous biopsy

This is a convenient and reliable method of diagnosis in patients in whom liver disease is detected for the first time. Both ultrasound and CT can be used to guide needles into focal lesions; ultrasound on the whole is more convenient and readily available and the technique of choice. CT should be reserved for those situations where ultrasound fails, particularly where the echo characteristics of the abnormal tissue are too similar to that of normal tissue or in areas of the liver which are difficult to display by ultrasound, notably those high under the dome of the diaphragm. Biopsy is contraindicated in haemangioma, or where there is clotting or platelet dysfunction. The detailed technique is beyond the scope of this chapter and the reader is referred to specialized texts.

Guided needle biopsy is an accurate technique and can be expected to provide a conclusive diagnosis in up to 95% of cases. Failure usually results from poor needle localization or when the tumour is necrotic. Fine-needle aspiration to provide material for cytology is suitable in most tumour types, but large cutting needles should be used to provide specimens for histology if the patient is thought to have disease that is difficult to diagnose cytologically. The most important example is lymphoma.

Percutaneous biopsy is an invasive procedure and should only be carried out if it is believed that the results will influence management. The main risks from liver biopsy are local pain, haemorrhage, and peumothorax but these are rarely severe enough to require active treatment.

Percutaneous drainage

This technique is worth considering when there are symptoms from pressure effects due to metastases that have undergone necrosis or those which are primarily cystic. Both ultrasound and CT are convenient for guidance and drainage may be by either single aspiration or indwelling catheter (Golding & Husband, 1984).

Interventional angiography

The mean survival time for patients with untreated

liver metastases varies from 50 to 150 days (Jaffe *et al.*, 1968). Such a poor prognosis has spurred the angiographer to develop selective and super-selective catheterization in a bid to improve treatment, either by local infusion of chemotherapeutic agents, or embolization (Chuang *et al.*, 1983).

The vascularity of hepatic metastases varies considerably, but approximately 90% of the blood supplied to them comes from the hepatic artery, providing more than 95% of the oxygen requirements. Normal liver receives 75% of its blood supply and 50% of its oxygen requirements from the portal vein. This distribution provides the rationale of embolization and local infusion. Detailed knowledge of the arterial anatomy is necessary before embarking on these techniques and it is important to check that the portal vein is patent before embolization. Selective angiography reveals the vascular anatomy so that specialized guide wires and shaped catheters may be used to obtain superselective catheterization, allowing the drug or emboli to be delivered as close as possible to the metastases.

The most common indication for hepatic embolization is severe pain. It is also sometimes used to reduce the perfusion of vascular lesions before surgery, or when there is residue from an incomplete resection. The most commonly used embolic materials are gelatin sponge cubes, polyvinyl alcohol particles, and homologous lyophilized dura mater, with or without steel coils to provide additional certainty of long-lasting occlusion. Initial peripheral occlusion lessens the development of arterial collaterals to the tumour.

Portal venous obstruction is an absolute contraindication for hepatic embolization, and hepatic cirrhosis or high serum alkaline phosphatase are relative contraindications (Chuang & Wallace, 1983, Powell-Tuck *et al.*, 1984). Care must be taken to prepare the patient for embolization and to take steps to combat the postembolization syndrome (Clouse & Lee, 1984).

Hepatic embolization and/or selective chemotherapy may make a dramatic difference to the patient's symptoms and this is particularly evident in carcinoid syndrome (Maton *et al.*, 1983). The exact technique employed and the longer-term results are still being assessed, but Chuang & Wallace report a median survival time from the time of first embolization of 11.5 months as compared with 11 weeks for untreated metastases.

The impact of radiology on management

Patients with hepatic metastases often have a limited life expectancy and in many cases no effective treatment is available. Once liver disease has been demonstrated, therefore, it is important that no further diagnostic or treatment techniques are used needlessly in these patients. Before starting a procedure the radiologist should have a clear idea of how the result is likely to effect the management of the patient, particularly in the case of interventional techniques or follow-up examinations in patients with progressive disease.

None the less, in the situations described in this chapter the radiologist may have a key role in the management of the patient and a chance to contribute positively to improving the patient's quality of life. As therapeutic agents and regimes improve it is probable that this role will become increasingly important in the future.

Acknowledgements

We are grateful to Dr B.J. Shepstone for his advice and for the examples of scintigrams, and to Miss J. Edmonds for secretarial assistance.

References

Alderson, P.O., Adams, D.F., McNeill, B.J. *et al.* (1983) Computed tomography, ultrasound, and scintigraphy of the liver in patients with colon or breast carcinoma: a prospective comparison. *Radiology*, **149**, 225–230.

Barnett, P.H., Zerhouni, E.A., White, R.I. Jr. & Siegelman, S.S. (1980) Computed tomography in the diagnosis of cavernous hemangioma of the liver. *American Journal of Roentgenology*, **134**, 439–447.

Bekerman, C., Hoffer, P.B. & Bitran, J.D. (1984) The role of gallium-67 in the clinical evaluation of cancer. *Seminars in Nuclear Medicine*, **XIV(4)**, 296–323.

Berland, L.L., Lawson, T.L., Foley, W.D., Melrose, B.L., Chintapalli, K.N. & Taylor, A.J. (1982) Comparison of pre- and postcontrast CT in hepatic masses. *American Journal of Roentgenology*, **138**, 853–858.

Bernardino, M.E., Thomas, J.L., Barnes, P.A. & Lewis, E. (1982) Diagnostic approaches to liver and spleen metastases. *Radiologic Clinics of North America*, **20(3)**, 469–485.

Burgener, F.A. & Hamlin, D.J. (1983) Contrast enhancement of hepatic tumors in CT: comparison between bolus and infusion techniques. *American Journal of Roentgenology*, **140**, 291–295.

Carrasquillo, J.A., Rogers, J.V., Williams, D.L., Shuman, W.P., Olson, D.O & Larson, S.M. (1983) Single-photon emission computed tomography of the normal liver. *American Journal of Roentgenology*, **141**, 937–941.

Chuang, V.P. (1983) Hepatic tumor angiography: A subject review. *Radiology*, **148**, 633–639.

Chuang, V.P. & Wallace, S. (1983) Interventional approaches to hepatic tumor treatment. *Seminars in Roentgenology*, **XVIII**, 127–135.

Chuang, V.P., Soo, C.S., Carrasco, C.M. & Wallace, S. (1983) Superselective catheterization techniques in hepatic angiography. *American Journal of Roentgenology*, **141**, 603–611.

Clark, R.A. & Matsui, O. (1983) CT of liver tumors. *Seminars in Roentgenology*, **XVIII**, 149–162.

Clouse, M.E. & Lee, R.G.L. (1984) Management of the posthepatic artery embolisation syndrome. *Radiology*, **52**, 238.

DeLand, F.H. & Goldenberg, D.M. (1985) Diagnosis and treatment of neoplasms with radionuclide-labeled antibodies. *Seminars in Nuclear Medicine*, **XV(1)**, 2–11.

DeLand, F.H. & Wagner, H.N. Jr. (1983) Nuclear medicine in hepatic mass lesions. *Seminars in Roentgenology*, **XVIII(2)**, 106–113.

Drum, E.D. & Beard, J.M. (1976) Scintigraphic criteria for hepatic metastases from cancer of the colon and breast. *Journal of Nuclear Medicine*, **17**, 677–680.

Ell, P.J. & Khan, O. (1981) Emission computerised tomography: clinical applications. *Seminars in Nuclear Medicine*, **11**, 50–60.

Freeny, P.C., (1983) Angiography of hepatic neoplasms. *Seminars in Roentgenology*, **XVIII**, 114–122.

Finlay, I.G., Meek, D.R., Gray, H.W., Duncan, J.G. & McArdle, C.S. (1982) Incidence and detection of occult hepatic metastases in colorectal carcinoma. *British Medical Journal*, **284**, 803–805.

Gilbert, H.A. & Kagan, A.R. (1976) Metastases: incidence, detection and evaluation without histological confirmation. In Weiss, L. (ed) *Fundamental Aspects of Metastasis*, pp. 385–405. North-Holland Publishing Company.

Ginaldi, S., Bernardino, M.E., Jing, B.S. & Green, B. (1980) Ultrasonographic patterns of hepatic lymphoma. *Radiology*, **136**, 427–431.

Golding, S.J. & Husband, J.E. (1984) Percutaneous drainage of malignant cysts. *Clinical Radiology*, **35**, 475–478.

Green, B., Bree, R.L., Goldstein, H.M. & Stanley, C. (1977) Gray-scale ultrasound evaluation of hepatic neoplasms; Patterns and correlations. *Radiology*, **124**, 203–208.

Halvorsen, R.A., Korobkin, M., Ram, P.C. & Thompson, W.M. (1982) CT appearances of focal fatty infiltration of the liver. *American Journal of Roentgenology*, **139**, 277–281.

Healy, J.F. & Sheena, K.S. (1963) Vascular patterns in metastatic liver tumours. *Surgery Forum*, **14**, 121–122.

Jaffe, B.M., Donegan, W.L., Watson, F. & Spratt, J.S. (1968) Factors influencing survival in patients with untreated hepatic metastases. *Surgery, Gynecology and Obstetrics*, **127**, 1–11.

Knopf, D.R., Torres, W.E., Faiman, W.J. & Sones, P.J. Jr. (1982) Liver lesions: comparative accuracy of scintigraphy and computed tomography. *American Journal of Roentgenology*, **138**, 623–627.

Mansfield, C.M. & Park, C.H. (1985) Contribution of radionuclide imaging to radiation oncology. *Seminars in Nuclear Medicine*, **XV(1)**, 28–45.

Marchal, G.J., Baert, A.L. & Wilms, G.E. (1980) CT of noncystic liver lesions: bolus enhancement. *American Journal of Roentgenology*, **135**, 57–65.

Maton, P.N., Camilleri, M., Griffin, G., Allison, D.J.,

Hodgson, H.J.F. & Chadwick, V.S. (1983) Role of hepatic embolisation in the carcinoid syndrome. *British Medical Journal*, **287**, 932–935.

Matsui, O., Kadoya, M., Suzuki, M., Inoue, K., Itoh, H., Ida, M. & Takashima, T. (1983) Work in progress: Dynamic sequential computed tomography during arterial portography in the detection of hepatic neoplasms. *Radiology*, **146**, 721–727.

Milder, M.S., Larson, S.M., Bagley, C.M., DeVita, V.T., Johnson, R.E. & Johnston, G.S. (1973) Liver-spleen scan in Hodgkins disease. *Cancer*, **31**, 826–834.

Moinuddin, M., Allison, J.R., Montgomery, J.H., Rockett, J.F. & McMurray, J.M. (1985) Scintigraphic diagnosis of hepatic hemangioma: Its role in the management of hepatic mass lesions. *American Journal of Roentgenology*, **145**, 223–228.

Moss, A.A., Schrumpf, J., Schnyder, P., Korobkin, M. & Shimshak, R.R. (1979) Computed tomography of focal hepatic lesions: A blind clinical evaluation of the effect of contrast enhancement. *Radiology*, **131**, 427–430.

Moss, A.A., Goldberg, H.I., Stark, D.B., Davis, P.L., Margulis, A.R., Kaufman, L. & Crooks, L.E. (1984) Hepatic tumours: magnetic resonance and CT appearance. *Radiology*, **150**, 141–147.

Ohtomo, K., Itai, Y. & Iio, M. (1986) Magnetic resonance imaging of the liver. In Kressel, H.Y. (ed.) *Magnetic Resonance Annual*, pp. 197–212. Raven Press, New York.

Powell-Tuck, J., McIvor, J., Reynolds, K.W. & Murray-Lyon, I.M. (1984) Prediction of early death after therapeutic hepatic arterial embolisation. *British Medical Journal*, **288**, 1257–1259.

Prando, A., Wallace, S., Bernardino, M.E. & Lindell, M.M. (1979) Computed tomographic arteriography of the liver. *Radiology*, **130**, 697–701.

Roche, A., Schmit, P., Medina, F., Raynaud, A. & Lacombe, P. (1982) The value of portal study in determining etiology of hepatic masses in the adult. *Radiology*, **143**, 387–393.

Rossi, P., Simonetti, G., Passariello, R., Tempesta, P., Pesce, B., Pavone, P. & Castrucci, M. (1985) Digital coeliac arteriography. *Radiology*, **154**, 229–231.

Scatarige, J.C., Fishman, E.K., Saksouk, F.A. & Siegelman, S.S. (1983) Computed tomography of calcified liver masses. *Journal of Computer Assisted Tomography*, **7(1)**, 83–89.

Scheible, W., Gosink, B.B. & Leopold, R.G. (1977) Gray-scale echographic patterns of hepatic metastatic disease. *American Journal of Roentgenology*, **129**, 983–987.

Scherer, U., Santos, M. & Lissner, J. (1979) CT studies of the liver *in vitro*: a report on 82 cases with pathological correlation. *Journal of Computer Assisted Tomography*, **3**, 589–595.

Schreve, R.H., Terpstra, O.T., Ausema, L., Lameris, J.S., metastases. A prospective study comparing liver enzymes, scintigraphy, ultrasonography and computed tomography. *British Journal of Surgery*, **71**, 947–949.

Stark, D.D., Felder, R.C., Wittenberg, J. *et al.*, (1985) Magnetic resonance imaging of cavernous hemangioma of the liver: Tissue-specific characterisation. *American Journal of Roentgenology*, **145** 213–222.

Steiner, R.E. (1986) Magnetic resonance imaging of the body. In Steiner R.E. & Sherwood, T. (eds) *Recent Advances in Radiology and Medical Imaging 8*, pp. 61–84. Churchill Livingstone, Edinburgh, London, Melbourne

& New York.

Thomas, J.L., Bernardino, M.E., Vermess, M. *et al.*, (1982). EOE-13 in the detection of hepatosplenic lymphoma. *Radiology*, **145**, 629−634.

Vermess, M., Doppman, J.L., Sugarbank, P.H. *et al.* (1982). Computed tomography of the liver and spleen with intravenous lipoid contrast material: Review of 60 examinations. *American Journal of Roentgenology*, **138**, 1063−1071.

Weill, F.S. (1978) *Ultrasonography of Digestive Diseases*, pp. 113−132. C.V. Mosby, St Louis.

Weinreb, J.C., Brateman, L. & Maravilla, K.R. (1984) Magnetic resonance imaging of hepatic lymphoma. *American Journal of Roentgenology*, **143**, 1211−1214.

Williamson, B.W.A., Blumgart, L.H. & McKellar, N.J. (1980) Management of tumors of the liver. Combined use of arteriography and venography in the assessment of resectability especially in liver tumors. *American Journal of Surgery*, **139**, 210−215.

Wong, K.L., Lai, C.L., Wu, P.C., Hui, W.M., Wong, K.P. & Lok, A.S.K. (1985) Ultrasonographic studies in hepatic neoplasms: Patterns and comparison with radiological contrast studies. *Clinical Radiology*, **36**, 511−515.

Zeman, R.K., Paushter, D.M., Schiebler, M.L., Choyke, P.L., Jaffe, M.H. & Clark, L.R. (1985) Hepatic imaging: current status. *Radiologic Clinics of North America*, **23(3)**, 473−487.

Zornoza, J. & Dodd, G.D. (1980) Lymphoma of the gastrointestinal tract. *Seminars in Roentgenology*, **XV(4)**, 272−287.

15: The Radiological Investigation and Management of Carcinoid and other Neuroendocrine Tumours

D.J. ALLISON, A.P. HEMINGWAY AND A. KENNEDY

Introduction

During the past 25 years or so many clinical syndromes have been described that are associated with the hypersecretion of individual peptides from neuroendocrine tumours. Originally it was thought that each tumour had only a single peptide product, e.g. that an 'insulinoma' only produced insulin, but it is now known that most of these tumours (which arise predominantly in the pancreas) secrete several peptides, varying in their degree of biological activity, and that even for each peptide several different molecular forms may be produced. The various tumour syndromes are still named after the secreted peptide whose biological activity dominates the clinical picture in any given case (Friesen, 1982). Most neuroendocrine tumours are derived from cells of the islet cell tumour series first described by Pearse (Bloom & Polak, 1981). This system consists of cells that contain intrinsic amines or have the capacity to take up amine precursors and transform them into amines by intracellular decarboxylation. Islet-cell tumour cells probably originate from neuroectoderm, they are located in a variety of sites throughout the body including the pancreas and gut, either within specialized tissues such as the pancreatic islets or in a more dispersed form. For each peptide produced there is a distinctive cell type and the peptides have vital normal functions. Tumours of one cell type producing predominantly one hormone have fairly characteristic clinical features (see Table 15.1), and several tumours can appear in different sites in the body to constitute one of the various multiple endocrine neoplasia (MEN) syndromes.

The diagnosis of an islet-cell tumour is suspected on clinical grounds and confirmed by measuring elevated levels of the appropriate hormone in the serum. Although many pancreatic endocrine tumours contain more than one cell type and hormone, the symptoms are predominantly related to

one hormone but the dominant hormone may change with time. Although neuroendocrine tumours are relatively uncommon they are important for the radiologist since, even when malignant, they tend to be slow-growing and the patient may suffer from the effects of the hypersecreted hormone for many years if untreated. The localization of the primary tumour(s) and metastases when present is a task for the radiologist; a task that may be extremely rewarding for in some instances removal of the primary tumour can be curative, and the localization of secondary deposits in the case of malignant metastatic lesions may assist in directing palliative therapy to the most appropriate sites.

As the site of origin and clinical behaviour of carcinoid tumours is somewhat different from the other neuroendocrine tumours occurring in the abdomen, the radiology of the carcinoid syndrome is correspondingly different and this tumour type is considered separately from the others that are discussed together later under Pancreatic neuroendocrine tumours.

Carcinoid tumours

Clinical features

Carcinoid tumours arise primarily in either the bronchus or the gastrointestinal tract, and the present description will be confined to a consideration of the tumours occurring in the abdomen. Primary gut tumours may manifest themselves prior to metastasizing by giving rise to haemorrhage, obstruction or intussusception, but they are frequently discovered incidentally at laparotomy. Only a small proportion of carcinoid tumours are malignant and it is not until they have metastasized to the liver that the 'carcinoid syndrome' is produced.

Those primary carcinoid tumours (slowly growing tumours of enterochromaffin cells) that metastasize and produce the carcinoid syndrome usually arise in the ileum, but can originate anywhere in the small intestine or in organs derived from embryonic foregut (bronchus, stomach, pancreas, and thyroid). The syndrome has also been produced by ovarian and testicular teratomas. Unlike the tumours arising in the ileum, primary appendicular carcinoids are usually benign and do not metastasize, whereas large gut carcinoids may metastasize, but do not produce the syndrome. In total only about 10% of patients with carcinoid tumours exhibit the syndrome, which is due to the secretion into the circulation of serotonin (5-hydroxytryptamine) and other vasoactive substances including histamine, bradykinin, and adrenocorticotrophic hormone (ACTH). Bronchial and gonadal carcinoids drain directly into the systemic venous circulation and can produce the syndrome without metastasizing. The association between metastatic carcinoid tumours and the symptoms of flushing, wheezing, diarrhoea, telangiectasia, and cardiac valvular lesions was made in the early 1950s.

The primary intestinal tumours can themselves give rise to problems of haemorrhage, obstruction, and intussusception. The diagnosis of the syndrome is made by measuring an elevated level of 5-hydroxyindoleacetic acid (5-HIAA; the metabolite of 5-HT) in the urine. A level of greater than 25 mg 5-HIAA in 24 h is abnormal provided that bananas and tomatoes have not been ingested in excess and that certain drugs have not been taken. Cutaneous flushing, the commonest clinical feature of the syndrome, usually involves the face and neck and can be accompanied by lacrimation and periorbital oedema. Attacks can be provoked by alcohol, excitement, exercise, eating, and adrenaline. Intestinal hypermotility can be accompanied by explosive diarrhoea or chronic diarrhoea with malabsorption. Bronchoconstriction, although uncommon, can be severe. Cardiac features include endocardial fibrosis of the right heart giving rise to pulmonary stenosis and tricuspid incompetence.

Radiological diagnosis

PRIMARY TUMOURS

Carcinoid tumours of the appendix are a common incidental finding at laparotomy, they are benign, usually asymptomatic, and have no distinctive radiological features.

Primary carcinoid tumours should enter the differential diagnosis of any tumour-like lesion discovered on barium examination of the upper gastrointestinal tract. They are uncommon in the colon, but should be considered if a lesion is not typical of, say, a carcinoma.

The deliberate hunt for a primary carcinoid tumour occurs once the diagnosis of the syndrome (and hence hepatic metastases) has been made.

Barium studies

Barium studies of the upper gastrointestinal tract should be performed first. Gastric carcinoids appear as lobulated tumours of the mucosa. There are no pathognomonic features and the definitive diagnosis is made by endoscopic biopsy. A number of abnormalities may be detected on small-bowel enema studies if a primary lesion is present. They include concentric or eccentric luminal narrowing (Fig. 15.1) secondary to fibrosis, and a desmoplastic reaction in the mesentery, stricture formation, intraluminal filling defect (Fig. 15.2), and occasionally intussusception (Jeffrey et al., 1984).

Computerized tomography

This is usually carried out to assess the extent of any hepatic metastases present (Fig. 15.3) and may well reveal the presence of thickening in the mesenteric folds which occurs as a result of the intense desmoplastic reaction in the region of the primary tumour; presumably due to local hormonal changes.

Angiography

This is rarely used simply as a means of locating a primary lesion, although a superior mesenteric study in the presence of a small-bowel carcinoid can show distinctive appearances. In the region of the tumour there is increased tortuosity of the vessels with local changes in calibre of a concertina-like nature secondary to a mesenteric fibrotic reaction (Fig. 15.4). Occasionally there is also a dense vascular blush within the tumour itself.

SECONDARY TUMOURS

Primary carcinoid tumours can of course metastasize to virtually any site within the body, including liver, lungs (Fig. 15.5) and bone (Fig. 15.6). Bone

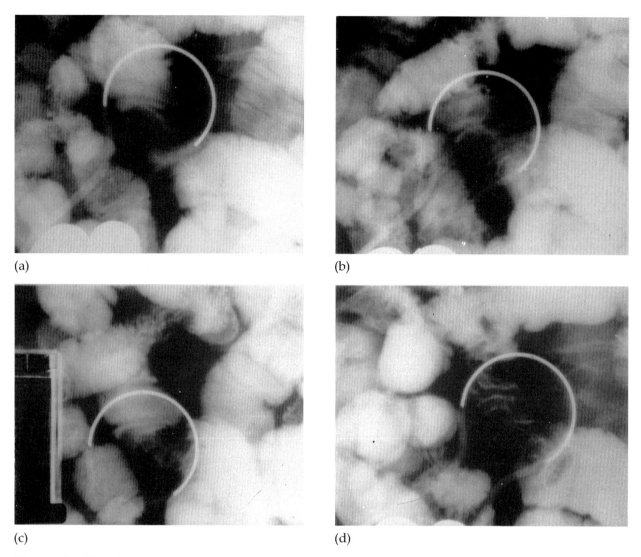

(a)

(b)

(c)

(d)

Fig. 15.1 Small bowel enema. Several 'spot films' of an area of constant luminal narrowing associated with a primary carcinoid tumour.

metastases are commonly sclerotic rather than lytic. The characteristic clinical syndrome occurs following the development of actively secreting secondary deposits and is most commonly associated with hepatic metastases.

Following the clinical diagnosis of carcinoid syndrome it is important to determine the size and extent of such metastases, as this information will significantly affect the mode of treatment. A solitary metastasis or metastases confined to one lobe of the liver can be resected surgically. Multiple diffuse small lesions can be managed by chemotherapeutic agents, whereas multiple large lesions or lesions that do not otherwise respond may be suitable for embolization (see below).

Useful investigations in detecting metastases include plain radiography (chest and bone lesions), ultrasound, isotope scintigraphy, computerized tomography, magnetic resonance imaging, and angiography.

Ultrasound

This, the least invasive of the sophisticated imaging modalities (and probably the cheapest), may alone provide all the information necessary for treatment decisions.

The lesions are characteristically hyperechoic and well-defined. The advantage of ultrasound is that not only can the parenchymal lesions be detected, but detailed information regarding vascular anatomy and involvement of vessels by the

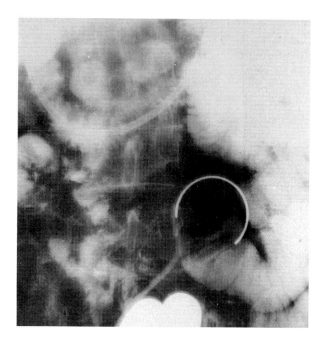

Fig. 15.2 Small bowel enema. The primary carcinoid tumour seen as an intraluminal filling defect.

tumour can be obtained (Gibson & Hemingway, 1988).

The detection of normal anatomical arterial variations (e.g. an accessory right hepatic artery) is important if surgery or embolization are contemplated. Portal-vein compression and occlusion in-

volving either the main vein or any of the major branches may render a tumour inoperable or unsuitable for embolization. It is also possible to assess the patency of the hepatic veins and inferior vena cava, particularly in the presence of large tumour masses. With modern ultrasound equipment the quality of information obtainable is of such high standard that no further imaging may be necessary prior to a treatment decision. Ultrasound is also particularly useful in assessment of progress during treatment.

Isotope scintigraphy

Although highly sensitive in proving that space-occupying lesions are present in the liver, very little anatomical or vascular information can be obtained by hepatic scintigraphy. [131]Iodine MIBG (Metaiodobenzyl-guanidine) is useful in the localization and treatment of some of these tumours but this has proved to be of only limited value. The technique is no greater than 50% specific and remains very expensive. It should be borne in mind, however, for 'difficult' lesions.

Computerized tomography (CT)

Carcinoid metastases may be hypo- or isodense prior to contrast enhancement, after which they become hyperdense. CT can detect lesions less

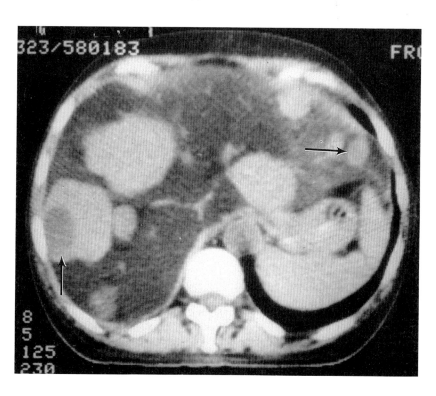

Fig. 15.3 CT scan. There is fatty infiltration of the liver with metastatic deposits (arrows) in some of the areas of normal liver.

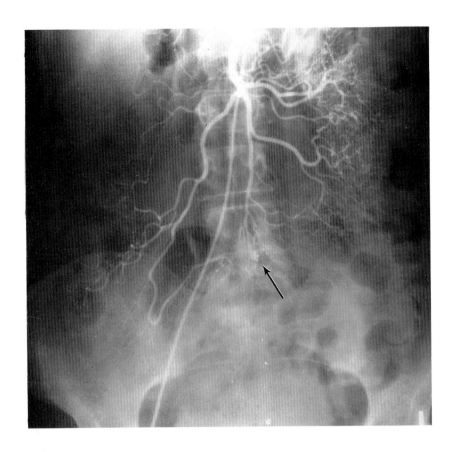

Fig. 15.4 Superior mesenteric arteriogram. The vessels in the region of the tumour show a 'corkscrew' pattern (*arrow*) secondary to fibrosis in the mesentery.

than 1 cm in size and is invaluable in determining the extent of disease. Extrahepatic involvement of lymph nodes and peritoneum can also be demonstrated, along with skeletal and lung secondaries. CT, like ultrasound, is very useful in following the progress of disease after treatment.

Magnetic resonance imaging (MRI)

Although this modality can detect liver metastases its role in the routine imaging of these lesions is at present superfluous. In future years the spectroscopic aspects of MRI may prove useful.

Angiography

This remains one of the most useful imaging modalities in metastatic carcinoid tumours (Gibson & Hemingway, 1988), and is performed for a variety of reasons:
- To confirm the presence of metastases.
- To determine the extent of metastatic involvement.
- To delineate arterial anatomy prior to surgery or embolization.
- To assess portal-vein patency prior to surgery or embolization.

- In conjunction with therapeutic arterial embolization.

Although details of angiographic technique have been dealt with in Chapter 5 it is worth emphasizing one or two technical points related to diagnostic angiography. It is important to perform selective hepatic arteriography and not to rely on coeliac axis injection alone (Fig. 15.7). On a number of occasions we have been able to demonstrate small (less than 5 mm) lesions on selective hepatic studies that could not be detected on a more general injection of contrast medium into the coeliac axis. This is because in a coeliac axis injection there is both hepatic arterial and portal venous opacification of the liver parenchyma in the late phase, whereas in the more selective arterial injections there is no portal-vein filling (portogram) to obscure small lesions. Any normal variants in hepatic arterial supply, such as an accessory right hepatic artery, should be demonstrated. It is crucial to demonstrate adequately not only the main portal vein but also the major right and left trunks. It may be necessary to perform an oblique study (left posterior oblique) in order to visualize the left portal vein adequately. Digital subtraction angiography has greatly facilitated the demonstration of portal venous anatomy. In the presence of a large

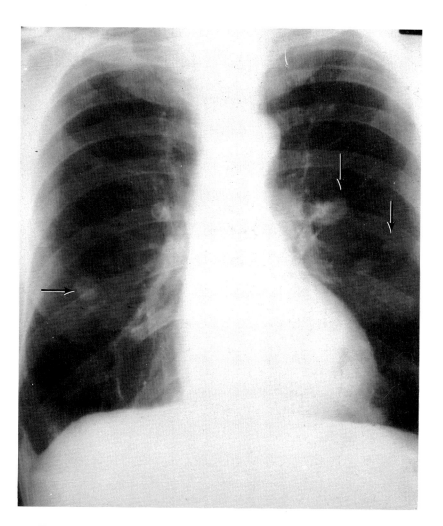

Fig. 15.5 Chest radiograph. Multiple lung metastases (*arrows*) in a patient with the carcinoid syndrome.

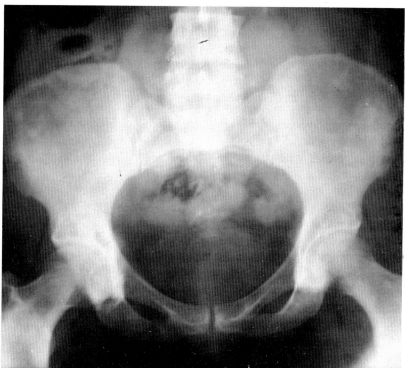

Fig. 15.6 Pelvic radiograph. Typical sclerotic bone metastases that may be seen in the carcinoid syndrome.

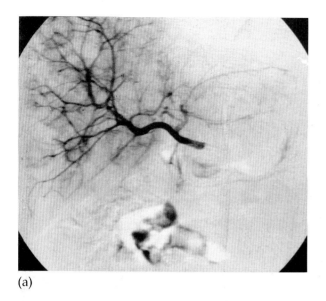

(a)

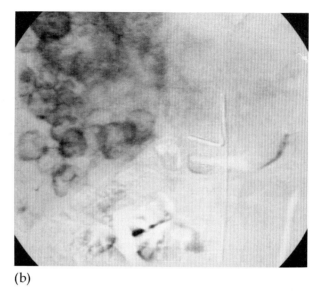

(b)

Fig. 15.7 Selective hepatic arteriogram. (a) The arterial phase shows multiple vascular metastases in the liver of a patient with the carcinoid syndrome. (b) These are more clearly seen in the capillary phase.

tumour mass (and when surgical resection is contemplated) it is also important to demonstrate the inferior vena cava in both the AP and lateral projections to exclude tumour invasion, and if the hepatic veins have not been seen clearly on ultrasound, tumour invasion should be excluded by selective venography prior to surgical resection (Fig. 15.8).

The radiological management of hepatic carcinoid metastases by embolization is discussed later in this chapter.

Pancreatic neuroendocrine tumours

Pancreatic endocrine tumours, unlike the carcinoid tumours discussed above, which usually arise outside the pancreas, commonly present with symptoms of excess hormone production prior to their metastasizing to the liver. Once a clinical and biochemical diagnosis has been made, radiological examinations are directed initially at localizing the primary tumour, as well as determining whether or not spread has occurred (Gunther, 1985). Surgical resection of a primary lesion prior to spread is very successful in curing the syndrome.

Clinical features

Neuroendocrine pancreatic tumours have several clinical features in common: they tend to be slow-growing, and often ultimately prove fatal because

of the systemic effects of peptide hypersecretion rather than local tumour bulk. With the exception of the insulinoma, 90% of which are benign, most of the tumours tend to be malignant and metastases within the abdominal cavity have frequently occurred by the time of diagnosis (Kloppel, 1983, Creutzfeld, 1980). Excision of a solitary primary tumour is often curative in the case of insulinomas, and may give years of disease-free life in other more aggressive types of tumour. In the case of metastatic disease, treatment options include surgery to reduce tumour bulk, cytotoxic chemotherapy, hepatic arterial or portal embolization, and palliative pharmacological therapy with the new long-acting somatostatin analogue octreotide SMS 201–995.

Although it is well-recognized that multiple peptide hypersecretion may occur from virtually any neuroendocrine tumour, the clinical picture is commonly dominated at any given time by the action of one particular hormone, and a list of the common clinical symptoms associated with islet-cell tumour hormone production is given in Table 15.1 (Adapted from Bloom, 1981).

A detailed description of these disease syndromes is beyond the scope of this article and for further information the reader is referred to specialist publications such as those by Bloom & Polak (1981), Shearman & Finlayson (1982) and Lai *et al.* (1988).

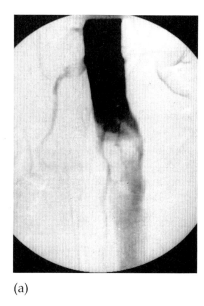

(a)

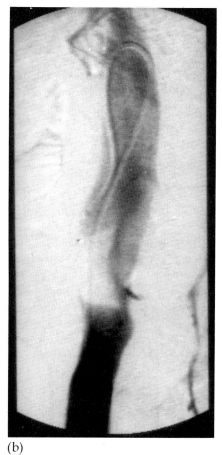

(b)

Fig. 15.8 Inferior vena cavagram. AP (a) and lateral (b) films show that the inferior vena cava has been invaded by carcinoid metastases.

Table 15.1 Clinical features associated with some abdominal neuroendocrine tumours

Clinical features	Pancreatic apudoma
Hypoglycaemia	Insulinoma
Diarrhoea	Carcinoid
	Gastrinoma
	Vipoma
Peptic ulceration	Gastrinoma
	Insulinoma etc., in MEA
Hyperglycaemia	Glucagonoma
	Somatostatinoma
	Corticotrophinoma
	Catecholamine-apudoma
Hypokalaemia	
Acidotic	Vipoma
Alkalotic	Corticotrophinoma
Migratory dermatitis	Glucagonoma
Flushing	Vipoma
	Carcinoid

Radiological investigation

The radiological investigation of islet-cell tumours is reviewed in detail by Rossi *et al.*, 1989.

PRIMARY TUMOURS

Since all the tumours alluded to above usually arise in the pancreas and spread either locally or to the liver, the radiological techniques used in their localization are common to all tumour types.

Plain films

Pancreatic apudomas may calcify, particularly glucagonomas (Breatnach *et al.*, 1985, Imhof & Frank, 1977) and vipomas (authors' unreported observation in several cases). The appearances are non-specific but, in a patient with no history of chronic pancreatitis to confuse the picture, may direct investigations to the correct site in the pancreas.

Ultrasound

Both the liver and pancreas should be examined. Technical considerations are covered in Chapter 2. Although pancreatic primary lesions may be very small and beyond the resolution of even the most sophisticated ultrasound machines, there are reports of tumours as small as 7 mm being localized (Kuhn *et al.*, 1982). They may ocasionally be large or multiple or diffuse infiltration of the pancreas by tumour may be present, all of which can be assessed ultrasonically. Two recent advances have improved the accuracy and usefulness of ultrasound — one being endoscopic ultrasound (Fig. 15.9), the other intraoperative ultrasound. Both of these techniques may allow better resolution of fine pancreatic detail (Shawker & Doppman 1988, Galiber *et al.*, 1988, Norton *et al.*, 1987, Gorman *et al.*, 1986).

Ultrasound is currently, without doubt, the least invasive means of detecting hepatic metastases and is very sensitive, though there are no specific features on ultrasound that distinguish these endocrine secondary tumours from other tumour types and it is the clinical syndrome that suggests the diagnosis. In a patient with symptoms suggestive of an endocrine tumour the demonstration of hepatic metastases clearly profoundly influences that patient's subsequent management.

Isotope scintigraphy

Isotope scintigraphy is of no value in detecting the primary pancreatic lesion and though liver metastases are readily detected, other modalities offer additional advantages including greater sensitivity and specificity. [131]Iodine-MIBG has not fulfilled its early promise of specific tumour localization in these patients.

Computerized tomography

In an early evaluation of CT in the detection of islet cell tumours (Dunnick *et al.*, 1980), a primary tumour was identified in 32% of cases; hepatic metastases were detected in 40%. Those pancreatic primaries that were identified were large. Further refinement in CT hardware and software has greatly improved the sensitivity of the technique in detecting pancreatic lesions, but it is by no means infalliable (Gunther, 1985, Rossi *et al.*, 1985, Krudy *et al.*, 1984, Stark *et al.*, 1984). Very small lesions are lost owing to the partial volume effect, and diffuse infiltration may be impossible to detect. If an islet-cell tumour is suspected, 5 mm slices through the pancreas should be made with and without intravenous contrast enhancement. Further refinements of technique include dynamic intravenous CT and the injection of contrast medium into a selectively positioned coeliac axis cath-

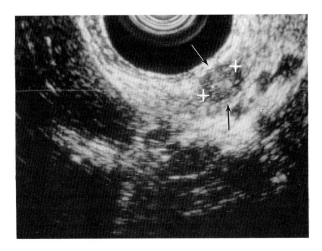

Fig. 15.9 Endoscopic ultrasound. A 1.4 cm hypoechoic insulinoma (*arrows* and *crosses*) in the pancreas. (Courtesy of Dr W. Lees, Middlesex Hospital, London.)

eter during CT imaging — 'angio-CT' (Fig. 15.10) (Fink *et al.*, 1985). CT is of course excellent at conforming the presence of hepatic metastases of all sizes and is useful in charting their progress during and after treatment.

Magnetic resonance imaging

As with carcinoid tumours, MRI is not used at present in the routine investigation of pancreatic islet-cell tumours, but spectroscopy may prove to be of value in the future.

Arteriography

Despite advances in other imaging methods, highly selective visceral arteriography is still of value in detecting primary pancreatic islet-cell tumours. The examination should commence with a general coeliac axis arteriogram. It is important to include arterial, capillary and venous phases in this study (Fig. 15.11). This will not only delineate the arterial anatomy prior to more selective studies but will on occasion reveal the primary tumour. It is advisable to use a low-osmolality or non-ionic contrast medium for these examinations because if superselective studies are required it is very easy to exceed contrast volume limitations. Following the coeliac-axis study, a selective splenic arteriogram (Fig. 15.12), and indirect splenoportogram are performed in both anteroposterior projection and the LAO projection to unfold the tail of the pancreas. It is useful to distend the stomach with gas, and prevent motility with Buscopan

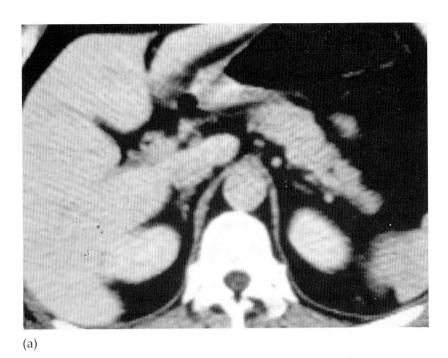

(a)

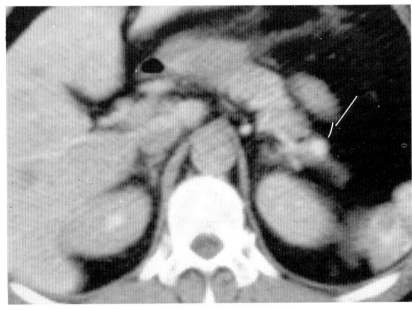

(b)

Fig. 15.10 Angio-CT. (a) Unenhanced scan. No definite abnormality is seen. (b) Enhanced scan. After injection of contrast medium through a catheter placed selectively in the coeliac artery, a well-defined enhancing lesion is seen in the tail of the pancreas (*arrow*). This was confirmed to be an insulinoma at surgery.

(hyoscine 2-butylbromide) for these two sequences. The distended stomach acts as a window through which the opacified pancreas can be visualized. There then follows a selective hepatic arteriogram (to detect intrahepatic metastases) and a selective gastroduodenal arteriogram (Fig. 15.13) to detect lesions in the pancreatic head. This examination is then followed by a superior mesenteric arteriogram as some lesions in the head will only be revealed on this study. It is occasionally necessary to perform selective pancreaticoduodenal, dorsal pancreatic, and arteria pancreatica magna studies to confirm or exclude the presence of a tumour.

Although there is no intrinsic pathological reason why islet-cell tumours should vary in their radiological appearances, it has been the authors' experience that some features are associated with particular tumour types. Insulinomas and glucagonomas are usually intensely vascular with a

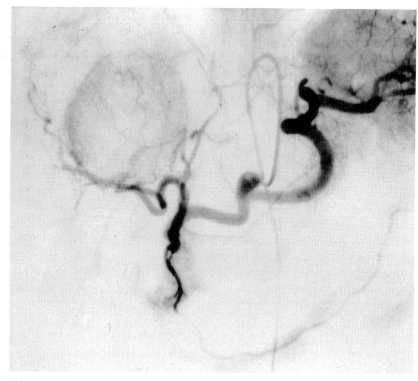

(a)

Fig. 15.11 (a) Coeliac axis arteriogram. Arterial phase. A large vascular metastasis in a patient with the carcinoid syndrome.

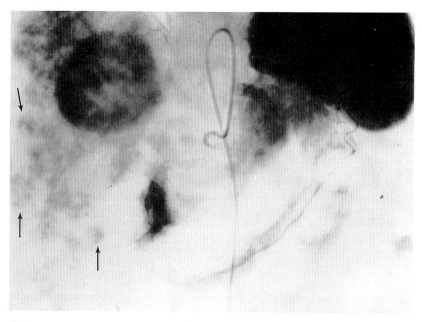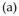

(b)

Fig. 15.11 (b) Capillary phase. The large metastasis is more clearly seen and several smaller metastases (*arrows*) are also identified.

very distinctive tumour blush (Figs 15.12, 15.13). Gastrinomas on the other hand are usually more difficult to find than either of the previous tumours (Maton *et al.*, 1987), and vary considerably in their degree of vascularity. Vipomas, like gastrinomas, may be relatively avascular but frequently exhibit a prominent 'marker' draining vein owing to the intense vasodilator properties of vasoactive intestinal polypeptide.

Trans-hepatic portal venous sampling

This may be performed under either local or general anaesthesia depending on the patient's age,

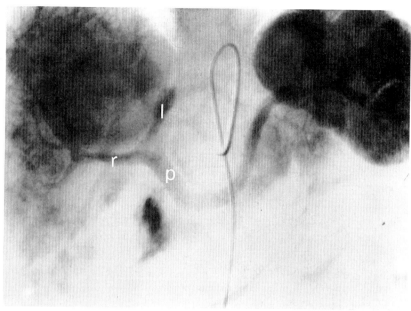

Fig. 15.11 (c) Venous phase. The main portal vein (p) and its right (r) and left (l) branches are patent.

(c)

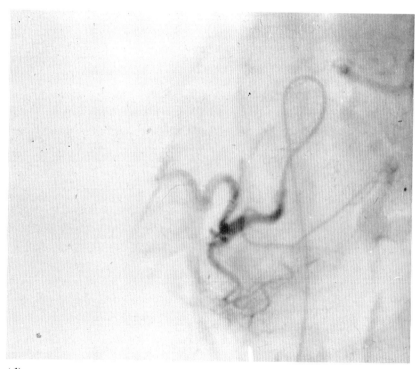

Fig. 15.11 (d) Postembolization arteriogram. This shows that the arterial supply to the liver has been obliterated.

(d)

general health, etc. It is a long procedure and often uncomfortable and therefore tends to be performed under general anaesthesia. The principle of the technique is that a catheter is introduced percutaneously into the intrahepatic portal vein, and then steered under fluoroscopic control into not only the main mesenteric and portal branches, but also into the numerous pancreatic draining veins.

From each catheter position a blood sample is taken, labelled and 'mapped' on a chart of the venous system. The samples are then analysed for levels of the appropriate hormone(s). It is critical that the samples are handled correctly, as many require to be kept at certain temperatures or/and centrifuged to prevent hormone degradation. High levels of hormone can then be matched with the

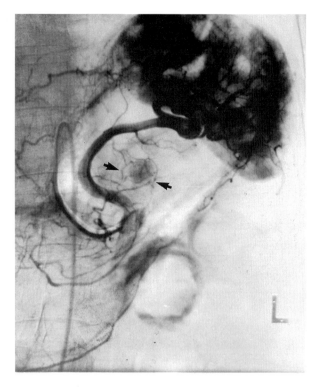

Fig. 15.12 Selective splenic arteriogram. This insulinoma (*arrows*) exhibits a typical dense parenchymal 'blush'.

(Allison, 1982) and it is technically demanding to perform (Roche *et al.*, 1982). Improvements in CT and ultrasound localization have largely replaced it except in difficult cases.

Secondary tumour localization

The principles of selective hepatic arteriography and indirect portography are the same as in the localization and detection of carcinoid metastases. Islet-cell tumour secondaries are usually highly vascular, but if small, very high-quality angiography or digital subtraction techniques may be needed to identify them.

Hepatic embolization

Therapeutic hepatic embolization (Fig. 15.11) is the deliberate occlusion of branches of the hepatic artery (or occasionally the portal vein), by emboli injected through a selectively sited catheter (Allison *et al.*, 1977, Allison, 1978a, Chuang & Wallace 1980, Blumgart & Allison, 1982, Yamada *et al.*, 1983). The object of this mode of therapy in cases of hepatic tumour is to render the neoplasm ischaemic, thereby inhibiting the growth and spread of tumour tissue and in the case of carcinoid and islet-cell tumours to reduce hormone production and secretion (Fig. 15.12).

site of acquisition on the map (Rossi *et al.*, 1989), thus locating the likely site of the hormones. There are numerous sources of error in this technique

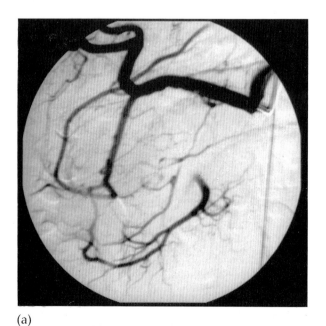

(a)

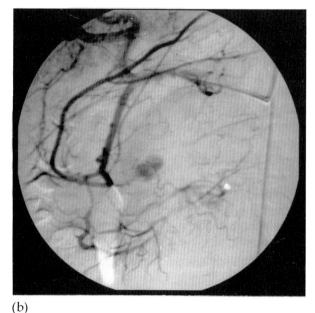

(b)

Fig. 15.13 Selective gastroduodenal arteriogram. The early arterial phase (a) looks normal in this study, but the characteristic blush of a small islet-cell tumour is clearly seen in a slightly delayed film (b).

Portal venous blood accounts for approximately 70% of the total liver blood flow in man and normal liver cells can apparently survive on portal venous blood alone. This fact makes the liver a particularly suitable organ for arterial embolization, since its dual blood supply protects it from infarction (Allison, 1983). Despite the fact that most tumour cells presumably arrive in the liver via the portal circulation, they commonly obtain their blood supply for growth from the arterial circulation; this means that embolization of the hepatic artery can induce selective necrosis of metastatic hepatic tumours while leaving normal liver relatively unaffected.

It might be supposed that surgical ligation or division of the hepatic artery would produce the same end result as embolization and achieve it in a more permanent manner (Murray-Lyon et al., 1970). There are a number of reasons, however, why embolization is preferable to simple arterial ligation. Firstly, even a simple surgical operation usually requires general anaesthesia and an abdominal incision: both factors adding increased risks in patients in whom massive hepatomegaly could compromise respiratory excursion, leading to pulmonary collapse and/or infection in the postoperative period. In the case of hepatic endocrine metastases, hormones may be produced that affect the cardiovascular and respiratory systems, posing difficult problems for the anaesthetist (Dery, 1971, McDermott & Hensle, 1974, Allison, 1982). Secondly, mainstem hepatic arterial ligation is not an effective means of producing vascular occlusion because of the potentially large number of collateral arterial routes to the hepatic circulation (Michels, 1953, Nebesar et al., 1969, Mays & Wheeler, 1974, Sivula & Sipponen, 1976, Allison, 1985). Michels (1953) has shown that at least 26 potential collateral pathways exist and these may continue to feed a tumour in the liver following ligation of the main hepatic artery. Arteriography performed shortly after main arterial occlusion demonstrates the existence of such collaterals, and these can grow rapidly in size and number over a period of days or weeks.

In a properly conducted embolization procedure the problem posed by collaterals can be obviated by showering the peripheral arterial tree in the tumour and surrounding liver with minute emboli so that no vascular bed exists for collateral vessels to supply. By the same token it is important that the radiologist should not embolize the principal arteries with large emboli alone; this will only produce the same result as surgical ligation and may leave blood flow to the tumour virtually unimpaired. Some of the above-mentioned drawbacks of surgical ligation relative to embolization may be overcome if the surgical procedure is accompanied by a thorough surgical arterial devascularization of the liver. This is a major procedure, however, and does not avoid one of the major disadvantages of ligation, which is that it precludes any subsequent attempts to embolize the liver should the tumour recur or new deposits appear. The renewed blood supply in such cases is often derived from unusual vessels that may be difficult or impossible to catheterize selectively in the presence of a ligated mainstem artery. With the embolization method the procedure can be repeated as often as is considered necessary or desirable.

All patients undergoing hepatic arterial embolization should be given adequate premedication in a dose suitable for age and weight. Antibiotics (against aerobic and anaerobic organisms) should be administered with the pre-medication and continued for 6–10 days after the embolization. It is very important to keep the patient well hydrated before, during, and after the procedure, to minimize the toxic effects, not only of the hormones released, but also of the contrast medium and breakdown products released by tumour necrosis. Embolization is usually performed under local anaesthesia and antiemetics. Patient reaction to hepatic embolization varies considerably from individual to individual, but it is sometimes necessary to administer analgesics intravenously during the procedure once the hepatic artery is occluded.

Patients suffering from the carcinoid syndrome may experience very dramatic cardiovascular effects during and after the procedure as the large areas of hormone-producing tissue are destroyed. To minimize these effects it is essential that the patient is placed on adequate doses of appropriate blocking agents for at least 48 h prior to the procedure and that these are continued throughout the immediate postembolization period.

The effects of embolization should be monitored by regular recordings of temperature, white cell count, hormone levels and ultrasound of the liver.

Most hepatic embolization procedures are followed by the postembolization syndrome (fever, elevated WBC, and pain) which can last for several days (Hemingway & Allison, 1988) (Fig. 15.14). A persistent fever should, however, be regarded as indication of infection and blood cultures taken.

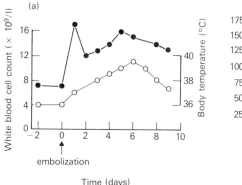

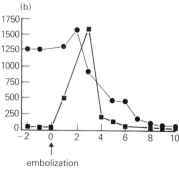

Fig. 15.14 Postembolization changes in a patient with carcinoid syndrome. Hepatic artery embolization (a) (○) Body temperature and (●) white cell count. (b) (■) Serum GOT (AST) (IU/c) and (●) urinary 5-HIAA (μmol/24 h) levels.

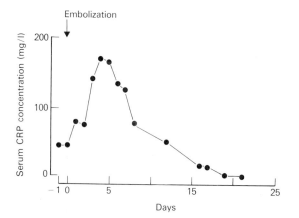

Fig. 15.15 Effect of hepatic embolization on C-reactive protein. Serum C-reactive protein changes following an uncomplicated hepatic embolization in a patient with metastatic carcinoid disease.

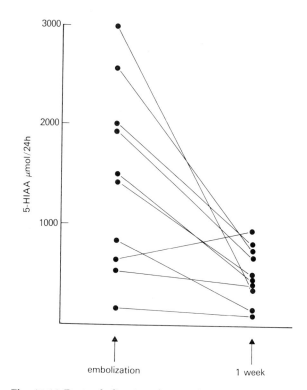

Fig. 15.16 Postembolization changes in tumour metabolites. Urinary 5-HIAA (5-hydroxyindoleacetic acid) levels pre- and postembolization in 10 patients with metastatic carcinoid disease.

Estimation of serum C-reactive protein levels is also useful; in an uncomplicated embolization they reach a peak at about 4 days, declining to normal levels at about 10 days (Fig. 15.15). If the levels stay elevated or continue to rise, this indicates infection (Hind & Pepys, 1984, Hind *et al.*, 1985).

Gas within the infarcted tumour is readily recognizable on ultrasound, CT, and even plain films, and the reasons for its presence are the subject of controversy (Hennessy & Allison, 1983, Carroll & Walter, 1983), though it is certain that it does not necessarily signify infection. The presence of a fluid level on an erect film suggests abscess formation. After extensive hepatic embolization many patients have an ileus for a few days and therefore require intravenous fluids to prevent dehydration.

The most severe complications such as gall bladder necrosis (De Jode *et al.*, 1976), sepsis, and shock lung, occur in those patients who are least

well prior to the procedure, and the possible occurrence of these complications must be weighed against the fact that there may be no other form of treatment suitable for that patient.

In general, the embolization of liver tumours does not confer any significant improvement in the duration of survival for patients with metastatic disease. The principal indication for liver embolization, therefore, is the amelioration of symptoms, and the technique can be dramatically successful in achieving this end in patients suffering from the distressing humoral effects of peptide hyper-secretion (Fig. 15.16). (Allison *et al.*, 1977, Allison *et al.*, 1985, Chuang & Wallace, 1983, Clouse *et al.*, 1983, Jaffee *et al.*, 1968, Maton *et al.*, 1983).

References

Allison, D.J. (1978a) Therapeutic embolization. *British Journal of Hospital Medicine*, **20**, 707–715.

Allison, D.J. (1978b) Therapeutic embolization and venous sampling. In Taylor, S. (ed.) *Recent Advances in Surgery*. 27–64. Churchill Livingstone, Edinburgh.

Allison, D.J. (1982) The non-surgical management of meta-static endocrine tumours to the liver. In Wilkins, R.A. & Viamonte, M. (eds) *Interventional Radiology*, pp. 191–208. Blackwell Scientific Publications, Oxford.

Allison, D.J. (1983) Interventional radiology. In Steiner, R.E. (ed.) *Recent Advances in Radiology and Medical Imaging*, Vol. 7, pp. 139–170. Churchill Livingstone, Edinburgh.

Allison, D.J. (1985) Interventional radiology. In Grianger, R.G. & Allison, D.J. (eds) *Diagnostic Radiology: an Anglo-American Textbook of Imaging*, pp. 2121–2165. Churchill Livingstone, Edinburgh.

Allison, D.J., Hennessy, O. & Jordan, H. (1985) Therapeutic embolization of the hepatic artery: a review of 75 pro-cedures. *Lancet*, **i**, 595–599.

Allison, D.J., Modlin, I.M. & Jenkins, W.J. (1977) Treat-ment of carcinoid liver metastases by hepatic artery em-bolization. *Lancet*, **ii**, 1323–1325.

Bloom, S.R. & Polak J.M. (eds) (1981). *Gut Hormones*, 2nd edn. Churchill Livingstone, Edinburgh.

Blumgart, L.H. & Allison, D.J. (1982) Resection and em-bolization in the management of secondary hepatic tu-mours. *World Journal of Surgery*, **6**, 32–45.

Breatnach, E.S., Han, S.Y., Rahatzad, M.D. & Stanley, R.J. (1985) CT evaluation of glucagonomas. *Journal of Computer Assisted Tomography*, **9**, 25–29.

Carroll, B.A. & Walter, J.P. (1983) Gas in embolized tu-mours: an alternative hypothesis for its origin. *Radiology*, **147**, 441–444.

Chuang, V.P. & Wallace, S. (1980) Hepatic artery emboli-zation in the treatment of hepatic neoplasms. *Radiology*, **140**, 51–58.

Chuang, V.P. & Wallace, S. (1983) Interventional approaches to hepatic tumor treatment. *Seminar in Roentgenology*, **18**, 127–135.

Clouse, M.E., Lee, R.G., Duszlak, E.J. *et al.* (1983) Peripheral artery embolization for primary and secondary hepatic neoplasms. *Radiology*, **147**, 407–411.

Creutzfeld, W. (1980). Endocrine tumors of the pancreas: Clinical, chemical and morphological findings. In Fitzgerald, P.J. & Morrison, A.B. (eds) *The Pancreas*, pp. 208–230. Williams & Wilkins, Baltimore.

De Jode, L.R., Nicholls, R.D. & Wright, P.L. (1976) Ischaemic necrosis of the gallbladder following hepatic artery em-bolization. *British Journal of Surgery*, **63**, 621.

Dery, R. (1971) Theoretical and clinical consideration in anaesthesis for secreting carcinoid tumours. *Canadian Anaesthetists Society Journal*, **18**, 245.

Dunnick, M.R., Doppman, J.C., Mills, S.R. & McCarthy, D.M. (1980). Computed tomographic detection of non

beta pancreatic islet cell tumors. *Radiology*, **135**, 117–120.

Fink, I.J., Krudy, A.G., Shawker, T.H. *et al.* (1985) Demon-stration of an angiographically hypovascular insulinoma with intra-arterial dynamic CT. *American Journal of Roentgenology*, **144**, 555–557.

Friesen, S.R. (1982). Tumors of the endocrine pancreas. *New England Journal of Medicine*, **306**, 580–590.

Galiber, A.K., Reading, C.C., Charboneau, J.W. *et al.* (1988) Localization of pancreatic insulinoma: comparison of pre- and intra-operative US with CT and angiography. *Radio-logy*, **166**, 405–408.

Gibson, R.N. & Hemingway, A.P. (1988) Radiological anat-omy of the liver and biliary tract. In Blumgart, L.H. (ed) *Surgery of the Liver and Biliary Tract*, pp. 3–37. Edinburgh, Churchill Livingstone.

Gorman, B., Charboneau, J.W., Meredith James, E. *et al.* (1986) Benign pancreatic insulinoma: pre-operative and intra-operative sonographic localization. *American Journal of Roentgenology*, **144**, 929–934.

Gunther, R.W. (1985) Ultrasound and CT in the assessment of suspected islet cell tumors of the pancreas. *Seminars in Ultrasonography, Computerized Tomography and Magnetic Resonance*, **6**, 261–275.

Hemingway, A.P. & Allison, D.J. (1988) Complications of embolization: analysis of 410 procedures. *Radiology*, **166**, 669–672.

Hennessy, O.F. & Allison, D.J. (1983) Intrahepatic gas fol-lowing embolization. *British Journal of Radiology*, **56**, 348–350.

Hind, C.R.K. & Pepys, M.B. (1984) The role of serum C-reactive protein measurement in clinical practice. *Internal Medicine for the Specialist*, **5**, 112–151.

Hind, C.R.K., Thomas, A.M.K., Pepys, M.B. & Allison, D.J. (1985) Serum C-reactive protein response to therapeutic embolization: possible role in management. *Clinical Radiology*, **36**, 179–183.

Imhof, H. & Frank, P. (1977) Pancreatic calcifications in malignant islet cell tumors. *Radiology*, **122**, 333–337.

Jaffee, B.M., Donegan, W.L., Watson, F. *et al.* (1968) Factors influencing survival in patients with untreated hepatic metastases. *Surgery, Gynecology and Obstetrics*, **127**, 1–11.

Jeffrey, M.A., Barter, S.J., Hemingway, A.P. & Nolan, D.J. (1984) Primary carcinoid tumours of the ileum: radio-logical appearances. *Clinical Radiology*, **35**, 451–455.

Kloppel, G. (1983) Pathologie der endokrinen Tumoren des Pankreas. In Kummerle F. & Ruckert, K. (eds) *Chirurgie des endocrinen Pankreas*. pp. 1–43. Thieme, Stuttgart.

Krudy, A.G., Doppman, J.L., Jensen, R.T. *et al.* (1984) Localization of islet cell tumors by dynamic CT: compari-son with plain CT, arteriography, sonography and venous sampling. *American Journal of Roentgenology*, **143**, 585–589.

Kuhn, F.P., Gunther, R., Ruckert, K. & Beyer, J. (1982) Ultra-sonic demonstration of small pancreatic islet cell tumours. *Journal of Clinical Ultrasound*, **10**, 173–175.

Lai, J., Ch'ng, C., Polak, J. & Bloom, S.R. (1988) Endocrine aspects of liver tumours. In Blumgart, L.H. (ed) *Surgery of the Liver and Biliary Tract*, pp. 1191–1217. Churchill Livingstone, Edinburgh.

McDermott, W.V. & Hensle, T.W. (1974) Metastatic carci-noid to the liver treated by hepatic dearterialization. *Annals of Surgery*, **180**, 305.

Maton, P.N., Miller, D.L., Doppman, J.L. *et al.* (1987) Role of selective angiography in the management of patients with Zollinger–Ellison syndrome. *Gastroenterology*, **92**, 913–918.

Maton, P.M., Camilleri, M., Griffin, G., Allison, D.J., Hodgson, H.G.F. & Chadwick, V.S. (1983) Role of hepatic arterial embolization in the carcinoid syndrome. *British Medical Journal*, **287**, 932–935.

Mays, E.T. & Wheeler, C.S. (1974) Demonstration of collateral arterial flow after interruption of hepatic arteries in man. *New England Journal of Medicine*, **290**, 993.

Michels, N.A. (1953) Collateral arterial pathways to the liver after ligation of the hepatic artery and removal of the celiac axis. *Cancer*, **6**, 708.

Murray-Lyon, I.M., Dawson, J.L., Parsons, V.A., Rake, M.O., Blendis, L.M. & Laws, J.W. (1970) Treatment of secondary hepatic tumours by ligation of hepatic artery and infusion of cytotoxic drugs. *Lancet*, **ii**, 172.

Nebesar, R.A., Knorblith, P.L., Pollard, J.J. & Michels, N.A. (1969) *Coeliac and Superior Mesenteric Arteries*. J. & A. Churchill, London.

Norton, J.A., Cromack, D.T., Shawker, T.H. *et al.* (1987) Intra-operative ultrasonographic localization of islet cell tumors, a prospective comparison to palpation. *Annals of Surgery*, 207, 160–168.

Polak, J.M. (ed) (1981) *Endocrine Tumours: The Pathobiology of Regulatory Peptide-Producing Tumours*. Churchill Living-stone, Edinburgh.

Roche, A., Raisonnier, A. & Gillou-Savouret, M.C. (1982) Pancreatic venous sampling and arteriography in localizing insullinomas and gastrinomas: Procedure and results in 55 cases. *Radiology*, **145**, 621–627.

Rossi P, Allison D. J. *et al.* (1989) Endocrine tumours of the pancreas. *Radiologic Clinics of North America*, (in press).

Rossi, P., Baert, A., Pasariello, R., Simonetti, G., Pavone, P. & Tempesta, P. (1985) CT of functioning tumors of the pancreas. *American Journal of Roentgenology*, **144**, 57–60.

Shawker, T.H. & Doppman, J.L. (1988) Intra-operative US (editorial). *Radiology*, **166**, 568–569.

Shearman, D.J. & Finlayson, N.D. (eds) (1982). *Diseases of the Gastrointestinal Tract and Liver*. Churchill Livingstone, London.

Sivula, A. & Sipponen, P. (1976) The effect of hepatic dearterialization and re-dearterialization on carcinoid liver metastases. *Annales Chirurgiae et Gynaecologiae*, **65**, 168.

Stark, D.D., Moss, A.A., Goldberg, M.I. & Deveney, W. (1984) CT of pancreatic islet cell tumors. *Radiology*, **150**, 491–494.

Yamada, R., Sato, M., Kawabata, M., Nakatsuka, H., Nakamura, K. & Takashima, S. (1983) Hepatic artery embolization in 120 patients with unresectable hepatoma. *Radiology*, **148**, 397–401.

16: Paediatric Liver Disease

H. CARTY

Investigation

The techniques employed in investigation of the liver in adult practice are applicable in paediatric practice. Ultrasound is the primary imaging investigation. The combination of ultrasound, isotope, and CT imaging have virtually precluded the use of oral and intravenous cholecystography in children. Care must be taken in all investigations in children to ensure a warm environment and to keep heat loss to a minimum, especially in neonates who are very susceptible to rapid temperature change (Bush *et al.*, 1978). Simple measures such as reducing the exposed area and wrapping unexposed parts in blankets and polythene sheeting suffice. During angiographic procedures contrast and flushing solution volumes must be carefully monitored, as must blood loss, to prevent circulatory overload.

Neonatal jaundice

Neonatal jaundice is a common clinical problem. The causes are many and include septicaemia, haemolysis, physiological jaundice, exchange transfusion, and congenital enzymatic defects. When the jaundice persists beyond the first 4 weeks without an identifiable cause and has an obstructive pattern biochemically, the two most likely diagnoses are biliary atresia and neonatal hepatitis. Biliary atresia is commoner in females but neonatal hepatitis is commoner in males.

Biliary atresia is a disease in which there is extrahepatic obliteration of the bile ducts to a variable degree. The types are classified into correctable, 12%, and non-correctable (88%). Correctable types are those in which the intrahepatic ducts are patent and there is sufficient patent extrahepatic bile duct to permit an anastomosis with the gut. With extrahepatic atresia there is associated intrahepatic proliferation of the small bile ducts, and periportal fibrosis. At the time of diagnosis there is a variable degree of cirrhosis, which becomes progressive unless bile drainage is established surgically. Other anomalies are reported in association with biliary atresia. These include duodenal atresia, preduodenal portal vein, polysplenia, situs inversus, left-sided inferior vena cava, and azygos continuation of the inferior vena cava (Choulot *et al.*, 1979, Brun *et al.*, 1985).

Neonatal hepatitis has a clinical picture similar to biliary atresia. The children are usually term babies with normal birth weight, and have hepatomegaly and obstructive jaundice both clinically and biochemically. In neonatal hepatitis the bile ducts are patent but there is parenchymal disorganization with infiltration of the liver by multinucleated giant cells. There is increase in free iron, intracellular and intracanalicular bile retention, inflammatory infiltration, and fibrosis of the portal tracts. There is usually a degree of cirrhosis present at diagnosis but this is not as severe as in atresia and can be reversible as the disease resolves. Neonatal hepatitis is thought to have numerous different causes but the term 'neonatal hepatitis' is usually reserved for those infants in whom no cause for their disease is identified (Gellis, 1975). Infecting organisms known to be associated with neonatal hepatitis include viruses, protozoa, and spirochaetes, but in most children no organism is isolated. All children with neonatal hepatitis should be screened for metabolic defects, as these cause an identical picture. The metabolic disorders include galactosaemia, fructosaemia, tyrosinaemia, α_1-antitrypsin deficiency, cystic fibrosis, Gaucher's disease, Wolmen's disease, Zellweger's syndrome, and Dubin–Johnson syndrome (Mowat, 1979a).

It may well be that biliary atresia and neonatal hepatitis have a common cause, and biliary atresia represents the severe end of the spectrum, where sclerosing cholangitis causes obliteration of the extrahepatic ducts (Landing, 1974).

Children with neonatal hepatitis or biliary

237

atresia are usually presented for investigation be-tween the ages of 4—7 weeks, when concern grows as the jaundice fails to resolve. The first investi-gation is an ultrasound examination of the liver and gall bladder, which should be done just before a meal. In normal children the gall bladder is easily seen in these circumstances. If not seen with contact scanning, a water bag should be used as the gall bladder can be very superficial. High-frequency probes (5—75 MHz) are essential for good paediatric ultrasound.

Demonstration of a normal gall bladder at ultra-sound virtually excludes biliary atresia (Abramson *et al.*, 1982). The gall bladder may not be seen in some children with neonatal hepatitis, for un-known reasons. Children with biliary atresia usually have no gall bladder visible at ultrasound, but a small number may have a small (<1.5 cm long) often thick-walled gall bladder visible (Abramson *et al.*, 1982, Brun *et al.*, 1985). Failure to visualize a gall bladder in a jaundiced neonate is a strong pointer to a diagnosis of biliary atresia; this is our experience. We have never seen a gall bladder on ultrasound in a child with biliary atresia. In neonatal hepatitis the gall bladder is usually visible. The presence of the common bile duct is then sought. If this is seen it also virtually

excludes a diagnosis of biliary atresia, but in some normal infants it may not be visualized.

Attempts have been made to identify a charac-teristic sonographic pattern of the liver in the neonatal jaundiced states, but these have been un-successful (Blane *et al.*, 1983).

Other anatomical abnormalities are noted if pre-sent. Ultrasound is followed by hepatobiliary scintigraphy. The agent normally used nowadays is a ^{99m}Tc-labelled compound of one of the deriva-tives of iminodiacetic acid (IDA) (Leonard *et al.*, 1982). These are extracted by the hepatocytes and excreted into the biliary system. In jaundiced in-fants it is imperative to give phenobarbitone 5 mg/kg per day for 5 days to potentiate the uptake and excretion of the ^{99m}Tc IDA in these compro-mised livers. (Majd *et al.*, 1981). The radiopharma-ceutical usually appears in the small bowel in 30 min in normal patients, but in infants with severely compromised livers excretion can be very delayed, and images which are only possible up to 24 h with ^{99m}Tc compound must be taken to avoid false-negative examination. Delayed imaging is possible with ^{131}I rose bengal but the poor-quality images, long half-life (8 days), and high beta emission make it unsatisfactory for children. Improved accuracy of diagnosis in distinguishing

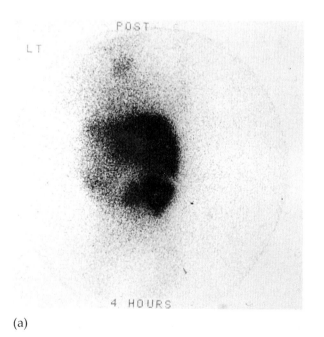

(a)

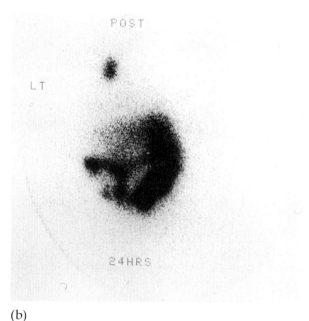

(b)

Fig. 16.1 Seven-week-old female with jaundice since birth. Diagnosis was neonatal hepatitis. (a) ^{123}I bromsulphthalein image at 4 h; (b) 24 h. At 4 h there is radiopharmaceutical in the bowel, which has increased at 24 h. On both images there is retention of bromsulphthalein in the liver, indicating liver damage due to hepatitis. There is some free iodine in the preparation and this is taken up in the thyroid.

atresia from neonatal hepatitis can be achieved with the use of clearance curves as well as images (Leonard *et al.*, 1982). Excretion of HIDA from the liver into the bowel indicates a patent biliary tree and excludes a diagnosis of biliary atresia. Further radiological investigation is not required, but a liver biopsy may be necessary to establish the extent of disease. Non-visualization of tracer in the intestine does not distinguish between biliary atresia and neonatal hepatitis and further investigation is necessary.

Recently, ^{123}I bromsulphthalein, which is an excellent hepatobiliary agent (Serafini *et al.*, 1975) has been available and in a small series of eight patients it has been completely predictive and is now our agent of choice (Figs 16.1, 16.2).

Non-visualization of the gall bladder by ultrasound and failure of excretion of radiopharmaceutical into the bowel lead to a presumptive diagnosis of biliary atresia, but this requires further confirmation by cholangiography and biopsy. Percutaneous cholangiography is possible in the neonate (Carty, 1978). In biliary atresia, extensive lymphatic drainage is seen but no ducts are entered (Fig. 16.3). The procedure is always followed by a liver biopsy. Clotting factors must be satisfactory before commencement of the procedure.

In severe neonatal hepatitis and in the correctable forms of biliary atresia a gall bladder may be seen ultrasonically, but no excretion of radionuclide takes place. Percutaneous transhepatic cholangiography in these children can be achieved either by the conventional approach (Chaumont, 1982) or preferably by percutaneous cholecystography (Brunelle, 1984). Alternatively, operative cholangiography is performed, and is the first step at laparotomy. In neonatal hepatitis a patent system is demonstrated but it may be smaller than normal. The pattern seen on cholangiography in biliary atresia depends on the nature of the atresia. It should be noted that even cholangiography is not 100% accurate in distinguishing biliary atresia from hepatitis, and the final diagnosis is by a combination of imaging and histology (Smith,

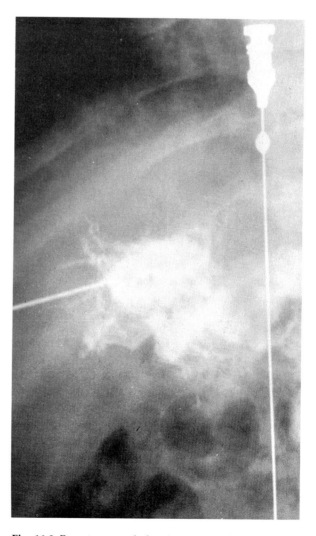

Fig. 16.3 Percutaneous cholangiogram in infant with biliary atresia. There is pooling of contrast due to failure of clearance by the liver following test injections. No ducts are demonstrated. Multiple irregular lymphatics are filled.

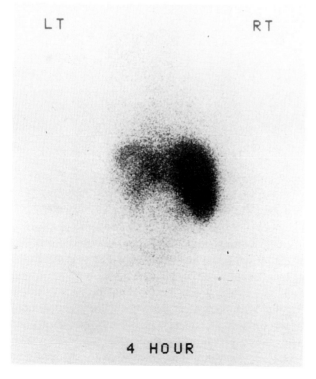

Fig. 16.2 Eight-week-old male infant with biliary atresia. There is no excretion of bromsulphthalein at 4 h, and delayed images at 24 h were unchanged.

1982). Correctable lesions occur in approximately 12% of children with biliary atresia (Smith 1982). The Kasai procedure of portoenterostomy is used to establish drainage in the vast majority of cases (Kasai *et al.*, 1968).

Postoperatively, radionuclide imaging with ^{99m}technetium-HIDA or ^{123}iodine-bromsulphthalein provides an excellent assessment of the success of the drainage procedure. The patency of the anastomosis may also be demonstrated by percutaneous transhepatic cholangiography (Fig. 16.4.).

The results of the Kasai procedure vary from poor to excellent, and are dependent on the timing of the procedure. Success is greater if the operation is done before 10 weeks (Altman, 1978). The quality of life with successful portoenterostomy is good for a number of years. Eventually, cirrhosis destroys the liver and portal hypertension becomes established. When this occurs the child presents with recurrent upper gastrointestinal bleeding from varices that may be massive, splenomegaly, and ultimately liver failure. Radiological investigation may be necessary to determine the bleeding point. It may be necessary to use all the techniques of splenoportography, angiography and radionuclide studies to localize it (Fig. 16.5).

Less dramatic, but nevertheless important, complications of chronic liver disease in children are failure to thrive, rickets, and in some children chronic lung disease due to biliary cirrhosis. Regular X-rays of the hand and wrist in these children will often detect the rickets before it is clinically apparent (Fig. 16.6).

The pulmonary infiltrate is visible on X-ray as a fine, recticular pattern in small-volume lungs. Pulmonary function is further compromised from restriction of respiratory movement by the enlarged abdomen, which is due to a combination of liver enlargement and ascites, present in many of these children (Fig. 16.7).

Hypertrophic osteoarthropathy has been described in two children with biliary atresia (Rothberg & Boal, 1983). It is a recognized complication in adults with liver disease.

Biliary hypoplasia

In addition to neonatal hepatitis and biliary atresia

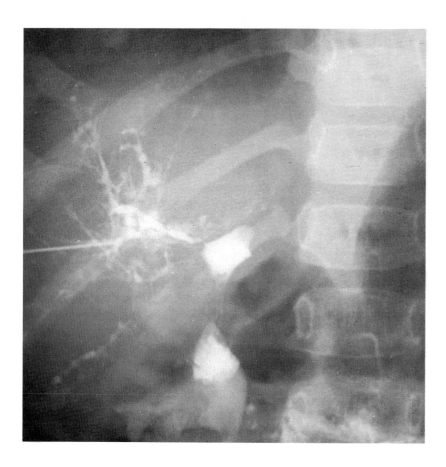

Fig. 16.4 Percutaneous cholangiogram after Kasai operation. There is good drainage at the anastomosis. The intrahepatic ducts are irregular and have the appearance of sclerosing cholangitis.

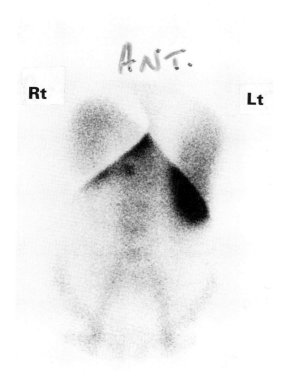

Fig. 16.5 Six-year-old girl who had had Kasai procedure as a neonate. Presented with severe upper gastrointestinal haemorrhage. Bleeding point was not identified at endoscopy. A sulphur colloid dynamic scan shows a bleeding focus in the duodenum.

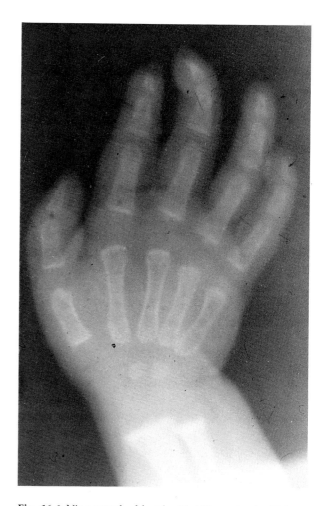

Fig. 16.6 Nine-month-old girl with biliary atresia. Rickets is present at the wrist.

there are a smaller group of children who have a similar clinical picture but have a patent but very hypoplastic biliary tree at cholangiography. Histologically there is cholestasis and features of hepatitis. Many of these children will progress to cirrhosis and liver failure from hepatic fibrosis (Smith, 1982, Mowat, 1979b) (Fig. 16.8).

Choledochal cyst

About 5% of children who present with obstructive jaundice in the neonatal period may have a congenital choledochal cyst as the causative lesion (Smith, 1982) although most children with choledochal cysts present later in childhood. Choledochal cysts are discussed in detail in Chapter 21.

Cholestasis associated with intravenous feeding

A clinical picture of obstructive jaundice similar to that seen in biliary atresia and neonatal hepatitis

may occur in infants on prolonged intravenous alimentation (Touloukian & Seashore, 1975). The liver is normally echogenic on ultrasound. The gall bladder is normal, thus excluding a diagnosis of atresia. Patency of the biliary tree is confirmed by radionuclide scanning. Histologically there are variable degrees of cholestasis and hepatocellular drainage. The diagnosis is made on the combination of negative investigation plus the relevant clinical history.

Inspissated bile syndrome

This is a rare condition in which the obstructive jaundice is due to a bile plug inspissated in the distal common bile duct. There are scattered reports in the surgical literature describing this condition but none has described the ultrasonic and radionuclide appearances. The author has personal

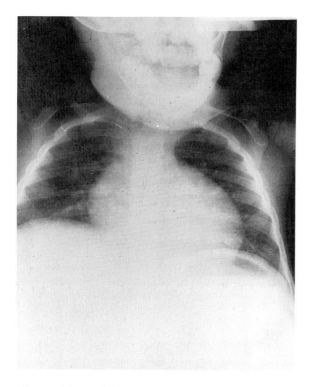

Fig. 16.7 Same child as in Fig. 16.6 at 3 years. She complained of severe dyspnoea. The lungs are of small volume and there is restriction of diaphragm movement due to massive abdominal enlargement. She had both an enlarged liver and ascites.

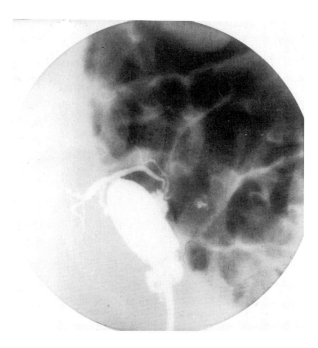

Fig. 16.8 Four-month-old male infant with jaundice. Operative cholangiogram shows a patent but small common hepatic and common bile duct. Even though there was patency, any attempt to clamp or remove the draining tube to the gall bladder resulted in a rapid and severe increase in jaundice and ill health. Death from hepatic failure occurred at 4 years.

experience of one case, but prior to the availability of ultrasound and radionuclides. A percutaneous cholangiogram performed prior to liver biopsy showed a dilated biliary tree with no flow of contrast into the duodenum (Fig. 16.9). However, within 10 h of the examination the child passed a coloured stool and rapidly lost her jaundice. Presumably the hyperosmolar contrast, plus increased pressure on the system, dislodged the plug. This accords well with the surgical experiences (Cook & Rickham, 1978).

Hepatic pulmonary angiodysplasia

There is a well-documented association of hepatic cirrhosis, cyanosis, finger clubbing, and right-to-left shunting at pulmonary level (Sang Oh et al., 1983). The pulmonary lesions appear as multiple spidery vessels evenly distributed throughout the lungs on the plain chest radiograph. At angiography the pulmonary arteries are small, tapered, and empty rapidly into dilated pulmonary veins

with right-to-left shunting. Levin describes a further variant with facial and skeletal abnormalities in addition to the hepatic and pulmonary changes (Alagille et al., 1975, Levin et al., 1980).

Bile duct dilatation and immunodeficiency syndrome

Hepatomegaly in children with immune deficiency syndrome is most commonly due to infective hepatitis or abscess. There is also a well-established association with sclerosing cholangitis (Isenberg et al., 1976, Naveh et al., 1983, Garel et al., 1985). This has been described in both single and combined deficiency. There is one report in association with immunodeficiency and cartilage–hair hypoplasia. (Garel et al., 1985). The discovery of hepatomegaly clinically leads to referral for ultrasound. Bile duct dilatation is present at ultrasound. At percutaneous transhepatic cholangiography multiple stenoses of the ducts are present, as seen in primary sclerosing cholangitis.

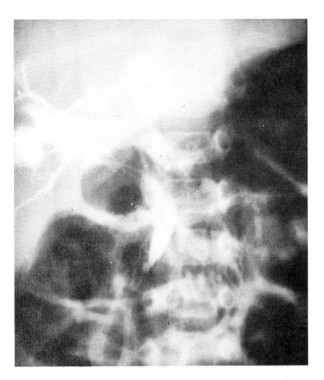

Fig. 16.9 Eight-week-old infant. Percutaneous transhepatic cholangiogram. The bile ducts and common bile duct are normal but there is no flow of contrast into the duodenum. Within 10 h of the examination the child passed a coloured stool and rapidly lost her jaundice. The presumptive diagnosis was inspissated bile syndrome.

Hepatic abscess

Hepatic abscesses in children most frequently occur as a complication of generalized septicaemia or as a complication of surgery or trauma. They are frequently multiple. The common infecting organisms are the staphylococcus and *E. coli*. Symptoms will often be masked by the primary problem, but include fever, hepatomegaly and jaundice. Premature infants with prolonged intravenous catheterization, or who have had necrotizing enterocolitis or surgery in the neonatal period are at risk, as are children with immunodeficiency states, and defects of leukocyte chemotaxis.

The lesion is usually first discovered at ultrasound examination and most frequently is echolucent but contains debris. Successful percutaneous drainage is possible in children. The abscesses are also easily visible on CT and appear as cold defects on sulphur colloid radionuclide scanning. Amoebic abscesses and hydatid cysts also occur in children from endemic areas. They have identical features to those seen in adult life.

Fatty infiltration of the liver

Fatty infiltration of the liver has a variety of causes. These include cystic fibrosis, Reye's syndrome, acute starvation and severe malnutrition states, malabsorption syndrome, steroid therapy, glycogen storage disease, and hepatitis. This leads to increased liver radiolucency on plain abdominal radiographs. An unusual clarity of the lateral border of the right kidney, an interface between the abdominal wall muscle, blurring of the medial margin of the properitoneal fat stripe, and fat—water interface are the described radiographic appearances (Melhem 1976, Yousefzadeh *et al.*, 1979). At ultrasound the liver may be unusually bright due to fatty infiltration. In severe cases the macroscopic appearance of a white biopsy specimen is characteristic.

Wilson's disease

Hepatolenticular degeneration is an inborn error of copper metabolism. It is inherited as an autosomal recessive trait. The disease is characterized by degeneration in the central nervous system, cirrhosis of the liver, and renal abnormalities. The presence of Kayser—Fleischer rings at the corneal limbus is diagnostic. Bony manifestations in the adult include osteoporosis, osteomalacia, and osteoarthritis. Bony manifestations in childhood will appear as rickets (Yu-Zhang *et al.*, 1985).

Hepatic calcification

Calcification occurs in the child's liver. The cause of the calcification is usually fairly obvious, i.e. tumour, abscess cavity, tuberculosis, histoplasmosis, and parasites in children from endemic areas. Perihepatic calcification can occur in meconium peritonitis. Rare infective causes of calcification include intrauterine infections and chronic granulomatous disease (McNulty, 1977). Intrahepatic calculi have been reported in Caroli's disease, and calcification is also reported in thrombi in both the portal vein and hepatic artery, but all are extremely rare. Calcification can also occur in the inferior vena cava at the level of the suprarenal gland and can cause confusion with hepatic vascular calcification. The condition is asymptomatic and usually discovered fortuitously. The plain film appearance is characteristic (Kassner *et al.*, 1976).

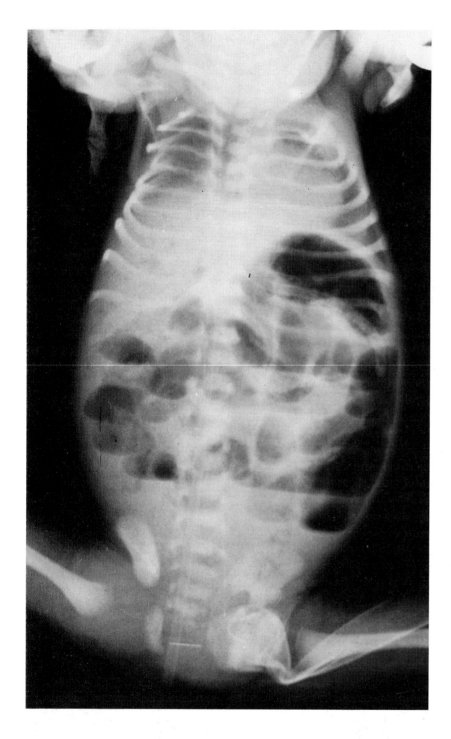

Fig. 16.10 Infant with necrotizing enterocolitis. There is portal venous air. The characteristic branching pattern is seen.

Subcapsular haematoma of the liver in the newborn

Subcapsular haematoma is a rare but well-recognized complication in the neonatal period. Children at risk include large babies with a history of difficult delivery, infants with erythroblastosis, and babies who have received cardiac massage. The children usually present in the 2nd–5th day of life with sudden onset of shock, anuria, and often abdominal distension. If the haematoma ruptures, a haemoperitoneum develops. Ultrasound is usually diagnostic. A fluid-filled band containing a few echoes is seen surrounding the liver (Cohen *et al.*, 1982).

Hepatic air

Air in the liver as seen on a plain abdominal radiograph is usually in either the biliary tree or in the portal venous system. Gas in the biliary tree in children is almost always postoperative and occurs following anastomosis between the biliary tree or gall bladder and bowel lumen. Air in the portal venous system has a characteristic branching pattern with the branches extending to the periphery of the liver (Fig. 16.10) It is seen most commonly in children with severe necrotizing enterocolitis, but is also described in association with infection with gas-forming organisms, ingestion of corrosives, bowel obstruction, and umbilical catheterization.

Congenital hepatic fibrosis

Patients with congenital hepatic fibrosis almost invariably present in childhood, though affected individuals may live well into adult life. Presentation is usually in the first decade, often with hepatosplenomegaly discovered fortuitously at routine clinical examination. Other children will present with haematemesis from varices. Rarely, presentation is with liver failure or septicaemia. The histological pattern is very characteristic. Broad bands of connective tissue are present in a portal or periportal distribution and these contain ectatic and dysplastic small bile ducts. Congenital hepatic fibrosis most commonly occurs in association with the autosomally recessive infantile poly-

cystic disease, but the renal lesion is usually silent and only minimal at presentation, as only 10–20% of the renal tubules may be involved, and is discovered during the investigation of the hepatic disease. Renal failure is a later problem. Congenital hepatic fibrosis is also seen without infantile polycystic kidneys and is found in Ivermark's syndrome (dysplastic kidneys and hepatic fibrosis), Heckel's syndrome (encephalocoele, cleft lip and palate polydactyly, and cysts in kidney), and rarely in association with the adult form of polycystic renal disease (Silverman & Roy, 1983). It may also occur as an isolated lesion and is sometimes familial.

Initial investigation is ultrasound of the liver, spleen, and kidneys. The ultrasonic findings in the liver will depend on the degree of cirrhosis and fibrosis. In the early stages the liver is simply enlarged but otherwise normal. As the cirrhosis develops the ultrasonic pattern will alter to that of cirrhosis, and multiple nodules may be seen. The kidney, however, will often appear unusually bright due to the numerous small cysts (Figs 16.11, 16.12). The definitive diagnosis is made by liver biopsy.

Further radiological investigation may be required to identify bleeding points as portal hypertension and varices develop.

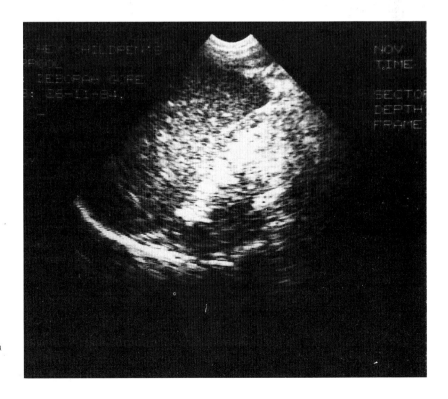

Fig. 16.11 Congenital hepatic fibrosis. The kidney is intensely bright due to the numerous small cysts. This is the typical pattern seen at ultrasound in infantile polycystic kidneys.

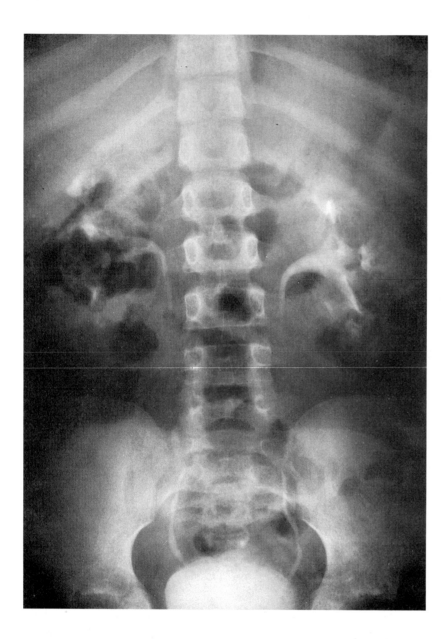

Fig. 16.12 Same child as in Fig. 16.11. Intravenous pyelography. Persistent retention of contrast is present in the renal tubules. These are the classical changes of mild infantile polycystic disease.

Portal hypertension in childhood

The clinical manifestations and presenting complaint of portal hypertension in childhood include splenomegaly, melaena, haematemesis, hypersplenism, hepatomegaly, cutaneous portasystemic shunts, ascites, and malabsorption. Portal hypertension exists when the portal venous pressure rises above 20 cm water. The rise in pressure may occur through (a) pre- or extrahepatic obstruction to venous flow in the portal vein or one of its tributaries, (b) intrahepatic disease, or (c) posthepatic disease with hepatic venous thrombosis leading to a rise in portal venous pressure. More rarely, increased flow through the liver such as

occurs in arteriovenous malformation will also lead to a rise in portal pressure.

Extrahepatic portal hypertension occurs from obstruction of the portal or splenic vein (Fig. 16.13). There are some documented cases in association with sepsis and the use of umbilical venous catheters in the neonate, but this, though traditionally quoted as the cause, is in fact rare, and most cases are idiopathic. Most children present with splenomegaly or gastrointestinal bleeding.

Intrahepatic portal hypertension is a sequel of cirrhosis, which itself is the result of disorders such as neonatal hepatitis and biliary atresia, cholestasis, congenital hepatic fibrosis (Fig. 16.14), cystic fibrosis, chronic hepatitis, schistosomiasis,

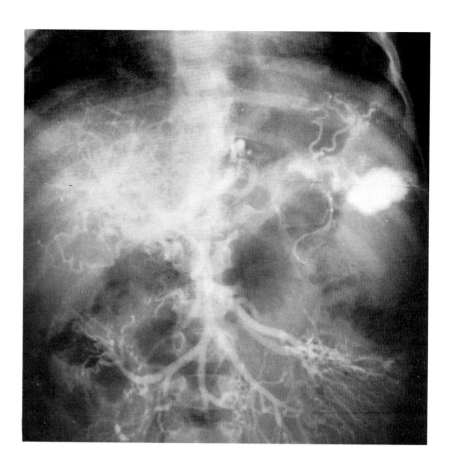

Fig. 16.13 Splenoportogram. Twelve-year-old male with incidental finding of enlarged spleen. The portal vein is occluded and replaced by collaterals.

and veno-occlusive disease, to name but a few causes. These children will tend to show features of chronic liver disease and will frequently have an appropriate history.

Post-hepatic portal hypertension is due to obstruction of the hepatic vein either in the main channel — Budd—Chiari syndrome, or in the intrahepatic venules—veno-occlusive disease. These causes are very rare in children. Hepatic-vein thrombosis is most commonly due to malignancy.

Extrahepatic cases of portal hypertension occur more frequently in paediatric practice than in adults, where intrahepatic disease tends to dominate.

Investigation of children with portal hypertension will depend on the mode of presentation. If the child presents with a life-threatening haemorrhage, then angiography and radionuclide studies will be required to identify the bleeding point if this is not seen at endoscopy. Most frequently initial investigation is by plain abdominal X-ray and ultrasound. At ultrasound the liver and spleen are usually normal in texture but enlarged. Varices may be visible in the hilum of the spleen. The normal portal vein is replaced by collaterals, which may cause a mass effect (Grand & Remy, 1979), and in severe hypertension the ductus venosus (Fig. 16.15) becomes visible. Ascites is noted if present. Barium studies will show varices but will underestimate their true extent and may fail to demonstrate fundal lesions in the stomach. The choice of splenoportography or angiography to demonstrate portal venous anatomy, the extent of the varices, and the patency of the splenic vein, is a local one and will depend on local experience. Both procedures may be required for full delineation of the anatomy. This must always be fully displayed before surgery. In general, the demonstration of the portal venous anatomy is poorer with arterial studies than with splenoportography, and portal venous pressures cannot be measured, but information about the superior mesenteric vein and the arterial anatomy can be obtained that cannot be seen at splenoportography. Splenoportography must never be performed without first confirming that the clotting time is normal.

Hepatic venography is carried out by passing a catheter via the femoral vein and inferior vena

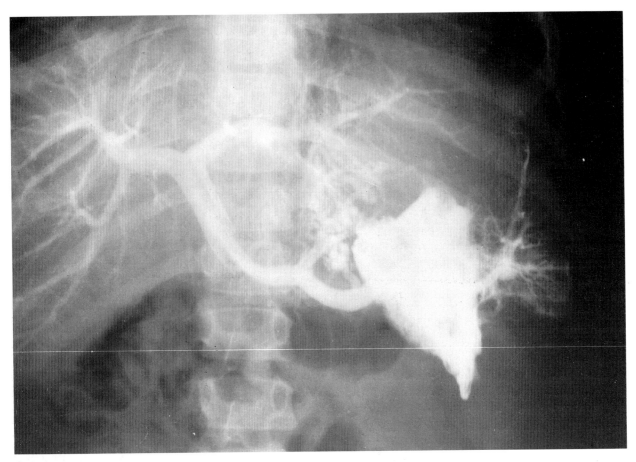

Fig. 16.14 Same child as in Figs 16.11 and 16.12. Splenoportogram. Extravasation of contrast occurred during injection. The portal vein and intrahepatic veins are patent. There is a cluster of varices arising from the left gastric vein.

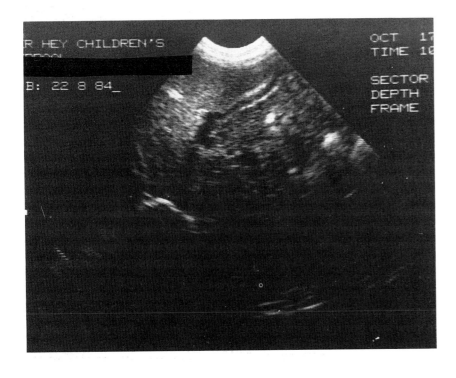

Fig. 16.15 Infant with portal hypertension. The ductus venosus is patent.

cava into the hepatic vein. Contrast is injected to assess the vein's patency and the wedge pressure is measured. Hepatic venous occlusion has been detected by ultrasound in adults but there are no reported childhood cases yet (Makuuchi *et al.*, 1984).

Veno-occlusive disease of the liver

This is an important cause of portal hypertension in children from endemic areas and is thought to be due to a toxin in 'bush tea' made from certain plants. The disease was originally described in Jamaica but similar cases have been seen in South Africa, India, and in Egyptian children. Sporadic idiopathic cases are seen in the US and Britain. Radiological investigation will demonstrate varices but will also show patency and normal structure of the main hepatic veins, and the portal and splenic veins. The diagnosis is made at biopsy. Veno-occlusive disease is also reported in association with chemotherapy for leukaemia and in association with congenital immune deficiency.

Inborn errors of metabolism and hepatomegaly

Numerous inherited disorders of metabolism have jaundice and/or hepatomegaly as part of the clinical problem. These include galactosaemia,

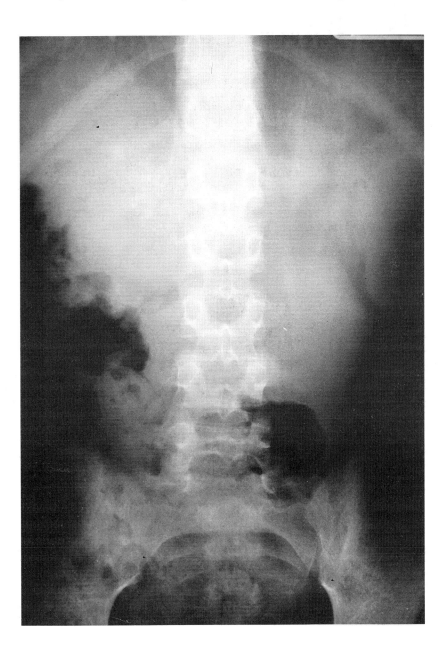

Fig. 16.16 Fifteen-year-old boy with cystic fibrosis. Pancreatic calcification is present. Note also abnormal bowel content and enlarged spleen.

diabetes, glycogen storage disease, lipid storage disorders, amino acid disorders, enzymatic defects in the urea cycle, porphyria, beta thalassaemia, and mucopolysaccharidoses (Mowat, 1979a and c). The association with the neonatal hepatitis syndrome has already been discussed. Radiology is not usually normally useful in primary diagnosis but may be important in monitoring the course of the disease and in detecting complications such as liver adenomas in glycogen storage disease (Brunelle *et al.*, 1984).

Cystic fibrosis

The existence of liver and gall bladder disease in patients with cystic fibrosis is now well-recognized. Up to 8% of affected adults have insulin dependent diabetes and 20% of adolescents have cirrhosis. Other complications include fatty infiltration of the liver, portal hypertension, gall stones, and micro gall bladder (Graham *et al.*, 1985). Pancreatic calcification also occurs (Fig. 16.16). While these complications increase with

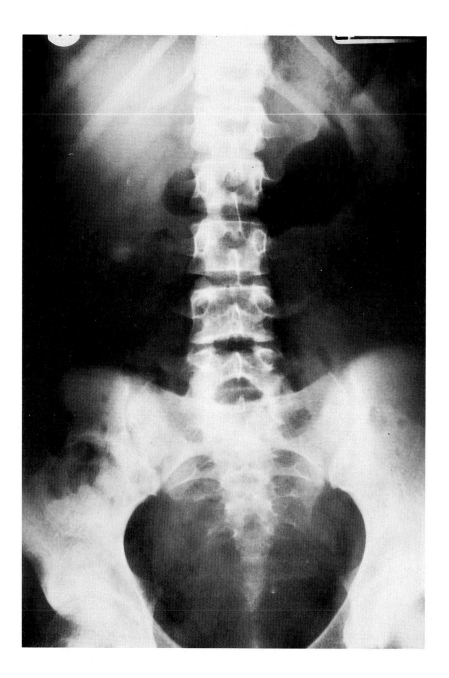

Fig. 16.17 Fifteen-year-old girl with total colectomy for Crohn's disease. Note ileostomy. She presented with a further episode of colicky abdominal pain. A plain abdominal film was taken to exclude obstruction. Gall stones were found incidentally and were probably the cause of the pain.

age, all are also encountered in childhood. The ultrasonic features in the liver are those of cirrhosis. The gall bladder wall is thickened and the whole gall bladder is small (1.5 cm long). Pancreatic calcification and gall stones may be seen on plain radiographs, detected ultrasonically, or be seen on CT.

Mucocutaneous lymph node syndrome: Kawasaki disease

Kawasaki disease is a febrile illness of unknown origin that occurs in children mainly under 5 years old. The general features include fever, rash, and lymphadenopathy. Serious cardiac complications include coronary artery aneurysm, myocardial infarction, pericardial effusion, and congestive failure. One further well-described association is hydrops of the gall bladder, and it may be the presenting complaint in association with the rash. The children have fever, abdominal pain, and tenderness. Ultrasound of the abdomen is diagnostic — a huge, tense gall bladder with a normal thickness wall is found (Haden et al., 1984, Grisoni et al., 1984).

Cholelithiasis in paediatrics

Gall stone disease is rare in paediatric practice. About 20% are said to be associated with haemolytic disorders (Smith, 1982) but most occur in children and have no underlying cause. In areas with a large endemic population with sickle-cell disease a higher incidence may be found. The signs and symptoms in older children are similar to those in adults. The difficulty in making the diagnosis is simply one of failure to think of it. Radiological investigation is by plain abdominal film and by ultrasound. Cholecystography, oral or intravenous, is no longer indicated in the primary investigation.

Gall stones also occur in children with cystic fibrosis and in children who have disturbance of the enterohepatic circulation due to terminal ileal disease, e.g. Crohn's disease (Fig. 16.17) or ileal resection of congenital atresia.

Neonatal cholelithiasis is extremely rare, but occurs and is usually not diagnosed until surgery for jaundice or perforation (Brill et al., 1982, Shaw et al., 1984) but occasionally calcified gall stones are seen on the plain abdominal radiograph.

Spontaneous perforation of the bile duct in infancy

Bile peritonitis may develop in infancy from spontaneous perforation of the bile duct. The clinical picture is one of irritability, vomiting, failure to thrive and low-grade fever in association with jaundice and acholic stools. The diagnostic clue lies in the discovery of ascites at ultrasound examination, and this may precede development of bile-stained hydrocoele or umbilical hernia. The site of perforation is usually demonstrated at operative cholangiography.

References

Abramson, S.J., Treves, S. & Teele, R.S. (1982) The infant with possible biliary atresia: evaluation by ultrasound and nuclear medicine. *Paediatric Radiology*, **12**, 1—5.

Alagille, D., Odievre, M., Gautier, M. & Dommergues, J.P. (1975) Hepatic ductal hypoplasia associated with characteristic facies, vertebral malformations, retarded physical, mental and sexual development and cardiac murmur. *Journal of Pediatrics*, **86**, 63—71.

Altman, Q.P. (1978) The portoenerostomy procedure for biliary atresia: A five year experience. *Annals of Surgery*, **188**, 351—362.

Blane, C.E., Jongeward, R.H. & Silver, T.M. (1983) Sonographic features of hepatocellular disease in neonates and infants. *American Journal of Roentgenology*, **141**, 1313—1316.

Brill, P.W., Winchester, P. & Rosen, M.S. (1982) Neonatal cholelithiasis. *Pediatric Radiology*, **12**, 285—289.

Brun, P., Gauthier, F., Boucher, D. & Brunelle, F. (1985) Ultrasound findings in biliary atresia in children. *Annales de Radiologie (Paris)*, **28**, 259—263.

Brunelle, F. & Chaumont, P. (1984) Percutaneous cholecystography in children. *Annales de Radiologie (Paris)*, **27**, 111—116.

Brunelle, F., Tamman, S., Odievre, M. & Chaumont, P. (1984) Liver adenomas in glycogen storage disease in children. *Pediatric Radiology*, **14**, 94—101.

Bush, G.H., Dangel, P. & Rickham, P.P. (1978) In Lister, J., Rickham, P.P., Irving, I. (eds) Neonatal respiratory physiology and respiratory complications. *Neonatal Surgery*, pp. 35—52. Butterworth, London.

Carty, H. (1978) Percutaneous fine needle cholangiography in jaundiced infants. *Annales de Radiologie (Paris)*, **21**, 149—154.

Chaumont, P., Martin, N., Riou, Y. & Brunelle, F. (1982) Percutaneous transhepatic cholangiography in extra hepatic biliary duct atresia in children. *Annales de Radiologie (Paris)*, **25**, 94—100.

Choulot, J.J., Gautier, M., Eliot, N. & Odievre, M. (1979) Les malformations associées à l'atrésie des voies biliares extra-hépatiques. *Archives Francáis de Pediatrie (Paris)*, **36**, 19—24.

Cohen, J.Y., Garel, L., Sorin, B., Roze, J.C. & Mouzard, A. (1982) Subcapsular hematomas of the Liver in the Newborn. *Annales de Radiologie (Paris)*, **25**, 34—40.

Cook, R.C.M. & Rickham, P.P. (1978) In Lister, J., Rickham, P.P. & Irving, I. (eds) The liver and biliary tract. *Neonatal Surgery*, pp. 483–497. Butterworth, London.

Garel, L., Brunelle, F., Fischer, A., Sirinelli, D. & Sauvegrain, J. (1985) Bile duct dilatation and immunodeficiency in children. *Annales de Radiologie (Paris)*, **28**, 249–255.

Gellis, S.S. (1975) Atresia. *Pediatrics*, **55**, 8–9.

Graham, N., Manhire, A.R., Stead, R.J., Lees, W.R., Hodson, M.E. & Batten, J.C. (1985) Cystic fibrosis: ultrasonographic findings in the pancreas and hepatobiliary system correlated with clinical data and pathology. *Clinical Radiology*, **36**, 199–203.

Grand, M.P. & Remy, J. (1979) Ultrasound diagnosis of extrahepatic portal vein obstruction in childhood. *Pediatric Radiology*, **8**, 155–159.

Grisoni, E., Fisher, R. & Izant, R. (1984) Kawasaki syndrome: Report of four cases with acute gall bladder hydrops. *Journal of Pediatric Surgery*, **19**, 9–11.

Haden, M.A., Alford, B.A. & Young, L.W. (1984) Hydrops of the gall bladder secondary to Kawasaki disease. *American Journal of Diseases of Children*, **138**, 985–986.

Isenberg, J.N., Hanson, R.F., Williams, J.C., Zavoral, J., Page, A.R. & Sharp, H.L. (1976) Immunodeficiency xanthomas and obstructive liver disease. *American Journal of Medicine*, **61**, 393–400.

Kasai, M., Kimura, S., Asakura, Y., Suzuki, H., Taira, Y. & Ohasi, E. (1968) Surgical treatment of biliary atresia. *Journal of Pediatric Surgery*, **3**, 665–674.

Kassner, E.G., Baumstark, A., Kinkhabwala, M.N., Ablow, R.C. & Haller, J.O. (1976) Calcified thrombus in the inferior vena cava in infants and children. *Pediatric Radiology*, **4**, 167–171.

Landing, B.H. (1974) Considerations of the pathogenesis of neonatal hepatitis, biliary atresia and choledochal cyst — the concept of infantile obstructive cholangiopathy. *Progress in Pediatric Surgery*, **6**, 113–139.

Leonard, J.C., Hitch, D.C. & Manion, C.V. (1982) Use of ^{99m}Tc diethyl IDA clearance curves in the differentiation of biliary atresia from the other forms of neonatal jaundice. *Radiology*, **142**, 773–776.

Levin, S., Zarws, P., Milner, S. & Schmaman, A. (1980) Arteriohepatic dysplasia: Association of liver disease with pulmonary arterial stenosis as well as facial and skeletal abnormalities. *Pediatrics*, **66**, 876–883.

McNulty, J.G., (1977) *Radiology of the Liver*. W.B. Saunders, Philadelphia.

Majd, M., Reba, R.C. & Altman, R.P. (1981) Effect of phenobarbital on ^{99m}Tc-IDA scintigraphy in the evaluation of neonatal jaundice. *Seminars in Nuclear Medicine*, **11**, 194–204.

Makuuchi, M., Hasegawa, H., Yamazaki, S., Moriyama, N., Takayasu, K. & Okazaki, M. (1984) Primary Budd–Chiari syndrome ultrasonic demonstration. *Radiology*, **152**, 775–779.

Melhem, R.E. (1976) The radiolucent liver. *Pediatric Radiology*, **4**, 153–156.

Mowat, A. (ed) (1979a). Inborn errors of metabolism. *Liver Disorders in Childhood*, pp. 162–202. Butterworths, London.

Mowat, A. (ed) (1979b). Intrahepatic biliary hypoplasia. *Liver Disorders*, pp. 69–71. Butterworths, London.

Mowat, A. (ed) (1979c). Conjugated hyperbilirubinaemia. *Liver Disorders in Childhood*, pp. 54–55. Butterworths, London.

Naveh, Y., Mendelsohn, H., Spira, G., Auslaender, L., Mandel, H. & Berant, M. (1983) Primary sclerosing cholangitis associated with immunodeficiency. *American Journal of Diseases of Children*, **137**, 114–117.

Rothberg, A.D. & Boal, D.K. (1983) Hypertrophic osteoarthropathy in biliary atresia. *Pediatric Radiology*, **13**, 44–46.

Sang Oh, K., Brinder, T.M., Bowen, A. & Ledesma-Medine, J. (1983) Plain radiographic, nuclear medicine and angiographic observations of hepatogenic pulmonary angiodysplasia. *Pediatric Radiology*, **13**, 111–115.

Serafini, A.N., Snoak, W.M. & Hupf, H.B. (1975) Iodine 123 Rose Bengal: An improved hepatobiliary imaging agent. *Journal of Nuclear Medicine*, **16**, 629–632.

Shaw, G.J., Spitz, L. & Watson, J.G. (1984) Extrahepatic biliary obstruction due to stone. *Archives of Disease in Childhood*, **59**, 896–897.

Silverman, A., & Roy, C.C. (eds) (1983a). Prolonged obstructive jaundice. *Paediatric Clinical Gastroenterology*, p. 552. C.V. Mosby Company, St Louis.

Silverman, A. & Roy, C.C. (eds) (1983b). Portal hypertension. *Paediatric Clinical Gastroenterology*, pp. 788, 792. C.V. Mosby Company, St Louis.

Smith, W.L. (1982) In Franken, E.A. (ed) Gastrointestinal Imaging in Pediatrics. *The Liver*, pp. 426–429. Harper & Row, Philadelphia.

Touloukian, R.J. & Seashore, J.H. (1975) Hepatic secretory obstruction with total parenteral nutrition in the infant. *Journal of Pediatric Surgery*, **10**, 353–360.

Yousefzadeh, D.K., Lupetin, A.R. & Jackson, J.H. (1979) The radiographic signs of fatty liver. *Radiology*, **131**, 351–355.

Yu-Zhang Xie, Xue-Zhe Zhang, Xian-Hao Xu, Zhen-Xin Zhang & Ying-Kum Eeng. (1985) Radiologic study of 42 cases of Wilson disease. *Skeletal Radiology*, **13**, 114–119.

17: Liver Transplantation

H.B. NUNNERLEY

Introduction

Liver transplantation for irreversible disease that has exhausted conventional medical and surgical treatment is now occurring with increasing frequency and in a larger number of centres. The European liver transplant registry reported recently that over 1200 patients had been transplanted in 32 centres (Bismuth *et al.*, 1987). Since 1984 the rate has more than doubled. It is of interest that the survival at 1 year is 44% and at 2 years is 41%, whereas the preoperative mortality was recorded at 30%. Similar figures are obtained from the USA. There the largest series is recorded in Pittsburg where 500 patients were transplanted between 1980 and 1985 (Tzakis *et al.*, 1987).

There has been a slight change in the indications for transplantation from the early days up to 1984 as compared with more recent years. Undoubtedly end-stage liver disease, cirrhosis of any type, with primary biliary cirrhosis predominating, is the most common cause. There has been a significant increase in children with biliary atresia now being transplanted and, indeed, in patients with acute hepatic failure, as well as the Budd–Chiari syndrome and patients with sclerosing cholangitis. There has, however, been a significant decline in the number of patients transplanted for malignant disease, because of the high incidence of recurrence following transplantation. The only patients with metastatic liver tumours now considered for transplantation are those with metastatic carcinoid tumour, which has a relatively benign biological behaviour. Children do particularly well, and those transplanted for biliary atresia show a survival at 30 days, 6 months, 1 year, and 2 years, respectively, of 87%, 77%, 74% and 68% (Bismuth *et al.*, 1987).

Preoperative evaluation

All patients referred for liver transplantation need very careful evaluation before undergoing such a complicated procedure. Apart from the general chemical and other tests, radiology plays a very important role in this. A large proportion of these patients, up to 75%, can be evaluated without invasive studies. Nuclear medicine studies play a role. Radionuclide liver spleen scans are helpful in assessing the size of, and the function remaining in, the liver and give some idea about the presence or absence of portal hypertension. Technetium sulphur colloid scans give information about the reticuloendothelial system within the liver, as well as the conjugating and bile excretion function (example, DIISIDA scans). These latter are of particular importance in children with biliary atresia and adults with primary biliary cirrhosis.

Ultrasound plays a vital part in preoperative assessment, gives an indication of the liver parenchyma, and localizes any focal lesion. One of the critical factors in the decision to transplant is the patency of the portal vein. Doppler ultrasound is of particular use here, and is successful in over 80% of patients. Thrombus can be detected and the flow, whether it is present, and its direction, can be noted. Infants who have had surgery such as portoenterostomy can be somewhat difficult patients in whom to determine the patency of the portal vein, because of technical problems. The size and patency of the inferior vena cava can also be well noted with ultrasound.

Computerized tomography also has a place. It is especially helpful in determining the presence and extent of ascites. In patients with tumours the extent of the tumour can be clearly mapped out and any extrahepatic extension of the tumour, particularly to the lymph nodes, can be noted.

Arteriography is of value in assessing the extent of malignant disease, including encasement of adjacent vessels. A number of patients are referred initially for possible resection of tumour, and if this is found to be impossible they are considered for possible transplantation. The arterial anatomy of the liver is variable, so it is of help, if an arterial study is being performed, to note the appropriate configuration in the patient, i.e. whether the hepatic artery arises in the conventional manner from the coeliac axis or whether there are branches from vessels such as the left gastric artery or more commonly the superior mesenteric artery.

The state of the portal venous system can be shown by the arterial method using digital subtraction angiography. It is possible to give a reasonable map of the portal venous system. The problems arise when there is extensive hepatofugal flow and most of the contrast medium passes via shunts into the venous system. If this is the case it is possible to puncture a branch of the portal vein within the liver with a fine needle (22 gauge Chiba) and inject contrast. Using digital subtraction techniques this gives a very clear picture of the main portal vein and its pattern.

In small children we have found it particularly helpful, if they still have a spleen, to do splenoportograms. We use a fine needle placed in the splenic pulp, and inject contrast, again using the digital subtraction technique. With a small amount, 10 ml of 110 mg per ml strength contrast medium, good visualization of the splenic and portal veins can be obtained.

The inferior vena cava can be readily demonstrated by injecting contrast via a femoral vein. If a patient has the Budd–Chiari syndrome, it is important to exclude a web at the upper end of the inferior vena cava; thus, in addition to contrast studies, pressure studies should be done in the inferior vena cava from below the level of the liver into the right atrium. If there is a sharp pressure gradient at the upper end, above the gradient one would expect from an enlarged liver, this would be supportive evidence for the presence of a web.

In patients with tumour, distant metastases in the lungs, pleura, and bones must be excluded if possible.

Early postoperative complications

Patients undergoing such major surgery as liver transplantation have the usual complications of major surgery. These include chest problems. One of the most frequent complications is that of a right pleural effusion as well as patchy collapse/consolidation at both bases. In the immediate postoperative period, bleeding can cause concern, as these patients may well have serious inherent clotting defects. It is important, except in cases of

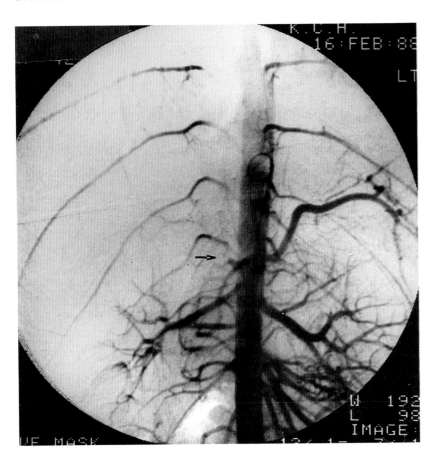

Fig. 17.1 Flush arteriogram showing occlusion of the hepatic artery at the anastomotic site.

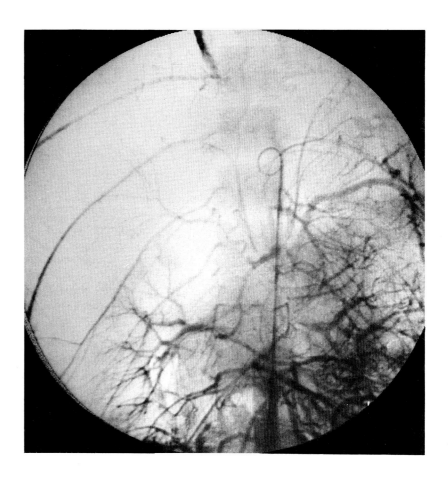

Fig. 17.2 Flush arteriogram showing compression of the hepatic artery in acute rejection.

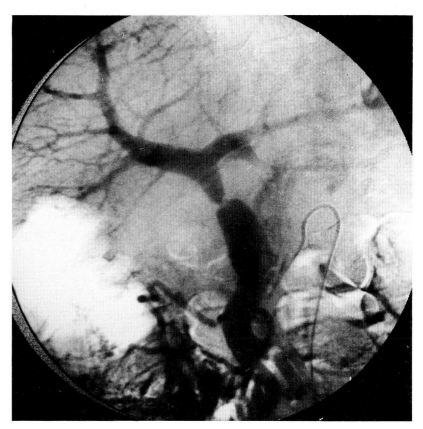

Fig. 17.3 Aortoportogram showing narrowing of the portal vein at the anastomosis.

acute liver failure, to transplant before liver function deteriorates to extreme levels. Many patients have some form of collection of fluid around the liver, which is readily demonstrated on ultrasound. In the earlier days these tended to be aspirated, but now they are noted and watched in postoperative ultrasound studies. It is possible to aspirate such collections and find out the nature — whether it is blood, bile, pus, or serous fluid. Leakage of bile from the biliary anastomosis is one of the commonest early problems.

General postoperative problems

It can be difficult, without radiological techniques, to distinguish rejection from other postoperative complications. Non-interventional techniques such as ultrasound should be used in the first instance. In this way any dilatation of the duct system can be diagnosed, as well as possible thrombosis in the portal venous system.

Arterial complications

One of the most serious complications following transplantation is thrombosis of the hepatic artery. Doppler ultrasound should give evidence of this. Angiography confirms the finding when it is very obvious that there is no flow within the liver on a flush aortic injection (Fig. 17.1) A tight stricture in the artery can also be seen when there is very little perfusion of the transplanted liver. In acute rejection the branches of the hepatic artery are compressed by the swollen liver, and this diminishes perfusion, though no actual narrowing is shown in the main hepatic artery (Fig. 17.2).

The portal vein

Thrombosis in the portal vein can be detected on ultrasound. If there is any doubt, this can be confirmed by aortoportography, preferably with DSA. Both thrombosis and narrowing of the portal vein can be demonstrated (Fig. 17.3).

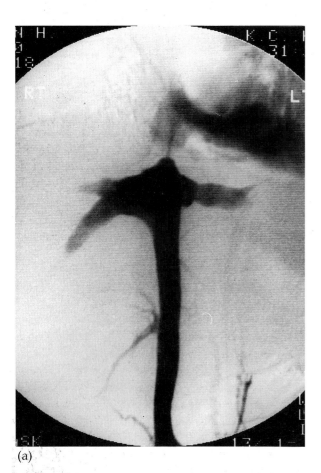
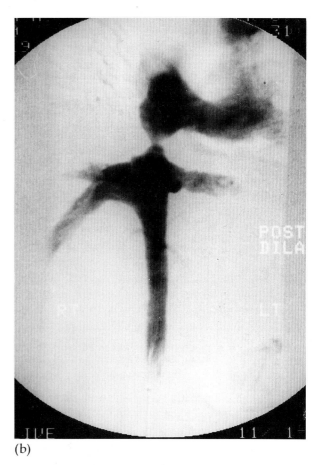

(a)   (b)

Fig. 17.4 Inferior vena cavogram (a) narrowing at the upper anastomosis; (b) dilatation following the use of an angioplasty balloon catheter.

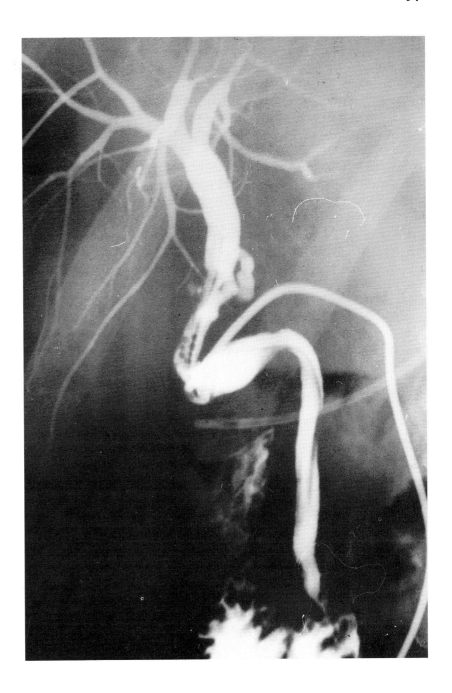

Fig. 17.5 Normal cholangiogram after liver transplantation with the donor gall bladder as a conduit.

Inferior vena cava

Problems with the inferior vena cava can be well shown on ultrasound. It is possible to get thrombosis within the inferior vena cava. It is also possible to get narrowing of the inferior vena cava at the sites of the anastomoses. In one patient we have been able to dilate such a stenosis with an angioplasty balloon catheter (Fig. 17.4 a,b) (Reading *et al.*, 1987) on two occassions, thereby largely relieving a very extensive oedema of the legs which had developed.

Problems in the biliary system

In our experience as radiologists this has been one of the more frequent problems that we have been asked to diagnose and treat. To assess complications of the biliary system one has to know the surgical procedure very accurately. For a period (1976–1987) in the Cambridge–King's series, an anastomosis using the donor gall bladder as a conduit between the donor and recipient common bile duct was used (Fig. 17.5). More recently use has been made of a straight anastomosis with a T-

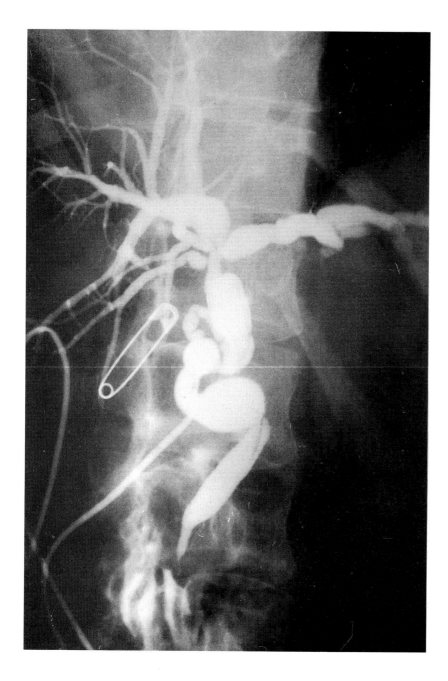

Fig. 17.6 Cholangiogram showing stricturing at the hilum.

tube through the anastomosis. Strictures can occur at any of the anastomoses. They are commonly seen in the hilum at the origins of the right and left ducts (Fig. 17.6). This is attributed to ischaemic change, because of the nature of the vascularization of the biliary tree. There can be leaks also at anastomotic sites. If there is not a fistula that leads to a collection of fluid detectable by ultrasound, the first abnormality noted is dilatation of the ducts which can also be diagnosed by ultrasound. Often, sludge and casts form within the biliary tree.

For actual visualization of the biliary system it is possible to do a tubogram if the T-tube is still present. Tubograms should be carried out with great care in liver transplant patients, as they are immunosuppressed and particularly susceptible to infection. The procedure should, therefore, be performed with full antibiotic cover, and then only if absolutely essential. Because of the nature of the anastomoses, the patient must sometimes be positioned very carefully, for example head down, and quite a large volume of contrast may be needed to sort out all the problems.

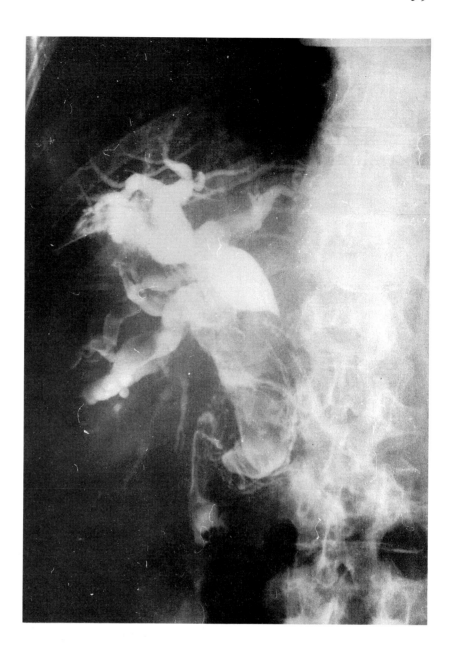

Fig. 17.7 Cholangiogram showing dilated ducts, with debris in the ducts and conduit.

If there is no access by T-tube, a percutaneous cholangiogram can be carried out in the usual manner, or alternatively a retrograde endoscopic cannulation of the recipient's duct can be performed. Often both tests are needed, as they are complementary. Again, antibiotics are required if the patient is not already receiving them. Interventional radiology can be of great help in sorting out some of these problems:

1 It is possible to place a pigtail drainage catheter in dilated intrahepatic ducts to drain them above a hilar stricture. The biliary tree may subsequently be perfused with heparinized saline to wash out some of the debris (Fig. 17.7).

2 It is also possible to pass a guide wire down the duct system to break up some of the casts and soft calculi, and enable them to be washed out of the duct system.

3 Over a guide wire, strictures may be dilated using first a catheter such as a Van Andel, and then angioplasty balloon catheters. At King's we have carried out a number of these procedures, even in quite small children.

4 A guide wire can be passed up by the endoscopic route and a stent inserted across the stricture.

Long-term complications

Following transplantation patients receive immuno-suppressants and steroids as part of their therapy, and are therefore particularly susceptible to infection. The possibility of problems such as liver abscesses, which can be diagnosed on ultrasound, should always be borne in mind. A recurrence of the original disease can occur, or the patient may develop cirrhotic changes in the transplanted liver. Recurrence of tumour in malignant disease may also occur.

As far as general effects are concerned, liver transplantation patients are especially susceptible to the changes of osteoporosis, with collapsed vertebrae, and infections within the bone. As immunosuppressed subjects they can get unusual lung infections and are notably susceptible to tuberculosis.

References

Bismuth, H., Castaing, D., Ericzon, B.G., Otte, J.B., Rolles, K., Ringe, B. & Sloof, M. (1987) Hepatic transplantation in Europe. *Lancet* **ii**, 674–676.

Reading, N.G., O'Grady, J.G., Williams, R. & Nunnerley, H.B. (1987) Balloon dilatation of an anastomotic stenosis of the inferior vena cava. *Journal of Interventional Radiology*, **2**, 81–82.

Tzakis, A.G., Gordon, R.D., Makowka, L., Esquivel, C.O., Todo, S., Iwatsuki, S. & Starzl, T.E. (1987) Clinical considerations in orthotopic liver transplantation. *Radiologic Clinics of North America*, **25**, N.2, 289–297.

Part 3
The Biliary System

18: The Gall Bladder

A. GRUNDY AND A.E.A. JOSEPH

Anatomy

The biliary tree starts blindly with the bile canaliculus. This has no wall proper to itself but is an intercellular space 0.1–0.5 μm diameter formed by the apposition of the edges of gutter-like grooves on the adjacent surfaces of neighbouring hepatocytes. They are located intralobularly and drain bile from the periphery of an acinar lobe toward the portal tract. The canaliculi form a complicated polygonal network with many anastomotic interconnections. They drain into periportal cholangioles or terminal ductules, which unite within the smallest portal tracts to form interlobular bile ducts. These are lined by a flattened cuboidal epithelium. The interlobular ducts anastomose freely and form larger septal or trabecular ducts. As the ducts become more confluent the epithelium becomes columnar and there is an increase in the connective tissue and smooth muscle in the wall.

There is considerable variation in the arrangement of the intrahepatic ducts. The ducts from the quadrate and caudate lobes of the liver usually drain into the main left hepatic duct close to the liver hilum. The duct from the posterior segment of the right lobe usually joins the right anterior segment duct proximal to the hilum. The most common variants are where the anterior or the posterior segment ducts from the right lobe of the liver drain into the left, rather than the right hepatic duct. The right and left main hepatic ducts emerge from the liver parenchyma and join to form the common hepatic duct. The proximal portion of the main hepatic duct is close to the liver hilum, although it is extrahepatic (Healey & Schroy, 1953).

As the common hepatic duct passes down in the hepatoduodenal ligament, the proximal part of the common hepatic duct lies anterior to the right branch of the portal vein and the distal hepatic duct lies anterior to the main portal vein (Fig. 18.1). The length of the common hepatic duct varies depending on the insertion of the cystic duct. This is variable but the average length is 3 cm. The common bile duct begins at the junction of the common hepatic duct and the cystic duct. The length of the common bile duct also depends on the variable insertion of the cystic duct but is usually about 8 cm in length. The common bile duct passes downwards and slightly posterior and to the left. It lies in the hepatoduodenal ligament or free edge of the lesser omentum, passing posterior to the duodenum to the right of the gastroduodenal artery. As it passes down towards the second part of the duodenum it usually lies in a groove on the posterior surface of the head of the pancreas, although it may occasionally be embedded in the substance of the pancreas.

The terminal portion of the common bile duct is

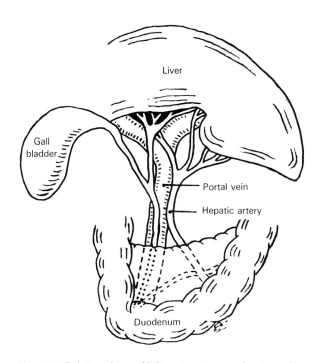

Fig. 18.1 Relationships of biliary tree to portal vein and hepatic artery.

closely associated with the terminal portion of the pancreatic duct in its intramural course through the wall of the descending duodenum. In about 60% of people the common bile duct and the terminal portion of the pancreatic duct form a common channel which may be up to 1 cm in length — the hepatopancreatic ampulla. The distal, constricted end of the ampulla opens into the descending part of the duodenum at the summit of the major duodenal papilla.

The exhahepatic ducts are lined by columnar epithelium. The submucosal tissues have abundant elastic fibres and in the common bile duct there are scattered bundles of smooth muscle running in longitudinal and transverse directions. As the common bile duct nears the duodenum, the smooth muscle layer becomes more prominent and in its intramural position condenses to form the sphincter of Oddi. Because of its lack of muscle fibres, the common bile duct is a passive conduit without peristaltic activity. The muscular activity of the smooth muscle fibres of the spincter of Oddi accounts for the clinical symptoms of biliary colic and spasm.

The gall bladder is a pear-shaped sac which lies under the right lobe of the liver. It extends from the right margin of the liver hilum to the inferior border of the right lobe of the liver under the sixth rib adjacent to the lateral margin of rectus abdominis. The gall bladder is attached to the underside of the liver by loose connective tissue. At the neck of the gall bladder the cystic artery lies embedded in this tissue. The gall bladder is covered on two-thirds of its surface by peritoneum, which occasionally may completely envelop it so that it lies suspended from the liver by a short mesentery. The volume of the gall bladder is usually 30–50 ml.

The end of the gall bladder is expanded to form the fundus. This is covered on all sides by peritoneum and extends below the inferior edge of the liver to lie up against the anterior abdominal wall. Posteriorly it is related to the hepatic flexure of the colon. The fundus blends with the body passing upwards posteriorly and to the left. The body tapers to form the neck which becomes continous with the cystic duct. The cystic duct passes backwards and downwards, running parallel with the common hepatic duct for a short distance before uniting with it. The mucosa of the cystic duct is thrown up into a series of crescentic folds, producing the spiral valve of Heister.

The wall of the gall bladder is 1 mm thick.

Histologically it consists of a single layer of tall columnar epithelial cells on a lamina propria. There is no muscularis mucosae nor a submucosa. The smooth muscle layer immediately beneath the epithelium consists of an irregular network of longitudinal, transverse, and oblique fibres. A dense connective tissue layer external to the muscle layer surrounds the gall bladder and in places is continuous with the interlobar connective tissue of the liver. The portion of the gall bladder not in direct contact with the liver is covered by peritoneum (Fawcett, 1986).

Physiology

Hepatic bile, secreted by the hepatocytes into the bile canaliculi, is a solution of bile acids, bilirubin, phospholipids, cholesterol, and electrolytes in water. The daily output is 700–1200 ml. The hepatic bile is modified as it passes downstream through the ductules and ducts by reabsorption or secretion of electrolytes and water. Bile formation and excretion may be impaired by hepatocellular disease or by obstruction to the intra- or extrahepatic ducts. Failure to excrete bile results in jaundice, the yellow coloration being due to bilirubin accumulating in blood and lymph.

About 80% of bilirubin is produced by breakdown of mature red cells by the reticuloendothelial cells of the liver and spleen. Circulating bilirubin released by the reticuloendothelial system is carried to the liver bound to albumin. In the hepatocyte the lipid-soluble bilirubin is conjugated with uridine disphosphate glucuronic acid, producing water-soluble bilirubin diglucuronide, which is then secreted into the bile canaliculi. Bilirubin remains conjugated in the bile and intestine until bacterial degradation in the colon deconjugates it and reduces it to urobilinogen, some of which is reabsorbed into the enterohepatic circulation.

Cholesterol is practically insoluble in water and is excreted into the bile in the form of micelles with bile salts and phospholipids. This is the only excretion pathway for cholesterol.

The primary bile acids, cholic and chenodeoxycholic acid, are synthesized from cholesterol in the liver and conjugated with taurine and glycine to form bile salts, which are secreted into the bile. In the small intestine they are essential for micelle formation in the digestion and absorption of lipids. In this process the bile salts are deconjugated and thereby conserved by reabsorption in the terminal ileum. A proportion of primary bile acids is converted by bacterial action in the gut into secondary bile acids. A proportion of cholic acid is converted to deoxycholic acid, which is absorbed and re-excreted. Small amounts of lithocholic acid are produced from chenodeoxycholic acid but are not normally absorbed.

In the gall bladder, hepatic bile is concentrated by the absorption of sodium chloride and bicarbonate together with water. This results in concentration of bile salts, cholesterol micelles, conjugated bilirubin, and other non-diffusable solutes. The volume of hepatic bile is thus reduced by 80−90%. Emptying of the gall bladder is primarily under the hormonal control of cholecystokinin — pancreazymin (CCK-PZ) present in the intestinal mucosa. When fat or essential amino acids enter the duodenum, CCK-PZ is released. CCK-PZ acts directly on the gall bladder muscle causing it to contract and at the same time relaxes the sphincter of Oddi.

Contrast agents

Oral cholecystographic agents are the only radiographic contrast agents based on an excretory function performed with an orally administered contrast agent. The contrast agent must be capable of being absorbed easily from the gut and excreted by the liver in high enough concentration for there to be prompt and intense radiographic visualization. Intravenous agents on the other hand only need to have pharmacological properties enabling them to be readily excreted by the liver.

Oral contrast agents are all based on aromatic tri-iodo alkanoic acid derivatives. Iopanoic acid (Telepaque) was first produced in 1952 with greater efficiency and safety than previous contrast agents. More recent agents have appeared based on this molecule: sodium and calcium ipodate (Biloptin and Solu-Biloptin). The ipodate salts are much more water soluble than iopanoic acid and intestinal absorption of these agents is more complete.

Intravenous agents are all based on a molecule consisting of two tri-iodinated benzene rings linked by a polymethylene chain of differing lengths. They are all highly soluble in water.

Oral agents are absorbed by passive diffusion across the gastrointestinal mucosa. Their solubility in the gut appears to be enhanced by the presence of bile salts.

Both oral and intravenous agents are carried in the blood bound to plasma albumin. The degree of protein binding is related to their toxicity. The protein binding may be important in reducing the renal excretion of these compounds. The oral agents, like bilirubin, are converted by the hepatocytes into a water-soluble glucuronide conjugate. This is brought about by the action of glucoronyl transferase. Conjugation produces a more water-soluble molecule for excretion in the bile. Intravenous agents are excreted unchanged by the hepatocytes.

Excretion of both oral and i.v. agents proceeds against a concentration gradient limited by a transport maximum. The rate of excretion increases in relation to plasma concentration until it reaches a maximum (transport maximum). Further increase in plasma concentration produces no further additional biliary excretion. The i.v. agents are all in themselves potent choleretics.

A proportion of excreted contrast agent is lost by bile flow directly into the duodenum, the majority of excreted contrast normally reaches the gall bladder, where it is concentrated by reabsorption of water across the gall bladder mucosa. The peak radiographic opacification of the gall bladder following iopanoic acid occurs at 19 h. The peak concentration of ipodate occurs at 12 h.

Imaging the gall bladder and bile ducts

Oral cholecystography has been the major method of imaging the biliary system since its introduction in 1924 by Graham & Cole. It has been regarded as an easy, safe and reliable method of imaging the biliary tree. However, with the advent of the more recent imaging techniques of ultrasound, nuclear medicine, and computerized tomography, its value as the first-line imaging modality is being reassessed. In many countries ultrasound has replaced oral cholecystography as the initial investigation in the biliary tree.

Oral cholecystography and ultrasound of the biliary system are complementary (DeLacey et al., 1984). The false-negative rate for calculi on oral cholecystography may be as high as 6−8% (Krook et al., 1980). The false-negative rate for ultrasound is probably less than 5%. Ultrasound is now regarded as the initial investigation of the biliary tree in most centres. If the ultrasound examination is normal but symptoms persist, then oral cholecystography should be performed. The outcome would depend on the underlying pathology giving rise to symptoms. In calculus disease the yield with ultrasound would be high, while adenomyomatosis is more difficult to detect on ultrasound.

Cystic duct calculi cannot be adequately assessed on ultrasound and the degree of calcification of gall stones can only be assessed by radiographic techniques.

Intravenous cholangiography has played a significant role in the assessment of the biliary tree, especially in the post-cholecystectomy patient, but is now becoming less important. There is a significant morbidity and mortality associated with i.v. cholangiography, when compared to other i.v. contrast studies such as i.v. urography. The improvement in direct cholangiographic imaging by endoscopic retrograde cholangiopancreatography and percutaneous transhepatic cholangiography is making i.v. cholangiography a less useful imaging method.

Indications for i.v. cholangiography now need reassessing. In the past the usual indications have been: (i) non-visualization of the gall bladder on oral cholecystography; (ii) evaluation of post-cholecystectomy symptoms; (iii) preoperative evaluation of the common bile duct prior to survey. (Scholz et al., 1976). All these indications can now be better and more safely assessed with other imaging modalities.

Oral cholecystography

The contrast agents at present available for oral cholecystography are sodium and calcium ipodate (Biloptin and Solu-Biloptin), iocetamic acid (Cholebrin) and iopanoic acid (Telepaque). Iopanoic acid is more widely used in North America than in Britain.

The contrast agent is administered on the evening prior to the examination. It must be absorbed from the small intestine, conjugated by the hepatocyte, and excreted into the bile. It then passes to the gall bladder to be concentrated. Maximum biliary levels occur at about 3 h following administration, but maximum gall bladder concentration occurs between 12 and 15 h. Sodium ipodate is usually given in a dose of six 3 g capsules, iocetamid acid and iopanoic acid are given as six 500 mg tablets on the evening prior to the examination. An additional early morning dose of contrast may be given on the day of the examination, enabling the examination to coincide with peak biliary levels of the agent and so improve visualization of the bile ducts. It may be that an additional dose is

not justified, however, since the visualization of the bile duct may be no better than that obtained following a fatty meal (McConnell et al., 1983).

The main contraindications to the oral cholecystographic agents are impaired renal and hepatic function. Oral cholecystographic agents all have a uricosuric effect, which may be responsible for the rare cases of acute renal failure that have been reported. Patients should not be dehydrated; in fact the state of hydration has little effect on the accuracy of the study (Bainton et al., 1973). It has often been assumed that the patient should have a low-fat diet prior to oral cholecystography, since fat in the diet will cause the gall bladder to contract and empty though Mauthe (1974) has shown there is probably no merit in this practice.

Minor side-effects from oral agents are noted by about 50% of patients. The commonest complaints are of transient mild nausea and abdominal discomfort. Diarrhoea and vomiting are exceptional although the incidence of side-effects is twice as common with iopanoic acid than ipodate or iocetamic acid (Owen & Lavelle, 1978, Reiner et al., 1980). Urticaria has been described rarely and there is one reported case of thrombocytopenia following iopanoic acid (Curradi et al., 1981).

As with any other contrast examinations it is good radiological practice to obtain a control film of the area of interest prior to contrast administration. The control film may demonstrate calcified calculi (Fig. 18.2), gall-bladder wall calcification (porcelain gall bladder, Fig. 18.3), air in the biliary tree or in non-opaque calculi (Mercedes−Benz sign, Fig. 18.4), or a soft-tissue mass of an enlarged gall bladder. Other pathology outside the biliary system may be found in about 5% of patients (Karned & LeVeen, 1978). Only 10−15% of biliary calculi contain enough calcium to make them visible on plain films (Berk, 1973).

Opaque calculi may be obscured following contrast administration in between 2 and 8% of patients (Karned & LeVeen, 1978, Twomey et al., 1983).

There is considerable divergence of opinion regarding the value of the plain film. Some authors believe that it is wrong to omit the plain film since 5−6% of calculi will be missed. (Twomey et al., 1983), whereas others hold that the plain film provides a decisive diagnosis in only 0.1% of patients and that the sensitivity of the examination would only drop by 0.43% if the plain film were omitted (Anderson & Madsen, 1979). The demonstration of calcified calculi may be relevant if

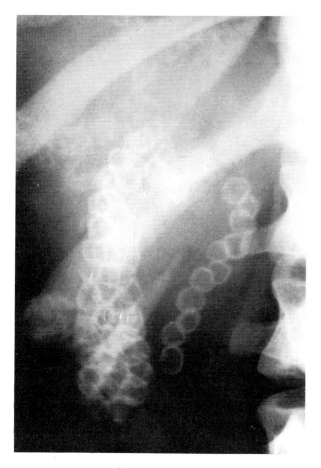

Fig. 18.2 Multiple faceted calcified calculi in the gall bladder and in the common bile duct.

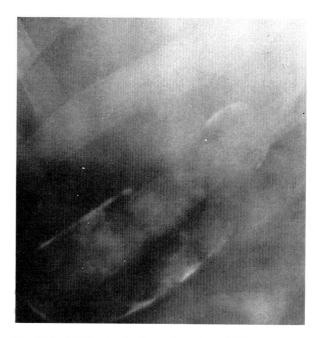

Fig. 18.3 Calcification in the wall of the gall bladder: porcelain gall bladder.

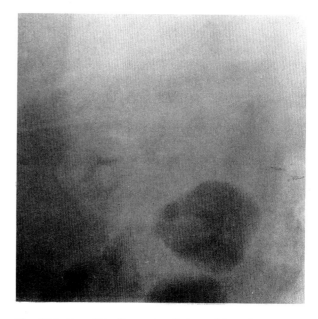

Fig. 18.4 Air within fissured gall stone: Mercedes—Benz

medical dissolution of gall stones is being considered.

The sequence of radiographs taken depends on the particular preference of the radiologist, but conventionally the prone 20—30° left anterior oblique and erect positions are obtained (Fig. 18.5). Fluoroscopy with compression may be indispensable, especially if no calculi have been seen on the standard views. The gall bladder can be freed of overlying bowel gas and compression can be applied to reduce gall bladder density and improve radiographic detail. A relatively low kV technique (70 kVp) will optimize contrast density.

In addition, tomography may be useful in improving the diagnostic accuracy of the examination (Stephens *et al.*, 1976, Pilbrow, 1980). It is of value in the interpretation of a non-visualized or poorly functioning gall bladder. Non-visualization of the gall bladder when the bile ducts are visible implies cystic-duct obstruction, or obliteration of the gall bladder lumen (McInick & LoCurcio, 1973). In the faintly opacified gall bladder non-opaque calculi

may be visualized (Fig. 18.6). Calcified stones may be lost amongst ribs and costal cartilage on standard views, and it may be possible to see occasional calcified stones in the absence of gall bladder obscured by bowel gas and in localizing small filling defects within the gall bladder. Tomography is unlikely, however, to add any extra information to an oral cholecystogram in which a

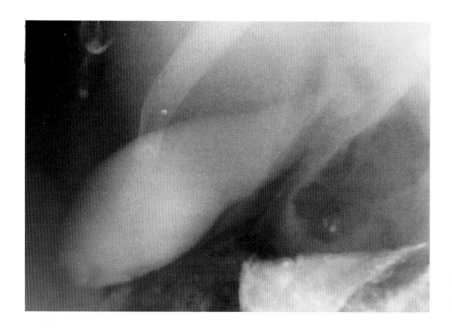

Fig. 18.5 Erect 15-h film from oral cholecystogram. (Note unabsorbed contrast media remaining in bowel.)

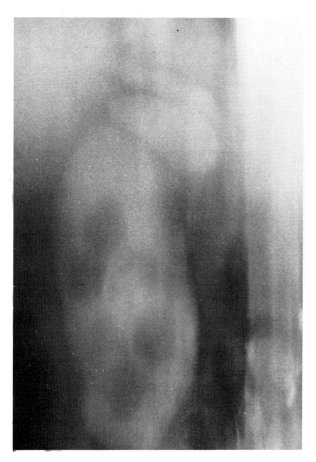

Fig. 18.6 Tomography at oral cholecystography revealing non-opaque calculi within gall bladder.

good fatty meal film has been obtained (Pilbrow, 1980).

The use of a fatty meal to stimulate gall bladder contraction is a time-honoured part of the oral cholecystogram for freeing the gall bladder from overlying bowel gas, for differentiating between calculi and fixed filling defects of the gall bladder wall, for demonstrating adenomyomatosis and the assessment of biliary dyskinesia, and for demonstrating the common bile duct (Fig. 18.7). More recently, cholecystokinin and its synthetic analogue ceruletide have been introduced.

Post-fatty meal films are essential to the diagnosis of adenomyomatosis on oral cholecystography. The gall bladder may look normal before the fatty meal in up to 28% of patients with adenomyomatosis (Gajjar *et al.*, 1984). There is little to choose between the various fatty meal preparations in their ability to produce gall bladder contraction (Harvey, 1977). The fatty meal causes release of cholecystokinin from the duodenal mucosa, resulting in contraction of the gall bladder usually within 30–60 min. The response to the fatty meal is variable. Cholecystokinin or ceruletide cholecystography has been suggested as a provocative test of function to reproduce symptoms in the patient with no obvious gall bladder pathology. The ability of the opacified gall bladder to contract against resistance, resulting in pain and the production of an abnormal contour of the gall bladder is the basis of the cholecystokinin test and may be useful to detect acalculous gall bladder disease that may benefit from cholecystectomy (Sykes, 1982, Rajagopolan & Pickleman, 1982).

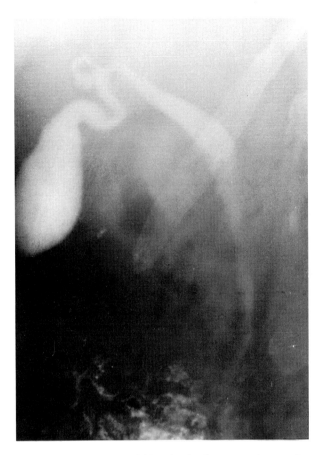

Fig. 18.7 Post-fatty meal film clearly demonstrating cystic duct and common bile duct.

Others believe that the fatty meal and cholecystokinin stimulation tests are of little value in assessing functional disorders of the biliary tract (McConnell *et al.*, 1983, Morewood & Whitehouse, 1985).

The synthetic peptide ceruletide is more potent than cholecystokinin in contracting the gall bladder and relaxing the sphincter of Oddi. Ceruletide has a more rapid onset of action than a fattymeal and it may cause the gall bladder to empty completely. These agents have the disadvantage of requiring an intramuscular injection.

An occasional problem encountered is that of the apparent non-functioning gall bladder on oral cholecystography. Extrinsic causes of non-function such as vomiting, pyloric stenosis, fasting, small-bowel disease, and liver disease must be excluded. Satisfactory studies can be obtained in up to 94% of patients with the conventional method of oral cholecystography (Nathan & Newman, 1981). If the gall bladder is unopacified and all extrinsic factors have been excluded, intravenous cholangi-

ography may show calculi in a diseased gall bladder (Mujahed *et al.*, 1974). Tomography may well avoid the necessity of a second examination. Failed cholecystography seems to be less of a problem with ipodate and iocetamic acid than with iopanoic acid.

The oral cholecystogram is regarded as a fairly accurate examination. Errors in interpretation are usually due to failure to free the gall bladder adequately from overlying gas or from poor opacification. In these circumstances tomography or spot filming with compression and the use of the fatty meal should be considered to improve the diagnostic yield of the examination.

Intravenous cholangiography

With the increasing availability of ultrasound, computerized tomography, percutaneous transhepatic cholangiography and endoscopic cholangiography, intravenous cholangiography is assuming far less importance than in the past. If ultrasound and/or computerized tomography is available, intravenous cholangiography makes very little difference to the diagnostic success (Rholl *et al.*, 1985).

There is a significant failure rate of intravenous cholangiography even in the presence of normal hepatic function. Up to 45% of examinations may not provide adequate visualization of the biliary tree and there may also be a diagnostic error rate of 40% even in adequate studies (Goodman *et al.*, 1980).

The potential uses to which intravenous cholangiography have been put include:
1 Post-cholecystectomy patients with recurrent symptoms.
2 The assessment of the acute abdomen to diagnose acute cholecystitis.
3 Demonstration of the common bile duct pre-operatively when the gall bladder has been shown to contain calculi on an oral study.
4 Demonstration of possible abnormality of the common duct when the oral study appears normal.
5 Further assessment of the non-functioning gall bladder on oral cholecystography (Scholz *et al.*, 1976).
Most of these clinical situations can now be better resolved wih other imaging methods, but i.v. cholangiography is still valuable where other imaging methods are not readily available.

The contrast agents are present in use in Britain

are meglumine ioglycamate (Biligram), meglumine iotroxate (Biliscopin) and meglumine iodoxamate (Endobil). The main contraindications to the use of these agents are hypersensitivity to iodinated intravenous agents, and impaired hepatic and renal function. There has been one reported case of a fatal reaction to ioglycamate in a patient with Waldenstrom's macroglobulinaemia (Bauer *et al.*, 1974). IgM paraproteins have been precipitated by ioglycamate. In view of this risk of intravenous cholangiographic agents it is inadvisable to use them in the patient with myeloma, and the precaution of measuring a patient's erythrocyte sedimentation rate (ESR) and obtaining a protein electrophoresis strip should be considered. In the UK survey of i.v. cholangiography with iodipamide (Biligrafin), intermediate reactions occurred in 1 in 700 patients, severe reactions occurred in 1 in 1600 patients, and death occurred in 1 in 5000 examinations. These reactions are about eight times that experienced from intravenous urographic agents (Ansell, 1970). Minor side-effects from these agents are not uncommon. An unpleasant taste, a feeling of heat, and occasional nausea and vomiting are not unusual. The incidence of side-effects depends on the rate of injection (Ansell & Faux, 1973). Rarer side-effects include severe hypotension and collapse with circulatory failure, ventricular fibrillation, and cardiac arrest.

The patient for i.v. cholangiography should not be dehydrated prior to the investigation. There is probably little value in dietary preparation, though a high fat diet will increase bile flow which in turn may dilute the contrast medium. All intravenous cholangiographic agents are potent choleretics. There is a transport maximum for the hepatocyte handling of these agents and it has been shown that the best opacification of the biliary tree can be obtained by a slow drip infusion technique. If ioglycamate is used, this can be infused in a dosage of 100 ml of 17% solution over 45 min or so to give optimum biliary opacification. The rate of infusion is important and the exact rate varies with the different agents. Too slow an infusion rate will fail to give optimal opacification and too fast a rate will increase the side-effects (Bell *et al.*, 1978).

RADIOGRAPHIC TECHNIQUE

A control film of the right upper quadrant should be performed with the same indications as with oral cholecystography. If possible the patient should remain on the radiographic table during the infusion of contrast. It is customary to obtain films in the prone left anterior oblique position of the right upper quadrant at the end of the infusion. If the common bile duct is seen at this stage, tomography at 0.5 cm intervals is necessary to demonstrate the duct in its entirety (Fig. 18.8). If the duct is not visible on the immediate film a further film should be taken after 30 min. At this point if the duct is not visible tomography can be employed. In order to visualize the gall bladder (if still present) films may need to be taken up to 4 h. Only if no contrast is seen in the gall bladder at this time can a diagnosis of cystic duct obstruction be made.

Recently there has been an interest in the techniques of glucagon-enhanced i.v. cholangiography as a means of improving the diagnostic yield, (Cannon & Legge, 1979, Jarrett & Bell, 1980, Evans & Whitehouse, 1980). Glucagon increases basal bile flow and also produces relaxation of the sphincter of Oddi. Its exact mechanism in improving the vizualization of the biliary tree is uncertain. Intravenous glucagon will produce an elevation of biliary iodine concentration within 3 min of injection but this returns to pre-injection levels at 5 min (Jarrett & Bell, 1980). Glucagon seems to improve duct visualization and especially gall-bladder filling in infusion studies. Glucagon may also be of value in differentiating between a filling defect at the lower end of the common bile duct to a stone at the ampulla, and a defect due to muscular constriction of the sphincter of Oddi.

Errors in interpretation

Most errors in interpretation of the i.v. cholangiogram are due to failure to adequately visualize the duct and failure to obtain adequate tomographic cuts. Confusion may occur if muscular spasm at the lower end of the duct is mistaken for a calculus. Occasionally a collection of contrast seen adjacent to the common bile duct may be seen and misinterpreted as gall bladder filling when in fact it is due to contrast refluxing into the duodenal cap (Fig. 18.9).

Ultrasound of the biliary tree

Ultrasound examination of the biliary tree has in the late 1970s been established as the first-line investigation. With the introduction of real-time high-resolution devices accuracy rates of over 95%

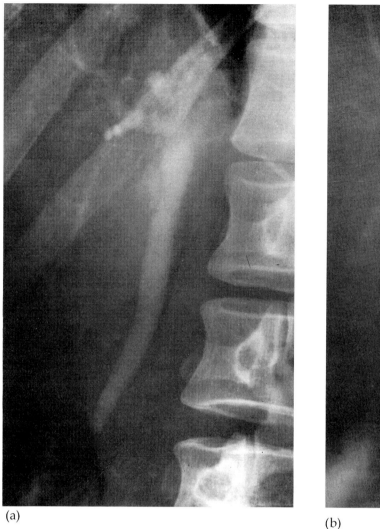

(a)

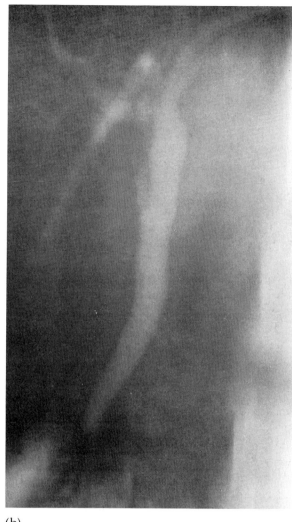

(b)

Fig. 18.8 Post-cholecystectomy. Intravenous cholangiography: prone oblique view (a) and tomography (b) demonstrating hepatic ducts and common bile duct, and cystic duct remnant.

are routinely achieved for the detection of gall stones. (Krook *et al.*, 1980, McIntosh & Penny, 1980). Rapidity and ease of the procedure compared to oral cystography has also significantly contributed to the decline in the use of the oral cholecystogram. It is regarded as an observer-dependent investigation, so close supervision by a physician is considered essential. The real-time images and the ease of conduction of the examination enables the operator to assess not only the biliary tree but also the liver and other adjacent organs such as the pancreas and kidney, which may be giving rise to the symptoms. Valuable clues might also be obtained by scanning the stomach, duodenum, and colon. Consequently,

neoplastic lesions or inflammatory lesions are not uncommonly detected.

EXAMINATION TECHNIQUE

Gall bladder

Examination of the biliary tree is best conducted with the patient in a fasting state, and periods of fasting of 4–8 h are recommended.

Imaging of the biliary tree is usually carried out initially with the patient supine. With static scanners it was customary to stress routine longitudinal and transverse scans, but with the use of real-time scanning, we now emphasize the fact that the organ is scanned in the plane in which it is best

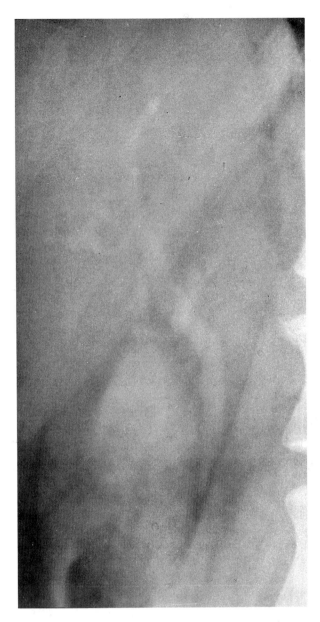

Fig. 18.9 Intravenous cholangiography: contrast in the duodenum projected adjacent to common bile duct mimicking the gall bladder.

demonstrated. Scanning is commenced subcostally in the right hypochondrium and the gall bladder is visualized as a fluid-filled pear-shaped organ nestling between the liver anteriorly and the kidney and the duodenum posteriorly. The posterior relationship of the duodenum is essential to recognize, since gas in the duodenum may mimic gall stones. (Fig. 18.10). The scan plane is then oriented to visualize the gall bladder in its longitudinal axis and in a plane at right angles. Scans are normally done in suspendend inspiration, but this is not always essential. Patients sometimes retract the anterior abdominal wall while taking a deep breath and it is often helpful to request the patient to 'push out' the abdominal wall; with the descent of the diaphragm and the liver, the gall bladder now becomes more accessible subcostally. These manoeuvres may still be inadequate to demonstrate the gall bladder subcostally and intercostal scans may then have to be performed. No examination of the gall bladder is complete without the patient's being turned into the left posterior oblique position, when the region of the neck of the gall bladder is often best demonstrated.

When the gall bladder is not readily visualized it may be helpful to identify the main lobar fissure as a linear echogenic region seen to extend from the right branch of the portal vein to the gall bladder (Callen & Filly, 1979).

Occasionally the hepatic flexure with loaded faeces may mimic a gall bladder full of calculi, or calcification in the gall bladder wall, especially when it is small and contracted, either physiologically or due to disease or agenesis. Less commonly a fluid-filled duodenum, particularly with duodenal obstruction, may mimic a pathologically thick-walled gall bladder. Care must be taken to avoid these errors. The former is avoided by noting the continuity of the hepatic flexure with the ascending and transverse colon. The duodenum will often show peristalsis and evidence of changing shape; a pathologically thick-walled gall bladder does not show any alteration in shape or size.

The long axis of the gall bladder may vary considerably in relation to the sagittal plane and may occasionally lie horizontally, with the fundus lateral to the right kidney.

In a normal distended gall bladder the wall appears as a single echogenic layer of 1–2 mm in thickness. In a physiologically contracted gall bladder, the wall is thickened and may measure 3–4 mm. An echogenic outer layer is recognized with a crenated inner, less echogenic layer (Fig. 18.11). A third echo-free between these two layers may sometimes be seen. The crenated layer represents the mucosa thrown into folds. These layers are, however, very uniform in appearance and thickness and serve to distinguish the physiologically contracted gall bladder from a diseased one.

Bile ducts

Examination of the bile ducts should aim to image the duct system from the confluence of the right and left hepatic ducts to the ampulla of Vater. The

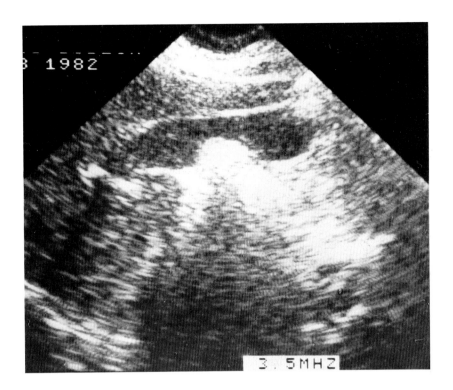

Fig. 18.10 Gas in duodenum mimicking a gall stone.

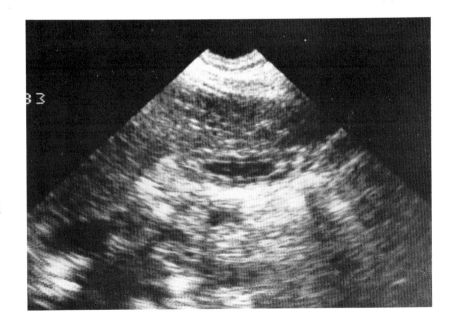

Fig. 18.11 Physiologically contracted gall bladder. Inner mucosal layer is smooth and continuous. The contracted muscular layer shows an echo-poor region giving rise to the double-wall effect. This is most obvious when a normally large gall bladder undergoes contraction.

intrahepatic bile ducts proximal to the right and left hepatic ducts are usually not demonstrated with the resolution capabilities of the currently available scanners. The common hepatic duct was seen in 98 of 100 normal individuals in one study (Cooperberg, 1978) and several other authors (Cooperberg, 1978, Dewbury, 1980), have shown that a part of the common bile duct could also be demonstrated in the majority of normal individuals. The distal common bile duct is less frequently visualized due to overlying duodenum.

Real-time sector scanners or linear array systems may be used for the examination of the bile ducts, but the yield from static scanners is lower. The supine or right anterior oblique projections, with varying degrees of obliquity may be employed.

The transducer may, however, be placed on the patient's abdomen to correspond to varying degrees of obliquity when the patient is unable to turn, but it is less satisfactory since the colon is often in the path of the beam.

The bifurcation of the main portal vein is identified, and parasagittal scanning usually shows the proximal common hepatic duct as a tubular structure lying anterior to the right branch of the portal vein. The right branch of the hepatic artery is usually seen in cross-section between the common hepatic duct and the portal vein. This portion of the bile duct is visualized in virtually every patient (Fig. 18.12). If the transducer is then rotated at right angles with the scanning plane now slightly oblique to the transverse plane, the right and left hepatic ducts may be visualized anterior to the confluence of the right and left branches of the portal vein. Moving the transducer caudally the union of the hepatic ducts, and then the common duct, may be visualized anterior to the portal vein. The degree of obliquity may occasionally be as much as a plane parallel to the lower costal margin.

With the patient in the anterior oblique position the whole length of the extrahepatic biliary tree may be visualized, but quite commonly only segments of the bile ducts may be seen in any one position of the probe.

ANATOMIC VARIATION

Confusion may arise from variation in the course of the right hepatic artery when it courses anterior to the common duct in about 15% of individuals. (Berland et al., 1982). Tracing the vessel to the rest of the hepatic artery and the coeliac axis usually resolves this problem. A transverse course of the mid-portion of the common duct may in the undilated duct be mistaken for the hepatic artery (Jacobson & Brodey, 1981). Continuity is usually easily established, particularly when scanning in the coronal plane with the patient in the right anterior oblique position.

Normal duct size

Measurement of the common duct is most commonly where the duct lies anterior to the right branch of the portal vein, or just distal to this when it courses through the free edge of the lesser omentum. Duct size is routinely measured with the patient in the right anterior oblique position.

In several studies that measured the size of the common duct on intravenous cholangiography, percutaneous cholangiography, and ERCP, the upper limit of normal of the common duct is quoted as 8—11 mm (Fromhold & Fromhold, 1973). On

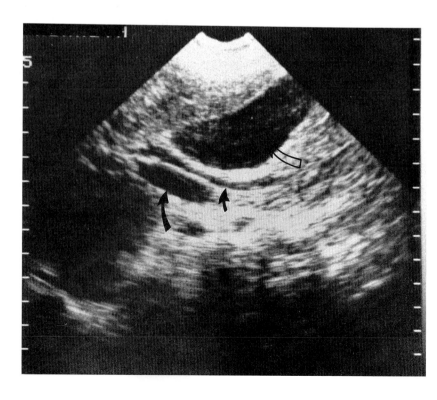

Fig. 18.12 Common bile duct (*small arrow*) anterior to portal vein (*large arrow*). Gall bladder (*open arrow*).

ultrasound examination, however, the range for the normal common duct has been lower, ranging from 4 to 8 mm (Cooperberg, 1978, Niederau et al., 1983). These measurements relate to the common duct when the gall bladder is in situ. We ourselves use an upper limit of 8 mm for the common duct. Very occasionally the duct may be seen to vary in calibre during an examination, but we have not observed a duct of more than 8 mm during the normal physiological process of filling. The normal range for the common duct after cholecystectomy is higher than with the gall bladder in situ. It is very uncommon to see a duct size of 4 mm and it usually measures between 8 and 10 mm (Sauerbrei, 1983). In the paediatric age group the duct increases in size from 1 mm to the adult size by about 16 years (Sauerbrei, 1983).

Discrepancies in measurement made at ultrasound or in radiographic examinations are mainly due to the magnification factor in radiographic procedures. This is usually a factor of 1.3. However, the echogenicity of the wall of the duct makes it appear thicker than it usually is and hence reduces the true size of the lumen. It is possible that the choleretic effect of contrast agents may cause slightly greater distension of the duct during cholangiographic procedures, and that pressure also causes distension during direct injection of contrast medium.

It is this group that poses problems as to whether there is superadded obstruction requiring further investigation. When associated with symptoms or altered liver function, but not otherwise further investigation would appear justifiable.

Intraoperative bile duct scanning

Few centres have facilities for intraoperative bile duct scanning. Claims have been made for an accuracy equivalent to that obtained with operative cholangiography (Sigel et al., 1981). The advantage would appear to be that it is less invasive and is a quicker procedure. Trained operators are obviously required. With the availability of small part scanners and higher-frequency probes of 7.5 or 10 MHz the technique is certainly feasible.

Biliary scintigraphy

[131]I-labelled rose bengal, introduced by Taplin and co-workers in 1962, found its greatest use in distinguishing obstructive from non-obstructive jaundice. Due to the high dose levels with ^{131}I,

technetium-labelled compounds were developed and pyridoxylidine-labelled amino acid complexes were introduced. These were soon followed by [99m]technetium-labelled chelates of iminodiacetic acid (IDA). A range of these components has been developed and evaluated, and diethyl HIDA and diisopropyl IDA (DISIDA) are currently in use. The earlier chelates of IDA had the disadvantage that the extraction efficiency and excretion was low in the presence of jaundice. Diethyl HIDA and DISIDA may be used even in the presence of moderately raised bilirubin. The pharmacokinetics of hepatobiliary scintigraphic agents are reviewed by Chervu et al., (1982).

The major applications for the use of biliary agents are now in the assessment of cystic duct patency, the evaluation of acute cholecystitis, and the evaluation of bile duct patency, particularly following biliary reconstructive surgery. It may also be used for the assessment of biliary leaks after surgery, and for hepatic clearance studies.

For the evaluation of cystic duct or bile duct patency 150 MBq of the biliary agent is injected i.v. with the patient in a fasting state, and serial images obtained at 10 min and every 30 min thereafter. A normal study shows prompt uptake of the agent in the liver with clearance of the blood pool activity in 5–10 min. The intrahepatic biliary radicles and the common duct are visualized shortly thereafter. The gall bladder is usually visualized at 1 h and activity should also be seen within the duodenum by this time.

Gall bladder filling may be delayed and studies may then have to be extended to 2–4 h, provided there is still activity left in the liver. Failure of the gall bladder to fill by 2–4 h is highly suggestive of cystic duct obstruction. Although this has been claimed to be highly specific in the diagnosis of acute cholecystitis, the claim must be viewed with suspicion; as with oral cholecystography and i.v. cholangiography there are patients with chronic cholecystitis in whom the gall bladder may not be demonstrated.

Activity is usually seen in the duodenum by 1 h. Delay, particularly in excess of 2 h, is indicative of obstruction.

References

Anderson, J.F. & Madsen, P.E.R.(1979) The value of plain radiographs prior to oral cholecystography. Radiology, 113, 309–310.

Ansell, G. (1970) Adverse reaction to contrast agents. Scope of the problem. *Investigative Radiology*, **5**, 374–384.

Ansell, G. & Faux P.A. (1973) Low dose infusion cholangiography. *Clinical Radiology*, **24**, 95–100.

Bainton, D., Davies, G.T., Evans, KT, Gravelle, I.H. & Abernethy, M. (1973) A comparison of two preparation regimes for cholecystography. *Clinical Radiology*, **24**, 381–384.

Bauer, K., Tragl, K.H. & Baur, G. (1974) Intravasale denaturierung von Plasma-proteinen bei einer IgM-paraproteinämie, ausgelöst durch ein intravenös verabreichtes lebergängiges Röntgenkontrasmittel. *Wiener Klinische Wochenschrift*, **86**, 766–769.

Bell, G.D., Frank, J., Fayadh, M., Smith, P.L.C. & Kelsey Fry, I. (1978) Ioglycamide studies in man. Radiological opacification of the bile duct. A comparison of a number of different methods. *British Journal of Radiology*, **51**, 191–195.

Berk, R.N. (1973) Radiology of the gall bladder and bile ducts. *Surgical Clinics of North America*, **53**, 973–1005.

Berland, L.L., Lawson, T.L. & Foley, W.D. (1982) Porta hepatis: Sonographic discrimination of bile ducts from arteries with pulser Doppler with new anatomic criteria. *American Journal of Roentgenology*, **138**, 833–840.

Callen, P.W. & Filly, R.A. (1979) Ultrasonographic localisation of the gall bladder. *Radiology*, **133**, 687–689.

Cannon, P. & Legg, D. (1979). Glucagon as a hypotonic agent in cholangiography. *Clinical Radiology*, **30**, 49–52.

Chervu, L.R., Nunn A.D. & Loberg, M.D. (1982) Radiopharmaceuticals for hepatobiliary imaging. *Seminars in Nuclear Medicine*, **12**, 5–17.

Cooperberg, P.L. (1978) High resolution real time ultrasound in the evaluation of the normal and obstructed biliary tree. *Radiology*, **129**, 477–480.

Curradi, F., Abbritti, G. & Agnelli, G. (1981) Acute thrombocytopenia following oral cholecystography with iopanoic acid. *Clinical Toxicology*, **18**, 221–224.

DeLacey, G., Gajjar, B., Twomey, B., Levi, J. & Cox, A.G. (1984) Should cholecystography or ultrasound be the primary investigation for gall bladder disease? *Lancet*, **i**, 205–207.

Dewbury, K.C. (1980) Visualisation of the normal biliary ducts with ultrasound. *British Journal of Radiology*, **53**, 774–780.

Evans, A.F. & Whitehouse, G.H. (1980) Further studies with glucagon enhanced cholangiography. *Clinical Radiology*, **31**, 663–665.

Fawcett, D.W. (1986) In Bloom & Fawcett (eds) *A Textbook of Histology*, pp. 708–713. W.B. Saunder Co, Philadelphia.

Fromhold, W. & Fromhold, M. (1973) *Alimentary Tract Radiology*, pp. 1264. Mosby, St Louis.

Gajjar, V., Twomey, B. & DeLacey, G. (1984) The fatty meal and acalculous gall bladder disease. *Clinical Radiology*, **35**, 405–408.

Goodman, M.W., Ansel, H.J., Vennes, J.A., Lasser, R.B. & Silvis, S.E. (1980) Is intravenous cholangiography still useful? *Gastroenterology*, **79**, 642–645.

Harvey, U.C. (1977) Milk chocolate as the fatty meal in cholecystography. *Clinical Radiology*, **28**, 635–636.

Healey, J.E. & Schroy, P.C. (1953) Anatomy of the bile ducts within the human liver. *Archives of Surgery*, **66**, 599–616.

Jacobson, J.B. & Brodey, P.A. (1981) The transverse common duct. *American Journal of Roentgenology*, **136**, 91–95.

Jarrett, L.N. & Bell, G.D. (1980) Effect of i.v. glucagon on the biliary secretion of a cholangiographic agent in man. *Clinical Radiology*, **31**, 657–661.

Karned, R.K. & LeVeen, R.F. (1978) Preliminary abdominal films in oral cholecystography: are they necessary? *American Journal of Roentgenology*, **130**, 477–479.

Krook, P.M., Allen, R.H. & Bush, W.H. Jr. (1980) Comparison of real time cholecystosonography and oral cholecystography. *Radiology*, **135**, 145–148.

McConnell, C.A., Whitehouse, G.H. & Evans, A.F. (1983) Gall bladder contraction and bile duct opacification in oral cholecystography: a comparison of different methods. *British Journal of Radiology*, **56**, 371–376.

McInick, G.S. & LoCurcio, J.B. (1973) The 'non-visualised' gallbladder. *Radiology*, **108**, 513–515.

McIntosh, D.M.F. & Penny, H.F. (1980) Gray-scale ultrasonography as a screening procedure in the detection of gall bladder disease. *Radiology*, **136**, 725–727.

Mauthe, K. (1974) The low fat meal in gall bladder examinations. *Radiology*, **112**, 5–7.

Morewood, D.J.S. & Whitehouse, G.K. (1985) Assessment of gall bladder function using ceruletide in oral cholecystography. *Gastrointestinal Radiology*, **10**, 97–105.

Mujahed, Z., Evans, J.A., Whalen, J.P. (1974) The non opacified gall bladder on oral cholecystography. *Radiology*, **112**, 1–3.

Nathan, M.H. & Newman, A. (1981) Conventional oral cholecystography versus single visit oral cholecystography. *American Journal of Roentgenology*, **94**, 495–499.

Niederau, C., Muller, J., Sonneberg, A. et al. (1983) Extrahepatic ducts in healthy subjects, in patients with cholelithiasis and in post cholecystectomy patients: a prospective ultrasound study. *Journal of Clinical Ultrasound*, **11**, 23–27.

Owen, J.P. & Lavelle, M.F. (1978) Comparative study of iocetamic acid and calcium ipodate in the visualisation of the gall bladder and common bile duct. *Clinical Radiology*, **29**, 535–540.

Pilbrow, W.J. (1980) Tomography of the biliary tract during oral cholecystography. A review of 200 cases. *Clinical Radiology*, **31**, 189–193.

Rajagopolan, A.E. & Pickleman, J. (1982) Biliary colic and functional gall bladder disease. *Archives of Surgery*, **117**, 1005–1008.

Reiner, R.G., Lawson, M.J., Davies, G.T., Tucker, W.G., Mileski, O., Read, T.R. & Kerr Grant, A. (1980) Fractionated dose cholecystography: a comparison between ioponoic acid and sodium ipodate. *Clinical Radiology*, **31**, 667–669.

Rholl, K.S., Smathers, R.L., McClennan, B.L. & Lee, J.K.T. (1985) Intravenous cholangiography in the CT era. *Gastrointestinal Radiology*, **10**, 69–74.

Sauerbrei, E. (1983) *Ultrasound Annual* 1983, pp. 1–46. Raven Press, New York.

Scholz, F.J., Larsen, C.R. & Wise, R.E. (1976) Intravenous cholangiography: recurring concepts. *Seminars in Roentgenology*, **11**, 197–202.

Sigel, B., Coelho, J.C.U., Apigos, D.G., Donahue, P.E., Wood, D.K. & Nyhus, L.M. (1981) Ultrasonic imaging during biliary and pancreatic surgery. *American Journal of Surgery*, **141**, 84–89.

Stephens, D.H., Carlson, H.C. & Gisvold, J.J. (1976) Tomography in problem cholecystography. *Radiologic*

Clinics of North America, **14**, 15—21.

Sykes, D. (1982) The use of cholecystokinia in diagnosing biliary pain. *Annals of the Royal College of Surgeons of England*, **64**, 114—116.

Twomey, B., DeLacey, G. & Gajjar, B. (1983) The plain radiograph in oral cholecystography — should it be abandoned? *British Journal of Radiology*, **56**, 99—100.

19: Direct Cholangiography

D.J. LINTOTT

Introduction

Direct cholangiography includes all techniques involving the introduction of water-soluble contrast media directly into the biliary system under fluoroscopic control. It produces the most accurate morphological demonstration of the biliary system, as the contrast volume and density, rate of injection, and positioning of the patient are all under the control of the operator. Contrast may be introduced in an antegrade direction by percutaneous trans-hepatic cholangiography (PTC) or retrogradely by endoscopic retrograde cholangiography (ERC).

The indications for direct cholangiography are as follows:

1 Investigation of cholestatic jaundice to confirm or exclude extrahepatic duct obstruction.

2 Investigation of abdominal pain that could be biliary in origin.

3 To confirm or exclude gall stones in the investigation of pancreatitis.

4 As a prelude to a therapeutic manoeuvre such as biliary drainage or sphincterotomy.

Operative cholangiography and postoperative T-tube cholangiography are used in specific circumstances almost exclusively for the detection or exclusion of duct stones.

Clinical assessment and biochemical testing may both be misleading in the differentiation of intrahepatic and extrahepatic cholestasis, and oral cholecystography and intravenous cholangiography contribute little in the presence of jaundice. Direct cholangiography permits the early differentiation of those patients amenable to surgical relief from those with intrahepatic cholestasis, in whom unnecessary surgery is associated with a 10% mortality. Surgeons no longer welcome or expect a 'blind date with jaundice' and no jaundiced patient need now be operated upon without previous confirmation of obstruction, demonstration of its level and, in most instances, its cause.

Ultrasound examination will confirm or exclude the presence of intrahepatic duct dilatation in virtually 100% of patients. The accuracy of ultrasound in determining the level and cause of biliary obstruction has increased greatly, especially if repeated or serial examinations are performed. It is more successful in the assessment of high rather than low obstructing lesions and accuracy figures of 95% for the level and 88% for the cause of obstruction have been reached (Gibson *et al.*, 1986). Small stones at the lower end of the common duct may be impossible to detect because of overlying gas, and conversely a duct packed full of stones may give misleading ultrasonic appearances. It is now well-recognized that extrahepatic obstruction may be present in the absence of duct dilatation (Muhletaler *et al.*, 1980) and also that postcholecystectomy patients may show an increase in duct calibre even in the absence of current obstruction (Hamilton *et al.*, 1982). Patients with sclerosing cholangitis or widespread intrahepatic metastases may have obstruction without significant duct dilatation.

Therefore the assessment of duct calibre alone on a single occasion may not be a reliable discriminator between extrahepatic and intrahepatic cholestasis, any more than is the finding of stones in the gall bladder. There will, of course, be many cases with unequivocal ultrasound findings, but, as a general rule, in the presence of cholestatic jaundice some form of direct-contrast cholangiography will be required either to complete the diagnosis or to determine management.

Computerized tomography provides similar and in some instances more detailed information to ultrasound, especially in respect of obstructing lesions at the lower end of the common duct. However, as it is not as widely available or as easily performed it is unlikely to replace ultrasound as the primary imaging technique in the investigation of the jaundiced patient.

General principles of direct cholangiography

In any technique of direct-contrast cholangiography certain principles apply that influence the conduct of the examination and the interpretation of radiographs. These principles are discussed below and specific examples are illustrated later.

Effect of gravity upon contrast flow

Contrast media are heavier than bile. The pattern and sequence of duct opacification are therefore gravity dependent, and determined by the site of contrast injection and the position of the patient. The normal course of the common extrahepatic duct is downwards and backwards from the porta hepatis to the duodenum. In the prone position, at ERC, contrast will flow towards the porta hepatis and the lower end of the duct may not be seen clearly until the table is tilted or the patient turned supine. Also, as the left intrahepatic ducts are situated more anteriorly than the right they fill preferentially with the patient prone. In the supine position, for PTC or T-tube cholangiography, it is often necessary to turn the patient on to the left side or even prone to demonstrate the left intrahepatic branches.

Volume of contrast medium

Underfilling of the duct system can produce misleading appearances and lead to potential diagnostic errors. The initial flow of contrast down the dependent wall of a dilated duct produces a 'trickle' artefact, giving a falsely narrowed impression of duct calibre. Incomplete mixing and layering can produce transient filling defects, and underfilling of the intrahepatic branches can produce an erroneous impression of parenchymal liver disease. Contrast may flow preferentially into the gall bladder or through a fistula, preventing complete duct opacification, and the injection of insufficient contrast medium into a grossly dilated duct system may give misleading information as to the level and nature of obstruction.

Although in many instances complete opacification of the whole biliary system is both desirable and readily obtainable, caution is necessary in the presence of obstruction not to introduce a larger volume of contrast medium than is required to make the diagnosis. Excessive injection of medium under pressure into an obstructed or infected duct system produces not only pain but may also precipitate life-threatening sepsis.

Concentration of contrast medium

Any standard water-soluble contrast medium may be used for direct cholangiography and only in exceptional circumstances will a non-ionic medium be indicated. The main consideration is the density of the medium, especially in the presence of duct dilatation. A dilute solution of contrast medium will mix more readily with bile and produce fewer mixing artefacts but, more importantly, contrast medium that is too dense may totally obscure small stones. The optimum concentration for routine use is approximately 150 mg iodine per ml depending upon the radiographic factors used. However, in the presence of gross duct dilatation even further dilution may be required to avoid 'whitewashing' stones.

Air bubbles

In all forms of direct cholangiography exceptional care should be taken not to introduce air bubbles. All connecting tubing, cannulae, and needles should be flushed with saline or contrast medium from the start, and particular care is necessary when changing syringes. If bubbles are inadvertently introduced, then the distinction from lucent stones has to be made. Using table tilt, all bubbles will float upwards and most stones will sink. However, small stones may sink very slowly or even float in contrast medium or may be reluctant to move, being adherent to the duct wall. Bubbles tend to move freely and rapidly within the ducts, are round and smooth in outline, and tend to coalesce in a characteristic way, thereby changing in number, size and shape. Bubbles can often be flushed out of the duct with the patient tilted head downwards. If, however, air is present within the duct system at the start of an examination, due to previous surgery or fistulation, it is often impossible to displace all of it with contrast medium (Fig. 19.1). In such instances the presence of small, round lucent stones cannot be excluded with certainty.

Duct calibre

The assessment of the calibre of the extrahepatic common duct depends upon the technique used to demonstrate it. The upper limit of normal at

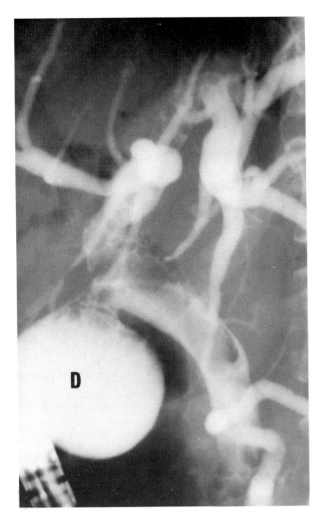

Fig. 19.1 Gas in bile ducts following choledochoduodenostomy (D = duodenal cap).

intravenous cholangiography has long been accepted as 10 mm, but this figure overestimates the true diameter due to radiographic magnification and also to a choleretic effect of the injection in some patients. On the other hand, ultrasound tends to underestimate true duct calibre (Sauerbrei et al., 1980). At ERC the duct calibre can be accurately measured by direct comparison with the endoscope but is dependent upon both the volume and pressure of injection. Duct measurement at ERC tends to be consistently higher than at intravenous cholangiography (Belsito et al., 1977). Taking all these factors into consideration it is therefore possible to obtain normal duct measurements of, for example, 4 mm at ultrasound and 12 mm at ERC in the same patient. This difference may be even more marked in patients who have had an episode of duct obstruction and dilatation in the past with the production of an unusually

distensible or 'floppy' duct. Duct measurements at PTC tend to be unreliable, as the magnification factor is not known.

In any discussion on duct calibre it is essential to recognize the fact that obstruction and dilatation are not synonymous. Ultrasound studies have shown that the bile duct is capable of doubling or halving its size in a matter of days (Mueller et al., 1982), and it is not infrequent to demonstrate stones causing obstruction in normal or only minimally dilated ducts. Also, in sclerosing cholangitis there may be severe obstruction without duct dilatation.

Anatomical variants

Important congenital abnormalities are dealt with elsewhere but it is not uncommon to find minor variants of branching at the porta hepatis or accessory ducts, usually from the right lobe. The site of insertion of the cystic duct is also variable. It may pursue a parallel course with the common hepatic duct over some distance and be inserted low down and medially (Fig. 19.2). This may not be apparent at surgery and a long cystic duct stump is not infrequently encountered at postcholecystectomy cholangiography. Occasionally the cystic duct has an ectopic insertion (Fig. 19.3).

Percutaneous trans-hepatic cholangiography

Percutaneous trans-hepatic cholangiography (PTC) was first performed by Huard & Do-Xuan-Hop (1937) but the first descriptions in the West appeared 15 years later (Carter & Saypol, 1952, Leger et al., 1952). Although the change from a rigid needle to a catheter/needle combination increased the safety of the procedure, PTC remained for the next 20 years or so a useful but potentially hazardous technique, which always had to be followed by surgery if biliary obstruction were demonstrated. In 1974 Kunio Okuda and his colleagues from Chiba University in Japan (Okuda et al., 1974) published their experience with 314 patients using a fine 23 gauge needle, first described by Tsuchiya (1969). The narrow calibre and flexibility of this 'Chiba' needle greatly increased both the safety and the success of the technique. Not only did the demonstration of biliary obstruction no longer have to be followed by immediate surgery but also the demonstration of

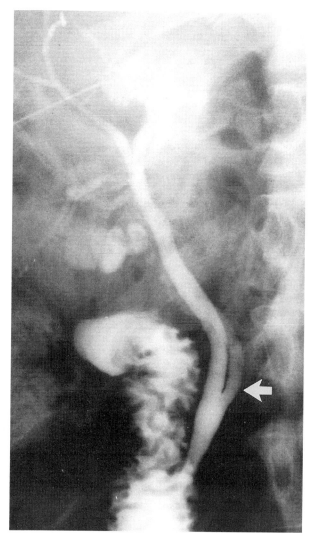

Fig. 19.2 Normal cholangiogram showing low and medial cystic duct insertion (*arrow*).

non-obstructed and non-dilated duct systems was made possible.

Although invasive, PTC is a simple technique readily available in most hospitals. The materials are inexpensive and no special expertise is required. It is therefore now in widespread use as a primary radiological procedure, and world-wide experience has shown it to be a simple and accurate technique, with a low complication rate, for the demonstration of the biliary system.

Contraindications

1 Any bleeding tendency or coagulation defect is potentially dangerous. As biliary obstruction and severe liver damage both impair the production of coagulation factors, the prothrombin time should be measured. A value of greater than 3 s above the control should be corrected with vitamin K injection before undertaking PTC.

2 Patients with known contrast-medium hypersensitivity should be investigated by other means. Jaundiced patients should be tested for hepatitis B surface antigen (HBsAg) and appropriate precautions taken if positive.

3 In the presence of active cholangitis, PTC should be performed with caution. Appropriate antibiotic cover and the maintenance of adequate hydration of the patient are essential, and only the smallest volume of contrast required to establish the diagnosis should be injected to reduce the risk of septic shock. However, the establishment of biliary drainage in such patients may be life saving.

4 The procedure will be more difficult to perform, and therefore more likely to produce complications, in patients in a poor general condition who cannot lie still or hold their breath. Gross ascites makes the procedure more difficult and hazardous and preliminary paracentesis is advisable.

Technique

PTC is usually performed under local anaesthetic. It is undertaken in close co-operation with clinical colleagues and with the informed consent of the patient. The platelet count and prothrombin time are measured beforehand and corrected if necessary.

It is important to retain the patient's co-operation throughout the procedure and it can frequently be performed without sedation. If mild sedation is considered desirable the choice and dose should be influenced by the possibility of disturbed liver metabolism. Only children and very unco-operative adults require general anaesthetic.

In view of the high incidence of infected bile in the presence of obstruction, especially when due to stones and when incomplete (Scott, 1971), there is general agreement that antibiotic cover is desirable. This may be given prophylactically although some workers prefer to await confirmation of obstruction and bacteriological examination of the aspirated bile. A single intravenous dose before the procedure may be sufficient but in the presence of obstruction or clinical evidence of infection more prolonged administration is required until the obstruction is relieved or the signs of infection have resolved.

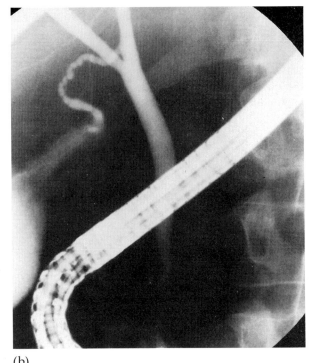

(b)

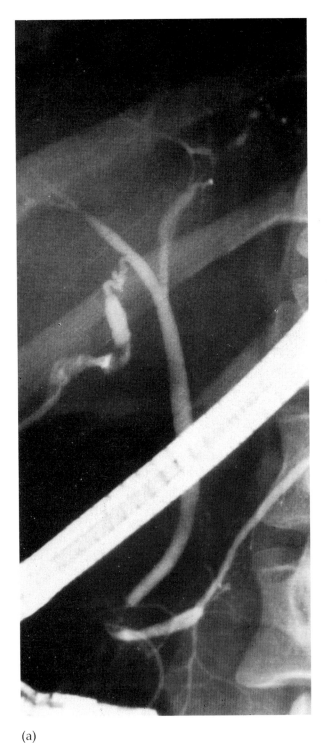

(a)

Fig. 19.3 Ectopic cystic duct origins: (a) from right hepatic duct (b) from left hepatic duct.

The standard approach involves a lateral puncture of the right lobe of the liver although in certain circumstances anterior puncture of the left lobe may be indicated. Chiba needles in general use are thin-walled flexible stainless steel, 22 gauge, 15–20 cm in length, with a short bevel (Fig. 19.4).

Following routine aseptic preparation a point is chosen below the pleural reflection on deep inspiration, observed fluoroscopically, in the mid-axillary line usually at a height of 11–12 cm from the table top, depending upon the patient's build. The tissues down to the liver capsule are infiltrated with local anaesthetic and a small incision is made in the skin. The patient is instructed to stop breathing in mid-inspiration and the Chiba needle is

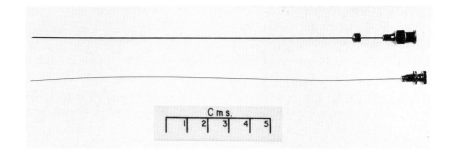

Fig. 19.4 Chiba needle with stilette removed. Note short bevel.

advanced briskly through the liver substance, under fluoroscopic control, in a plane parallel to the table top. A brisk passage of the needle through the liver substance is more likely to result in successful duct puncture than a hesitant or intermittent advance. The needle tip is aimed towards a point a few cm to the right of the spine, half-way between the dome of the diaphragm and the duodenal cap. When the needle is in position the patient resumes gentle breathing.

Water-soluble contrast medium (approximately 150 mg iodine per ml) is then injected under fluoroscopic control whilst slowly withdrawing the needle. This concentration of contrast medium is easy to inject and mixes freely with bile; it also avoids too dense parenchymal staining or 'whitewashing' small duct stones. As soon as a bile duct is entered the characteristic branching pattern with slow centrifugal flow towards the hilum is seen. As the movement of contrast medium in the ducts is gravity dependent, various positional manoeuvres, such as tilting the patient feet downwards, or sitting up after removal of the needle, are used to established the exact level and configuration of any obstructing lesion. Under normal circumstances, with the patient supine, contrast flows freely down to the lower end of the common duct (Fig. 19.5). However, in high-grade obstruction with gross dilatation, contrast medium tends to pool in dilated intrahepatic branches and may give the erroneous impression of obstruction at the porta hepatis when in fact it is lower down. This pitfall can be avoided by rotating and tilting the patient as described or by arranging delayed films. It is, however, important to avoid the injection of excess contrast medium into an obstructed duct system as this will greatly increase the risk of septic shock, which will not necessarily be prevented by prophylactic antibiotics.

Carcinoma of the head of the pancreas often produces anterior displacement of the lower end

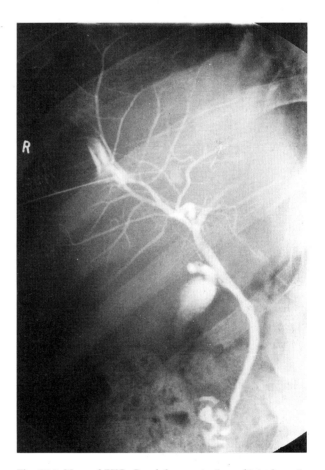

Fig. 19.5 Normal PTC. Good demonstration of intrahepatic and extrahepatic ducts with contrast flow into the duodenum and gall bladder. Slight parenchymal staining is seen from a previous needle pass.

of the common duct and the exact level of obstruction may not be shown with the patient supine. In the presence of obstructing lesions at or near the porta hepatis it must be established whether the left lobe is in communication with the right or separately obstructed, as this may determine whether a drainage procedure is possible.

If a bile duct is not punctured on the initial pass,

repeated attempts may be made with slight variations in craniocaudal angulation, but without withdrawing the needle from the liver substance. It is best to start slightly high (cranially) and work downwards (caudally) so that any initial contrast extravasation does not obscure detail of ducts subsequently opacified. There is no limit to the number of passes permitted as this is not related to the incidence of serious complications (Harbin *et al.*, 1980, Ariyama, 1983). However, after about 20 unsuccessful attempts, both the patient and the operator begin to find the procedure tedious.

Contrast injection into liver parenchyma produces a persistent amorphous stain, and injection into vascular structures results in rapid flushing away of contrast medium in a direction appropriate to the vessel entered. Lymphatic vessels show as narrow, irregular channels passing downwards and medially but without the typical branching pattern of bile ducts (Fig. 19.6). Periportal extravasation produces a characteristic static branching stain (Fig. 19.7), readily distinguishable from normal bile duct configuration.

In addition to fluoroscopic observation, spot radiographs are exposed as required during the procedure, supplemented by delayed films if indicated. Following the procedure the patient is placed on bed rest, with monitoring of pulse, blood pressure, and temperature for 12–24 h.

Success rate

The success of PTC in opacifing the biliary system is directly related to the presence of duct dilatation and the number of attempts made (Jaques *et al.*, 1980). Harbin *et al.* (1980) reviewed 2005 examinations from 31 centres in North America and found an overall success rate of 97.8% in the presence of duct dilatation, rising to 99% when 12 or more needle passes were made. In the same series, the success of puncturing non-dilated duct systems was 70.2%. Ariyama (1983), reviewing 2515 cases from 11 sources, found success rates of 98% and 82%, respectively. Therefore, in the presence of established duct dilatation, PTC will be successful in virtually every case. In addition, its success in demonstrating non-dilated duct systems compares favourably with that achieved by ERC.

Complications

Although serious complications are infrequent, those that can occur may require early surgical intervention. The examination should therefore

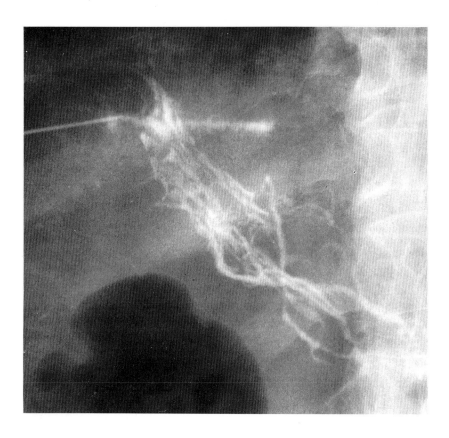

Fig. 19.6 PTC. Lymphatic channels.

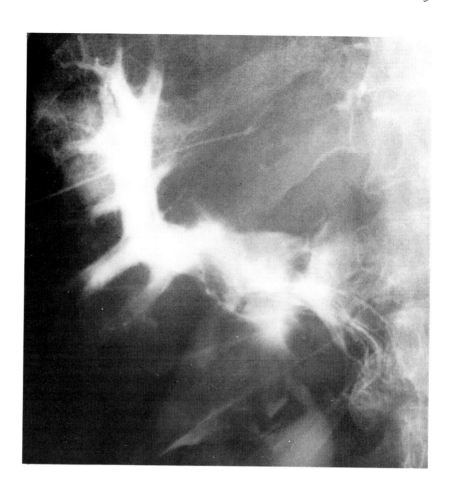

Fig. 19.7 PTC. Extravasation around portal vein. Some lymphatic channels are also opacified towards the hilum.

never be performed in a unit where this is not available. The incidence of complications in the two large multicentre reviews by Harbin *et al.* (1980) and Ariyama (1983) totalling 4750 procedures is shown in Table 19.1.

Sepsis

Cholangitis is the most frequent and serious complication and is related to the high incidence of infected bile in the presence of obstruction (Scott, 1971). This is most likely if the obstruction is due to a benign cause, e.g. stone or stricture, and if it is incomplete. Total neoplastic obstruction is only rarely associated with biliary infection. In the two large series quoted, serious septic complications were invariably associated with the presence of obstruction. The introduction of infected bile into the blood stream can produce a spectrum of clinical effects from fever, with or without rigors, to severe hypotension and shock. Although appropriate antibiotic prophylaxis will greatly reduce the incidence, it may not prevent development of septic shock.

Table 19.1 Complications of PTC

References	Harbin *et al.*, 1980	Ariyama, 1983	Totals
No. of procedures	2005	2745	4750
Sepsis	28	46	74 (1.6%)
Bile leak	29	24	53 (1.1%)
Bleeding	7	6	13 (0.3%)
Deaths	4	3	7 (0.1%)

Bile leak

Intraperitoneal bile leak is also much more likely to occur in the presence of obstruction but the main causative factor is inadvertent puncture of the extrahepatic ducts or gall bladder. If this occurs in the presence of obstruction, then the surgical team should be alerted immediately. On the other hand, evidence of a small intraperitoneal bile leak may be an incidental finding at subsequent laparotomy in the absence of any associated clinical symptoms or signs.

Bleeding

Intraperitoneal bleeding is usually related to a coagulation defect but is also more likely if the although these usually produce little clinical disturbance. Haemobilia may result from the procedure and produces a characteristic appearance of mixing artefacts and filling defects on the contrast films (Fig. 19.8).

Other complications

Miscellaneous other complications include pneumothorax, intrahepatic arteriovenous fistulae, and contrast reactions.

Despite the serious nature of these complications, their overall incidence is low and is comparable with those resulting from ERCP, e.g. serious complications 3% and deaths 0.15%, as shown by Bilbao *et al.* (1976).

Endoscopic retrograde cholangiography

Endoscopic cannulation of the papilla of Vater was first described in America (McCune *et al.*, 1968). However, it was not until specialized duodenoscopes developed in Japan (Oi *et al.*, 1969) became generally available that endoscopic retrograde cholangiopancreatography (ERCP) became widespread. The technique is now in use world-wide for the investigation of both biliary and pancreatic systems (Cotton, 1977) but the emphasis of this chapter will be on endoscopic retrograde cholangiography (ERC) as a means of producing a direct-contrast cholangiogram.

Although ERC is essentially a radiological examination, its success depends upon endoscopic expertise and is best performed as a joint exercise by a radiologist and a gastroenterologist. The indications for and advantages of direct-contrast cholangiography in the investigation of jaundice and biliary symptoms have been described previously and apply in general to both ERC and PTC. However, the endoscopic approach can provide additional useful information in respect of the appearance of the papilla, with the ability to take biopsies, and from demonstration of pancreas.

Contraindications

Any contraindication to or condition preventing upper gastrointestinal endoscopy will preclude ERC. These include oesophageal stenosis, gastric

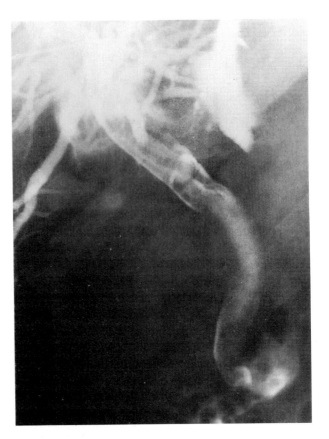

Fig. 19.8 Haemobilia. Irregular dilution of contrast medium and mixing artefacts produced by bleeding into the duct system at PTC.

outflow obstruction, and severe cardiopulmonary disease. Previous gastric surgery or resection may make the procedure difficult or even impossible, although an expert endoscopist can often succeed in the presence of a Polya-type gastrectomy. Special precautions are necessary when there is a risk of contamination, e.g. in patients known to be HBsAg or HIV positive and those with active pulmonary tuberculosis.

Patients with known or suspected contrast-medium sensitivity should preferably be investigated by other means, but if ERC is considered essential full prophylactic measures should be instituted. However, the risk from contrast reactions is probably less than at PTC. Active cholangitis is not a contraindication but appropriate antibiotic cover is essential and care must be taken not to inject excess contrast medium into an obstructed duct system. The establishment of biliary drainage by sphincterotomy in such patients is beneficial. Contraindications in respect of the pancreas are dealt with elsewhere.

Technique

ERCP requires a team approach and should be performed in the radiology department. Fluoroscopic equipment of high quality is required for optimum results and the room used should be large enough to accommodate the necessary personnel and apparatus (Goldberg *et al.*, 1976). Patients are prepared as for any upper gastrointestinal endoscopic examination and informed consent is obtained. The type and amount of premedication and sedation used varies according to local practice and clinical indications. Prophylactic antibiotics are given if specifically indicated but are not usually required for a routine diagnostic study. It is beyond the scope of this chapter to describe the endoscopic technique in detail but, using a side-viewing endoscope the duodenum is entered, the patient turned prone and a control radiograph is exposed. The papilla of Vater is then identified, any abnormality of it noted, and it is cannulated. Duodenal ileus produced by i.v. hyoscine-n-butylbromide (Buscopan) or glucagon assists cannulation and glyceryl trinitrate sublingual spray may help to relax the sphincter of Oddi.

Water-soluble contrast medium is injected under fluoroscopic control. A low concentration (approximately 150 mg/ml) is used for cholangiography to avoid 'whitewashing' small stones within a dilated duct. Spot radiographs should always be taken during filling as stones may be most clearly visible at this stage. In the presence of duct obstruction only sufficient contrast medium to establish the diagnosis should be injected, because of the risk of sepsis. In the absence of obstruction attempts should be made to achieve complete filling of intrahepatic ducts and gall bladder (Fig. 19.9).

In the prone position the porta hepatis is below the level of the ampulla and contrast medium therefore flows freely towards the liver away from the lower end of the common duct. In the presence of dilatation this initial contrast flow along the dependent wall of the duct can produce a 'trickle' artefact, giving a falsely narrowed impression of calibre. Only after complete opacification and uniform mixing of contrast medium with bile is the true duct calibre revealed. Also, if the duct is unusually distensible or 'floppy', possibly resulting from a previous episode of obstruction, the calibre on completion of injection may appear greater than that observed after removal of the cannula (Fig. 19.10). In the prone position, the left hepatic duct is dependent and fills first. The right

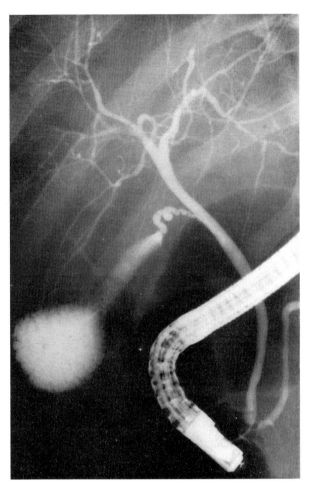

Fig. 19.9 Normal ERC with complete opacification of the biliary system. Contrast medium is also present in the pancreatic duct.

ducts may not be fully demonstrated until the patient is turned supine (Fig. 19.11).

The lower end of the common duct is often best demonstrated after removal of the cannula and with the patient supine, possibly with additional table tilt. In the event of achieving only 'flash filling' this may be the only position to demonstrate pathology here (Fig. 19.12). Fluoroscopic observation and spot radiographs of the intramural segment with the patient supine are an essential part of the procedure. Complete intrahepatic filling may be impossible due to free and preferential contrast flow into the gall bladder.

Care should be taken to avoid the introduction of air bubbles although these can usually be differentiated from stones by their gravitational response. Some patients, such as those who have had endoscopic sphincterotomy or surgery to the lower end of the bile duct, will have gas in the

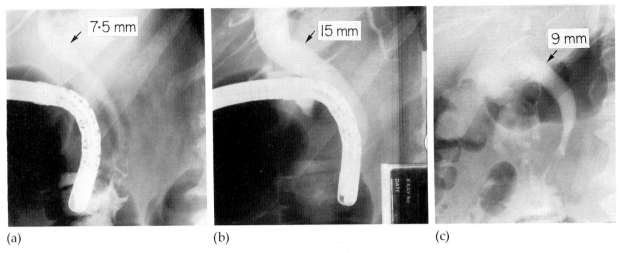

Fig. 19.10 ERC technique. (a) During filling a trickle of contrast medium along the dependent wall of a dilated duct gives an erroneous impression of duct calibre. (b) and (c) Note the difference in calibre on completion of injection and after removal of the cannula due to duct distensibility.

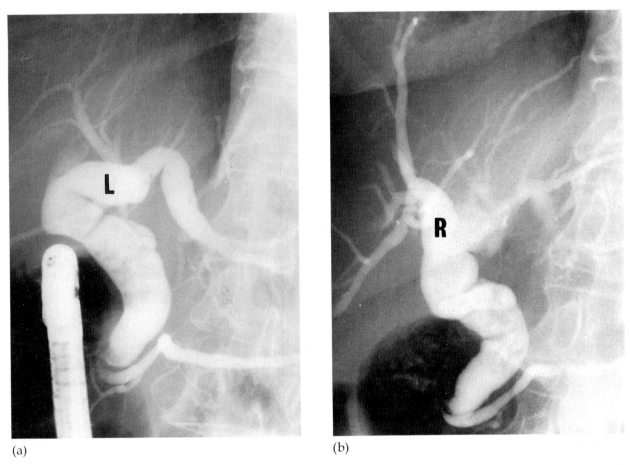

Fig. 19.11 ERC technique. (a) In the prone position, the left (L) hepatic duct fills preferentially. (b) In the supine the right (R) duct is opacified. Multiple small stones are present in the common duct.

ducts at the start of the examination and a modification of technique is required to obtain a cholangiogram. The cannula is advanced as high as possible into the common duct, preferably up to the porta hepatis, the patient is tilted steeply head downwards and the system flushed rapidly with

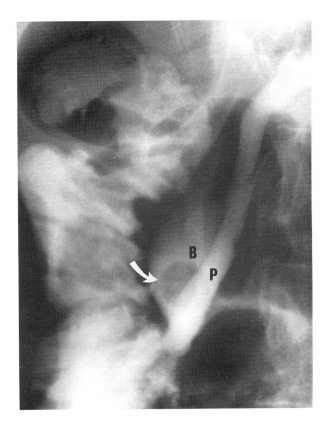

Fig. 19.12 ERC technique. 'Flash filling' of the common duct (B). Only when this patient was turned supine and tilted feet downwards was a duct stone revealed (*arrow*). The pancreatic duct (P) has also been opacified.

dilute contrast medium. In this way bubbles are expelled into the duodenum and an adequate contrast cholangiogram can usually be obtained.

Emptying times of the common duct are very variable and it is difficult to assess their diagnostic significance. Apart from the presence of obvious obstructing lesions, emptying times will be affected by the medication given, the duration and difficulty of cannulation and the presence of the gall bladder.

Sufficient radiographs are exposed during and on completion of contrast injection to ensure a diagnostic result. As the procedure is so labour intensive it is essential to avoid compromising the result by obtaining too few films. Also, as the patients are sedated and occasionally restless, detail on some films may be lost by movement blur. On the other hand, radiation exposure of patients, staff and the endoscope should be kept to a minimum. Late films are occasionally required, usually to confirm or exclude the presence of stones in the

gall bladder, although this information is usually known beforehand from ultrasound examination.

The success rate of ERC is directly related to the skill and experience of the endoscopist. Retrograde cholangiography is usually more difficult than pancreatography, but in experienced hands success rates in excess of 80% are achieved. Causes of failure include pathology in the region of the papilla, the presence of periampullary diverticula, and previous gastric surgery.

Complications

Complications of ERC include those related to endoscopy and medication in addition to those resulting from duct cannulation and contrast injection.

Endoscopy and medication

These are similar to those of any upper gastrointestinal endoscopic procedure and include perforation, inhalation of vomit, cross-infection, and drug reaction.

Cannulation and contrast injection

Sepsis is the most serious and when it occurs it is almost invariably in the presence of duct obstruction. Only the minimum volume of contrast medium required for diagnosis should be injected and the temptation to obtain outstanding or dramatic radiographs should be resisted. Trauma to the papilla during cannulation or submucosal contrast injection may interfere with the interpretation of radiographs but are not usually of clinical significance. Contrast reactions are uncommon but the indications for the examination should be reconsidered and precautions taken in any patient known or suspected of being at risk.

Bilbao *et al.* (1976) showed that both complications and success rates of ERCP were related to the experience of the operators. In an assessment of over 10 000 examinations from 222 centres in North America, 8 of the 15 deaths recorded resulted from cholangitis (Table 19.2). The overall incidence of serious complications (3%) and deaths (0.2%) are comparable with those resulting from PTC (Table 19.1).

Comparison of PTC and ERC

The choice between these two methods of direct

Table 19.2 Complications of ERCP (from Bilbao *et al.* 1976)

10 435 Cases	No.	Deaths
Pancreatitis	94	—
Cholangitis	72	8
Drug reaction	51	—
Pancreatic sepsis	25	5
Instrumental injury	16	2
Aspiration pneumonia	8	—
Miscellaneous	4	—

cholangiography will be determined to some extent by local availability and practice. If ERC is not readily available, then PTC will be performed more frequently than in a hospital with an active endoscopy unit. PTC, although invasive, is usually a quick and simple procedure. Materials are inexpensive and no special expertise is required. On the other hand, ERC is a labour intensive exercise, the success of which is dependent upon the experience of the operator, and it involves expensive equipment with team organization.

In the presence of total extrahepatic biliary obstruction the information obtained from the demonstration of the ducts above the obstruction by PTC is usually of more use in treatment planning than that obtained from showing the unobstructed lower end using ERC. However, ERC may provide additional evidence from endoscopic examination of the duodenal loop and papilla, possibly supplemented by biopsy, and by demonstration of the pancreas. PTC is the method of choice in many postgastrectomy patients in whom ERC may be difficult or unsuccessful. Both techniques may be used as a prelude to biliary drainage procedures, but relief of stone obstruction by sphincterotomy obviously requires the endoscopic approach. Difficulties in retrograde cannulation may be overcome by a combined approach, using both techniques, as in the trans-hepatic placement of a guide wire or catheter to assist endoscopic sphincterotomy or stent insertion.

There is no overall difference between PTC and ERC in their success in demonstrating non-dilated bile ducts or in the incidence of serious complications and mortality.

Operative cholangiography

Operative cholangiography was first described by Mirizzi (1937) but despite its obvious advantages it took many years to become generally accepted in England (Love, 1952, Le Quesne, 1960).

On clinical assessment alone, 5–10% of patients at cholecystectomy will have unsuspected duct stones. Pre-exploratory operative cholangiography is therefore used during biliary surgery to confirm or exclude the presence of duct stones and to determine whether or not duct exploration is required. Also, the confident demonstration of normality will prevent unnecessary duct exploration with its increased morbidity and mortality (Chapman *et al.*, 1964). Operative cholangiography will in addition demonstrate any anatomical variations of duct anatomy with surgical relevance. Postexploratory or completion operative cholangiography is used to confirm that all stones have been removed.

The success of operative cholangiography depends upon careful attention to details of technique and willing co-operation between surgeon and radiologist. Most biliary surgeons now perform operative cholangiography routinely, although not all do both pre-exploratory and post-exploratory examinations. Properly organized and performed it is simple, safe, and accurate and should add only about 10 min to the operating time. The availability nowadays of endoscopic sphincterotomy or T-tube extraction for the removal of retained stones should not deter the biliary surgeon from performing routine operative cholangiography. The only contraindication is known hypersensitivity to contrast media.

Technique

The examination can be performed either radiographically or fluoroscopically. The standard method involves the exposure of two or three radiographs following incremental contrast injections. The surgeon must of course wait for the films to be developed but they do subsequently form a permanent record. On the other hand, some surgeons feel that the use of a mobile image intensifier, possibly supplemented by a video recorder, gives them an equally accurate, and certainly quicker, assessment.

A fine cannula, pre-filled with saline or contrast, is inserted into the cystic duct, taking great care not to introduce air bubbles. If the cystic duct is too short or inaccessible, then the common duct is punctured directly. The patient, or the X-ray beam, is angled 10–15° to project the common duct off the spine and all radio-opaque instruments are

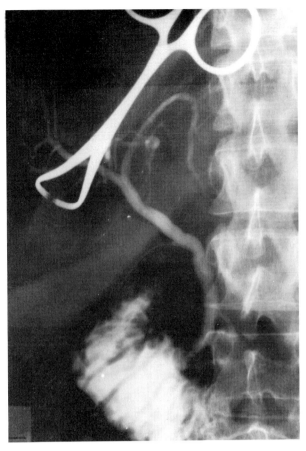

Fig. 19.13 Operative cholangiogram. Normal pre-exploratory examination fulfilling the five criteria (see text). The towel clip should have been removed.

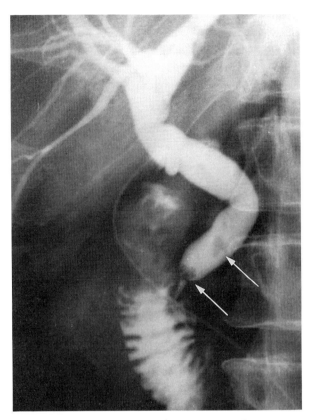

Fig. 19.14 Operative cholangiogram. Abnormal pre-exploratory examination. The common duct is dilated and contains two stones (*arrows*).

removed from the field. The use of a stationary grid is advantageous as many of these patients are overweight and the grid lines should be orientated crosswise to permit angulation. Dilute contrast medium (150 mg iodine/ml) is used to avoid obscuring small stones.

In the standard technique, radiographs are exposed following the injection of 2−3 ml, 6−8 ml and 10−12 ml of contrast medium. Larger volumes may be required if the duct system is obviously dilated. Some form of cassette tunnel or operating table designed for the purpose is required and care must be taken to maintain sterility of the operation site. Using an image intensifier the volume and rate of contrast medium injection are determined fluoroscopically.

Results

The five criteria for normality as defined by Le Quesne (1960) still hold good and are as follows:

1 Normal duct calibre, 12 mm being taken as the upper limit.
2 Free flow of contrast medium into the duodenum.
3 No excessive filling of intrahepatic ducts.
4 Demonstration of normal tapering intramural segment.
5 Absence of filling defects.
Examples of normal and abnormal examinations are illustrated (Figs 19.13, 19.14).

If the technique is meticulously performed and these criteria strictly applied then the accuracy will be over 90%. Difficulties in interpretation can result from the introduction of bubbles, too much or too little or too dense contrast medium, poor positioning of the patient, incorrect exposure, or movement blur. In many instances the films will be interpreted by the surgeon, but radiological advice should always be available if required.

Postexploratory or completion cholangiography

This is performed via the T-tube following duct

exploration. The general principles are similar to those of pre-exploratory cholangiography although a larger volume of contrast medium is usually required because of the dead space of the T-tube. The avoidance of air bubbles is more difficult and it is usual to irrigate the T-tube gently with saline during its insertion to exclude them.

The lower end of the common duct may be oedematous following exploration and instrumentation and therefore free contrast flow into the duodenum and a normal intramural segment may not be seen on postexploratory films. Their absence is therefore not significant at this stage and the only important diagnostic sign is the presence or absence of filling defects. Even these may be difficult to interpret as they may be due to blood clot following instrumentation rather than residual stones.

T-tube cholangiography

T-tube cholangiography is used to demonstrate the biliary duct system, usually prior to removal of the T-tube. It aims to confirm the absence of any retained duct stones and to show free contrast flow into the duodenum. It may also be used to investigate problems produced by blocking or displacement of the T-tube itself. Routine T-tube cholangiography is usually performed 7–10 days after operation.

Technique

The examination is performed in a standard fluoroscopy room. No preparation of the patient is required but the T-tube should be clamped beforehand to prevent air entering the system. Having cleaned the T-tube it is punctured, using a fine needle connected by flexible extension tubing of sufficient length to a syringe containing contrast medium. All air bubbles should be excluded from this system before insertion of the needle, and gentle suction should produce a bubble-free interface between bile and contrast medium in the tubing.

The patient is turned into a shallow right posterior oblique position, to project the common duct off the spine, and after a control radiograph has been exposed, contrast medium is injected slowly under fluoroscopic monitoring. Spot radiographs are exposed as required during the injection and early films are essential to demonstrate the lower end of the common duct before it is

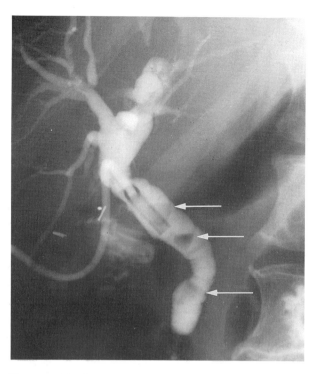

Fig. 19.15 T-tube cholangiogram. Three retained stones are clearly demonstrated (*arrows*).

obscured by contrast in the duodenum. Dilute water-soluble contrast medium (150 mg iodine/ml) is used to avoid the possibility of obscuring small stones (Fig. 19.15). Usually there is no discomfort to the patient unless too much contrast is injected too forcibly. A little contrast leak may be seen around the point of insertion of the T-tube into the duct but is of no significance and does not usually interfere with interpretation.

Stones may be missed if the whole duct system is not opacified (Fig. 19.16). As the left hepatic duct passes anteriorly from the porta hepatis it may be necessary to turn the patient on the left side or even prone to achieve complete filling. If contrast flow into the duodenum is particularly free then the patient may have to be tilted head downwards to demonstrate intrahepatic branches. On the other hand, if sphincter spasm is suspected, this can be relieved by an i.v. injection of glucagon or sublingual glyceryl trinitrate spray.

The distinction between stones and air bubbles can usually be made by their appearance, behaviour, and response to gravity (see p.281). Bubbles may often be flushed out of the duct with a rapid injection of dilute contrast medium or saline with the patient tilted steeply head downwards. If, however, genuine doubt persists then the T-tube

Jaundice due to stone obstruction is typically associated with duct dilatation (Figs 19.17, 19.18). However, dilatation may be minimal or even absent (Fig. 19.19). Very gross duct dilatation is more often due to neoplastic obstruction.

Stones, being common, may coexist with other lesions and therefore their demonstration does not necessarily establish a diagnosis. Patients with hepatocellular jaundice or intrahepatic cholestasis may have coincidental gall stones (Fig. 19.20) and there is an increased incidence in cirrhosis (*see* Fig. 19.46). Even stones within the duct may not be the primary lesion as they may be found in association with neoplastic obstruction (Fig. 19.21) or benign stricture.

At ERC a duct stone will only very rarely cause total obstruction to the retrograde flow of contrast medium. Total obstruction to retrograde filling of the common bile duct, with adequate cannulation, is almost always due to neoplasm (Fig. 19.21). In the author's experience of over 4500 ERCP examinations, the only exceptions to this rule have been when either a widely patent duct orifice (e.g. following sphincterotomy) or inadequate cannulation have resulted in free contrast medium reflux into

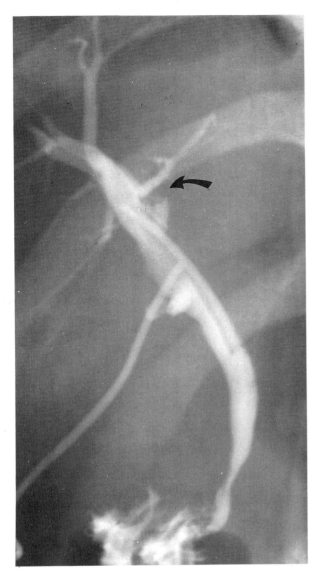

Fig. 19.16 T-tube cholangiogram. The left hepatic duct is not filled due to a round stone impacted in its orifice (*arrow*). This was missed at the time and subsequently removed by endoscopic sphincterotomy.

should be left in position and the examination repeated in a day or so.

Pathology

Stones

Gall stones are common and found in up to 20% of all patients, both male and female, in the older age groups. They may be single or multiple, large or small, round or facetted, lucent or opaque. The distinction between round, lucent stones and air bubbles has been discussed previously.

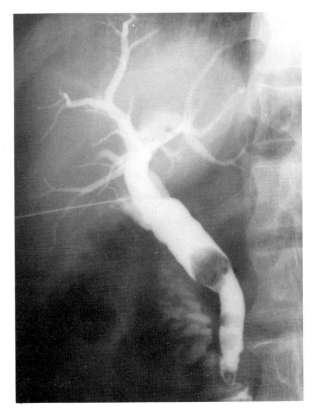

Fig. 19.17 Several large stones within a dilated common duct shown at PTC.

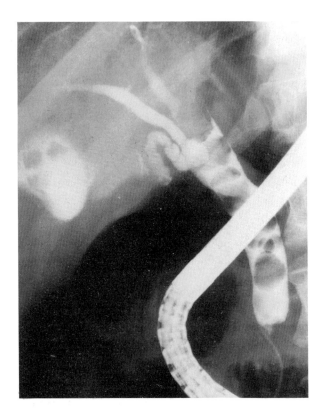

Fig. 19.18 Multiple stones in common duct and gall bladder shown at ERC.

the duodenum. This of course is not so at PTC, where the antegrade injection of contrast medium will cause further impaction of an obstructing stone. In such cases the characteristic concave configuration of the lower end of the contrast column usually indicates the cause.

Mirizzi's syndrome (Mirizzi, 1948) consists of partial obstruction of the common duct from extrinsic compression and inflammation caused by a stone impacted in the neck of the gall bladder or the cystic duct (Fig. 19.22). It is frequently associated with cholangitis and jaundice and may progress to fistulation.

Juxtapapillary diverticula are often encountered at ERC and, in addition to making cannulation more difficult, often cause deformity of the lower end of the contrast column producing a 'pseudo-stone' appearance (Lintott et al., 1981). The spurious nature of this appearance can usually be determined without difficulty by observing

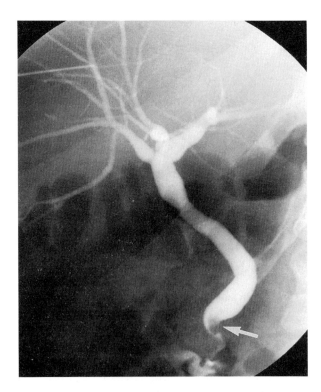

Fig. 19.19 Jaundice due to a stone (*arrow*) at the lower end of the common duct. Calibre of duct system within normal limits and intrahepatic branches 'non-dilated' at ultrasound.

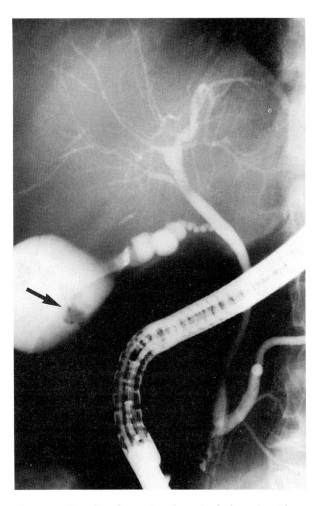

Fig. 19.20 Jaundice due to intrahepatic cholestasis with coincidental gall bladder stones (*arrow*).

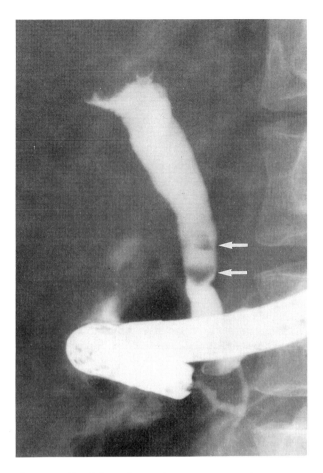

Fig. 19.21 Total duct obstruction on a retrograde cholangiogram due to metastatic nodes from a sigmoid carcinoma. In addition there are two small stones (*arrows*) within the duct below the obstruction.

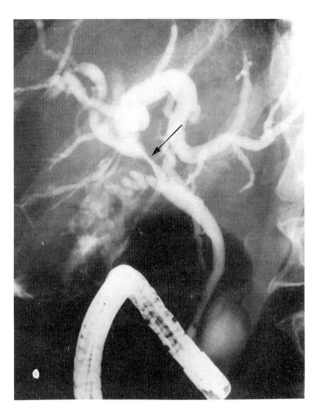

Fig. 19.22 Mirizzi's syndrome. Large gall bladder stone with surrounding inflammation causing extrinsic compression of the common hepatic duct (*arrow*) and proximal obstruction.

contraction and relaxation of the intramural segment on screening after removal of the cannula (Fig. 19.23).

Other intraduct filling defects may be due to blood clot, tumour fragments (Fig. 19.24), and parasites.

Postcholecystectomy syndrome

The postcholecystectomy syndrome is a poorly defined condition with a variety of possible causes. Persistence or recurrence of symptoms after cholecystectomy suggest the presence of a retained or reformed stone, but other biliary lesions such as stricture, fistula, or ampullary stenosis may be discovered. A long cystic duct stump has also been implicated but there is little evidence to support this. Non-biliary causes include pancreatitis and upper gastrointestinal digestive problems such as reflux oesophagitis and peptic ulceration.

Although duct dilatation is not caused by cholecystectomy (Le Quesne *et al.*, 1959) many postcholecystectomy patients without any retained stone or other obstructing lesion will have a duct calibre outside the normal range at ERC (Hamilton *et al.*, 1982). This is possibly a 'floppy duct' phenomenon due to previous obstruction, and it means that the measurement of calibre alone is of limited value in the investigation of postcholecystectomy patients (Fig. 19.25).

Benign stricture

Benign strictures may be traumatic, usually post-surgical, or inflammatory in origin.

Surgical trauma. Complete transection or ligation of the common duct at operation will be immediately obvious either at the time or in the early postoperative period (Fig. 19.26). Less severe duct damage may result in the subsequent development of a stricture, either at the site of interference or at a higher level as the result of devascularization

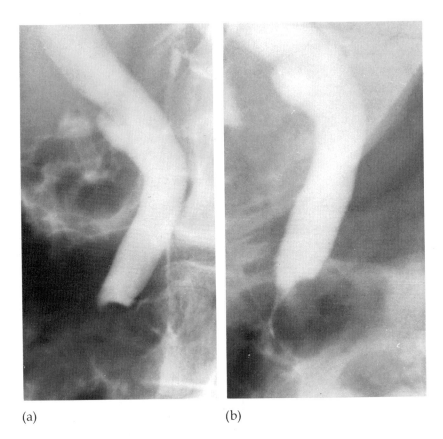

(a)　　　　　　　　　　　　　　(b)

Fig. 19.23 Pseudostone due to juxtapapillary diverticulum. (a) Concave filling defect mimicking a duct stone. (b) Relaxation of intramural segment showing normal configuration. No stone.

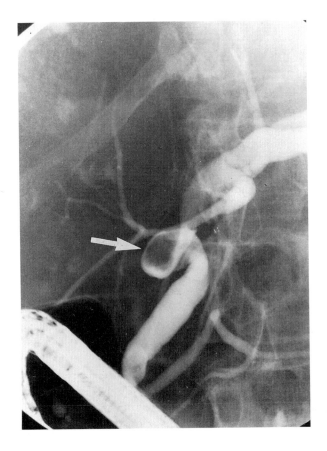

(Fig. 19.27). Slight narrowing or contour irregularity at the site of a previous T-tube insertion is not uncommon, but severe narrowing indicates operative damage. Benign strictures are typically associated with recurrent cholangitis. In the presence of high-grade or total obstruction, spontaneous fistulation into the duodenum may develop (Fig. 19.28).

Other trauma. Bile duct injury may also result from blunt or penetrating abdominal trauma (Fig. 19.29).

Pancreatitis. Strictures of the intrapancreatic portion of the common duct from chronic pancreatitis are typically long, either smooth or wavy, but incomplete (Fig. 19.30) (Sarles & Sahel, 1978). In acute pancreatitis the intrapancreatic segment may

Fig. 19.24 Intraduct filling defect (*arrow*) due to tumour fragment from metastatic colon carcinoma. During cholangiography this fragment was seen to move within the duct and at operation the whole of the right hepatic duct was occluded by necrotic tumour material lying free within the lumen.

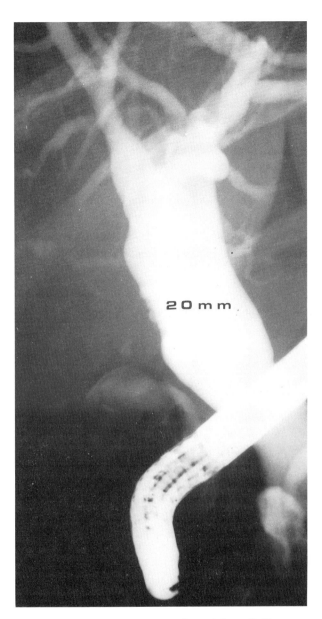

Fig. 19.25 Postcholecystectomy 'floppy' duct. Calibre 20 mm, but no stone or other cause of present duct obstruction demonstrated.

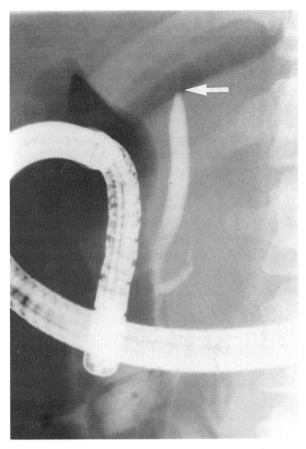

Fig. 19.26 Total common duct obstruction (*arrow*) due to inadvertent ligation at cholecystectomy.

be stretched and narrowed by surrounding inflammation (Fig. 19.31). In such cases it may be of importance to exclude an impacted stone as the cause of the attack.

Sclerosing cholangitis. Primary sclerosing cholangitis (PSC) is a condition of unknown cause characterized by diffuse fibrosis and multiple bile duct strictures usually affecting both the extrahepatic and intrahepatic ducts (Thorpe *et al.*, 1967). The four criteria usually considered essential for the establishment of the diagnosis of PSC are (i) diffuse involvement of extrahepatic ducts, (ii) absence of gall stones, (iii) no previous history of biliary surgery, and (iv) a chronic clinical course to exclude malignancy. It is now accepted, however, that PSC confined to the intrahepatic ducts is occasionally seen (Bhathal & Powell, 1969). There is a strong association with ulcerative colitis and possibly also with retroperitoneal fibrosis. The frequency of ulcerative colitis in patients with PSC varies from about one-quarter (Warren *et al.*, 1966) to about three-quarters (Chapman *et al.*, 1980). This difference probably reflects the greater accuracy of modern cholangiographic techniques. No association with Crohn's disease has been proved. In view of the increased incidence of cholangiocarcinoma in patients with ulcerative colitis it is not surprising that this malignancy may also develop in patients with long standing PSC.

The spectrum of cholangiographic appearances in PSC is wide and varied. Typically there are multiple strictures of both extrahepatic and intrahepatic ducts (Fig. 19.32) and often a beaded ap-

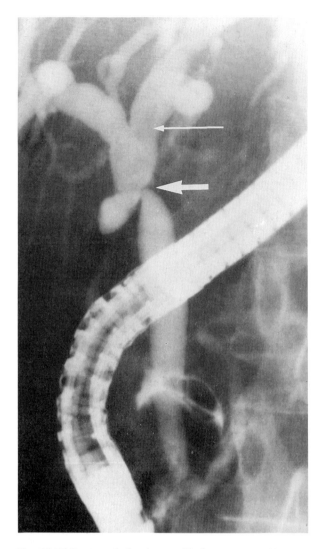

Fig. 19.27 Postsurgical stricture. Cholecystectomy 20 years ago. High common duct stricture (*thick arrow*) with a stone (*thin arrow*) in the upstream obstructed ducts.

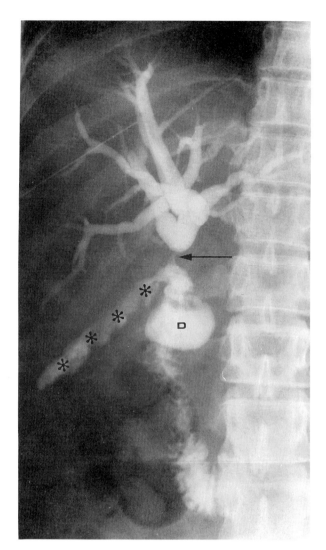

Fig. 19.28 Ligation of common duct at cholecystectomy (same case as Fig. 19.26). Spontaneous fistulation (*arrow*) has developed between the obstructed common duct and the duodenal cap (D). The asterisks indicate what remains of a previously huge intra-abdominal bile collection.

pearance with marginal sacculations (Fig. 19.33). As the duct involvement is diffuse, the degree of proximal dilatation is less than might be expected (Krieger *et al.*, 1970). If the gall bladder can be opacified it often shows normal distensibility (MacCarty *et al.*, 1983) but histological inflammatory changes may be found here also (Thorpe *et al.*, 1967).

Primary sclerosing cholangitis may be radiologically indistinguishable from diffuse cholangiocarcinoma (see Fig. 19.39) and the intrahepatic duct changes may be similar to those produced by severe parenchymal liver disease or diffuse metastases. Distinction is made on length of history, clinical details, and biopsy.

Chronic suppurative cholangitis, often with stones and with or without a history of surgery, can result in secondary sclerosing cholangitis with fibrosis and stricture formation, producing a similar radiological appearance.

Neoplastic obstruction

Pancreatic carcinoma. Carcinoma of the head of the pancreas causes low common duct obstruction, typically with an abrupt, rounded or slightly pointed configuration at PTC (Fig. 19.34). In addition, these tumours produce anterior and medial displacement of the lower end of the common duct

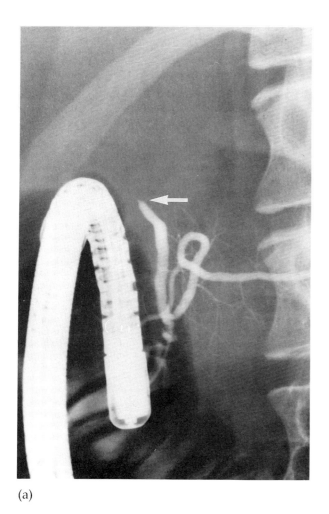

(a)

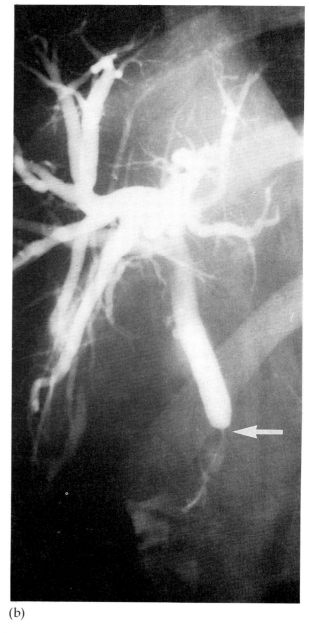

(b)

Fig. 19.29 Penetrating abdominal trauma, resulting from a fall through a plate glass window. ERC (a) and PTC (b) demonstrate a short, tight common duct stricture (*arrow*) with upstream dilatation. Normal pancreatogram.

(Fig. 19.35) and at PTC the patient may have to be tilted feet downwards or even turned prone to demonstrate the exact level and configuration of the obstruction. Stone obstruction typically produces a concave or 'claw' appearance, but occasionally confident distinction between stone and tumour may be difficult on the PTC appearances alone. Although contrast studies often indicate total obstruction, guidewires and catheters can almost always be negotiated through

the stricture during interventional drainage procedures.

At ERC, if biliary cannulation is possible, the obstruction is also typically abrupt and often total and associated with abnormalities of the pancreatogram. Adjacent obstruction of both biliary and pancreatic ducts at ERCP is termed the 'double duct' sign (Fig. 19.36) and is a strong indicator of a malignant lesion, especially if there is close proximity of the lesions and if biliary obstruction

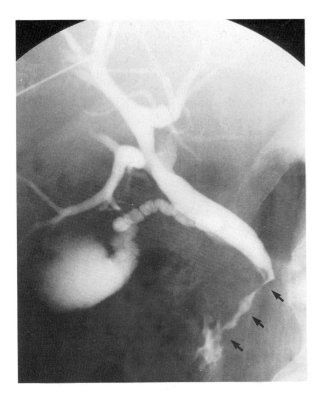

Fig. 19.30 Chronic pancreatitis. Typical long, wavy but incomplete stricture of the intrapancreatic portion of the common duct.

is total (Plumley *et al.*, 1982). It is possible to get adjacent stenoses of both ducts due to pancreatitis, but the presence of total biliary obstruction makes a malignant cause almost certain.

Ampullary neoplasm. Ampullary tumours, whether benign or malignant, often tend to present early with jaundice and the diagnosis is usually established endoscopically. Contrast studies demonstrate obstruction of both biliary and pancreatic ducts, often in the form of an irregular filling defect (Fig. 19.37).

Cholangiocarcinoma. The commonest manifestation of bile duct carcinoma is a focal stricture (Fig. 19.38), although in just over 10% of cases there is diffuse duct involvement (Anderson *et al.*, 1985) (Fig. 19.39). Occasionally the lesion may take the form of an intraluminal polypoid filling defect (Fig. 19.40) (Nichols *et al.*, 1983). Unfortunately the majority of these tumours involves the proximal extrahepatic ducts, making radical surgical treatment difficult or impossible. Although the overall prognosis is poor some of these tumours are slow growing, and prolonged survival may be possible

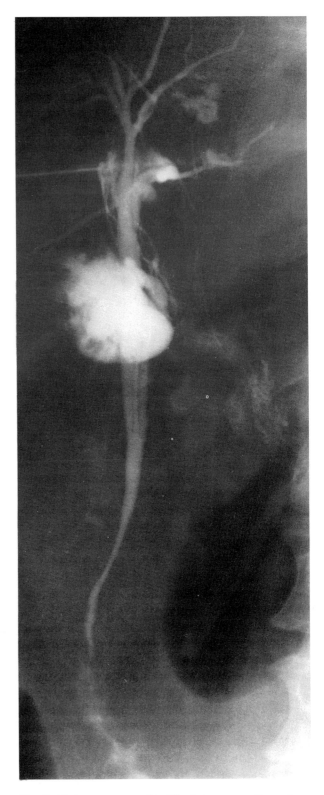

Fig. 19.31 Acute pancreatitis. The intrapancreatic portion of the common duct is stretched and narrowed by surrounding inflammation. (Courtesy W.B. Saunders & Co.)

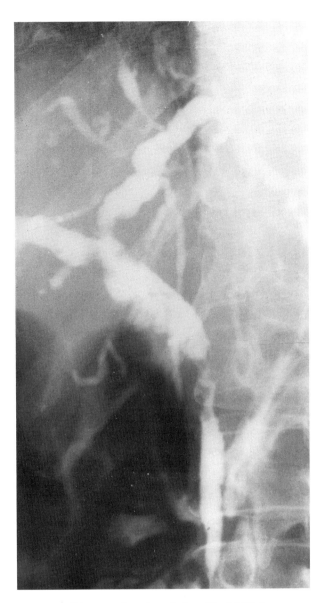

Fig. 19.32 Primary sclerosing cholangitis. Multiple irregular strictures of both extrahepatic and intrahepatic ducts.

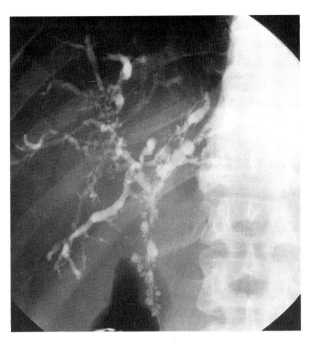

Fig. 19.33 Primary sclerosing cholangitis. Diffuse stricturing of the whole of the biliary system with a beaded configuration and prominent sacculations of the extrahepatic ducts. Note the absence of any duct dilatation.

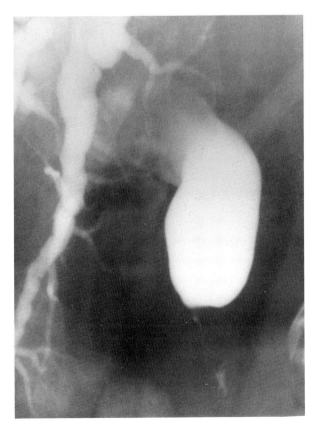

Fig. 19.34 Carcinoma of the head of the pancreas causing abrupt and virtually total common duct obstruction with a typical rounded configuration.

if jaundice is relieved. About one-quarter of cases have an association with gall stones, and the incidence of bile duct carcinoma is about 10 times more frequent in patients with ulcerative colitis than in the general population (Ritchie *et al.*, 1974).

Metastasis. Obstruction by metastatic nodes, usually from a gastrointestinal primary, typically causes high duct obstruction in the region of the porta hepatis (Fig. 19.41). PTC will determine the extent of intrahepatic spread and assist in the planning of any drainage procedure. It is essential therefore to demonstrate whether the right and

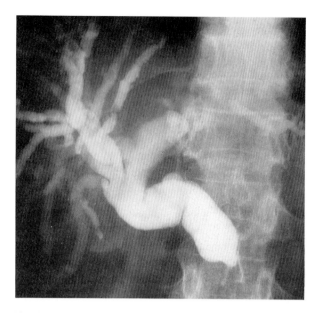

Fig. 19.35 Carcinoma of the head of the pancreas. Low common duct obstruction with marked medial displacement.

left hepatic ducts are in communication or separately obstructed (Fig. 19.42). Nodal deposits of lymphoma may also produce high duct obstruction (Fig. 19.43), which may respond dramatically to successful chemotherapy. As mentioned previously, total obstruction to the retrograde flow of contrast at ERC, assuming adequate cannulation, is almost invariably due to neoplasm, whether primary or metastatic, rather than stone.

Radiology plays an important role not only in the diagnosis of neoplastic bile duct obstruction but also in the assessment of the resectability of tumours or in the planning of palliative drainage procedures. Cholangiography will determine whether or not there is sufficient common duct above an obstruction for a bypass operation or whether the gall bladder is available, and in this

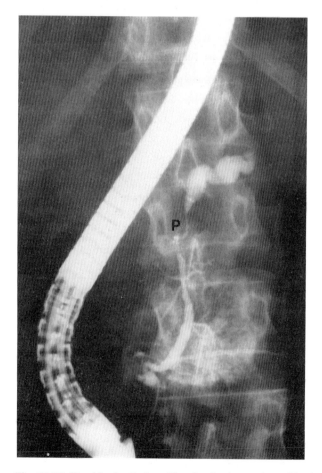

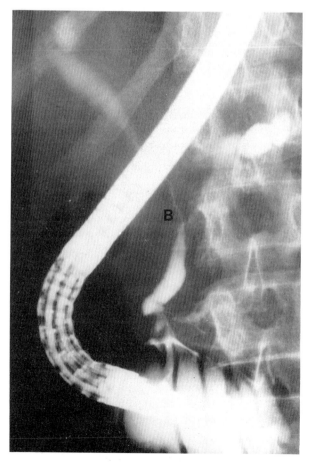

Fig. 19.36 'Double duct' sign. Neoplastic obstruction of both pancreatic (P) and bile (B) ducts at the same site.

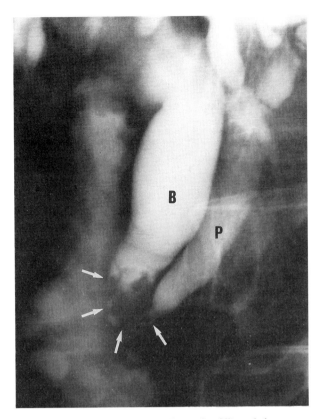

Fig. 19.37 Ampullary tumour. Irregular filling defect (*arrows*) at the ampulla causing obstruction of both bile (B) and pancreatic (P) ducts. (Courtesy of Churchill Livingstone.)

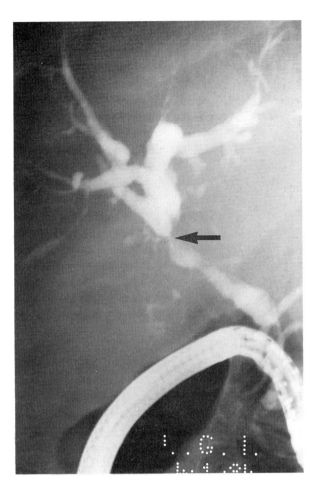

Fig. 19.38 Cholangiocarcinoma. High common duct stricture (*arrow*).

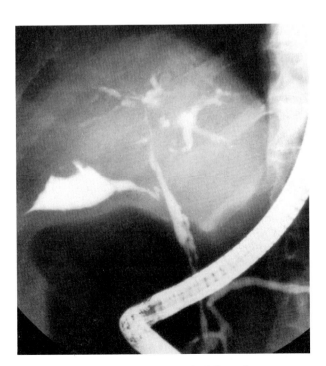

Fig. 19.39 Cholangiocarcinoma with diffuse duct involvement.

respect PTC usually provides more useful information than ERC. More and more palliative biliary drainage procedures are now performed endoscopically or trans-hepatically rather than surgically and direct cholangiography is an essential preliminary to these procedures. Ultrasound, CT, angiography, and possibly MRI all contribute to the assessment of tumour extent and resectability.

Intrahepatic lesions

Diffuse abnormalities of the intrahepatic ducts may be seen in a number of conditions. The cholangiographic appearances are frequently non-specific and the diagnosis will be made by other means, including biopsy.

Liver swelling due to oedema, fatty infiltration, or amyloid produces a generalized separation and attenuation of duct branches (Fig. 19.44).

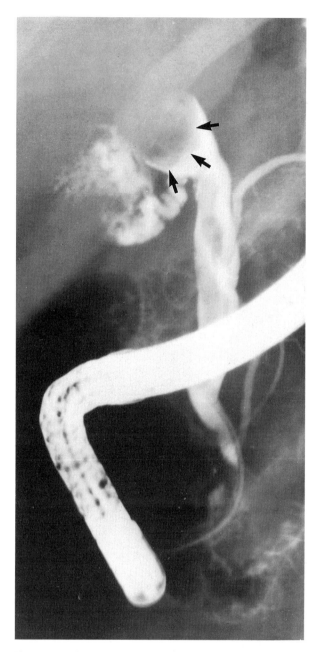

Fig. 19.40 Cholangiocarcinoma in the form of an intraluminal filling defect (*arrows*). Blood clots are present in the common duct below.

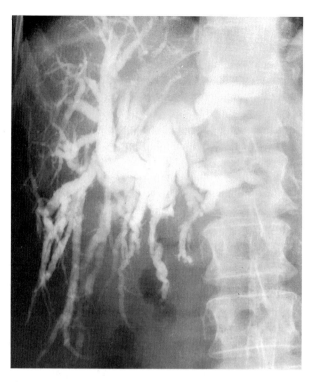

Fig. 19.41 Obstruction at the porta hepatis due to metastatic nodes causing gross intrahepatic duct dilatation.

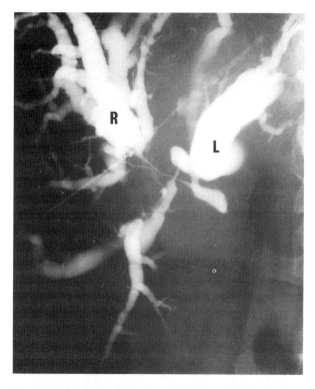

Fig. 19.42 Separate obstruction of right and left hepatic ducts due to metastatic deposits in the porta hepatis. (Courtesy W.B. Saunders & Co.)

Parenchymal liver disease may produce diffuse calibre irregularities (Fig. 19.45) and in advanced cirrhosis there is obvious shrinkage of the liver, with contraction and crowding of ducts (Fig. 19.46). In primary biliary cirrhosis a localized notch indenting the common hepatic ducts is seen in over 50% of cases (Fig. 19.47) (Hamilton *et al.*, 1983) and is considered to be due to lymph-node enlargement. A normal intrahepatic cholangiogram does not, however, exclude parenchymal

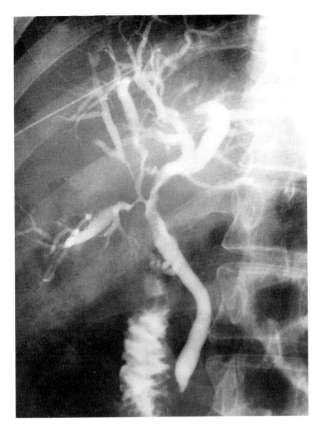

Fig. 19.43 Hodgkin's lymphoma with multiple duct encasement at the porta hepatis.

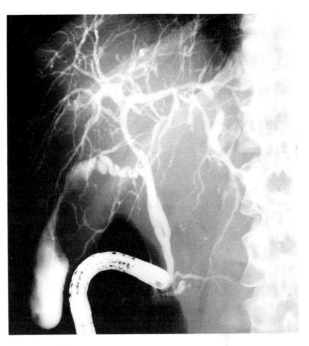

Fig. 19.45 Parenchymal liver disease (chronic active hepatitis) with diffuse minor calibre irregularities of intrahepatic branches.

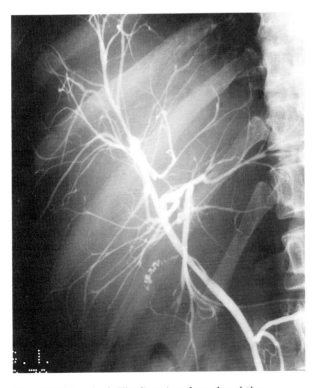

Fig. 19.44 Amyloid. The liver is enlarged and the intrahepatic branches are stretched and separated.

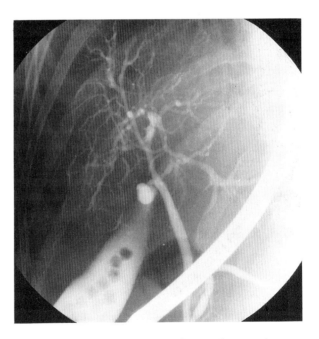

Fig. 19.46 Advanced cirrhosis with irregularity and crowding of intrahepatic ducts. Note gall bladder stones.

liver disease as one may be seen in patients with an abnormal liver biopsy.

The intrahepatic cholangiogram in metastatic liver disease will depend upon the size, number,

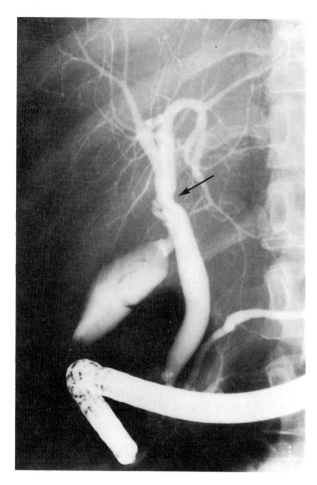

Fig. 19.47 Primary biliary cirrhosis. The intrahepatic cholangiogram is normal but there is a localized notch (*arrow*) indenting the common hepatic duct and thought to be due to lymph node enlargement.

and position of deposits (Fig. 19.48). Diffuse cholangiocarcinoma may also cause widespread intrahepatic duct abnormalities (see Fig. 19.39).

A wide spectrum of intrahepatic duct abnormalities may be seen in primary sclerosing cholangitis and in most cases the extrahepatic ducts are also abnormal (see Figs 19.32, 19.33). Secondary sclerosing cholangitis consequent upon chronic obstruction by stones or stricture, often with associated infection, can produce similar appearances, and in acute septic cholangitis multiple abscesses may be seen (Fig. 19.49). In the assessment of the intrahepatic cholangiogram it may be impossible, on radiological grounds alone, to distinguish confidently between diffuse malignancy, sclerosing cholangitis, and advanced cirrhosis. Also it is essential to guard against misinterpretation of artefactual appearances resulting from underfilling of the duct system (Fig. 19.50).

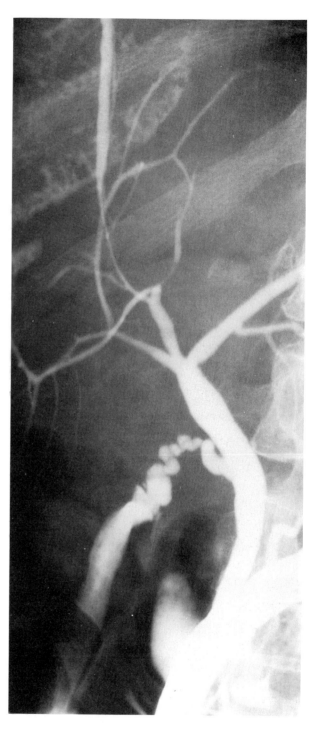

Fig. 19.48 Metastatic liver disease causing irregular narrowing and displacement of intrahepatic branches.

Localized intrahepatic lesions such as tumour, cyst, and absess will produce a mass defect with or without duct obstruction, according to their size and position and are dealt with in detail elsewhere.

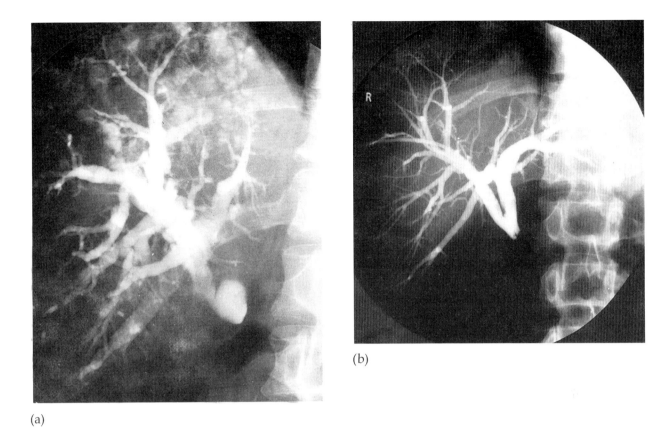

(b)

(a)

Fig. 19.49 Acute suppurative cholangitis in a patient with neoplastic common duct obstruction. (a) The intrahepatic ducts are dilated and numerous small abscess cavities are present. (b) One week after emergency external drainage, all of the abscesses have disappeared.

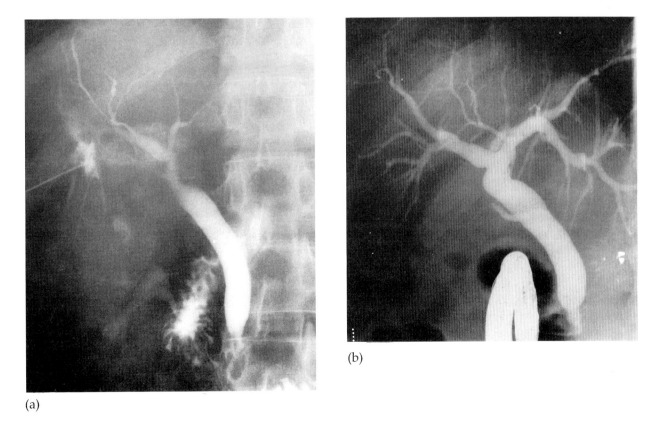

(b)

(a)

Fig. 19.50 (a) PTC. Underfilling of intrahepatic branches suggests the possibility of widespread infiltration. (b) ERC. Complete opacification demonstrates a normal intrahepatic cholangiogram.

References

Anderson, J.B., Cooper, M.J. & Williamson, R.C.N. (1985) Adenocarcinoma of the extrahepatic biliary tree. *Annals of the Royal College of Surgeons of England*, **67**, 139–143.

Ariyama, J. (1983) Percutaneous transhepatic cholangiography. In Margulis, A.R. & Burhenne, H.J. (eds) *Alimentary Tract Radiology*, pp. 2229–2241. C.V. Mosby, St Louis.

Belsito, A.A., Marta, J.B., Cramer, G.G. & Dickinson, P.B. (1977) Measurement of biliary tract size and drainage time. *Radiology*, **122**, 65–69.

Bhathal, P.S. & Powell, L.W. (1969) Primary intrahepatic obliterating cholangitis, a possible variant of 'sclerosing cholangitis'. *Gut*, **10**, 886–893.

Bilbao, M.K., Dotter, C.T., Lee, T.G. & Katon, R.M. (1976) Complications of endoscopic retrograde cholangio-pancreatography (ERCP). A study of 10,000 cases. *Gastroenterology*, **70**, 314–320.

Carter, F.R. & Saypol, G.M. (1952) Transabdominal cholangiography. *Journal of the American Medical Association*, **148**, 253–255.

Chapman, M., Curry, R.C. & Le Quesne, L.P. (1964) Operative cholangiography. An amendment of its reliability in the diagnosis of a normal, stone-free common bile duct. *British Journal of Surgery*, **51**, 600–601.

Chapman, R.W.G., Arborgh, B.A.M., Rhodes, J.M., Summerfield, J.A., Dick, R., Scheuer, P.J. & Sherlock, S. (1980) Primary sclerosing cholangitis: a review of its clinical features, cholangiography and hepatic histology. *Gut*, **21**, 870–877.

Cotton, P.B. (1977) Progress report ERCP. *Gut*, **18**, 316–341.

Gibson, R.N., Yeung, E., Thompson, J.N. *et al.* (1986) Bile duct obstruction: Radiologic evaluation of level, cause and tumor resectability. *Radiology*, **160**, 43–47.

Goldberg, H.I., Bilbao, M.K., Stewart, E.T., Rohrmann, C.A. & Moss, A.A. (1976) Endoscopic retrograde cholangio-pancreatography (ERCP): Radiographic technique. *American Journal of Digestive Diseases*, **21**, 270–278.

Hamilton, I., Lintott, D.J., Ruddell, W.S.J. & Axon, A.T.R. (1983) The endoscopic retrograde cholangiogram and pancreatogram in chronic liver disease. *Clinical Radiology*, **34**, 417–422.

Hamilton, I., Ruddell, W.S.J., Mitchell, C.J., Lintott, D.J. & Axon, A.T.R. (1982) Endoscopic retrograde cholangiograms of the normal and post-cholecystectomy biliary tree. *British Journal of Surgery*, **69**, 343–345.

Harbin, W.P., Mueller, P.R. & Ferrucci, J.T. (1980) Transhepatic cholangiography: complications and use-patterns of the fine needle technique. *Radiology*, **135**, 15–22.

Huard, P. & Do-Xuan-Hop (1937) La ponction transhepatique des canaux biliares. *Bulletin de la Societe Medico-Chirugicale de l'Indochine*, **62**, 1090–1100.

Jaques, P.F., Mauro, M.A. & Scatliff, J.H. (1980) The failed transhepatic cholangiogram. *Radiology*, **134**, 33–35.

Krieger, J., Seaman, W.B. & Porter, M.R. (1970) The roentgenologic appearance of sclerosing cholangitis. *Radiology*, **95**, 369–375.

Leger, L., Zara, M. & Arvay, N. (1952) Cholangiographie et drainage biliaire per ponction transhepatique. *Presse Medicale*, **60**, 936–937.

Le Quesne, L.P. (1960) Discussion on cholangiography. *Proceedings of the Royal Society of Medicine*, **52**, 852–855.

Le Quesne, L.P., Whiteside, C.G. & Hand, B.H. (1959) The common bile duct after cholecystectomy. *British Medical Journal*, **1**, 329–332.

Lintott, D.J., Ruddell, W.S.J. & Axon, A.T.R. (1981) Pseudo-stone at ERCP due to juxtapapillary diverticulum. *Clinical Radiology*, **32**, 173–176.

Love, R.J. McN. (1952) Modern trends in biliary surgery. *British Journal of Surgery*, **40**, 214–222.

MacCarty, R.L., LaRusso, N.F., Wiesner, R.H. & Ludwig, J. (1983) Primary sclerosing cholangitis: findings on cholangiography and pancreatography. *Radiology*, **149**, 39–44.

McCune, W.S., Shorb, P.E. & Moscovitz, H. (1968) Endoscopic cannulation of the ampulla of Vater. *Annals of Surgery*, **167**, 752–755.

Mirizzi, P.L. (1937) Operative cholangiography. *Surgery, Gynecology and Obstetrics*, **65**, 702–710.

Mirizzi, P.L. (1948) Sindrome del conducto hepatico. *Journal International Chirurgurie*, **8**, 731–777.

Mueller, P.R., Ferrucci, J.T., Simeone, J.F., Van Sonnenberg, E., Hall, D.A. & Wittenberg, J. (1982) Observations on the distensibility of the common bile duct. *Radiology*, **142**, 467–472.

Muhletaler, C.A., Gerlock, A.J., Fleischer, A.C. & James, A.E. (1980) Diagnosis of obstructive jaundice with non-dilated bile ducts. *American Journal of Roentgenology*, **134**, 1149–1152.

Nichols, D.A., MacCarty, R.L. & Gaffey, T.A. (1983) Cholangiographic evaluation of bile duct carcinoma. *American Journal of Roentgenology*, **141**, 1291–1294.

Okuda, K., Tanikawa, K., Emura, T. *et al.* (1974) Nonsurgical percutaneous transhepatic cholangiography — diagnostic significance in medical problems of the liver. *American Journal of Digestive Diseases*, **19**, 21–36.

Oi, I., Takemoto, T. & Kondo, T. (1969) Fiberduodenoscope direct observations of the papilla of Vater. *Endoscopy*, **1**, 101–103.

Plumley, T.F., Rohrmann, C.A., Freeny, P.C., Silverstein, F.E. & Ball, T.J. (1982) Double duct sign: reassured significance in E.R.C.P. *American Journal of Roentgenology*, **139**, 31–35.

Ritchie, J.K., Allan, R.N., Macartney, J., Thompson, H., Hawley, P.R. & Cooke, W.T. (1974) Biliary tract carcinoma associated with ulcerative colitis. *Quarterly Journal of Medicine*, **43**, 263–279.

Sarles, H. & Sahel, J. (1978) Progress report: cholestasis and lesions of the biliary tract in chronic pancreatitis. *Gut*, **19**, 851–857.

Sauerbrei, E.E., Cooperberg, P.L., Gordon, P., LI, D., Cohen, M.M. & Burhenne, H.J. (1980) The discrepancy between radiographic and sonographic bile duct measurements. *Radiology*, **137**, 751–755.

Scott, A.J. (1971) Bacteria and disease of the biliary tract. *Gut*, **12**, 487–492.

Thorpe, M.E.C., Scheuer, P.J. & Sherlock, S. (1967) Primary sclerosing cholangitis, the biliary tree and ulcerative colitis. *Gut*, **8**, 435–448.

Tsuchiya, Y. (1969) A new safe method of percutaneous transhepatic cholangiography. *Japanese Journal of Gastroenterology*, **66**, 438–455.

Warren, K.W., Athanassiades, S. & Monge, J.I. (1966) Primary sclerosing cholangitis. A study of 42 cases. *American Journal of Surgery*, **111**, 23–38.

20: Diseases of the Gall Bladder

A.E.A. JOSEPH AND A. GRUNDY

Gall stones

At least 25% of women and 20% of men will form gall stones during their lives. In the UK 122 gall bladders per 100 000 population are removed every year (Harding Rains, 1981). There may be an increased incidence of gall stones in patients taking oral contraceptives and the latter may also accelerate the development of gall bladder disease (Boston Collaborative Drug Surveillance Program, 1973, Royal College of General Practitioners, 1982).

Gall stones are formed from constituents of bile. In western communities about 10% of gall stones are composed purely of cholesterol and 80% of the remainder contain at least 70% cholesterol (Bouchier, 1976). Pure pigment stones are associated with haemolytic disorders. Most gall stones have a crystalline structure and are formed in the gall bladder. Crystalline stones found in the common bile duct probably originate from the gall bladder. Primary bile duct stones are more likely to be concretions of precipitated pigment and cholesterol. At least two factors are responsible for stone formation: increased secretion of biliary cholesterol, and a reduced secretion of bile acids in bile, associated with a smaller than normal bile acid pool (Bouchier, 1976). Reduction of bile acid content below a critical level will cause cholesterol to precipitate out of solution. This defect can be related to impaired production of bile acids from the liver, local conditions in the gall bladder and a defect in the enterohepatic circulation. Stasis in the gall bladder, particularly in the presence of infection, is followed by a fall in the bile pH allowing precipitation of cholesterol. Faceting of gall stones is due to unequal growth of crystals subsequent to pressure from adjacent stones. Stones may fracture spontaneously and fissures may form containing air, the Mercedes—Benz sign (Fig. 20.1).

The clinical features of gall stones depend on whether they remain in the gall bladder silently or whether they promote inflammation or move out of the gall bladder. Silent stones by definition are those found incidentally, but within 5 years of the finding of incidental stones, half the patients will have had symptoms due to stone migration (Harding Rains, 1981). Flatulent dyspepsia, nausea and abdominal distension are often associated with the presence of gall stones. Improvement in

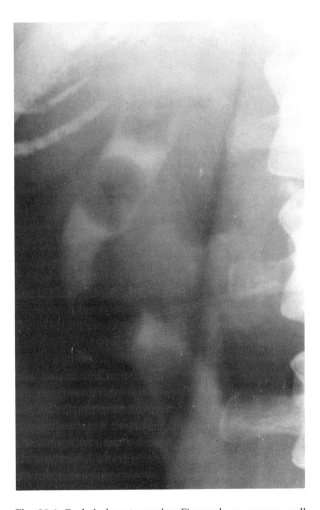

Fig. 20.1 Oral cholecystography. Fissured non-opaque gall stones containing air: 'Mercedes-Benz' sign.

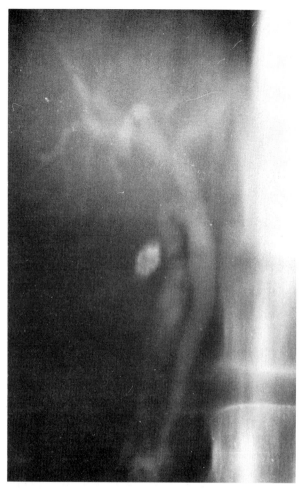

Fig. 20.2 Intravenous cholangiography. Calcific calculus impacted in the cystic duct with non-filling of the gall bladder.

patients' symptoms following cholecystectomy occurs in only 70% of patients (Johnson, 1975).

Movement of stones into the cystic duct or their impaction in the neck of the gall bladder will result in biliary colic that may last several hours. An attack of biliary colic may be followed by complete resolution, subsequent attacks of colic, or chronic cholecystitis. An impacted stone in the neck of the gall bladder will produce non-filling of the gall bladder on oral cholecystography or i.v. cholangiography (Fig. 20.2).

Most cases of acute cholecystitis are associated with stones. Gangrene and perforation of the gall bladder are more likely to occur when the infecting organism is *Clostridium welchii* or Klebsiella. The oedematous gall bladder is manifest by pain, pyrexia, and local tenderness and rigidity. In emphysematous cholecystitis, air may be visible on plain films within the gall bladder wall and within the gall bladder lumen and the bile ducts (Fig. 20.3). If the gall bladder is not removed in the acute situation the inflammatory reaction settles with the development of dense fibrosis, beginning within 10−20 days and taking up to 3 months to resolve, with the formation of adhesions to surrounding omentum, duodenum, and colon. Chronic cholecystitis resulting in adhesions between the gall bladder and duodenum or small bowel may be associated with erosion of a stone through the gut lumen and subsequent gall stone ileus.

Acute and chronic cholecystitis may in-

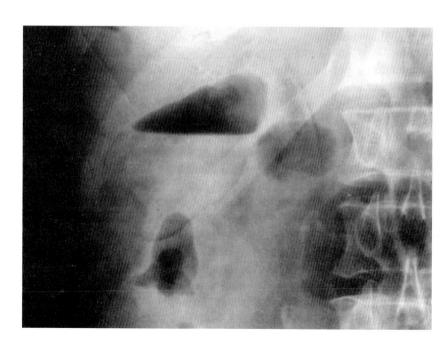

Fig. 20.3 Emphysematous cholecystitis. Air in the wall of the gall bladder and an air−fluid level within the gall bladder lumen. (Courtesy of Dr C.J. Dow, St. George's Hospital, London.)

frequently occur in the absence of calculi. Infecting organisms may reach the gall bladder via lymphatics from the colon, or via the blood stream from a distant focus.

Gall stones are readily demonstrated at oral cholecystography as filling defects within the contrast-filled viscus. They may be single or multiple and vary considerably in size. Typically gall stones are free to move about within the gall bladder and either float within the contrast (Fig. 20.4) or collect in the dependent part of the gall bladder (Fig. 20.5). The free mobility of gall stones differentiates them from fixed mural lesion such as excrescences of cholesterolosis or polyps.

In many centres an ultrasound examination has become the investigation of choice for the detection of gall stones. Several studies have established the sensitivity and specificity of ultrasound in the detection of gall stones (Crade *et al.*, 1978, Krook *et al.*, 1980, McIntosh & Penny, 1980). Calculi are recognized as echogenic structures within the gall bladder that change with position and show posterior shadowing. Posterior shadowing may not be a feature with all gall stones, the most common cause for this being the width of the beam in relation to the size of the calculus (Filly *et al.*, 1979). At the present time, no definite features can be attributed to the different gall stones to predict with any accuracy the composition of the calculi.

The gall bladder may be full of calculi and no bile-filled lumen may be recognized (Fig. 20.6). In this instance, an echogenic reflective layer is provided by the calculi packed within the gall bladder.

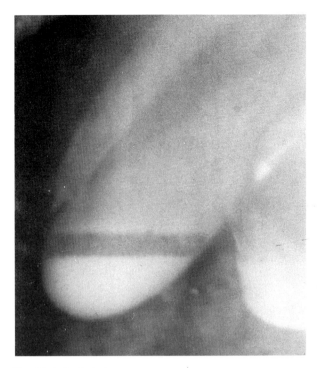

Fig. 20.4 Oral cholecystography. 'Floating' non-opaque calculi.

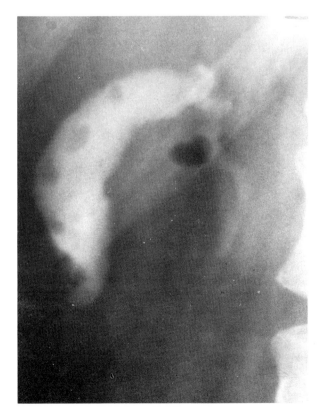

Fig. 20.5 Oral cholecystography. Prone oblique view. Multiple non-opaque calculi collecting in dependent part of the gall bladder.

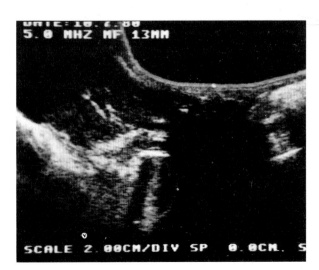

Fig. 20.6 Gall bladder full of calculi with posterior shadowing.

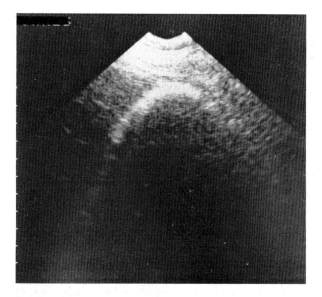

Fig. 20.7 Faecal-loaded hepatic flexure resembling a gall bladder full of calculi.

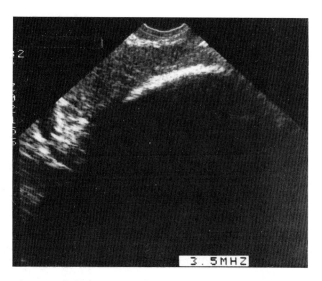

Fig. 20.8 Calcification in the wall of the gall bladder.

The acoustic shadow produced usually has clearly defined margins. The pitfall to be avoided, however, is not to misinterpret a loaded colon, which may closely mimic a gall bladder full of calculi (Fig. 20.7). Sometimes a thin layer of bile may be seen between the wall of the gall bladder and calculi. Calcification in the wall of the gall bladder may also mimic calculi (Fig. 20.8).

Ultrasound in acute and chronic cholecystitis

On ultrasound the wall of the gall bladder rarely exceeds 2 mm in thickness. In both acute and chronic cholecystitis, the wall may be thickened, but in acute cholecystitis a double-wall sign is frequently encountered (Fig. 20.9). Very occasionally a double wall may be encountered in chronic cholecystitis with marked hypertrophy of the muscular and fibrous layers (Joseph, 1983). Although initially the double-wall sign was thought to be highly diagnostic of acute cholecystitis, this sign may be seen in several conditions unrelated to intrinsic gall bladder disease. These include normal physiologically contracted gall bladder (Fig. 20.10), heart failure, renal disease, alcoholic liver disease, hepatitis, pericardial effusion, and infiltrative disorders such as multiple myeloma. Taken in the proper clinical context, however, the double-wall sign is extremely reliable. In 76 patients in whom a diagnosis of acute cholecystitis was made on ultrasound in our unit,

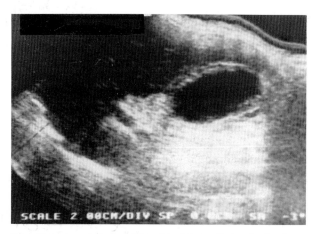

Fig. 20.9 Acute cholecystitis. Double-wall sign is clearly seen.

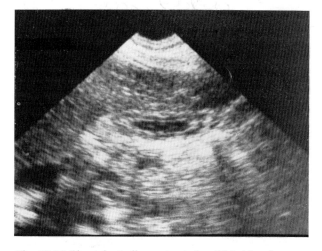

Fig. 20.10 Physiologically contracted gall bladder. Inner mucosal layer is smooth and continuous. The contracted muscular layer shows as an echo poor region giving rise to the double-wall effects. This is most obvious when a normally large bladder undergoes contraction.

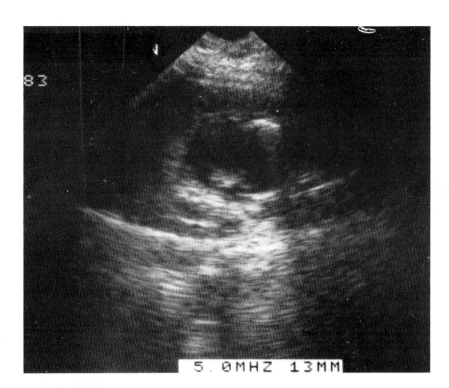

Fig. 20.11 Emphysematous cholecystitis showing focal increase in echogenicity in the wall, with reverberation echoes. Air may be seen more extensively in the wall and air may also be seen within the lumen in some cases.

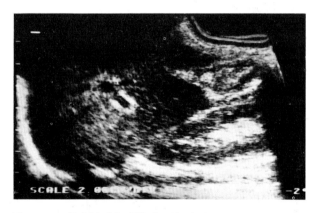

Fig. 20.12 Gall bladder filled with sludge.

this was confirmed at surgery with no false positives. One hundred per cent specificity has also been reported (Worthen *et al.*, 1981).

Although acute gangrenous cholecystitis is often associated with more severe clinical symptoms, when a discontinuous inner echogenic layer is observed in the presence of a double-wall sign, sloughing of the mucosal layer and a possible associated gangrenous cholecystitis should be considered. It is also worth noting that severe acute gangrenous cholecystitis may exist with minimal or no thickening of the gall bladder wall. A normal thickness gall bladder wall excludes neither acute nor chronic cholecystitis, since early

or mild forms may go unrecognized on ultrasound. Emphysematous cholecystitis is recognized on ultrasound by the production of classic reverberation echoes produced by gas (Fig. 20.11) (Blaquiere & Dewbury, 1982).

In addition to calculi, echogenic bile may be demonstrated in the gall bladder. Precipitated bile salts, cholesterol, and bile pigments are often layered out in the dependent portion of the gall bladder. Occasionally the gall bladder may be completely filled with echogenic bile (Fig. 20.12). The presence of echogenic bile or 'sludge' does not necessarily imply acute cholecystitis. Several other conditions that give rise to altered bile chemistry such as hepatitis and prolonged fasting may show this feature. Blood in the gall bladder could mimic sludge in the gall bladder (Fig. 20.13). Pus within the gall bladder may also layer out, simulating echogenic bile. Pericholecystic collections may be readily identified and occasionally perforation of the wall may also be seen. (Fig. 20.14).

Chronic cholecystitis with early changes may also show mild thickening of the gall bladder wall. As the condition progresses the wall may get thicker and the gall bladder become shrunken with the contraction of fibrous tissue. Gall stones are invariably seen. Occasionally small reverberation echoes may be seen arising from the wall of the gall bladder and probably have the same

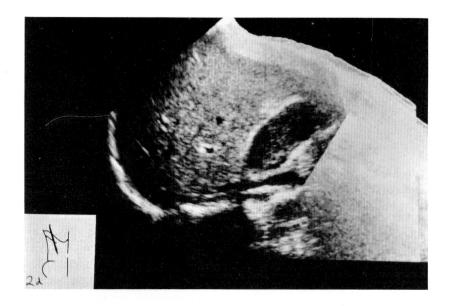

Fig. 20.13 Blood in the gall bladder in a patient with haemobilia following trauma. (Courtesy Dr K.C. Dewbury.)

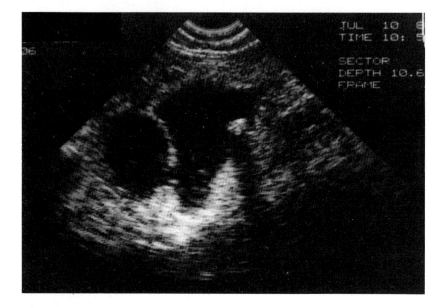

Fig. 20.14 Acute cholecystitis with pericholecystic collection, and perforation in the wall clearly visible. A calculus and sludge is noted. (Courtesy of Dr C.J. Dow.)

aetiology as the reverberation echoes seen in adeno-myomatosis. A double-wall appearance may also be seen due to marked hypertrophy of the muscular or fibrous tissue (Fig. 20.15). Marked thickening of the gall bladder wall may also be seen in patients with cystic fibrosis (Fig. 20.16).

Hepatobiliary scintigraphy may also be used in conjunction with an ultrasound examination for the diagnosis of acute cholecystitis. In most cases ultrasound examination is sufficient but if there is doubt, the demonstration of gall bladder filling by a scintigraphic agent will confirm that the cystic duct is patent and a diagnosis of acute cholecystitis would be unlikely. The failure of the gall bladder to fill, in the right clinical context, and a suggestive

ultrasound, would favour a diagnosis of acute cholecystitis (Fig. 20.17).

As part of the investigation of diarrhoea and pyrexia of unknown origin, we have seen a positive scan in a patient with bacterial cholecystitis due to Salmonella demonstrated by [111]Indium-labelled white cells. This was confirmed surgically, histologically, and bacteriologically.

Empyema of the gall bladder

In empyema of the gall bladder, the wall is thickened and the organ contains varying amounts of pus. At oral cholecystography or i.v. cholangiography, the gall bladder does not fill.

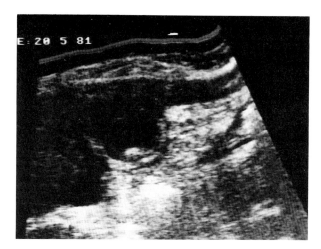

Fig. 20.15 Chronic cholecystitis with a thickened gall bladder wall. A double-wall sign is seen due to the markedly hypertrophied muscular and fibrous tissue.

Pus when present within the gall bladder may layer out, as does the material precipitated from bile. Pus often coexists with the precipitated material and on ultrasound two echogenic layers, one representing pus and the other the precipitated material, may sometimes be recognized. Experimentally, when pus is mixed with bile the layering phenomenon may be demonstrated (Joseph, 1983) (Fig. 20.18).

The relatively straight line interface may be associated with pus or sludge, but a wavy or mound-like appearance suggests sludge rather than pus. Rate of settling is not helpful in distinguishing sludge from pus, since this would depend on the viscosity of the bile within the gall bladder.

Limey bile and mucocele of the gall bladder

In this condition the gall bladder is filled with a cream of calcium carbonate caused by a change in the chemical constituents of bile. Calcium may also be deposited in the wall of the organ, producing the porcelain gall bladder. This is usually associated with stasis and partial obstruction of the cystic duct.

Obstruction of the cystic duct by a stone in the absence of infection may result in resorption of bile pigment from the remaining bile, and production of a large quantity of mucus. This causes distension and elongation of the gall bladder.

A few patients have symptoms of gall bladder disease and whose gall bladder is shown histologically to be abnormal, but who have normal contrast and ultrasound studies and who may be cured of their symptoms by cholecystectomy (Gough, 1977).

Hyperplastic cholecystoses

Jutras introduced the term hyperplastic cholecystoses for a group of conditions of the gall bladder separate from acute and chronic inflammatory states (Jutras *et al.*, 1960). The two major conditions are cholesterolosis and adenomyomatosis. Although grouped together, these conditions are

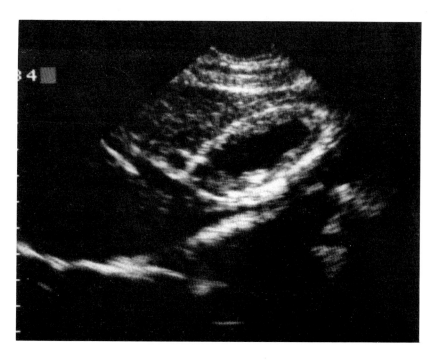

Fig. 20.16 Gall bladder in a patient with cystic fibrosis, showing marked thickening of the wall.

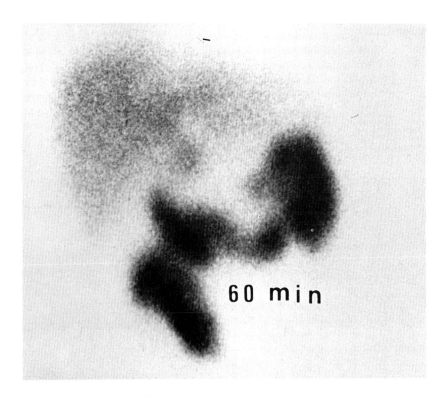

Fig. 20.17 ^{99m}Technetium HIDA scan showing failure of the gall bladder to fill, with good flow into the small bowel.

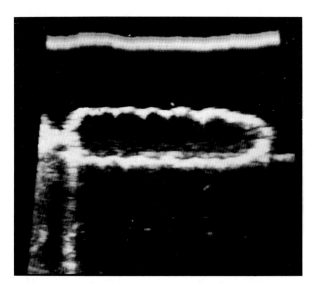

Fig. 20.18 Pus layering out with bile within a finger-stall.

distinct entities with different pathological and radiological appearances. Cholesterolosis is characterized by the deposition of various lipids in the wall of the gall bladder; adenomyomatosis is characterized by hyperplasia of the elements of the gall bladder wall. From a clinical point of view both these conditions may produce characteristic gall bladder symptoms of abdominal pain and dyspepsia and fatty intolerance in the absence

of gall stones. They do not produce a clearly recognizable clinical syndrome which can be differentiated from chronic cholecystitis and cholelithiasis. There are many patients in which these conditions are found coincidentally and who are asymptomatic.

Cholesterolosis

Cholesterolosis or 'strawberry gall bladder' is characterized by the deposition of lipids within macrophages in the lamina propria and epithelium of the gall bladder. The accumulation of lipids, mainly triglyceride, cholesterol or cholesterol precursors or cholesterol esters, produces excrescences on the surface of the gall bladder mucosa. With hyperaemia of the mucosa the appearances resemble a ripe strawberry. The abnormality is usually confined to the gall bladder. In about two-thirds of cases the excrescences are about 1 mm in diameter, giving the mucosa a uniformly coarse granular appearance. Larger, more discrete excrescences occur in the remainder and appear as polypoid masses (Berk *et al.*, 1983). Polypoid excrescences, unlike true adenomas, contain no glandular tissue or other stromal elements. These may occasionally break off and form a nidus for stone formation (Berk *et al.*, 1983). The cause of the lipid accumulation is unknown but the cholesterol is assumed to originate in the bile. Abnormal bile may be the cause of cholesterolosis or there may be abnormal excessive reabsorption of cholesterol through the gall bladder mucosa. There is no relationship between cholesterolosis and obesity, serum lipid levels, supersaturation of cholesterol in bile, or cholesterol gall stones. Stones are found in about 10–15% of patients with cholesterolosis. The majority of cases of cholesterolosis are of the diffuse variety which are not sufficiently prominent to be visible on oral cholecystography. Radiological diagnosis is only possible in a small number of cases. Polypoid excrescences may be detected particularly on post-fatty meal or compression filming (Fig. 20.19). Multiple filling defects, irregularity in size and uneveness in distribution, and fixity to the gall bladder wall form the basis of radiological diagnosis. Cholesterolosis

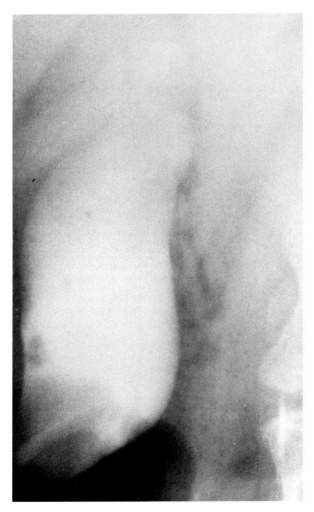

Fig. 20.19 Oral cholecystography. Solitary polypoid excrescence attached to the gall bladder wall: cholesterol polyp.

can nearly always be differentiated from cholelithiasis by determining that the radiolucent filling defects are fixed to the wall on radiographs obtained in different positions, whereas gall stones are usually free to move about and collect in the dependent part of the organ or float within the bile. Fixed filling defects in the gall bladder wall other than those due to cholesterolosis are uncommon.

Ultrasound findings are those of small echogenic masses attached to the wall of the gall bladder. These do not cast shadows and may appear to be finger-like rather than sessile masses. They may be indistinguishable from other polypoid structures arising from the gall bladder.

Adenomyomatosis

Adenomyomatosis is an abnormality of the gall bladder characterized by hyperplastic changes with overgrowth of the mucosa and thickening of the muscle wall. Intramural diverticula (Rokitansky–Aschoff sinuses) occur when the mucosa herniates through points of least resistance in the hypertrophied muscularis propria. Adenomyomatosis may be generalized, segmental, or localized. The localized form is usually found at the fundus. In most cases adenomyomatosis is not associated with cholesterolosis and there is no evidence of inflammatory change or neoplasia. In the early phase the intramural extension of the epithelium creates tubules and crypts which may be mistaken for true glandular structures. The muscle layer is up to three times the normal thickness. The channels connecting the diverticula with the gall bladder lumen may become obstructed, giving a false impression of cysts within the wall. In the segmental form a focal circumferential band of muscular hypertrophy divides the gall bladder into communicating compartments (compartmentalization). When confined to the fundus a nodule may be present which may be incorrectly referred to as an adenomyoma.

The aetiology of the muscular hyperplasia and formation of intramural diverticula is unknown. It has been postulated that excessive intramural pressure plays a role in its development.

The Rokitansky–Aschoff sinuses can be seen on contrast studies if they maintain their communication with the gall bladder lumen and if they are large enough to accumulate sufficient contrast medium (Fig. 20.20). Any portion of the gall bladder may be involved. The pools of contrast

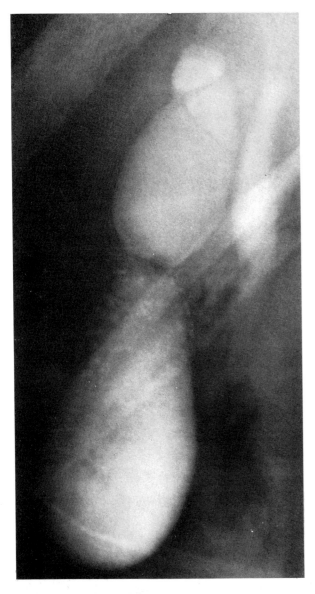

Fig. 20.20 Segmental area of adenomyomatosis in the body of the gall bladder. Small collections of contrast within Rokitansky−Aschoff sinuses, and compartmentalization of the gall bladder.

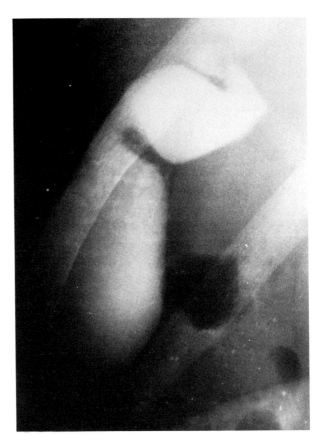

Fig. 20.21 Adenomyomatosis with a septum in the body of the gall bladder.

may be single or multiple, localized or generalized, and may vary in size from pin-point to 8−10 mm. Occasionally calcified concretions may be detected within the diverticula.

The segmental form of adenomyomatosis (Fig. 20.21) needs to be distinguished from congenital septae of the gall bladder such as the Phrygian cap. This is found at the fundus and is usually thinner and smoother than the septae associated with adenomyomatosis. As in the case with cholesterolosis, adenomyomatosis is often best demonstrated on films with the gall bladder con-

tracted. It may not be detected except on post-fatty-meal films (Gajjar *et al.*, 1984).

The localized form may show as a filling defect representing the sessile mass projecting from the wall into the lumen (Fig. 20.22). There may be central umbilication and evidence of diverticula around the base. A mound of adenomyomatosis may be stretched flat when the organ is fully distended and only evident on films following gall bladder contraction.

Ultrasound appearances may be very suggestive of adenomyomatosis. The wall of the gall bladder may be thickened and a double-wall appearance may be sometimes seen due to the muscular hypertrophy.

The segmental variety shows increased thickness of the wall and this region and other parts of the gall bladder wall may show small triangular-shaped reverberation echoes. These are probably produced by reverberations arising from the cystic spaces produced by the Rokitansky−Aschoff sinuses, or are due to the minute calculi formed within them (Raghavendra *et al.*, Fig. 20.23).

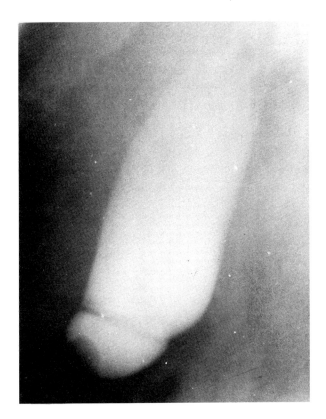

Fig. 20.22 Adenomyomatosis. Fundal adenomyoma and Phrygian cap deformity.

The localized form may be seen as an echogenic mass attached to the wall of the gall bladder in the fundus.

Tumours of the gall bladder

Benign tumours are more common than malignant tumours. Benign tumours may be found in 3% of removed gall bladders compared with carcinoma, which may be found in 1.3% of removed gall bladders (Ochsner & Ochsner, 1960).

Adenomata may occur anywhere in the gall bladder as single or multiple lesions up to 2 cm in diameter. They may be sessile or papillary. The rest of the organ may be normal or show changes of cholecystitis with or without calculi. Adenomata are potentially malignant. Adenomyomata, as found in adenomyomatosis, have been misconstrued as neoplastic. The majority of polyps seen in the gall bladder on contrast studies are cholesterol pseudopolyps, which appear as a yellow speck on the mucosa and are due to cholesterolosis.

Heterotopic tissue may also be found. Gastric tissue is the most common but pancreatic, hepatic, small intestinal, and even thyroid tissue have been reported (Curtis & Sheahan, 1969). Other benign tumours such as lipomata, leiomyomata, neurofibromata, and haemangiomata may rarely occur.

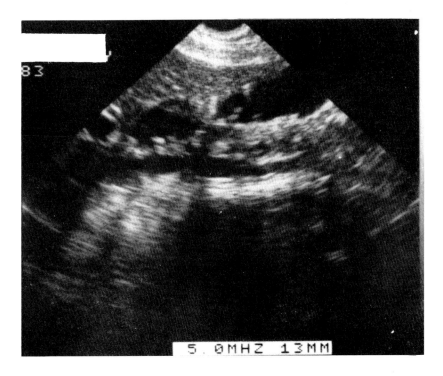

Fig. 20.23 Adenomyomatosis showing a thickened gall bladder with reverberation echoes arising from the wall.

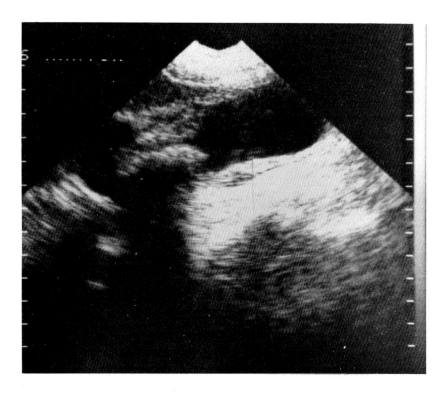

Fig. 20.24 Carcinoma of the gall bladder seen attached to the wall adjacent to a large calculus. Note heterogeneous echo pattern and non-dependent location of the mass.

Primary carcinoma of the gall bladder is a relatively rare condition with a uniformly bad prognosis. Tumours may be found incidentally at operation or as filling defects on oral cholecystography or ultrasound examination. It is a disease of the older age group and the majority of patients are women over 50 years of age. Gall stones are found in between 54 and 97% of patients with carcinoma of the gall bladder (Gazet, 1983). Adenocarcinoma accounts for 50–98% of primary carcinomata. Undifferentiated and squamous-cell carcinomata are less common. The common site is the fundus of the gall bladder. The tumours spread by local invasion of the liver and adjacent structures. Lymphatic spread occurs to nodes around the cystic duct and common bile duct, leading to pancreaticoduodenal nodes. Well-differentiated tumours tend to spread to the liver, whereas poorly differentiated tumours tend to spread by intraperitoneal seeding. There are no characteristic clinical features of gall bladder carcinoma. The mode of presentation may be with gall stones or they may present with malignant obstructive jaundice.

The ultrasound appearances are those of an echogenic mass, either partly or entirely filling the lumen of the gall bladder (Fig. 20.24). This has to be distinguished from sludge which may be raised up in mounds. Sludge is usually uniformly echogenic, whereas carcinoma has a more heterogeneous appearance and usually occupies a non-dependent position. There may be evidence of inflammation.

Occasionally a plain abdominal film may show a porcelain gall bladder, although the relationship of this to carcinoma is uncertain (Polk, 1966, Arianoff et al., 1973). Occasionally a functioning gall bladder on cholecystography may show a filling defect, but the majority of carcinomata have a non-functioning gall bladder in the absence of radio-opaque stones (Rabinov, 1966). Calcification of the gall bladder wall is readily demonstrated on ultrasound as a markedly echogenic layer. This is to be distinguished from calculi filling the gall bladder (see Fig. 20.8).

References

Arianoff, A.A., Vielle, G. & Dewulf, E. (1973) Le cancer de la vesicule. Apropos de 49 cas cholecystectomises. *Acta Gastroenterologica Belgica*, **36**, 310–331.

Berk, R.N., Van Der Vegt, J.H. & Lichtenstein, J.E. (1983) The hyperplastic cholecystoses: cholesterolosis and adenomyomatosis. *Radiology*, **146**, 593–601.

Blaquiere, R.M. & Dewbury, K.C. (1982) The ultrasound diagnosis of emphysematous cholecystitis. *British Journal of Radiology*, **55**, 114–116.

Boston Collaborative Drug Surveillance Program. (1973) Oral contraceptives and venous thromboembolic disease, confirmed gall bladder disease and breast tumours. *Lancet*, **i**, 1399—1404.

Bouchier, I.A.D. (1976) Disease of the alimentary system. Gallstones. *British Medical Journal*, **2**, 870—872.

Crade, M., Taylor, K.J.W. & Rosenfield, A.T. (1978) Surgical and pathologic correlation of cholecystosonography and cholecystography. *American Journal of Roentgenology*, **131**, 227—229.

Curtis, L.E. & Shehan, D.G. (1969) Heterotopic tissues in the gall bladder. *Archives of Pathology*, **88**, 677—683.

Filly, R.A., Morse, A.A. & Way, L.W. (1979) In vitro investigation of gall stone shadowing with ultrasound tomography. *Journal of Clinical Ultrasound*, **7**, 255—262.

Gajjar, B., Twomey, B. & DeLacey, G. (1984) The fatty meal and acalculous gall bladder disease. *Clinical Radiology*, **35**, 405—408.

Gazet, J.C. (1983) Primary carcinoma of the gall bladder. In *Carcinoma of the Liver, Biliary Tract and Pancreas*, pp. 82—103. Edward Arnold, London.

Gough, M.H. (1977) The cholecystogram is normal...but .... *British Medical Journal*, **1**, 960—962.

Harding Rains, A.J. (1981) Gall stones and cholecystitis. In Lord Smith de Sherlock, S. (eds) *Surgery of the Gall Bladder and Bile Ducts*, pp. 247—256. Butterworths, London.

Johnson, A.G. (1975) Cholecystectomy and gall stone dyspepsia. *Annals of the Royal College of Surgeons of England*, **56**, 69—80.

Joseph, A.E.A. (1983) *Clinics in Diagnostic Ultrasound: Ultrasound in Inflammatory Disease*. pp. 161—183. Churchill Livingstone, Edinburgh.

Jutras, J.A., Longtin, J.M. & Levesque, H.P. (1960) Hyperplastic cholecystoses. *American Journal of Roentgenology*, **83**, 795—827.

Krook, P.M., Allen, R.H., Bush, W.H. Jr. (1980) Comparison of real time cholecystosonography and oral cholecystography. *Radiology*, **135**, 145—148.

McIntosh, D.M.F. & Penny, H.F. (1980) Gray-scale ultrasonography as a screening procedure in the detection of gall bladder disease. *Radiology*, **136**, 725—727.

Ochsner, S.F., Ochsner, A. (1960) Benign neoplasms of the gall bladder: diagnosis and surgical implications. *Annals of Surgery*, **151**, 630—637.

Polk, H.C. (1966) Carcinoma and the calcified gall bladder. *Gastroenterology*, **50**, 582—585.

Rabinov, K. (1966). Primary carcinoma in a functioning gall bladder. *Gastroenterology*, **50**, 808—810.

Raghavendra, B.N., Subramanyam, B.R., Balthazar, E.J., Horii, S.C., Megibow, A.J. & Hilton, S. (1983) Sonography of adenomyomatosis of the gall bladder: radiologic—pathologic correlation. *Radiology*, **146**, 747—752.

Royal College of General Practitioners Oral Contraceptive Study (1982). Oral contraceptives and gall bladder disease. *Lancet*, **ii**, 957—959.

Worthen, N.J., Uszler, J.M. & Funamura, J.L. (1981) Cholecystitis: prospective evaluation of sonography and ^{99m}Tc HIDA cholescintigraphy. *American Journal of Roentgenology*, **137**, 973—978.

21: Obstructive Jaundice — A Diagnostic Approach

D.O. COSGROVE

Introduction

Jaundice, defined as an elevation of the serum bilirubin concentration above 17 μmol/l (1 mg/dl) is readily recognized clinically when the bilirubin level exceeds 60 μmol/l. It is caused by a disturbance at any point in the complex metabolic and excretory pathway of bile. A practical clinical classification is: (i) cases where the hyperbilirubinaemia is due to the liver's capacity being exceeded (overload, as in haemolysis), or impaired (hepatocellular) and (ii) cases where there is a disturbance of the removal of bile from the liver (obstructive or cholestatic). The obstructive group can be subdivided according to the level of the disturbance. It may occur at canalicular level in disorders affecting the hepatocyte surface (as in drug reactions, hepatitis and primary biliary cirrhosis), or at large-duct level due to a mechanical problem. Only this latter group is amenable to surgical correction.

The different groups are often not totally separable in clinical practice (Shenker et al., 1962); hepatitis for example often leads to transport failure at the damaged cell surface and this pattern may predominate in 'cholestatic hepatitis'. Likewise, chronic large-duct obstruction leads to hepatocellular damage with eventual secondary biliary cirrhosis. The goal of radiological investigation is to distinguish large-duct obstruction from other causes, to pin-point the site of the obstructing lesion and to determine its nature.

Causes of large-duct obstruction

The three common causes of biliary obstruction are stones, tumour, and inflammation (Schaffer & Popper, 1979). Because radiological investigation is directed to establishing the level of obstruction as well as confirming its nature, the causes can usefully be considered according to anatomical site (Fig. 21.1).

Porta. Because of the great metabolic reserve of the liver, both right and left hepatic ducts must be obstructed to cause jaundice, unless there is co-existent hepatocellular disease. Malignant conditions predominate; secondary deposits at the porta (Hardy et al., 1976), carcinoma of the gall bladder and cholangiocarcinoma of the upper biliary tree are typical examples. Strictures from inflammatory processes (sclerosing cholangitis, abscess) and surgical damage are occasional causes as are high-lying choledochal cysts. Gall stones rarely occur in the common hepatic duct except after cholecystectomy and in persistent infective oriental cholangitis.

Retroduodenal portion. This is the least common level for obstruction, pathological processes intrinsic to the biliary tree predominating. Typical causes are stricture due to surgery or instrumentation, chronic inflammation in sclerosing cholangitis, and cholangiocarcinoma.

Pancreatic. This is the commonest site, with the causes divided between tumour and impacted gall stones. The latter often produce an inflammatory mass which may dominate the radiological findings. Adenocarcinoma of the head of pancreas is the commonest tumour, with a predeliction for the over 50s, while ampullary adenocarcinoma has a peak incidence in the 6th decade. Other obstructing conditions include non-stone pancreatitis (traumatic, focal from penetrating peptic ulcers, annular pancreas), choledochocoele, cholangiocarcinoma, and rarely duodenal lesions (diverticula, tumours). Even rarer causes are foreign bodies such as ascaris worms, shed hydatid cysts, and blood clot.

Radiological techniques

The plain film may demonstrate the 10% of gall stones that are calcified, but is not of great help in

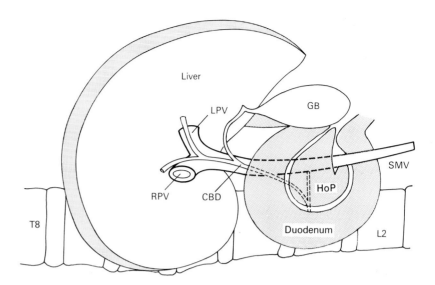

Fig. 21.1 The biliary tree. The biliary tree is viewed from the right with the right lobe of the liver largely removed. Obstruction to its three portions, supraduodenal, retroduodenal and intrapancreatic, is caused predominantly by different pathologies and with different frequencies. CBD = common bile duct; GB = gall bladder; HoP = head of pancreas; LPV = left portal vein; RPV = right portal vein; SMV = superior mesenteric vein. (Modified from Mueller, 1981 & Schneck, 1983.)

practice since this finding may be misleading, gall stones being a common incidental problem especially in the elderly. Stones in the common bile duct are very difficult to discern.

The intravenous cholangiogram (IVC), a somewhat fraught investigation even under ideal conditions (Ansell, 1970), relies on liver excretion of contrast (iodipamide) which is competitively inhibited by bilirubin. Therefore, excretion and duct visualization fail progressively with increasing jaundice, and the test is rarely useful at serum bilirubin levels above 80 μmol/l. Accuracy is unimpressive (Koenigsberg *et al.*, 1979). In a recent series of jaundiced patients, intravenous cholangiography failed to image the duct in 25% and missed duct stones in 63%; demonstration of the ampullary region is especially difficult and this is a serious failing in view of the frequency of lesions at this level (Ring *et al.*, 1983). Its use in the investigation of jaundice is outdated, though it may occasionally be helpful in mild or partial duct obstruction if other tests are unavailable (Ekelberg *et al.*, 1970).

Direct cholangiography

Percutaneous trans-hepatic cholangiography (PTC) gives superb anatomical delineation of both the intra- and extrahepatic biliary tree (Weichel, 1964, Ariyama, 1983) and its safety has been greatly improved with the widespread use of fine-gauge needles. The site of an obstructing lesion is readily demonstrated and the features allow the aetiology to be determined in 90% of cases. Impacted stones

produce a rounded or polygonal indentation at the site of obstruction, while the narrowing due to malignancy tends to be more extensive and irregular, often giving a 'rat-tail' appearance. Obstruction due to pancreatitis is characteristically extended and smooth and usually incomplete. (Harbin *et al.*, 1980). Less common conditions such as sclerosing cholangitis, Caroli's disease, and choledochal cysts are clearly displayed.

The technique involves the insertion of a fine (23 gauge) needle into the right lobe in the mid-axillary line under local anaesthesia with fluoroscopic control. When the ducts are dilated puncture is almost always successful, but ducts of normal calibre are more difficult to locate. PTC fails in 10% of this group, even when multiple punctures are used, though repeated failure suggests that the ducts are not dilated (Ariyama *et al.*, 1978). The technical skills required are easily learned and the apparatus is readily available.

The main drawback of PTC is its invasiveness, with attendant discomfort to the patient and risks of bacteraemia, haemorrhage, and bile leak (Mueller *et al.*, 1981). These have been greatly reduced by the introduction of fine-gauge needles. Nevertheless, bacteraemia follows in 1–2% of studies. It is a particular hazard where overt bacterial cholangitis pre-exists, as is the case in 75% of patients with gall stone obstruction. Avoidance of injection of excess contrast reduces the likelihood of bacteraemia and suitable antibiotic cover effectively deals with this risk. Bile leakage also occurs in 1–2% of cases but rarely produces clinically apparent peritonitis, provided that fine needles are used, unless the extrahepatic ducts are inadvertently punctured. Surgical correction may be required in this event, so the technique for PTC is designed to direct the needle away from the porta hepatis. Haemorrhage complicates PTC in 0.35% of cases; the risk is reduced by puncturing the liver capsule once for the several passes that may be required for successful cannulation. Patients with uncorrectable haemorrhagic diatheses should be avoided, and ascites is considered a contraindication.

A major advantage of PTC is the basis it forms for external biliary drainage, which may be essential in preparing patients in poor general condition for definitive surgery. It also has an important palliative role in advanced malignant disease for guiding drainage either externally or via an endoprosthesis.

Cannulation of the biliary tree via an endoscope (ERCP) is the alternative approach (Cotton, 1977). It also produces excellent delineation of the biliary tree, especially the lower portion. A flexible fibre-optic endoscope is passed, with the patient under light sedation and lying in the left decubitus position. Duodenal hypotension (achieved with atropine and glucagon) and turning the patient supine aid in visualization and cannulation of the papilla. The pancreatic duct is easily cannulated in 90% of studies (hence the usual title endoscopic retrograde cholangiopancreatography) and in fact in most patients is more easily found than the common bile duct, which in experienced hands can be cannulated in 80% of cases.

Its accuracy is about the same as that of percutaneous cholangiography, both being almost totally reliable in detecting duct obstruction and 90% reliable in distinguishing benign from malignant causes (Elias et al., 1976, Matzen et al., 1981). In contradistinction to PTC, non-dilated ducts are just as easily cannulated. In addition ERCP allows direct inspection of the papilla, with the possibility of biopsy and of endoscopic papillotomy and removal of impacted stones. Though moderately uncomfortable, the procedure is well tolerated and can be performed on an out-patient basis. There are few complications provided the injection of too much contrast is avoided, for this may precipitate pancreatitis or septicaemia. (Bilbao et al., 1976). Bleeding is not a problem, and a prolonged prothrombin time is not a contraindication. However, the technique is relatively difficult to perform, and inexperienced operators have higher failure rates.

Ultrasound

Ultrasound gives an excellent display of dilated intrahepatic ducts and the normal portions of the biliary tree at the porta hepatis can be imaged. Dilatation is demonstrable with a reliability of over 90% (Taylor et al., 1979). Failure to image caused by bowel gas preventing access — problems that affect the usefulness of ultrasound in other parts of the abdomen — do not apply here. As with any purely anatomical technique, there are difficulties in the unusual situation where the bile duct pressure and the duct calibre are disassociated. This may occur very early in an obstructive episode, or when the ducts are splinted as by a rigid liver in cirrhosis (Beinart et al., 1981). Ducts may be dilated though not under pressure after a resolved obstructive episode; the disparity may be extreme in cases of intermittent obstruction such as may be caused by a ball-valve calculus.

The clear display of the anatomy of the porta given by ultrasound allows a full evaluation of dilatation and the causative pathology at this level, nodes and tumour masses being readily detected. However the retroduodenal portion of the common bile duct is so often obscured by duodenal gas that obstructing lesions here cannot be detected reliably. The pancreatic portion is usually displayed and masses in the head of the pancreas are readily detected, provided that they are larger than 1–2 cm in diameter. The accuracy of ultrasound in the localization of obstruction is about 75% (Haubek et al., 1981).

The appearances of mass lesions are non-specific, malignant and inflammatory masses being indistinguishable unless signs of metastatic spread allow their nature to be inferred. In most cases biopsy is required for full evaluation and the most convenient approach is with ultrasound guidance. Smaller obstructing lesions such as strictures and ampullary tumours cannot be visualized. Stones in the common bile duct, though sometimes quite obvious, pose a diagnostic problem on occasions, since they may not show the distal acoustic shadowing typical of stones elsewhere, and therefore may simulate soft-tissue masses. Other causes of jaundice may be detectable, typical features of the intensely reflective liver together with signs of portal hypertension suggesting cirrhosis, or a poorly reflective liver with thickening of the gall bladder wall indicating hepatitis. The overall accuracy of ultrasound in the determination of the aetiology of obstruction is about 50% (Deitch, 1981).

Thus ultrasound provides a reliable assessment of duct calibre both within the liver and at the porta, with variable quality information below this. Its simplicity and safety are its advantages, with no discomfort or risks attached. Interpretation may be difficult, and thorough training in ultrasound techniques is a prerequisite.

Computerized tomography

The normal biliary tree is not visualized directly on computerized tomography (CT) but when dilated it can be demonstrated as a tubular pattern of lower attenuation radiating from the porta. In early cases the distinction between ducts and portal vessels is easier following contrast enhancement, when the branching pattern of dilated intrahepatic ducts is well seen against the higher density of the enhanced liver parenchyma, with an accuracy of 90% (Goldberg et al., 1978). Demonstration of the common bile duct requires rapid sequence scanning following a bolus injection to enhance the surrounding structures (Pedrosa et al., 1981, Baron et al., 1982). A series of contiguous slices at 5 mm spacing allows the duct to be traced down to the duodenum. Its calibre can be measured accurately and the site of an obstruction defined; it is often possible to determine the nature of the obstructing lesion using criteria similar to those for direct cholangiography.

Mass lesions in the head of the pancreas are easily delineated, though as with ultrasound the distinction between benign and malignant is unreliable and a biopsy is usually required; this may be guided by CT. Stones are more readily detected than on ultrasound though they remain a difficult problem especially when the ducts are not dilated (Shanser et al., 1978). Overall the accuracy of CT in determining the aetiology of biliary obstruction is about 70%. Thus CT gives information similar to that available from ultrasound, and it is less subject to technical failure (e.g. when dressings prevent ultrasonic contact) or operator error, although it is a more expensive technique.

Radionuclide scanning

Images of the biliary tree may be obtained using one of the family of iminodiacetic acid derivatives of which HIDA (dimethyliminodiacetic acid) is the prototype (Weissman et al., 1980a). The process of labelling with ^{99m}technetium is straightforward and scans are taken with a gamma camera over a 1–4-h period following injection. The information obtainable is similar to that available from intravenous cholangiography but the technique is simple and safe and gives images in the face of higher bilirubin levels. Newer scanning agents allow imaging with deeper jaundice; DISIDA (diisopropyl IDA) gives interpretable images with serum bilirubin levels up to 600 μmol/l with less confusion from renal excretion simulating transit into the gut. In patients with moderate jaundice due to hepatocellular failure, IDA scanning will show liver uptake followed by transit into the biliary tree and sequential concentration at the porta and common duct, with appearance of isotope in the duodenum by 1 h.

Total obstruction gives a diagnostic picture with activity moving into the duct system but failing to enter gut within 4 h. In partial obstruction there may be delayed transit that is difficult to distinguish from moderate hepatocellular failure, so that accuracy is reduced from over 90% in the typical obstructive pattern to about 80% (Fonseca et al., 1979). In severe liver-cell damage there is little or no hepatic uptake and the test fails.

Provided nuclear medicine facilities are available, IDA scanning is inexpensive, simple to perform and risk free, though it gives no information as to the cause of obstruction and cannot be used to guide biopsies. Its role therefore is as a screening study especially where ultrasound or CT are not available or where other studies are confusing. In cases of mild jaundice it can effectively eliminate medical causes and it has a special place following surgery to the upper gastrointestinal and biliary tracts, particularly where bypass procedures and enterostomies make endoscopy relatively difficult. Similarly, in conditions where the intrahepatic bile ducts do not dilate, as in sclerosing cholangitis, PTC may be difficult and IDA scanning can be used to exclude overlying obstruction.

The imaging approach to jaundice

The initial evaluation of the jaundiced patient will, of course, be clinical and biochemical. Many cases such as those with haemolysis, familial hyperbilirubinaemia, and unequivocal hepatitis will not need radiological investigation. Clinical evaluation is 85% accurate in distinguishing medical from surgical cholestasis though even experienced clinicians miss some cases of large-duct obstruction (Martin *et al.*, 1960). Thus, patients referred for radiological investigation have already been selected for the high probability of their having an obsctructive aetiology for their jaundice.

The choice of radiological test is governed by the same cost-effectiveness considerations that obtain elsewhere. The term 'cost' is taken in a wide sense to include not only financial consider-ations but also the cost to the patient of discomfort and delay. The definition of 'effectiveness' is not simple, since the local prevalence of the various diseases to be distinguished, as well as the level of expertise and the availability of specialized equip-ment, all need to be considered. No single strategy will serve all units in all parts of the world. How-ever, some general indications may be proposed.

Ultrasound is quick, simple, safe and acceptable, and has an excellent record for detecting large-duct obstruction with an accuracy over 90%. Provided that the requisite skills are available, it should be used as a first screening test for most patients (Fig. 21.2). It often provides additional information, which may be sufficient for definitive management, e.g. where a stone is clearly visual-ized in the common bile duct, or where a mass in the head of the pancreas is associated with liver metastases and a guided biopsy confirms carci-noma. Usually, however, when duct dilatation is demonstrated, ultrasound fails to reveal the cause (about 50% of cases) or does not provide the surgeon with sufficient information to proceed. It may indicate an obstruction in the lower common bile duct but be unable to demonstrate the ob-structing lesion or it may demonstrate a mass in the common bile duct but be unable to determine whether it represents tumour or biliary material.

Thus in the majority of cases demonstrated to be obstructive, further information is required, and this is best provided by direct cholangiography (Richter *et al.*, 1983). Both percutaneous trans-hepatic and endoscopic retrograde cholangi-ography give excellent anatomical detail and will confirm the obstructive nature of the jaundice and indicate the precise level in virtually every case, as well as suggesting the aetiology in over 80% of cases. PTC is cheaper and technically simpler, especially when there is duct dilatation, and will usually be chosen when the preliminary ultra-sound confirms this. It also allows preoperative drainage of the distended biliary tree. ERCP is less invasive but more liable to technical failure. If information on the pancreatic duct is also required,

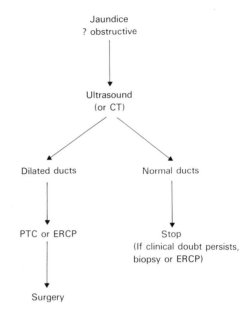

Fig. 21.2 Investigative pathway for suspected obstructive jaundice. Ultrasound and CT form the best initial screening study, ultrasound being preferred for its cost-effectiveness. Confirmed duct dilatation will usually need further investigation by direct cholangiography before surgery. PTC is usually more readily available but ERCP is equally useful. If the initial study is negative but clinical suspicion remains high (e.g. persistent biochemically obstructive jaundice), a liver biopsy or ERCP should be performed.

ERCP is preferred, and where a lesion at the ampulla may be treatable endoscopically this becomes the definitive procedure. When the patient's prothrombin time cannot be corrected, PTC is contraindicated. In practical terms the local expertise will determine which test is used first, and either is nearly always satisfactory. When one technique for direct cholangiography fails, gives incomplete information, or is equivocal, the other should be used.

When there is disagreement between the clinical impression and the initial ultrasound, there should be no hesitation in either repeating the study or passing on to direct cholangiography. No test is perfect and there are the occasions already referred to when duct dilatation does not occur or is delayed, and there are operator errors. With earlier patient referral for imaging, it is more common for the ultrasound scan to be negative but the patient's jaundice fail to resolve; often a repeat examination in a week or so will reveal duct dilatation. Ultra-sound may indicate another cause for the jaundice, such as the 'dark liver' of hepatitis, and thereby suggest that a biopsy is the most appropriate next test if there is clinical doubt. Continuing discrepancy between the clinical impression and the radiological findings should also lead to a Menghini liver biopsy.

The role of biliary scintigraphy is somewhat controversial (Weissmann *et al.*, 1980b). It may be used as a screening study, and where the result is clear-cut it is helpful; however, equivocal results are rather common so that ultrasound is generally preferred as a first imaging investigation in jaundice. The helpful ancillary information often provided by ultrasound and CT is not available from scintigraphy. In principle it might have a role in difficult cases, but in practice unless a test is in regular routine use, the background interpretative skill and confidence demanded by the difficult case will have been lost. For these reasons in most centres biliary scintigraphy is reserved for acute cholecystitis, where it is highly reliable, rather than jaundice.

Special situations

Evaluation pre and post-surgery

Where a pancreatic mass is delineated on ultrasound or CT, a biopsy is usually necessary, since none of the available tests can distinguish reliably between inflammatory and malignant processes. A biopsy is required even when metastases are demonstrated, since the primary may not be pancreatic; the possibility of lymphoma with its different management and better prognosis must be borne in mind.

The possibility of radical surgery may have been discounted on the ultrasound screening study because liver metastases, involved nodes, or invasion of the superior mesenteric or portal vessels have been demonstrated. If, however, a Whipple's resection is being considered, a CT scan will always be required because of the better display of local spread, vascular invasion, and nodal and liver involvement it provides. Most surgeons will also require a selective coeliac and possibly superior mesenteric arteriogram both to assess vascular involvement and to map this variable territory before complex radical resection (Stanley *et al.*, 1980).

IDA scanning plays a special role in evaluating bile duct patency in patients who develop jaundice after biliary surgery where there is no T-tube. The demonstration of free excretion of isotope into the duodenum excludes duct obstruction and prompts a search for hepatic causes of jaundice. In these patients, ultrasound can be very difficult technically (because of bowel gas, drainage tubes, etc.), and residual duct dilatation can be confusing on both ultrasound and CT. ERCP may be impossible if there has been gut surgery, and PTC may be contraindicated because of liver insufficiency.

Paediatric jaundice

Neonatal jaundice poses a major differential diagnostic problem, and radiology on the whole has not helped greatly in the important distinction between neonatal hepatitis and biliary atresia, both of which are thought to be manifestations of the same inflammatory process (Bill *et al.*, 1974). In the majority of cases of biliary atresia all the larger ducts are atretic, including those at the porta hepatis. In these cases conventional surgical anastamosis is precluded, but the surgical procedure whereby a loop of jejunum is attached to the denuded hepatic surface at the porta hepatis (portojejunostomy; the Kasai procedure) results in adequate biliary drainage in 90% of cases, provided that they are operated on within the first 2 months of life (Hays & Kimura, 1980). Thus the differential diagnosis is urgent. Ultrasound is useful where a normal biliary tree is demonstrated and sometimes an unexpected cause for obstruction is revealed, e.g. a choledochal cyst. The demonstration of one of the congenital anomalies associated with biliary atresia, e.g. asplenia, confirms a clinical impression. PTC will sometimes demonstrate persistent hepatic ducts in atresia.

Radiolabelled biliary agents can be used to demonstrate duct patency; [99m]technetium-labelled IDA derivatives give gamma camera images in which gut excretion can be demonstrated. A clear-cut positive result excludes atresia, but when liver function is severely depressed in hepatitis, the 12-h imaging period allowed by this short-lived isotope is inadequate. [131]I rose bengal is an alternative, but the small doses that must be used preclude imaging, and a faecal collection is required. Provided that a full 5-day collection can be obtained without urinary contamination, excretion of more than 5% of the tracer excludes atresia (Rosenthall, 1975).

Choledochal cysts produce jaundice by distortion of the biliary tree (Babbitt *et al.*, 1973). While in older children recurrent pain and jaundice are the common presentation, in neonates persistent jaundice raises the differential diagnosis of atresia or hepatitis. The diagnosis is usually straight-forward on ultrasound (Kobayashi & Ohbe, 1977), a cystic structure in the upper abdomen being associated with intrahepatic duct dilatation, though it may be difficult to demonstrate its point of origin from the bile duct. CT gives the same information but is not usually required. PTC will provide more detailed anatomy if this seems necessary.

Acknowledgements

Drs Elisabeth Bellamy and Hylton Meire provided valuable comments on the sections on CT scanning and Paediatric problems, respectively.

References

Ansell, G. (1970) Adverse reactions to contrast agents. *Investigative Radiology*, **5**, 374−378.

Ariyama, J. (1983) Direct cholangiography. In Herlinger, H., Lunderquist, A. & Wallace, S. (eds) *Clinical Radiology of the Liver*. Marcel Dekker, New York.

Ariyama, J., Shirakabe, H., Ohashi, K. & Roberts, G.M. (1978) Experience with percutaneous transhepatic chol-angiography using the Japanese needle. *Gastrointestinal Radiology*, **2**, 359−367.

Babbitt, D.P., Starshuk, R.J. & Clenett, A.R. (1973) Chole-dochal cyst: a concept of etiology. *American Journal of Roentgenology*, **119**, 57−60.

Baron, R.L., Stanley, R.J. & Lee, J.K.J. (1982) A prospective comparative evaluation of biliary obstruction using CT and ultrasound. *Radiology*, **145**, 91−98.

Beinart, C., Efrimides, S. & Cohen, B. (1981) Obstruction without dilatation: importance in the evaluation of jaundice. *Journal of the American Medical Association*, **245**, 353−356.

Bilbao, M.K., Dotter, C.T., Lee, T.G. & Katon, R.M. (1976) Complications of ERCP. *Gastroenterology*, **70**, 314−325.

Bill, A.H., Brennom, W.S. & Husby, T.L. (1974) Biliary atresia: new concepts of pathology, diagnosis and man-agement. *Archives of Surgery*, **109**, 367−380.

Cotton, P.B. (1977) Endoscopic retrograde cholangio-pancreatography. *Gut*, **18**, 316−341.

Deitch, E.A. (1981) The reliability and clinical limits of sonographic scanning of biliary ducts. *Annals of Surgery*, **194**, 167−170.

Ekelberg, M.E., Carlson, B.C. & McIlrath, D.C. (1970) Intra-venous cholangiography with an intact gall bladder. *American Journal of Roentgenology*, **110**, 235−240.

Elias, E., Hamlyn, A.N. & Jarvis, S. (1976) A random trial of percutaneous cholangiography with the Chiba needle versus endoscopic retrograde cholangiography for bile duct visualization in jaundice. *Gastroenterology*, **71**, 439−443.

Fonseca, C., Rosenthall, L. & Greenberg, D. (1979) Differ-ential diagnosis of jaundice by IDA hepatobiliary imaging. *Clinics in Nuclear Medicine*, **4**, 135−142.

Goldberg, H.I., Filley, R.A., Korobkin, M., Moss, A.A.,

Kressel, H.Y. & Callen, P.W. (1978) Capability of CT and ultrasonography to demonstrate the status of the biliary tree in patients with jaundice. *Radiology*, **129**, 731−750.

Harbin, W.P., Mueller, P.R. & Ferrucci, J.T. (1980) Trans-hepatic cholangiography. *Radiology*, **135**, 15−22.

Hardy, A.K.J., Wheatley, I.C., Anderson, A.E.I. & Bond, R.J. (1976) The lymph nodes of the porta hepatis. *Surgery, Gynecology and Obstetrics*, **143**, 225−230.

Haubek, A., Pederson, J.H., Burcharth, F., Gamelgaard, J., Hanke, S. & Willumsen, L. (1981) Dynamic ultrasound in the evaluation of jaundice. *American Journal of Roentgenology*, **136**, 1071−1082.

Hays, D.M. & Kimura, K. (1980) *Biliary Atresia: The Japanese Experience*. Harvard University Press.

Kobayashi, A. & Ohbe, Y. (1977) Choledochal cyst in infancy and childhood. *Archives of Disease in Childhood*, **52**, 121−130.

Koenigsberg, M., Weiner, S. & Walzer, A. (1979) The accuracy of sonography in the differential diagnosis of jaundice: a comparison with cholangiography. *Radiology*, **133**, 157−163.

Martin, E.B., Apostolakos, P.C. & Rosen, H. (1960). Clinical versus actuarial prediction in the differential diagnosis of jaundice. *American Journal of Medical Science*, **240**, 571−578.

Matzen, P., Haubek, A., Holst-Christensen, J., Leferstofte, J. & Juhl, E. (1981) Accuracy of direct cholangiography by endoscopic or transhepatic route in jaundice. *Gastro-enterology*, **81**, 237−245.

Mueller, P.R., Harbin, W.P., Ferrucci, J.T., Wittenberg, J. & van Sonnenburg, E. (1981) Fine needle transhepatic cholangiography. *American Journal of Roentgenology*, **136**, 85−91.

Pedrosa, C.S., Casanova, R. & Jezana, A.H. (1981) CT in obstructive jaundice. *Radiology*, **139**, 635−645.

Richter, J.M., Silverstein, M.D. & Schapiro, R. (1983) Suspected obstructive jaundice: a decision analysis of diagnostic strategies. *Annals of Internal Medicine*, **99**, 46−51.

Ring, E.J., Herlinger, H. & Gordon, R.L. (1983) Radiology in jaundice. In Herlinger, H., Lunderquist, A. & Wallace, S. (eds) *Clinical Radiology of the Liver*, pp. 611−644. Marcel Dekker, New York.

Rosenthall, L. (1975) Differentiation of intrahepatic disease and extrahepatic biliary atresia in infants, In Rosenthall, E. (ed.) *The Applications of Radioiodinated Rose Bengal and Colloidal Radiogold in the Detection of Hepatobiliary Disease*, pp. 121−129. Warren Green, St Louis.

Schaffer, F. & Popper, H. (1979) Classification and mechanism of cholestasis. In Wright, R., Albati, K.G., Karran, S. & Milward-Sadler, G.H. (eds) *Liver and Biliary Disease*, 296−323. Saunders, London.

Schneck, C. (1983) The anatomical basis of abdomino-pelvic sectional imaging. In Joseph, A.E. & Cosgrove, D.O. (eds) *Ultrasound in Inflammatory Diseases*, pp. 13−42. Churchill Livingstone, New York.

Shanser, J.D., Korobkin, M., Goldberg, H.I. & Rohlfing, B.M. (1978) Computed tomographic diagnosis of obstruc-tive jaundice in the absence of intrahepatic duct dila-tation. *American Journal of Roentgenology*, **133**, 323−330.

Shenker, S., Balint, J. & Schoff, L. (1962) Differential diag-nosis of jaundice. *American Journal of Digestive Diseases*, **7**, 449−456.

Stanley, R.J., Sagel, S.S. & Evens, R.G. (1980) The impact of new imaging methods on pancreatic arteriography. *Radiology*, **136**, 245–250.

Taylor, K.J.W., Rosenfield, A.T. & Spiro, H.M. (1979) Diagnostic accuracy of gray-scale ultrasonography for the jaundiced patient. *Archives of Internal Medicine*, **13**, 60–63.

Weichel, K.-L. (1964) Percutaneous transhepatic cholangiography. *Acta Chirurgica Scandinavica* (Suppl.), **33**, 5–12.

Weissmann, H.S., Frank, M.S., Rosenblatt, L.A., Sugarman, L.A. & Freeman, L.M. (1980a) Role of cholescintigraphy in the evaluation of biliary disorders. *Gastrointestinal Radiology*, **5**, 215–222.

Weissmann, H.S., Rosenblatt, R., Sugarman, L.A. & Freeman, L.M. (1980b) The role of nuclear imaging in evaluating cholestasis. *Seminars in Ultrasound*, **1**, 134–245.

22: Interventional Radiology in Obstructive Jaundice

R. DICK

Introduction

Non-surgical treatments for biliary tract disorders have grown in range and popularity. A multi-disciplinary approach is required, the best units having achieved harmony between surgeons, endoscopists, and interventional radiologists. Their aim is the same; to re-establish the unobstructed flow of non-infected bile into the bowel in order to lower serum bilirubin levels, remove pruritus, and improve both liver function and patient well-being. The method chosen for an individual patient will depend upon available expertise, pathological anatomy, and the clinical status of the patient. Unquestionably percutaneous interventional biliary radiology provides a useful alternative or adjunct to surgery in certain situations (Pogany *et al.*, 1985). Great care is required during any interventional study of the biliary tract. Surgical cover must be provided throughout all procedures, some of which require several sessions, as the danger of possible haemorrhage, cholangitis and other complications always exists.

Trans-hepatic catheters can now be placed anywhere in the biliary system. They will pass through obstructing lesions in 75% of high, and 93% of low lesions (Summerfield & Dooley, 1986). The design of large-bore (8 or 9 Fr.) drainage catheters has been improved so that stability in the ducts can be assured, and if capped externally, antegrade drainage into the duodenum will ensue. Long-term indwelling endoprostheses may be inserted either percutaneously (Coons & Carey, 1983) or endoscopically (Cotton, 1982). These avoid the problems associated with management of external biliary catheters and provide palliation in those patients with intolerable symptoms from inoperable malignancy obstructing the biliary tract.

The percutaneous trans-hepatic cholangiogram (PTC) remains the gold standard on which the interventional biliary radiologist plans later manoeuvres. Technically successful cholangiograms

should be possible in nearly all patients (*see* Chapter 19). Should a major percutaneous procedure be planned after the PTC, it is wise to administer a combination of sedative—hypnotic (10 mg diazepam) and narcotic—analgesic (100 mg pethidine) intravenously before commencing the PTC. General anaesthesia is only necessary in children, or in adults who are to have repeated balloon dilatations of benign strictures, such as patients with multiple intrahepatic strictures in primary sclerosing cholangitis. Antibiotics are not given routinely prior to duct catheterization, and it is desirable to obtain bile for culture before antibiotics are selected. If there has been a history of cholangitis or rigors, mezlocillin 2 g is given as a bolus intravenously for 2 h before the procedure. Occasionally an aminoglycoside and metzanidazole are also given.

Percutaneous trans-hepatic external biliary drainage

Catheterization of dilated intrahepatic bile ducts is possible in at least 98% of patients (Burcharth, 1982). It may be requested to relieve duct obstruction whilst a plan of management is formulated (definitive operation if patient improves, endoprosthesis if not), or it may be performed as an emergency in the patient with acute suppurative cholangitis. Surgical mortality for this condition is 50—75% compared with 10—17% for percutaneous trans-hepatic external biliary drainage (Kadir *et al.*, 1982). Drainage decompresses ducts and provides organisms for culture. Much care is needed in such patients to prevent formation of biliary—blood fistulae. Wires and catheters must be manipulated carefully, and contrast injected slowly (Fig. 22.1).

A decreasing number of surgeons favour percutaneous trans-hepatic external biliary drainage for 10—14 days before planned surgery. Early results (Denning *et al.*, 1981) suggested that this decreased

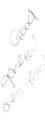

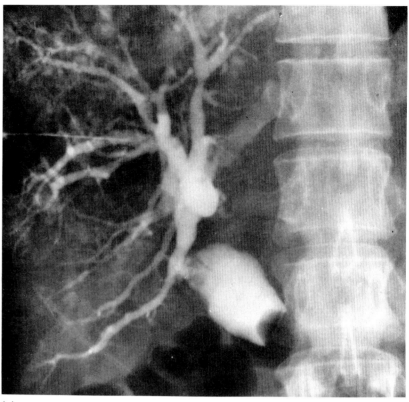

(a)

Fig. 22.1 (a) PTC in patient with acute suppurative cholangitis. Note calculus obstructing common bile duct. Numerous small microabscesses can be seen adjacent to small bile ducts in the hepatic parenchyma. (b) Same patient. Percutaneous drainage performed with resolution of abscesses 3 days later. *Arrows* indicate calculus in common duct.

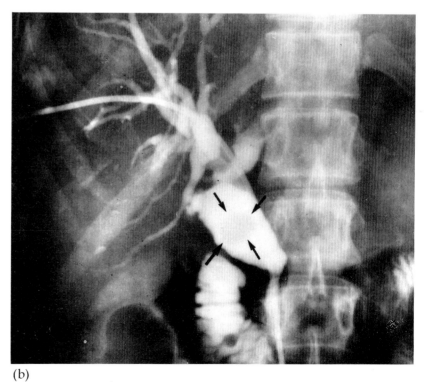

(b)

the 30-day postoperative mortality rate, but a more recent paper (Hatfield *et al.*, 1982) has shown no benefit. The final use for this technique is as a purely palliative exercise in patients with advanced biliary-tract cancer who are decompressed for the short period of their terminal disease (Fig. 22.2).

Technique

Percutaneous Trans-hepatic external biliary drainage

Equipment required is shown in Fig. 22.3. Careful study of the PTC is required before commencing duct catheterization. One method uses the initial thin cholangiogram needle for access, and makes a pass with a second thin needle-puncture into a selected large duct (Cope, 1983). A very thin guide wire (0.018–0.021 in. diameter) is passed through the needle, then sequentially larger dilators, catheters, and wires are exchanged until adequate sized catheters are in place. Although the concept of this method is ingenious, many feel it is difficult to achieve consistency, particularly with ascites, cirrhotic parenchyma, or tortuous bile ducts (Moore & Clark, 1984). Real-time ultrasound guidance has also been successful in aiding catheterization (Makuuchi *et al.*, 1980). This is usually too cumbersome for an intercostal approach to right lobe ducts, but may be most useful in locating left lobe ducts for an anterior subcostal approach. With all percutaneous techniques, direct radiation to the operator's hands must be avoided. Careful coning of the beam by the radiographer is required, and the operator should wear radiation-resistant sterile gloves.

The more traditional means of percutaneous trans-hepatic external biliary drainage involved selection of an appropriate tributary of the right hepatic duct after studying the PTC. A duct just above and behind the hilum is identified. Lateral screening helps locate the chosen duct in both planes, but is not essential. A needle-sheath set (Surgimed) is used to puncture this duct, bile is taken for culture and a moveable core 0.035 in. 'J'-tipped guide wire is passed into a larger down-stream duct. The J tip allows entry of the wire into the duct if the puncture is not quite central in the duct, whilst should the wire travel cephalad, it can be made floppy and its tip advanced to a peripheral duct, where it stops. The next segment of guide wire advanced through liver must pass caudally into the common hepatic duct; this segment may then be stiffened, so ensuring that the sheath will follow. If this technique fails,

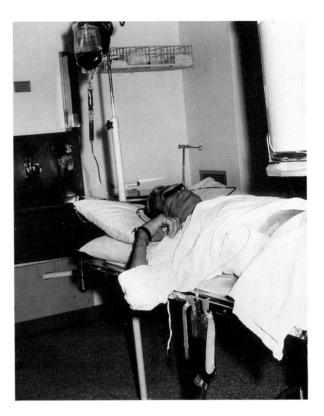

Fig. 22.2 Percutaneous trans-hepatic external biliary drainage performed in an elderly patient with inoperable obstructive jaundice. Bile is being returned to his gut via a nasogastric tube.

a steerable Lunderquist wire (William Cook, Europe) is used to enter the distal ducts. Once the sheath is pointing downstream, a heavy-duty or a rigid guide wire is introduced, enabling exchange of sheath to a definitive drainage catheter, usually a 6 Fr. pigtail. More satisfactory drainage will occur with a large 8.3 Fr. Ring Lunderquist catheter. Arterial dilators up to 9 Fr. size should be used through the liver before introducing the catheters (Fig. 22.4).

Complications

The two major risks are damage to bile duct and blood vessels with subsequent bile leakage and haemorrhage. These are common in the learning phase but rare with experience (Dooley *et al.*, 1986).

If care is taken with catheterization, then septicaemia occurs only in a minority, usually in those with infected bile. Patients with benign disease are more prone to bile infection with organisms including *E. coli*, *Streptococcus faecalis*, Klebsiella,

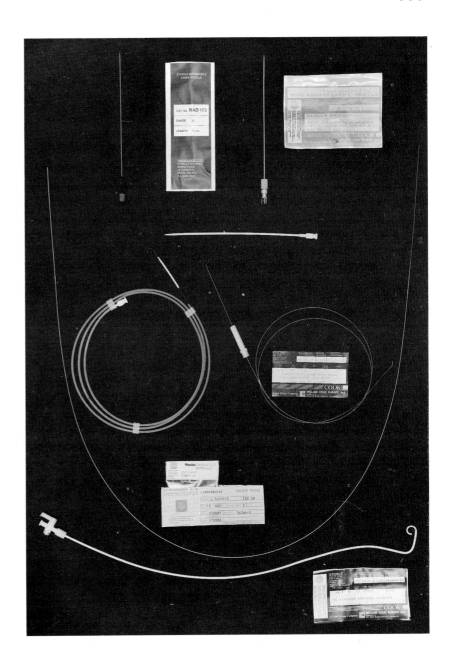

Fig. 22.3 Equipment for percutaneous trans-hepatic external biliary drainage. From above, and left to right. Thin cholangiogram needle, sheathed needle, dilator, J wire, steerable wire, rigid 'coathanger' wire, Ring—Lunderquist 8.3. Fr. drainage catheter.

and anaerobes. Appropriate antibiotics are given once bile culture results are known.

Dehydration and renal failure are major complications of external bile drainage if scrupulous fluid balance is not maintained, whilst later colonization of the biliary tract with bacteria is common. Catheter displacement occurs in 13%, despite careful fixation to the skin and good ward care.

Percutaneous trans-hepatic external—internal biliary drainage

This method avoids significant water and salt loss and allows thorough irrigation of both catheter and ducts. Wherever possible, the end of the pigtail catheter should be passed beyond the obstructing lesion into normal duct or bowel beyond. Stability of the catheter is thus assured, whilst should the catheter have negotiated a malignant stricture, cytology should be performed on the first 24 h drainage fluid (Fig. 22.5). In one series the sensitivity of exfoliative cytology of bile was found to be 34–50%, with no false positive results (Mura *et al.*, 1983). Where the clinical decision on a patient with malignant obstructive jaundice is to insert a percutaneous endoprosthesis, 48 h of percutaneous trans-hepatic external—internal biliary drainage is beneficial to clear the bile of blood or sludge. This

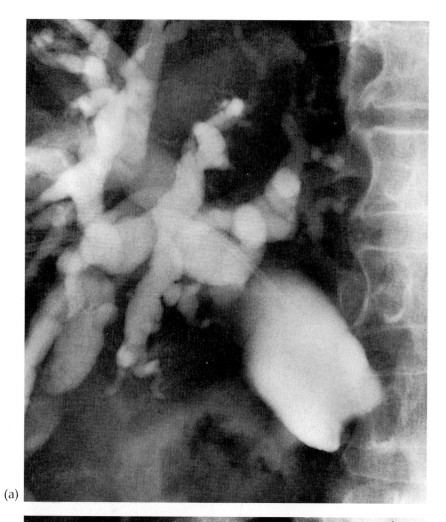

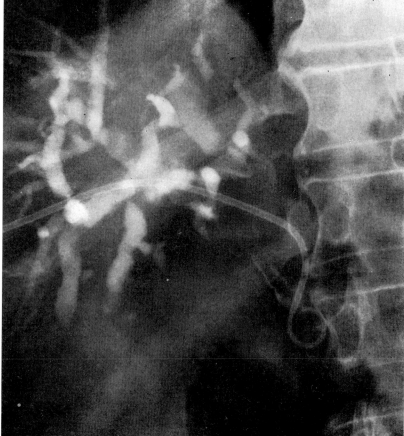

Fig. 22.4 (a) Percutaneous trans-hepatic external biliary drainage above a carcinoma of pancreatic head, which has grown into common duct. (b) After 24 h drainage, the ducts have decompressed.

(a)

(b)

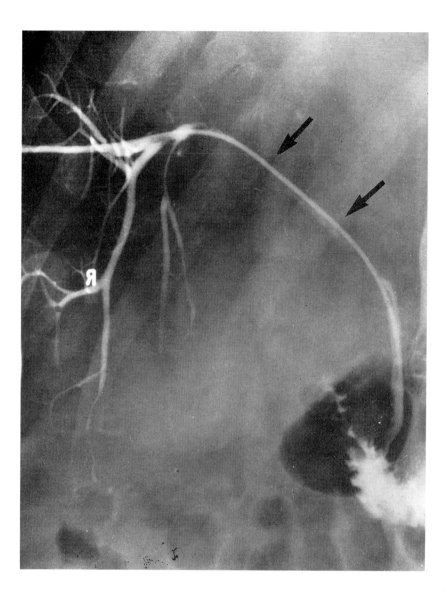

Fig. 22.5 Percutaneous trans-hepatic external–internal biliary drainage in a patient with ankylosing spondylitis (note spine) and sclerosing cholangitis. *Arrows* show catheter through a long stricture. Cytology of bile revealed cholangiocarcinoma cells.

method also allows a catheter to be anchored across a benign stricture between episodes of balloon dilatation.

The technique may be instituted as readily from the left hepatic ducts as the right (Fig. 22.6), the anterior approach having fewer complications (Jaques *et al.*, 1982). Some patients with hilar strictures require separate drainage of both systems, though effective palliation of jaundice may be achieved when only 30% of the liver is decompressed (Mueller *et al.*, 1982).

Percutaneous trans-hepatic endoprosthesis

A great variety of plastic tubes or 'stents' are available for bypassing benign or malignant biliary obstruction at any level. They range in materials, lengths, shapes, and internal diameters, their outer diameters usually being 10 or 12 Fr. Commonly available endoprostheses are shown in Fig. 22.7. The percutaneous insertion mostly depends upon the ability of the prosthesis to be 'railroaded' into place coaxially over an inner catheter which has in turn been positional over a heavy-duty guide wire. Preliminary dilatation of the stricture using a stiff dilator of matching size to the prosthesis is always essential. The procedure may be difficult and is usually painful. Ten milligrams of diazepam and 100 mg pethidine intravenously are recommended before commencement. General anaesthesia is occasionally required and should always be considered if especially requested by the patient (Fig. 22.8).

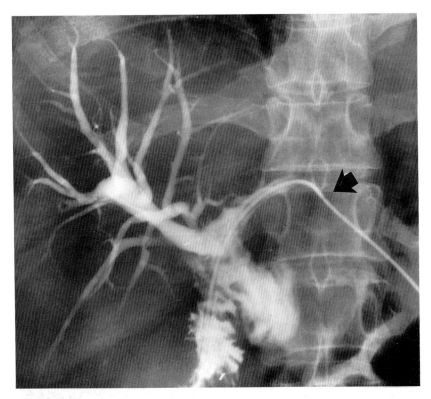

Fig. 22.6 Percutaneous trans-hepatic external−internal biliary drainage performed from left hepatic duct in patient who has balloon dilatation and surgery to biliary−enteric benign stricture. *Arrow* = site of catheter entry to skin.

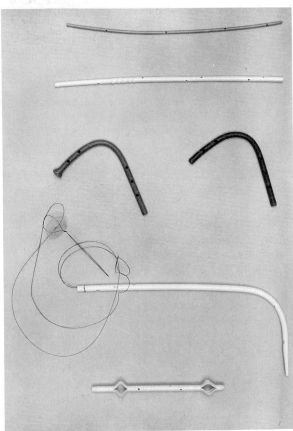

Fig. 22.7 Commonly available percutaneous endoprostheses. From top: Burcharth types 1 and 2; Lunderquist−T-wman with and without proximal flared tip; Carey−Coons; Miller.

Accurate placement of both upper and lower ends of a biliary endoprosthesis is essential (Fig. 22.8). It is wise to place metal skin markers on the skin of the right hypochondrium (or over the epigastrium for a left-sided approach) opposite the intended upper and lower ends of the final prosthesis. These are useful as the contrast cholangiogram often fades during the insertion procedure.

Results and complications

Experience with commercially available endoprostheses has not always matched conceptual promise. Although success rates for insertion exceed 95%, many prostheses have sludged after 8 months (Dick *et al.*, 1986). Small-bore Teflon prostheses with side holes have been replaced with longer, wider-bore models containing many side holes without an increase in the number of acute complications (Teplick *et al.*, 1982). The Coons & Carey (1983) 12 Fr. stent made of a soft 'Percuflex' polymer (Radiologic, UK) has many side holes and readily shapes itself within the bile ducts. Unfortunately its length means that invariably the lower end lies well around the duodenal loop, increasing the risk of intestinal content reflux into bile ducts and subsequent cholangitis (Fig. 22.9).

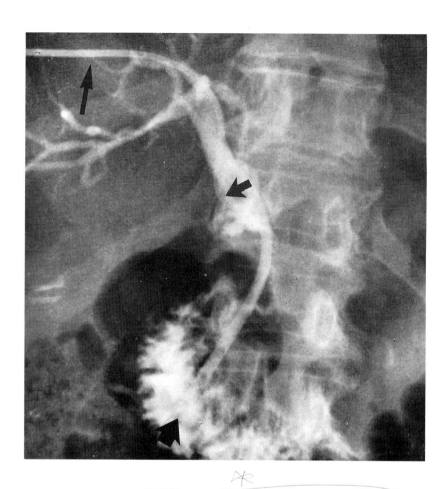

Fig. 22.8 PTE. The Lunderquist prosthesis lies well positioned through a pancreatic cancer. Pigtail temporary drainage catheter above (*thin arrow*). Lower end of prosthesis (*thick arrow*).

Common prob

Many early endoprostheses migrated (Moore & Clark., 1984). With newer, larger models distal migration can be corrected using a Gruntzig balloon catheter inflated within the endoprosthesis (Honickman *et al.*, 1982), or by pulling upon the suture sling attached to the proximal end of a prosthesis such as the Carey–Coons. Proximal malpositioning is corrected by advancing the outer pusher against the upper end of the prosthesis.

Table 22.1 lists the complications of percutaneous trans-hepatic endoprostheses. Serious complications are rare, and not significantly increased compared with those of external–internal biliary drainage (Teplick *et al.*, 1982). The most worrying are haemobilia, cholangitis and septicaemia, the last two requiring active management. A one-stage procedure is not advised, since haemobilia associated with tract dilatation may compromise prosthesis function. It is recommended that initial percutaneous trans-hepatic internal–external drainage be performed, followed by endoprosthesis insertion 48 h later, after which saline is gently irrigated through the system for 24 h. After a final cholangiogram to check patency

Table 22.1 Complications of percutaneous trans-hepatic endoprostheses

Common
Cholangitis/septicaemia
Early haemobilia

Rare
Bleeding into peritoneum
Marked haemobilia
Guide wire perforation of bowel
Pleural effusion (right)
Infection or tumour deposit at skin entry site
External biliary leak

and position of the endoprosthesis, the external tube is removed and the patient discharged.

Follow-up is clinical. Should there be signs of returning cholestasis a plain abdominal film may be taken to demonstrate air in biliary ducts (Fig. 22.10) or a hepatobiliary scan ([99m]technetium HIDA) may be performed. Once an endoprosthesis is shown to be malfunctioning or occluded, although percutaneous reboring is feasible, the

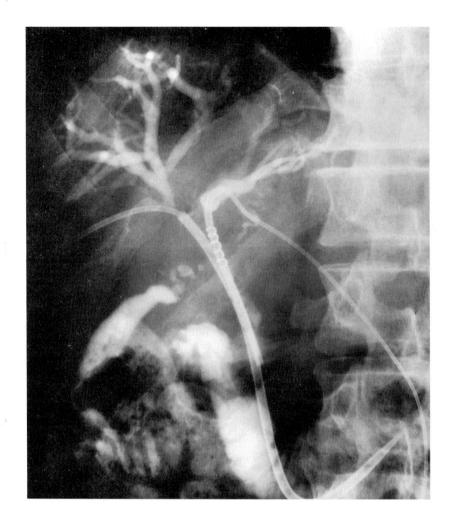

Fig. 22.9 Patient with cholangiocarcinoma (Klatskin tumour). Carey–Coons endoprosthesis from the right, Burcharth type 2 from the left, each with external catheters for 24 h flushing and final check cholangiogram.

prosthesis is best removed endoscopically (Fig. 22.11). A replacement can then be inserted endoscopically or percutaneously. Occasionally, surgical removal is necessary.

Undoubtedly the main indications for endoprostheses is to relieve the intolerable symptoms associated with malignant, obstructive jaundice, and in this it succeeds. An indwelling stent has great psychological advantage over an external tube, and requires no patient or nursing management. Many patients with cancer die before malfunction of the stent occurs. Cholangitis must be controlled by appropriate use of antibiotics on an individual basis. Of great concern are the occasionally reported metastases to skin after a trans-hepatic approach to a pancreatic or biliary malignancy (Baumgarten & von Rottkay, 1984, Dick *et al.*, 1986); this complication cannot occur with endoscopically placed endoprostheses. In the author's view the benefits of endoprostheses undoubtedly outweigh the difficulties of insertion and the unavoidable complication rate.

Percutaneous trans-hepatic balloon dilatation of biliary strictures

Dilatation of a benign or occasionally malignant stricture involving ampulla, common bile or hepatic duct and biliary–enteric anastomosis is an attractive alternative to further surgery in many patients (Ring & Kerlan, 1984) particularly those with benign disease who may have had up to 15 previous major biliary tract operations. Patency rates of 7 years have been reported (Molnar & Stockum, 1978).

The stricture or strictures must first be negotiated with a guide wire, the torque controlled formable tipped Lunderquist wire (Fig. 22.3) being passed across the narrowing, usually in less than 10 min screening time. A drainage catheter follows; then after the wire is removed, contrast must be injected to check that the catheter tip lies in normal duct or bowel below the site of disease. A heavy-duty (Coon's; Radiologic, UK) or a rigid wire is now inserted, and the catheter replaced with a

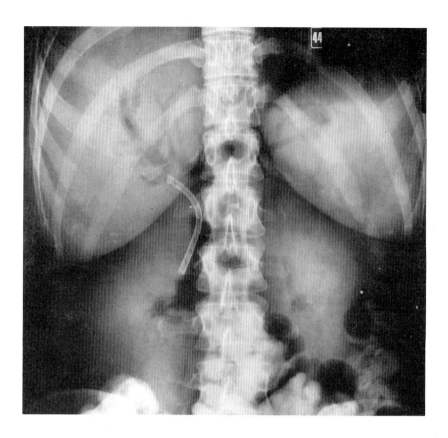

Fig. 22.10 Percutaneous trans-hepatic endoprosthesis was performed 4 years previously in this patient with a benign biliary stricture. Plain abdomen shows much air in ducts in both lobes of the liver.

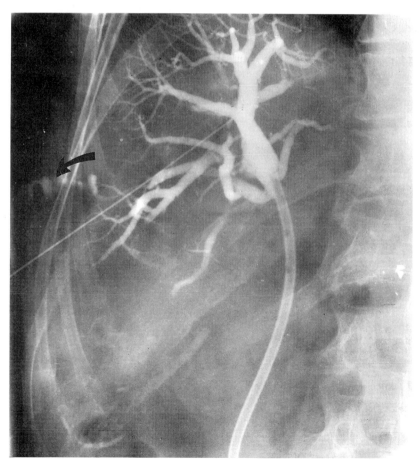

Fig. 22.11 PTC demonstrates blocked Carey−Coons prosthesis. It had been inserted only 3 months previously through an extensive carcinoma of gall bladder that had involved pancreas and liver hilum. Patient presented with external biliary fistula (*arrow*) at site of initial prosthesis.

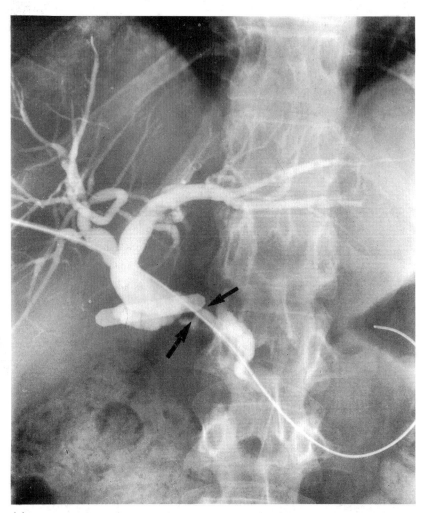

(a)

Fig. 22.12 Transplanted liver of 12 months. Benign biliary stricture at site of previous T-tube insertion. (a) *Arrows* indicate stricture through which a wire has been passed. Note metal skin marker opposite stricture in case cholangiogram should fade.

low-profile balloon catheter, which is dilated across the stricture. Benign strictures are invariably short, so a slightly longer balloon length is chosen, balloon diameter being 8–10 mm. Even though this diameter is in excess of the 'normal' common duct diameter, it is wise to over-dilate to prevent recurrence (Fig. 22.12).

Pain during this procedure may be considerable, particularly when scar tissue is dilated, and an anaesthetist should be present to titrate analgesia and if necessary to administer a general anaesthetic. No standard times for leaving the balloon dilated have been formulated. In the UK serial dilatations for 10 min periods over several days are favoured. An inflation handle is essential. In Scandinavia and the USA inflation may be maintained for 24 h. It is probably unnecessary to follow balloon dilatation with endoprosthesis insertion, though some favour this for a period of 6–12 months (Moore & Clark, 1984). In the absence of

stenting, dilatations may need to be repeated every 6 months, especially if intrahepatic strictures associated with sclerosing cholangitis are being attacked, and both patient and radiologist will require much patience. If general anaesthesia is not used, measures to decrease the pain of transhepatic procedures include intraductal lignocaine (15 ml of 2%) and intercostal nerve blocks using Marcain (Ferrucci *et al.*, 1983).

Interventional management of special problems affecting the biliary tract

Congenital cystic disease of ducts

In Caroli's disease or choledochal cyst there are selective dilatations of the intra- and extrahepatic ducts, respectively. Patients are prone to formation of calculi and to attacks of cholangitis. Imaging the duct abnormalities by US, CT, or cholangiography

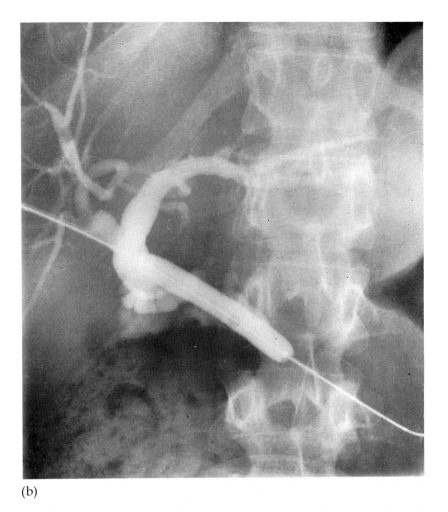

(b)

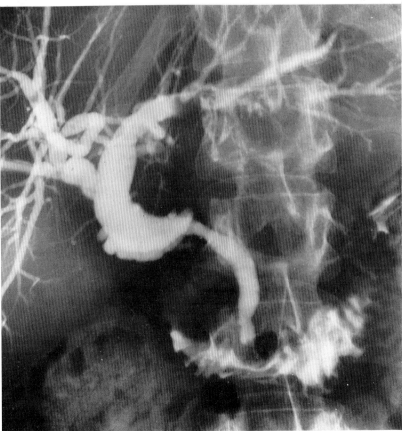

Fig. 22.12 (b) Balloon dilatation of stricture (Olbert 8 mm balloon). (c) Stricture ablated post-dilatation. Six months follow-up — no recurrene.

(c)

plays a vital role both in diagnosis and in treating some of the complications. Trans-hepatic or trans-T-tube access to ducts allows calculi to be removed by Dormia basket at multiple sessions, or ducts to be irrigated and antibiotics instilled (Fig. 22.13). Imaging may show other abnormalities such as congenital hepatic fibrosis and renal abnormalities (medullary cystic disease) which are all part of the spectrum of fibropolycystic liver disease (Summerfield *et al.*, 1986). Most importantly, imaging may pin-point a developing cholangiocarcinoma.

Biliary atresia

This has been discussed in Chapter 20. Although a fine-needle (Surg 25) cholangiogram has a useful role in showing the type of atresia, interventional percutaneous procedures are at present unable to help.

Biliary lavage for primary sclerosing cholangitis

This chronic inflammatory condition of bile ducts is becoming more common. Percutaneous or endoscopic infusion of 100 mg hydrocortisone in 1 litre of saline may be administered daily for 2 weeks. Whilst unmistakable radiological and clinical improvement occurs, no controlled trial is available, and it is probably more likely to benefit a patient with acute disease than one with established fibrosis. A trans-hepatic tube can be introduced into a peripheral duct and checked daily. Alternatively, an endoscopic catheter may be left astride the common hepatic duct and an occlusal balloon inflated here for the period of intrahepatic duct irrigation.

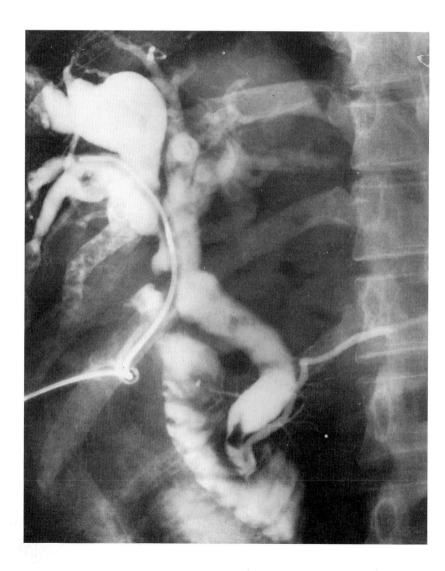

Fig. 22.13 Twenty-four-year-old patient with Caroli's disease. Multiple calculi lie within the ectatic clubbed ducts. A steerable wire and catheter has been introduced via T-tube track to remove stones.

Stomal access to diseased biliary ducts

Although intra- and extrahepatic bile duct strictures can be dilated trans-hepatically using balloon catheters introduced from both right and left sides (Martin *et al.*, 1981a), an easier access was described by Suruga *et al.* in 1982. This entails forming a skin access stoma in the Roux-en-Y loop of jejunum used for a hepaticojejunostomy anastomosis. Both radiologist and endoscopist then have access to bile ducts for non-operative management of recurrent biliary problems (Fig. 22.14). Repeated balloon dilatations may be performed, as well as lavage of the intrahepatic ducts when necessary (Russell *et al.*, 1986).

Cholangiocarcinoma

Combined external and internal irradiation may help the tumour mass regress and result in more effective chemotherapy. Internal therapy is given with [192]iridium (6000r over 4 days), which is administered by replacing the mandril of a transhepatically introduced guide wire with a measured length of iridium (Fig. 22.15). The highly concentrated dose is delivered to a 1 cm circumference of

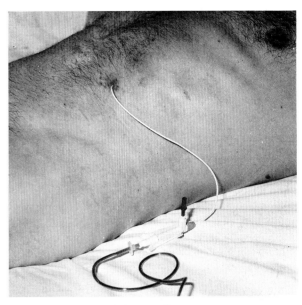

Fig. 22.14 Stoma in abdomen allowing percutaneous access to the bile ducts. When the catheter is removed, the skin heals, surgical clips marking the site for future forays. Preferably the stoma is on the right side, with a straight course to the liver hilum.

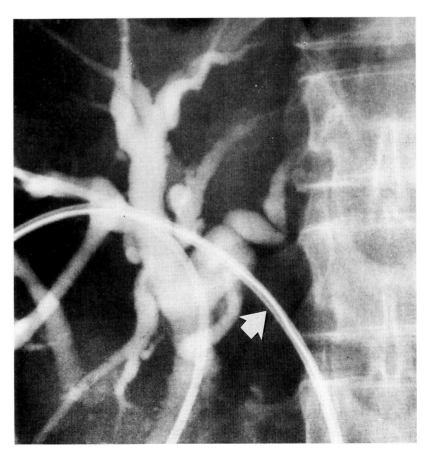

Fig. 22.15 Cholangiocarcinoma. *Arrow* indicates iridium wire inside conventional wire and catheter.

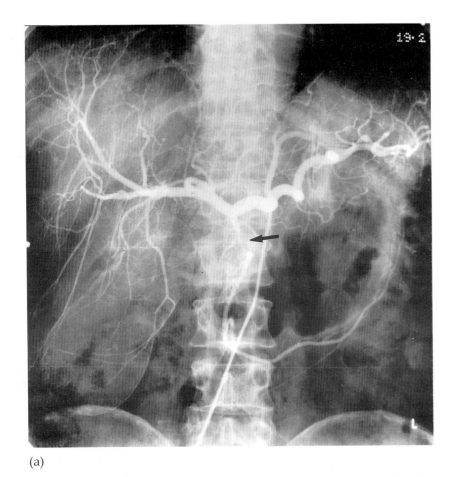

(a)

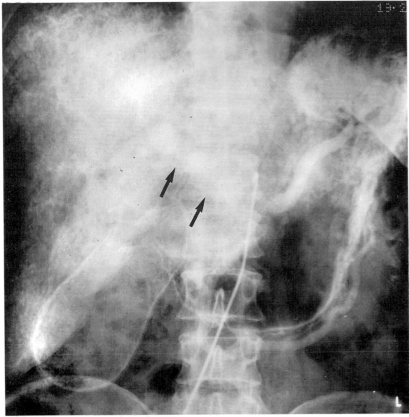

(b)

Fig. 22.16 Sixty-five-year-old restauranteur with carcinoma of head of pancreas. Is it operable? (a) Coeliac arteriogram. *Arrow* indicates encased gastroduodenal artery. (b) Venous phase. *Arrows* show two filling defects in portal vein. Note distended gall bladder.

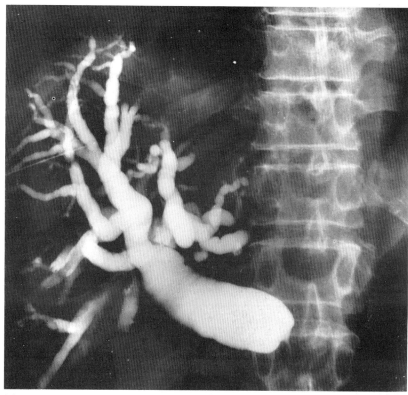

Fig. 22.16 (c) PTC on same patient. Obstruction corresponds to pathology shown in (a) and (b). Inoperable.

(c)

tumour, with limited radiation effects to surrounding healthy tissues. Good results are reported (Karani *et al.*, 1985) and the procedure has a low morbidity. At the end of the course, an endoprosthesis may be left across the stricture. In a patient with a cholangiocarcinoma at the confluence of ducts (Klatskin tumour) this may be done from both sides.

Minicholecystostomy

Cholecystectomy in geriatric patients has a mortality of 8–10% (Burhenne & Stoller, 1985). An alternative approach is a percutaneous cholecystostomy under local anaesthesia in this group to treat calculus disease in both gall bladder and ducts. All gall bladder calculi are removed in one sitting after 7 days, and in 80% the cystic duct may be negotiated. Results are promising, with low morbidity and no mortality. A cholecystectomy is a future possibility. Diagnostic percutaneous aspiration of the gall bladder under ultrasound guidance to establish diagnosis in the ill septic patient with acute cholecystitis is also described (McGahan & Walter, 1985).

Angiography

Most malignant tumours causing obstructive jaundice are poorly vascularized (carcinoma of pancreas, cholangiocarcinoma). Arteriography is useful for demonstrating operability or, in many cases, inoperability. Major arterial encasement, or portal-vein or inferior vena canal involvement firmly point to a non-operative course of management (Fig. 22.16). Occasionally benign tumours (biliary cystadenoma) or cysts such as hydatids compress the bile ducts and can be treated surgically.

Primary liver cancer (hepatoma) and metastases may present as cholestasis. Occasionally embolization will relieve pressure on ducts and jaundice will remit (Fig. 22.17). A mycotic aneurysm of the hepatic artery associated with septicaemia and jaundice has been reported and successfully embolized (Kibbler *et al.*, 1985).

Liver transplantation

Radiology can pin-point the cause of jaundice in this group, rejection, biliary obstruction, and infection being the usual differential diagnoses. As a

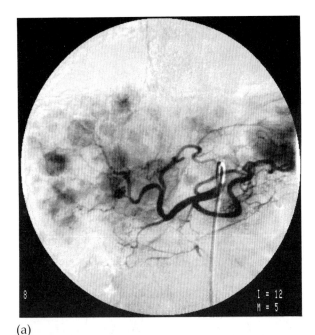

(a)

(b)

Fig. 22.17 DSA study in patient with multiple vascular metastases compressing bile ducts. (a) Arterial phase. (b) Post-embolization. Jaundice regressed.

result of patient immunosuppression, cholangitis may be due to a mix of organisms, including fungi. Percutaneous catheter procedures may be the only means to eradicate infection in ducts over a very long period. Choledochoscopes are introduced percutaneously after the trans-hepatic tract is dilated, to enable piecemeal removal of calculi and fungus material, and if necessary to help find an obstructed major hepatic duct (Fig. 22.18).

Biopsy procedures

Biopsies are amongst the most frequent techniques performed by the diagnostic radiologist A biopsy in the hepatobiliary—pancreatic system is well tolerated and has low morbidity. Jaundiced patients often have coagulopathies and low platelet counts (60 000/mm^3 or less). Both should be corrected as much as possible before biopsy.

The choice of biopsy needle depends upon the information required. For example, if US suggests an echogenic mass at the porta hepatis, a fine-needle aspiration biopsy (FNAB) is indicated. However, a patient who develops cholestasis after a bone marrow or liver transplant will often require a large-needle cutting biopsy (LNCB) to provide the type of histological specimen necessary to decide between rejection, hepatitis, drug reaction, cirrhosis, etc.

A thin-walled 22 gauge needle may safely be directed at any mass under fluoroscopic, US, or CT control. Minimal preparation is required (a short fast), and minimal analgesia, with the patient returning home after a short rest. Some thin needles have a mandril with a furled end (Surgimed) which will loosen cells prior to their aspiration. Repeat imaging is undertaken to check that the needle tip lies within the lesion and vigorous suction performed with a 20 ml luerlock syringe and tap. Whilst maintaining suction, the tap is closed prior to withdrawal of the syringe and attached needle, to prevent suction of non-representative cells during extraction. Ideally a cytologist is available to examine slides immediately in the imaging suite and to advise on the adequacy of the specimen.

FNAB can only confirm the presence of a suspected malignancy; it cannot exclude it. In one series (Ferrucci *et al.*, 1980) FNAB was positive for malignancy in 82% of patients. Only 3% had complications, the most serious being seeding of pancreatic carcinoma along the needle track. This complication is rare, and undoubtedly FNAB has negligible morbidity (Holm *et al.*, 1985).

LNCB is best performed with a Trucut needle (William Cook, Europe). Imaging allows the needle to be directed to a safe part of the liver, avoiding the right pleural recess and lower liver border, whilst if a focal lesion is present, the needle can be

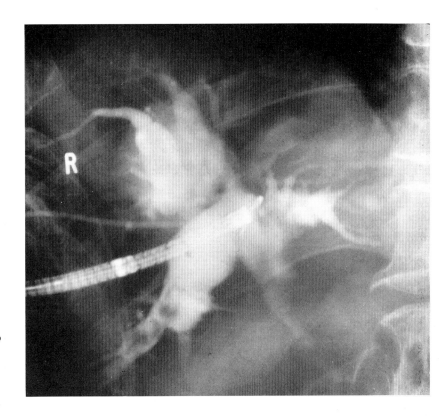

Fig. 22.18 Transplanted liver of 4 years. Dilated ducts with filling defects (right lobe inferiorly) and obstructed common hepatic duct. After trans-hepatic dilatation, a choledochoscope has been introduced 17 Fr.) This confirmed fungi within ducts and found the orifice of the common hepatic duct so that internal/external drainage could be performed after the intrahepatic ducts had been treated with irrigation and antifungal agents.

accurately guided to this site. The interventional radiologist should embolize the needle track with Gelfoam fragments in all jaundiced patients to prevent bile or blood leak.

In patients with grossly compromised clotting, the transvenous method of LNCB remains safest for obtaining tissue. The internal jugular vein is punctured in the neck by an approach from behind the sternomastoid on the ipsilateral side. When the head is turned to the opposite side, the skin site chosen is where the external jugular vein crosses the sternomastoid (Fig. 22.19). Any needle which takes a 0.038-in. guide wire may be used to aspirate from the internal jugular; then a catheter is guided into a right hepatic vein over the wire. Either a modified Ross trans-septal needle (Colapinto & Blendis, 1985) or a Trucut needle on a flexible coaxial cable (Bull *et al.*, 1983) are used to obtain tissue. Should bleeding follow the biopsy, it will occur into the patient's own venous circulation. Puncture of the capsule of the liver from within must be avoided. Should it occur in a small liver, firm manual compression of the upper abdomen must be undertaken for 20 min.

A final method of obtaining tissue is by brush biopsy performed through a trans-hepatic catheter. Bile should also be examined for exfoliated tumour

cells in the first 24 h of external drainage. Unfortunately, with very long periods of drainage, tumour cells have access to the trans-hepatic track, the peritoneal cavity, and the skin surface (Miller *et al.*, 1983).

Percutaneous extraction of retained gall stones

Using a surgically created T-tube track, it is possible to remove duct calculi under fluoroscopic control using steerable catheters or choledochoscopes in conjunction with wire baskets. Less frequently a patient has had an emergency cholecystostomy. Thirty per cent of these will have bile duct stones (Mason, 1985) and it is often possible to negotiate the cystic duct with a J-tipped guide wire and preshaped catheter. Prior to removing any stones via the cystic duct and cholecystostomy, it is usually necessary to dilate the cystic duct with a balloon catheter to at least 15 mm.

T-tube track extraction of retained gall stones was first reported by Mondet (1962) who used pliable forceps, Lagrave *et al.* (1969) first describing the use of a basket. For the confirmation of retained stones after biliary surgery a high-quality T-tube cholangiogram performed 7–10 days after surgery

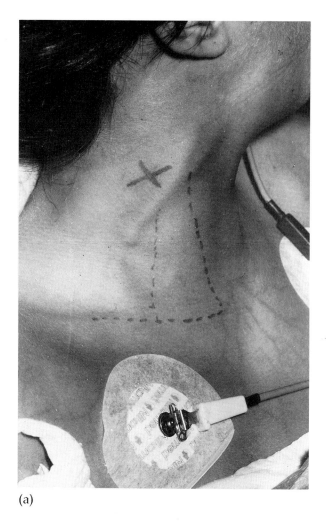 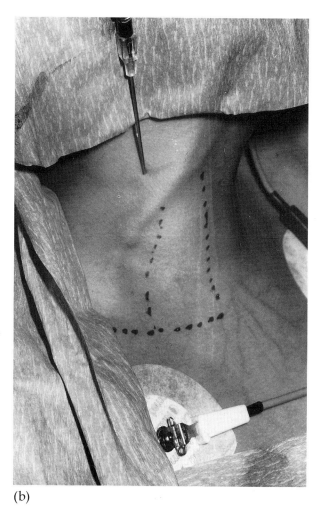

(a)   (b)

Fig. 22.19 Transjugular liver biopsy. (a) Approach to the right internal jugular vein is from behind the sternomastoid (*dotted line*). (b) Catheter inserted into internal jugular vein.

remains a most important examination. Contrast density should be no more than 150 mg iodine/ml. The entire biliary tree must be filled (including the left lobe) and a delay of 2–3 s should be allowed after injection before exposure is made, to allow any moving stones to settle (Fig. 22.20).

Eighty-five per cent of retained stones are situated in the extrahepatic bile ducts. This is fortunate for the radiologist as intrahepatic stones are considerably more difficult to purchase with a basket. Once stones are confirmed, 4–5 weeks should elapse before instrumentation, although this time may be shortened if a very large-calibre tube (18 Fr. or more) is present with a straight exit to skin. Ideally all T-tubes should exit laterally and be at least 14 Fr. They should certainly never be less in diameter than the stones removed at the time of cholecystectomy.

Technique

For the 5-week waiting period, patients may return home with a bile drainage bag. The T-tube is then removed and a surgically clean procedure commenced. A steerable catheter is introduced without anaesthetic into the T-tube track (Fig. 22.21) and negotiated so that the tip lies adjacent to the stone. A basket is chosen with a diameter the size of the duct, and introduced closed within its sheath down the steerable catheter. When just beyond the catheter tip the basket is opened and the catheter slightly withdrawn. Short excursions of the basket will engage the stone in the basket (Fig. 22.22). Next, both basket and stone are withdrawn until resistance caused by their meeting the catheter is felt. The relationship of basket, stone, and steerable catheter are kept constant with one hand, and all

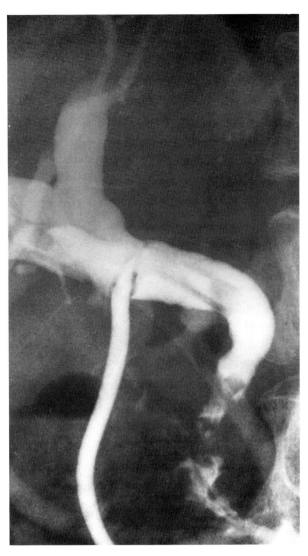

Fig. 22.20 T-tube cholangiogram indicates stone at lower end of common bile duct. Although the T-tube is large, its exit is unfortunately anterior.

are removed as an entity with the other hand. The procedure is repeated until all stones are removed (possibly over several sessions). With each entry to the track, contrast is injected ahead of the steerable catheter to prevent the creation of a false passage.

It is mandatory to keep access to the track until cholangiograms show with total certainty that there are no residual stones. A Foley balloon catheter keeps the track open between sessions. To ensure that the duct is finally free of stones films must be taken, as the resolution of fluoroscopy alone is insufficient to demonstrate all stones.

The success rate for T-tube track stone removal ranges between 70 and 95% (Burhenne, 1974).

Increasing experience greatly improves the rate. A complication rate of 5–10% is inherent in the technique. Serious complications such as track perforation and pancreatitis are rare; fever is not uncommon, and can occur with any manipulative techniques in the bile ducts. The mortality rate of endoscopic sphincterotomy, the alternative method for removal of stones from the common duct is 1% (Cotton, 1984). Clearly if there is T-tube access to retained stones in the bile ducts, then the percutaneous approach is the prime choice.

Electrohydraulic lithotripsy

Initially this was developed in the USSR as an industrial technique to fragment rocks. It has been tried successfully in the biliary tract in jaundiced patients who have multiple chronic diseases which have prevented a conventional approach to cholelithiasis (Lear *et al.*, 1984). Since the shock waves are caused by water vaporization it is critical that the tip of electrode is surrounded by water and not against the bile duct wall, since local heating and penetration have occurred experimentally. Martin *et al.* (1981b) have found in dogs that 80% of biliary calculi have fragmented. Once fragmented, pieces may be flushed through into duodenum or removed piecemeal.

Endoscopic management of biliary obstruction

Since the endoscopic approach to the biliary and pancreatic duct systems was first described by McCune *et al.* in 1968, many interventional procedures have developed to supplement the information obtained from basic pancreatograms and cholangiograms. Endoscopic sphincterotomy using a diathermy has been widely used, the commonest indication being to release calculi in the common duct, when a T-tube is not present in the duct. Stones either pass spontaneously (Fig. 22.23) or are removed with a basket which may also be guided into the cystic duct. Eight per cent of procedures are complicated by cholangitis (the same figure as for a surgical biliary–bowel anastomosis). Endoscopic sphincterotomy has also been used to treat acute cholangitis, acute pancreatitis, and as the sole surgical treatment for small ampullary tumours, especially in the elderly. In acute pancreatitis, early surgery has a 30-day mortality rate of 21%, compared to 5% endoscopic sphincterotomy. Sphincterotomy is also performed prior

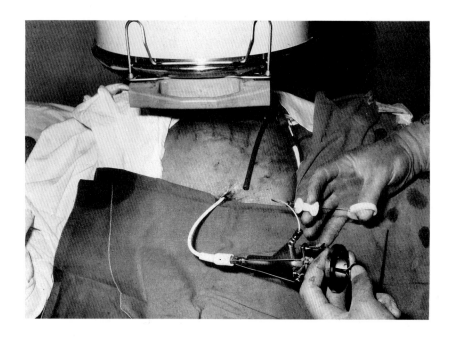

Fig. 22.21 A 16 Fr. T-tube has been removed from its lateral exit (ideal) and a steerable catheter is in the track. Basket and sheath have entered the side port.

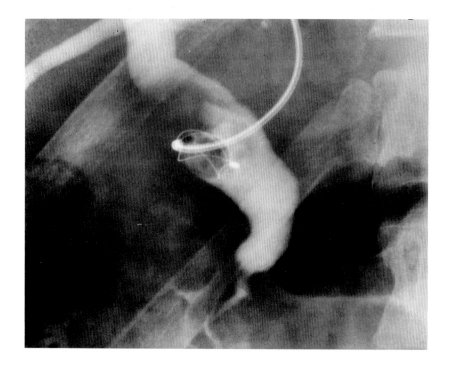

Fig. 22.22 Stone has been engaged in the basket. Same patient as in Fig. 22.20

to passing a nasobiliary tube for the infusion of therapeutic agents in sclerosing cholangitis (Fig. 22.24), or for the insertion of iridium wire to treat cholangiocarcinoma. The role of the radiologist in all these procedures is important in advising on the anatomy of ducts, in interpreting the pathology, and in recording the information. In some centres radiologists in addition to physicians and surgeons are becoming experienced endoscopists.

An endoprosthesis may be placed in the right and/or left biliary duct systems following endoscopic sphincterotomy (Huibregtse & Tytgat, 1982). Conditions treated include carcinoma of the pancreatic head, cholangiocarcinoma (Fig. 22.25), chronic pancreatitis with strictured common bile duct, and acute cholangitis, the stent in the latter condition providing drainage of infected bile into bowel. In an elderly patient with common duct stones, a prosthesis is a very satisfactory method to treat intermittent obstruction. Although the gall

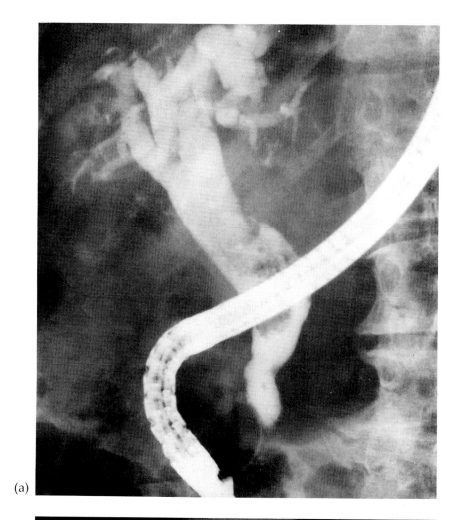

(a)

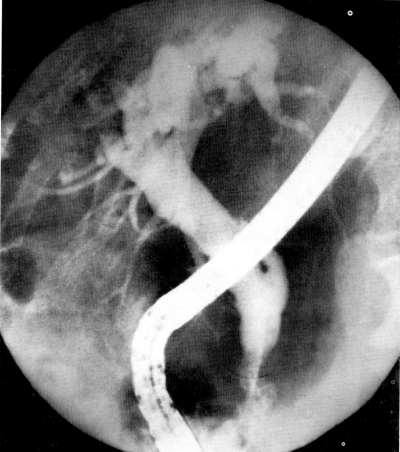

Fig. 22.23 Endoscopic retrograde
cholangiogram in 75-year-old.
(a) Multiple stones in dilated
common bile duct. Endoscopic
sphincterectomy performed.
(b) Repeat study after 1 week. The
stones have passed into the bowel.

(b)

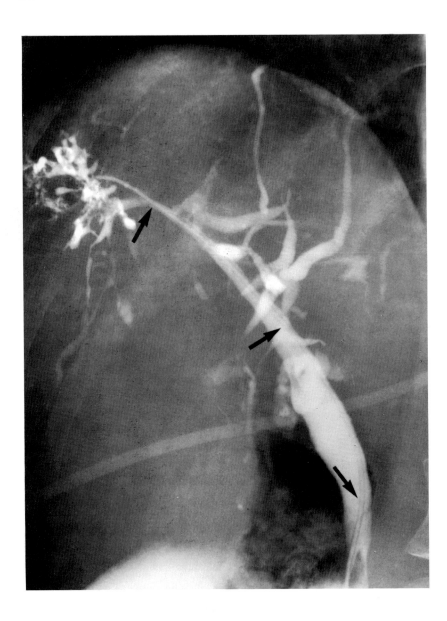

Fig. 22.24 Endoscopic nasobiliary cholangiogram in patient with sclerosing cholangitis (*arrows* = catheter). Saline and corticosteroids are being infused into grossly abnormal ducts peripherally in right lobe.

bladder is invariably diseased as well, it may be possible to avoid a cholecystectomy.

No endoprosthesis has yet been developed that will remain patent in the long term. An 8 Fr. size will remain patent for a median time of 12 weeks. Prostheses of up to 10 Fr. may currently be inserted endoscopically, and a 12 Fr. has been developed, the limitations on larger models being the size of the endoscope itself.

When endoscopic and percutaneous expertise is available at the same hospital, it is clear that the range of treatments available to the patient with obstructive jaundice is multiple. It is wise to try the endoscopic method first, the comparable advantages and disadvantages of each method being shown in Table 22.2. Even though it may appear logical that a percutaneous approach is best for hilar obstructions and an endoscopic for low obstructions, the second-choice procedure will usually succeed if the first fails, and Cotton (1986, personal communication) has achieved relief of cholestasis in 70% of patients with hilar cholangiocarcinoma when an endoscopic prosthesis was inserted into one lobe of the liver only. Patients with benign disease should respond well to any interventional procedure, provided it is done with care and under antibiotic cover. Fouteh & Sivak (1985) are performing endoscopic balloon dilatation of the extrahepatic ducts with promising results.

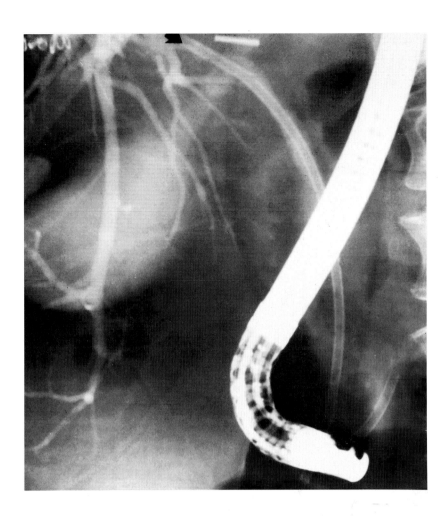

Fig. 22.25 Endoscopic biliary stent (*arrowed*) inserted via endoscope. A blocked percutaneous stent has been removed (bottom right hand corner). Note clip at liver hilum (previous surgery) and wire coils (top left) used to embolize liver tract following earlier biopsy (cholangiocarcinoma).

Table 22.2 Comparison of percutaneous trans-hepatic and endoscopic transpapillary insertion of endoprosthesis

	Percutaneous	Endoscopic
Cost of catheter set	£60–£80	£60–£80
Skill	+++	++++
Success rate (%):		
Overall	85	75
Hilar	75	65
Periampullary	95	85
Previous gastric surgery	Irrelevant	May make impossible
Blockage	Yes	Yes
Ease of replacement	Depends on size and position	Easy
Complications:		
Bile peritonitis	+	–
Haemorrhage	+	+
Septicaemia/cholangitis	+	+
Pancreatitis	–	+
Displacement	+	+

Percutaneous cholecystostomy

Percutaneous puncture of the gall bladder, under ultrasound, cholecystographic or CT control is becoming more widespread in application. Previously, cholecystostomy has been a surgical procedure, but now it is more frequently performed by radiologists (Wiener & Flynn, 1988). Indications include empyema of the gall bladder, underlying carcinoma of the pancreatic head, the dissolution of gall stones using solvents, and the direct removal of them via an operating endoscope. Dissolution is performed by circulating methylterbutyl ether through the gall bladder, whose contained stones must be of cholesterol type. Using a trans-hepatic approach, complications are few, and the average time for stone dissolution in 47 of 48 patients treated successfully in one series was 7.7 h (Thistle, 1987). An expected recurrence rate in

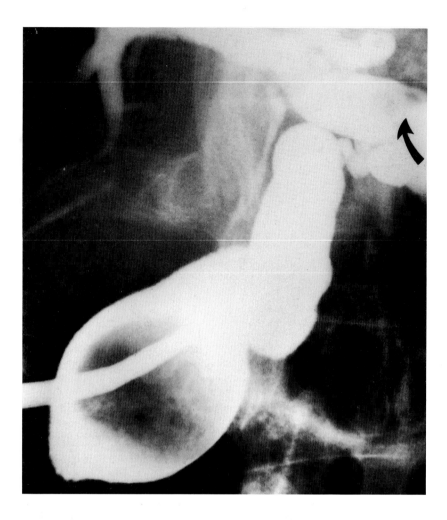

Fig. 22.26 Cholecystostomy with Foley catheter in gall bladder fundus. There are no residual calculi in gall bladder or cystic duct but stones in dilated bile duct (*arrow*) will need removal by cystic duct approach or sphincterotomy.

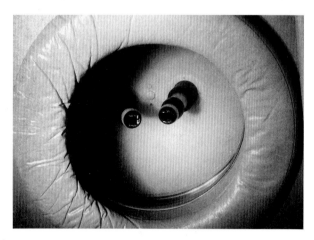

Fig. 22.27 Wolf lithotripter. Photograph shows water-filled bowl into which the patient's right hypochondrium is advanced. The bowl contains over 2000 piezoceramic crystals which generate the shock wave, whilst the two ultrasonic probes are for localization.

40% of patients over 2 years may limit this method and the direct transperitoneal removal of stones from otherwise normal gall bladders may be a more attractive option (Kellett *et al.*, 1988). If the remaining gall bladder and cystic duct could be ablated, then residual anxieties concerning stone recurrence or even the very rare gall bladder neoplasm in these patients should prove groundless (Fig. 22.26).

Other exciting developments involving both imaging and/or interventional skills are the use of pulsed dye laser to fragment stones in the gall bladder or bile ducts, and piezoceramic lithotripsy (Hood *et al.*, 1988). The latter is well-tolerated and safe (Fig. 22.27), but in patients where disintegration of stones is incomplete percutaneous cholecystolithotomy may prove complementary.

References

Baumgarten, C. & von Rottkay, P. (1984) Subcutaneous seeding of a gastric carcinoma metastasis along a trans-hepatic biliary tract — another case. *British Journal of Radiology*, **57**, 542.

Bull, H.J., Gilmore, I.T., Bradley, R.D., Marigold, J.H. & Thompson, R.P. (1983) Experience with transjugular liver biopsy. *Gut*, **24**, 1057−1060.

Burcharth, F. (1982) Nonsurgical drainage of the biliary tract. *Seminars in Liver Disease*, **2**, 78−85.

Burhenne, H.J. (1974) The technique of biliary duct stone extraction. *Radiology*, **113**, 567−572.

Burhenne, J.H. & Stoller, J.L. (1985) Minicholecystectomy and radiologic stone extraction in high-risk patients. *American Journal of Surgery*, **149**, 632−635.

Colapinto, R.F. & Blendis, L.M. (1983) Liver biopsy through the transjugular approach. Modification of instruments. *Radiology*, **148**, 306.

Coons, H.G. & Carey, P.H. (1983) Large-bore, long biliary endoprosthesis (biliary stents) for improved drainage. *Radiology*, **143**, 89−94.

Cope, C. (1983) Stiff fine needle guidewire for catheterisation and drainage. *Radiology*, **128**, 822−823.

Cotton, P.B. (1982) Dyodenoscopic placement of biliary prostheses to relieve malignant obstructive jaundice. *British Journal of Surgery*, **69**, 510−513.

Cotton, P.B. (1984) Endoscopic management of bile duct stones (apples and oranges). *Gut*, **25**, 587−597.

Denning, D.A., Ellison, E.C. & Carey, L.C. (1981) Preoperative percutaneous transhepatic biliary decompression lowers operative mobidity in patients with obstructive jaundice. *American Journal of Surgery*, **141**, 61−64.

Dick, R., Platts, A., Gilford, J., Reddy, K. & Irving, J.D. (1986) The Carey−Coons percutaneous biliary endoprosthesis; a 3 centre experience in 87 patients. *Clinical Radiology*.

Dooley, J.S., Dick, R., George, P., Kirk, R.M., Hobbs, K.E.F. & Sherlock, S. (1986) An evaluation of percutaneous external bile drainage with the results of a randomised controlled trial of preoperative drainage.

Ferrucci, J.T. Jr, Adson, M.A. & Mueller, P.R. (1983) Advances in the radiology of jaundice: a symposium and review. *American Journal of Radiology*, **141**, 1−20.

Ferrucci, J.T. Jr, Wittenberg, J. & Mueller, P.R. (1980) Diagnosis of abdominal malignancy by radiologic fine-needle aspiration biopsy. *American Journal of Radiology*, **134**, 323−330.

Fouteh, P.G. & Sivak, M.V. Jr (1985) Therapeutic endoscopic balloon dilatation of the extrahepatic biliary ducts. *American Journal of Gastroenterology*, **80**, 575−580.

Hatfield, A.R.W., Terblanche, J. & Faraar, S. (1982) Preoperative external biliary drainage in obstructive jaundice. *Lancet*, **ii**, 896−899.

Holm, H.H., Torp-Pedersen, S., Larsen, T. & Juul, N. (1985) Percutaneous fine needle biopsy. *Clinics in Gastroenterology*, **14**, 423−449.

Honickman, S.P., Mueller, P.R. & Ferrucci, J.T. Jr (1982) Malpositioned biliary endoprosthesis. Retrieval using a vascular balloon catheter. *Radiology*, **144**, 423−425.

Hood, K.A., Keightley, A., Dowling, R.H., Dick, J.A. & Mallinson, C.N. (1988) Piezo-ceramic lithtripsy of gallbladder stones; Initial experience in 38 patients. *Lancet*, **i**, 1322−1324.

Huibregtse, K. & Tytgat, G.N. (1982) Palliative treatment of obstructive jaundice by transpapillary introduction of large bore bile duct endoprosthesis; experience in 45 patients. *Gut*, **23**, 371−375.

Jaques, P.F., Mandell, V.S. & Delaney, D.J. (1982) Percu-

taneous transhepatic biliary drainage; advantages of the left lobe subxiphoid approach. *Radiology*, **145**, 534−536.

Kadir, S., Baassiri, A. & Barth, K.H. (1982) Percutaneous biliary drainage in the management of biliary sepsis. *American Journal of Radiology*, **138**, 25−29.

Karani, J., Fletcher, M., Brinkley, D., Dawson, J.L., Williams, R. & Nunnerley, H. (1985) Internal biliary drainage and local radiotherapy with Iridium-192 wire in treatment of cholangiocarcinoma. *Clinical Radiology*, **35**, 603−606.

Kellet, M.J., Wickham, J.E.A. & Russell, R.C.G. (1988) Percutaneous cholecystolithotomy. *British Medical Journal*, **296**, 453−316.

Kibbler, C., Cohen, D., Cruickshank, J., Kushawana, S., Morgan, M. & Dick, R. (1985) Use of CAT scan in the diagnosis and management of hepatic artery aneurysms. *Gut*, **26**, 752−756.

Lagrave, G., Plesses, J.L. & Pougeard-DuGimbert, G. (1969) Lithiase biliare residuelle extraction a la sonde de Dormia par le drain de Kehr. *Mémoires de l'Académie de Chirugie*, **95**, 430−435.

Lear, J.L., Ring, E.J. & Macoviak, J.A. (1984) Percutaneous transhepatic electrohydraulic lithotripsy. *Radiology*, **150**, 589−590.

McCune, W.S., Short, P.E. & Moscovitch, H. (1968) Endoscopic cannulation of the ampulla of Vater. A preliminary report. *Annuals of Surgery*, **167**, 752.

McGahan, J.P. & Walter, J.P. (1985) Diagnostic percutaneous aspiration of the gall bladder. *Radiology*, **155**, 619−622.

Makuuchi, M., Banai, Y. & Ito, T. (1980) Ultrasonically guided percutaneous transhepatic bile drainage. *Radiology*, **136**, 165−169.

Martin, E.C., Fankuchen, E.I. & Schultz, R.W. (1981a) Percutaneous dilatation in primary sclerosing cholangitis. Two experiences. *American Journal of Radiology*, **137**, 603−605.

Martin, E.C., Wolff, M. & Neff, R.A. (1981b) Use of the electrohydraulic lithotriptor in the biliary tree in dogs. *Radiology*, **139**, 215−217.

Mason, R. (1985) Percutaneous extraction of retained gall stones. In Buist, T. (ed.) *Clinics in Gastroenterology*, pp. 403−419. W.B. Saunders, London.

Miller, G.A., Heaston, D.K. & Moore, A.V. (1983) Peritoneal seeding of cholangiocarcinoma in patients with percutaneous biliary drainage. *American Journal of Radiology*, **141**, 561−562.

Molnar, J. & Stockum, A.E. (1978) Relief of obstructive jaundice through percutaneous transhepatic catheters — a new therapeutic method. *American Journal of Radiology*, **122**, 356−367.

Mondet, A. (1962) Tecnica de la extraccion incruenta de los calculos en la litiasis residual del coledoco. *Bulletin Sociedad Cirujia (Buenos Aires)*, **46**, 278.

Moore, P.T. & Clark, R.A. (1984) An update of interventional biliary radiology. *Seminars in Ultrasound, CT and MR*, **5**, 349−368.

Mueller, P.R., van Sonnenberg, E. & Ferrucci, J.T. Jr (1982) Percutaneous biliary drainage: technical and catheter related problems in 200 procedures. *American Journal of Radiology*, **136**, 901−906.

Mura, S., Mueller, P.R. & Ferrucci, J.T. Jr (1983) bile cytology: a routine addition to percutaneous biliary drainage. *Radiology*, **149**, 846−847.

Pogany, A.C. & Kerlan, R.K. Jr (1985) Percutaneous biliary drainage. *Clinics in Gastroenterology*, **14**, 387−402.

Ring, E.J. & Kerlan, R.K. (1984) Interventional biliary radiology. *American Journal of Radiology*, **142**, 31–34.

Russell, E., Yrizarry, J.M., Huber, J.S. *et al.* (1986) Percutaneous transjejunal biliary dilatation; alternative management for benign strictures. *Radiology*, **159**, 209–214.

Summerfield, J.A. & Dooley, J.S. (1986) In Thomas, H.C. & Jones, E.A. (eds) *Recent Advances in Hepatology*, Vol. 2. Churchill Livingstone, Edinburgh.

Summerfield, J.A., Nagafuchi, Y., Sherlock, S., Cadafalch, J. & Scheuer, P.J. (1986) A clinical and histological review of 51 patients. *Journal of Hepatology*, **2**, 145–156.

Suruga, K., Nagashimak, K.S., Miyano, T. & Kitahardt, I.N.

(1982) A clinical and radiological study of congenital biliary atresia. *Journal of Pediatric Surgery*, **7**, 655–659.

Teplick, S.K., Maskin, P.H. & Goldstein, R.C. (1982) A new biliary endoprosthesis made from commonly available catheter material. *American Journal of Radiology*, **139**, 615–617.

Thistle, J.L. (1987) Direct contact dissolution of gallstones. *Seminars in Liver Disease*, **7**, 311–316.

Wiener, H.M. & Flynn, J.D. Jr. (1988) Cholecystostomy case report and literature review. *Journal of the American Osteopathic Association*, **2**, 251–4.

23: Congenital Cystic Dilatation of the Biliary Tract

K.C. TAN AND E.R. HOWARD

Introduction

Choledochal cyst may be defined as a rare congenital dilatation of the common bile duct that is associated not infrequently with a congenital or acquired dilatation of the intrahepatic ducts. Although it was Vater who first reported it in 1748, it was left to Douglas to describe it in detail in a 17-year-old girl in 1852. Since then more than 3000 cases have been reported in the literature. It is most frequently observed in females and is more common in Oriental races especially in people of Japanese origin. The condition predisposes to cholangitis, gall stones and carcinoma, as well as to jaundice and portal hypertension. Without surgical treatment it is universally fatal.

Aetiology

It is usually accepted that choledochal cysts are congenital in origin but the mechanism of their formation remains in doubt. More than 60% of cases are diagnosed before the tenth year of life and there have been recent reports of its observation in fetuses by antenatal sonography (Dewbury et al., 1980, Frank et al., 1981).

Babbitt (Babbitt, 1969) suggested that a congenital malformation of the junction of pancreatic and bile ducts could allow a reflux of pancreatic juice that might cause recurrent cholangitis and eventual fibrosis of the wall of common bile duct. A cholangiographic study of 22 cases reported by Ono (Ono et al., 1982) showed abnormal pancreaticobiliary junctions on 15 occasions and several other studies have revealed common pancreaticobiliary channels greater than 0.5 cm in length. It has been suggested that this anatomic anomaly is the result of faulty budding of the primitive main pancreatic duct more proximally from the common bile duct. The terminal portion of the pancreatic duct therefore lies proximal to the sphincteric muscles of the ampulla of Vater, allowing free reflux of pancreatic juice.

The abnormally long 'common channels' that have been demonstrated on cholangiography distal to the terminal portions of pancreatic and common bile ducts may be important in the aetiology of choledochal cysts (Miyano et al., 1981); the high amylase content of some cysts, the well documented complication of pancreatitis, and the experimental evidence support this concept. However about 30% of cysts do not have a 'common channel' and neither do they contain high levels of pancreatic enzymes. Although the 'common channel' theory remains attractive, developmental factors may still be important; Lilly (Lilly, 1979) has pointed out that abnormal distal anatomy may be only one manifestation of a disordered embryology that may have affected the whole extrahepatic ductal system.

Pathology

The size of the cysts varies enormously, the smallest measuring 1.0–2.0 cm and the largest filling almost the entire abdomen. Characteristically the dilatation starts 1.0–2.0 cm above the duodenum and ends abruptly just below the bifurcation of the common hepatic duct. The cuboidal epithelium of the cyst wall may be intact but in many cases it is ulcerated to such a degree that only small patches of viable cells remain. The wall of the cyst may vary from 2.0–7.5 mm in thickness. Liver histology in a case of uncomplicated cyst may show little change apart from some inflammatory cell infiltration of portal tracts and some periportal fibrosis. Proliferation of bile ductules is a feature in infancy and may be associated with interlobular cholestasis in the neonatal period when it may be confused with the more common biliary atresia.

Several classifications have been proposed but

the scheme prepared by Alonso-Lej (Alonso-Lej *et al.*, 1959) is most commonly used. They divided the cysts as follows: Type I cystic; Type II diverticulum; and Type III choledochocoele (dilatation of intraduodenal common bile duct). Type IV includes cases with both extra and intrahepatic cysts. Todani (Todani *et al.*, 1977) modified it further by dividing Type I cysts into cystic, fusiform or segmental types and added a Type V for cases in which the dilatation was confined to the intrahepatic ducts (Fig. 23.1).

Presentation

Choledochal cyst may present in early infancy; the youngest in our series underwent surgery at 1 month of age. The majority of cases are diagnosed

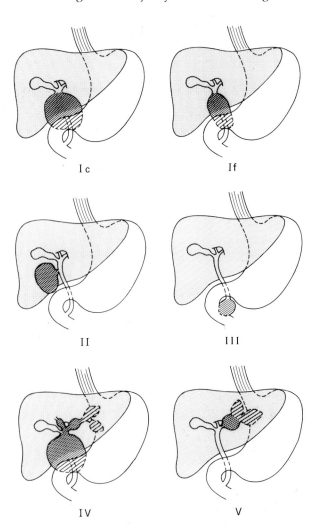

Fig. 23.1 Classification of bile duct cysts. Ic: cystic dilatation, If: fusiform dilatation, II: diverticulum, III: choledochocoele, IV: combination of both extra and intrahepatic cysts, V: dilatation confined to intrahepatic ducts.

in childhood before 10 years of age but occasional cases have been reported as late as the eighth decade.

The order of frequency of the classic signs of jaundice, pain and right hypochondrial mass varies from series to series. The occurrence of all three symptoms and signs in the same patients (classic triad) also varies from 13–63% of reported series (Alonso-Lej *et al.*, 1959). Obstructive jaundice is typically intermittent and is the main feature in infancy, while a mass is a more common finding in later childhood. Jaundice accompanied by fever (cholangitis) is reported more often in adults. Occasionally patients may present with one of the complications such as cholecystitis, pancreatitis, or haematemesis from portal hypertension.

The differential diagnosis of a cyst presenting with a mass in the right hypochondrium includes mucocoele of the gall bladder, hepatic cysts and tumour, neoplasms and cysts of the pancreas and suprarenal gland, kidney lesions, and the rare spontaneous perforation of the bile duct in infancy.

Intrahepatic cystic dilatation

The aetiologic relationship of classical choledochal cysts to intrahepatic cysts and Caroli's disease is unclear (Caroli *et al.*, 1958). Recent cholangiographic observations have revealed at least three types of intrahepatic dilatation:
1 Dilatation secondary to long standing extrahepatic obstruction, which rapidly returns to normal after excision of the cyst (Fig. 23.2).
2 Cystic dilatation of one or more segments of the primary branches of the intrahepatic ducts with normal peripheral ducts. It may be possible to decompress these at the time of extrahepatic cyst excision (Fig. 23.3).
3 Multiple cysts, either saccular or cylindrical, throughout the biliary tree. These may be restricted to one segment and may be amenable to segmental hepatic resection (Fig. 23.4).

Diagnostic studies

The diagnosis of choledochal cyst is frequently delayed as the symptoms are non-specific and variable, and the 'classic triad' is seldom seen. Radiologic studies have always played an important role in its diagnosis. With improving imaging methods in recent years the incidence of correct diagnosis before surgery has been more than 80% (Saito & Ishida, 1974) as compared to about 40%

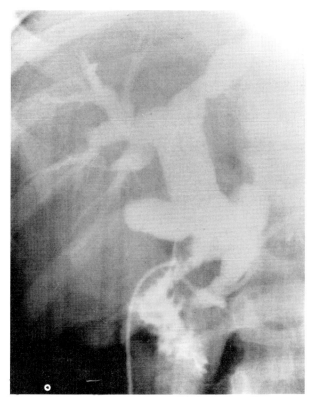

Fig. 23.2 Fusiform dilatation of the common bile duct (Type If) with secondary intrahepatic duct dilatation. Intraoperative cholangiogram in a 3-year-old female child who had suffered several attacks of painless jaundice.

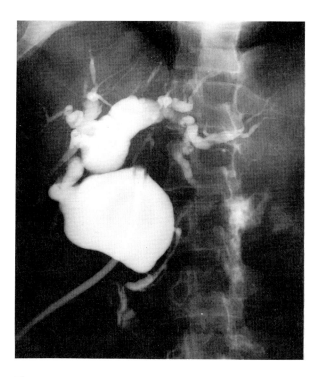

Fig. 23.3 Cystic dilatation of the common bile duct (Type Ic). In addition there is a segmental dilatation of the left hepatic duct. Operative cholangiogram in a 40-year-old woman with a short history of painless jaundice.

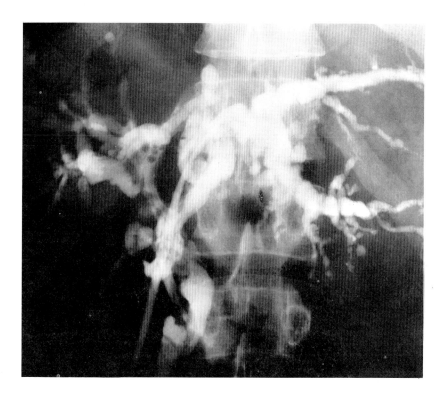

Fig. 23.4 Intrahepatic cystic dilatation (Type IV) in a 39-year-old male patient who presented with severe cholangitis. The dilated ducts contain considerable amount of debris. There was no distal obstruction at the ampulla of Vater. (T-tube cholangiogram.)

previously (Lee *et al.*, 1969). In our series of 21 new patients a correct diagnosis was made pre-operatively in 20 (96%).

The plain radiograph of the abdomen may show an area of soft tissue density continuous with the liver in the right hypochondrium, displacing the gas-filled loops of bowel (Fig. 23.5). Opaque calculi or gas within the cyst have been reported. The cyst wall is rarely calcified.

A barium meal will confirm the gut displacement, with the first and second parts of the duodenum moved anteriorly and to the left. The duodenal loop is usually elongated and stretched with mucosal flattening. It may show oesophageal varices from biliary cirrhosis or from extrahepatic portal vein compression.

Oral and intravenous cholangiography may reveal a cast (Fig. 23.6), but in most cases opacification is poor and the diagnosis may be missed.

Percutaneous transhepatic cholangiography (PTC) and endoscopic retrograde cholangiopancreatography (ERCP) give good visualization of both extrahepatic cyst and intrahepatic ductal anatomy, but they are invasive and difficult to perform in children.

Hepatobiliary scintigraphy with [99m]technetium provides good images and is considered by some to be the investigation of choice (Paramsothy & Somasundaram, 1981). An initial filling defect in the liver followed by a gradual increase in the concentration of radioactivity in the cyst on serial scans is pathognomonic (Fig. 23.7). Scintigraphy is also useful for demonstrating the patency of bile duct–bowel anastomosis after surgery.

Ultrasonography is particularly valuable in the diagnosis of choledochal cyst. Size, contour and position can all be determined and the diagnosis is made if a dilated common duct or hepatic ducts

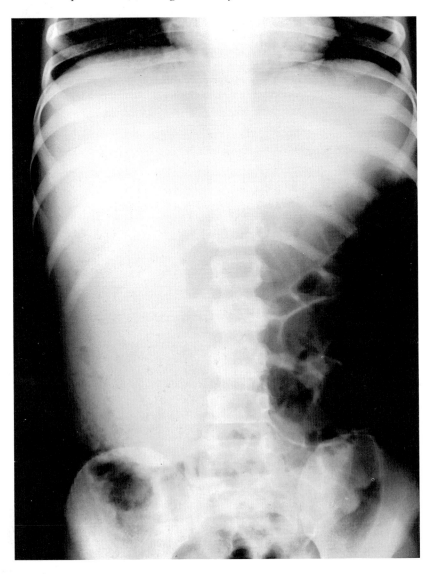

Fig. 23.5 Plain abdominal X-ray of a 7-year-old female child. Opaque mass in the right side of the abdomen representing a large choledochal cyst.

can be demonstrated to enter the cystic mass (Fig. 23.8). High-resolution, real-time scanning is very accurate in determining the anatomy of the intra-hepatic ducts and the confluence of the extra-hepatic ducts.

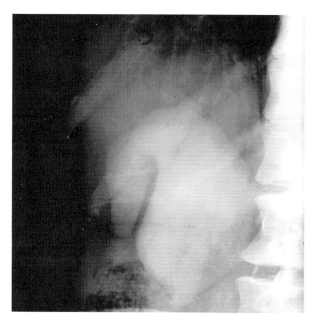

Fig. 23.6 Oral cholecystogram showing cystic dilatation of the common bile duct (Type Ic) and gall bladder in a 50-year-old woman who presented with recurrent right hypochondrial pain.

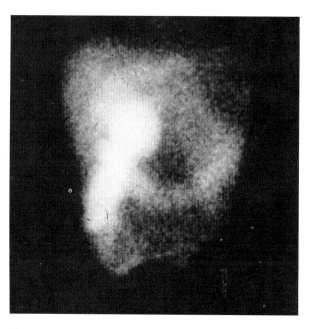

Fig. 23.7 Radionuclide scan which revealed a cystic dilatation of the common bile duct in a jaundiced 4-year-old male child.

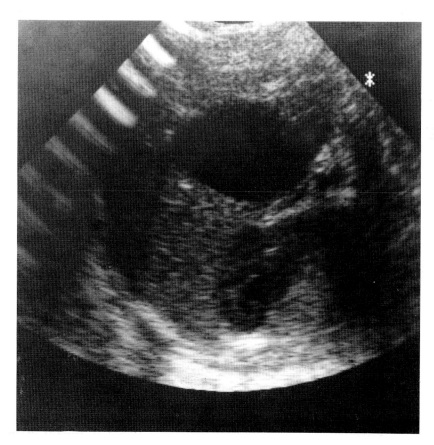

Fig. 23.8 Ultrasound scan of the right hypochondrium which shows a cystic dilatation of the common bile duct in a 2-year-old female child who presented with one episode of painless jaundice.

Computerized tomography (CT) also gives a clear demonstration of the size, extent and the cystic nature of the lesion (Fig. 23.9). It has been reported to be useful in differentiating between congenital and acquired dilatation of the intrahepatic ducts and also when associated carcinoma is suspected (Araki *et al.*, 1980, Cholankeril *et al.*, 1982). In choledochal cyst, significant intrahepatic duct dilatation is limited to the central parts of the duct system, whereas in acquired disease the dilatation tapers gradually towards the periphery.

Operative cholangiogram is useful in defining the type of cyst, the relationship of the common duct with the pancreatic duct and its patency into the duodenum, and the status of the intrahepatic bile ducts (see Fig. 23.3). These findings are important in the planning of the immediate operative procedure.

Surgical treatment

Previously biliary drainage via a choledochocystojejunostomy used to be a popular form of treatment. However the complication and re-operation rate were unacceptably high (Flannigan, 1975). Complete excision of the cyst and reconstruction by Roux-en-Y hepaticojejunostomy is now the treatment of choice (Howard, 1985) and good results have been obtained consistently (Jones *et al.*, 1971, Somasundaram *et al.*, 1985). The operation is relatively safe and we have no mortality in our series of 18 patients. Cyst excision eliminates a reservoir for bile stasis and stone formation and the possibility of continuing reflux of pancreatic juice into the biliary system with resultant cholangitis. The possibility of malignant change, which has been estimated to be twenty times higher than for the general population, is also eliminated.

Acknowledgement

Figures 23.2, 23.3 and 23.6 were reproduced from Howard (1985), with kind permission of the author and Appleton-Century-Crofts.

References

Alonso-Lej, F., Rever, W.B.Jr. & Pessagno, D.J. (1959) Congenital choledochal cyst, with a report of 2 cases and an analysis of 94 cases. *International Abstracts of Surgery*, 108, 1–30.

Araki, T., Itai, Y. & Tasaka, A. (1980) CT of choledochal cyst. *American Journal of Radiology*, 135, 729–734.

Babbitt, D.P. (1969) Congenital choledochal cysts: New etiological concept based on anomalous relationships of common bile duct and pancreatic bulb. *Annals of Radiology*, 12, 231–240.

Caroli, J., Couinaud, C., Soupault, de R., Porcher, P. & Eteve, J. (1985) Une affection nouvelle sans doute congénitale des voies biliaires. La dilatation kystique unilobaire des canaux hepatiques. *Semaine des Hôpitaux de Paris*, 34, 136–143.

Cholankeril, J.V., Ketyer, S. & Joshi, R. (1982) Demonstration of choledochal cyst by computed tomography. *Computerized Radiology*, 6(2), 340–344.

Dewbury, K.C., Aluwihare, M., Birch, S.J. & Freeman, N.V. (1980) Prenatal ultrasound demonstration of a choledochal cyst. *British Journal of Radiology*, 53, 906–907.

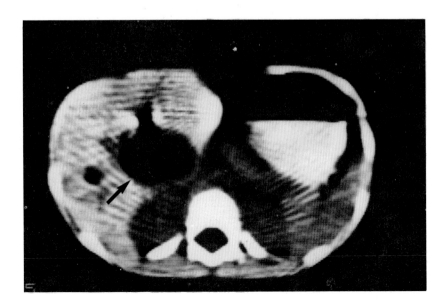

Fig. 23.9 Computerized tomography of the right hypochondrium showing a choledochal cyst (Type Ic) in a 4-year-old male child. Gastrograffin can be seen in the stomach.

Flannigan, D.P. (1975) Biliary cysts. *Annals of Surgery*, **182**, 635—643.

Frank, J.L., Hill, M.C., Chirathival, S., Sfakianakis, G.N. & Marchildon, M. (1981) Antenatal observation of a choledochal cyst by ultrasonography. *American Journal of Radiology*, **137**, 166—168.

Howard, E.R. (1985) In Schwartz, E. (ed) *Maingot's Abdominal Operations*, 8th edn, 1789—1808. Appleton-Century-Crofts, Norwalk, Connecticut.

Jones, P.G., Smith, E.D., Clarke, A.M. & Kent, M. (1971) Choledochal cyst: experience with radical excision. *Journal of Pediatric Surgery*, **6**, 112—120.

Lee, S.S., Mun, P.C., Kim, G.S. & Hong, P.W. (1969) Choledochal cyst, a report of 9 cases and a review of the literature. *Archives of Surgery*, **99**, 19—28.

Lilly, J.R. (1979) Surgery of coexisting biliary malformations in choledochal cyst. *Journal of Pediatric Surgery*, **14**(6), 643—647.

Miyano, T., Suruga, K. & Suda, K. (1981) The choledocho-pancreatic long common channel disorders in relation to the etiology of congenital biliary dilatation and other biliary tract disease. *Annals of the Academy of Medicine, Singapore*, **10**(4), 419—426.

Ono, J., Sakoda, K. & Akita, H. (1982) Surgical aspects of cystic dilatation of the bile duct. An anomalous junction of the pancreatico-biliary tract in adults. *Annals of Surgery*, **195**(2), 203—208.

Paramsothy, M. & Somasundaram, K. (1981) Technetium 99m-diethyl-IDA hepatobiliary scintigraphy in the preoperative diagnosis of choledochal cyst. *British Journal of Radiology*, **54**, 1104—1107.

Saito, S. & Ishida, M. (1974) Congenital choledochal cyst. *Progress in Pediatric Surgery*, **6**, 63—90.

Somasundaram, K., Wong, T.J. & Tan, K.C. (1985) Choledochal cyst—A review of 25 cases. *Australian and New Zealand Journal of Surgery*, **55**(5), 443—446.

Todani, T., Watanabe, Y., Narusue, M., Tobuchi, K. & Okajima, K. (1977) Congenital bile duct cysts: classification, operative procedures and review of 37 cases including cancer arising from choledochal cyst. *American Journal of Surgery*, **134**, 263—269.

Part 4
The Pancreas

24: Pancreatic Imaging — General Considerations

P.A. DUBBINS

The pancreas is an unpaired digestive gland that has exocrine and endocrine functions. It develops from two gut diverticula. The ventral diverticulum gives rise to the liver, gall bladder and bile ducts and contributes the uncinate process and part of the pancreatic head. The dorsal diverticulum is responsible for the remainder of the pancreatic head, the pancreatic body and tail (Wyburn, 1964).

The pancreas is a slender, soft, lobulated organ which extends from the epigastrium to the left hypochondrium about the level of the transpyloric plane lying in the retroperitoneum, behind the omental bursa and in front of the bodies of the first and second lumbar vertebrae (Fig. 24.1). This transpyloric axis is somewhat modified usually with the tail of the pancreas situated more cephalad than the head and being related to the hilum of the spleen and the upper pole of the left kidney. The splenic flexure may be superimposed on the tail of the pancreas but usually lies inferior to it (Fig. 24.2). Occasionally the axis of the pancreas is transverse, and more infrequently the tail may lie caudal to the head. The pancreas measures from

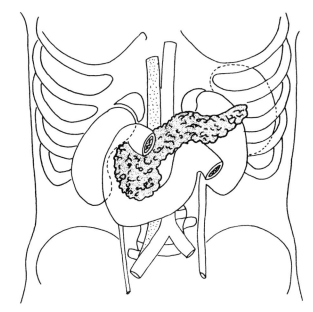

Fig. 24.1 Surface markings and anatomical relations of the pancreas. The transpyloric plane.

12.5 to 15 cm in length, is 3–5 cm in height and between 1.5 and 3.5 cm thick. The thickness of the pancreas varies between the head, neck, body and

Fig. 24.2 Anatomical relations of the pancreas (P), which lies with the head nestled in the 'C' loop of the duodenum (D). The right kidney (RK) forms a right posterolateral relation with the head of the pancreas, while the left kidney (LK) and the spleen (S) form a posterolateral relation to the tail. The splenic flexure (SF) and the stomach (not shown) are anterior relations of the tail and body of the pancreas. The superior mesenteric artery and vein (SMA) and (SMV) and their branches emerge inferiorly, posterior to the neck of the pancreas. GDA = gastroduodenal artery; RA = right adrenal gland; LA = left adrenal gland.

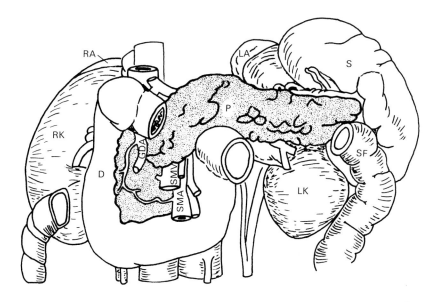

tail, but also varies with age, the pancreas becoming thinner with advancing years (Fig. 24.3, see also Figs 24.38, 24.45).

The head of the pancreas has a constant relationship to the 'C' loop of the duodenum, its right border being flattened as it nestles within the loop. (Figs 24.1, 24.2) Although the branch

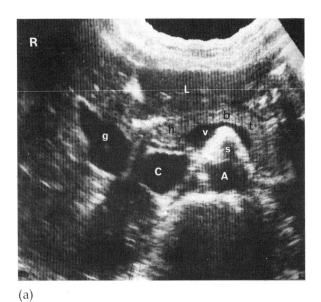

(a)

Fig. 24.3 (a) Transverse ultrasound scan in the transpyloric plane, demonstrating the relationship of the abdominal vasculature to the head, body and tail (h,b,t) of the pancreas. L = liver; g = gall bladder; C = inferior vena cava; A = aorta; s = superior mesenteric artery; v = splenic vein; R = right side.

vessels of the abdominal aorta are important anatomical relations of the pancreas, the relationship of the head of the pancreas to the second and third parts of the duodenum is its most constant landmark. The pancreatic neck lies immediately anterior to the confluence of the superior mesenteric and splenic veins. The body arches laterally and anteriorly and then merges into the tail which extends to the hilum of the spleen.

Anterior relations of the pancreas are the gastric body and antrum, and the duodenal cap. The left lobe of the liver may be related to the body and the gall bladder to the pancreatic head (Fig. 24.4, 24.5). The common bile duct enters the head of the pancreas after passing posteriorly to the first part of the duodenum in the free edge of the lesser sac into its cephalad and ventral margin (Fig. 24.6). It passes dorsally and inferiorly to join with the pancreatic duct of Wirsung as it enters the posteromedial aspect of the duodenum through the major papilla (Fig. 24.7). The pancreatic duct follows a variable course through the pancreas, receiving between 20 and 35 ductules as it travels from tail to head. The duct drains through two routes, the main duct of Wirsung into the major papilla and the accessory duct of Santorini to the anterior aspect of the duodenum via the minor papilla (Fig. 24.8). The accessory duct is occasionally rudimentary, may be occluded or on occasion may drain a portion of the pancreas completely

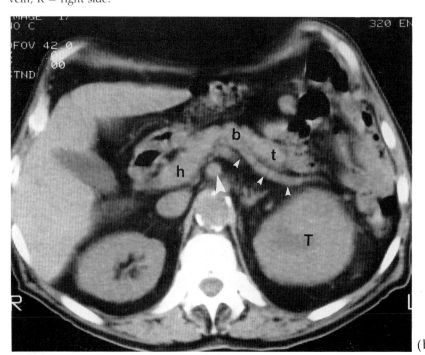

Fig. 24.3 (b) CT scan at a similar level in a different patient, showing the head, body and tail (h,b,t) of the pancreas and the relationship to the superior mesenteric artery (*large arrowhead*) and the splenic vein (*small arrowheads*). T = tumour in the upper pole of the left kidney. *Comment*: It is unusual to see the entire pancreas on a single CT scan. (b) (See text.)

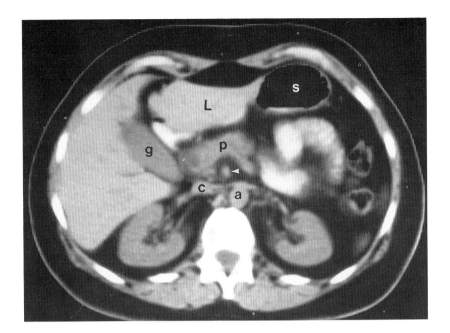

Fig. 24.4 CT scan showing the relationship of the pancreatic head to the gall bladder (g), the pancreatic neck and proximal body to the left lobe of the liver (L), and the position of the stomach (s) and small bowel. The inferior vena cava (c) the aorta (a), and the superior mesenteric artery (*arrowhead*) as posterior relations of the pancreas are shown.

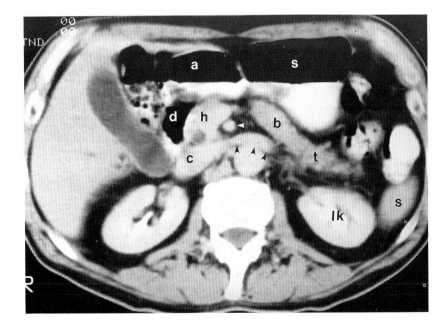

Fig. 24.5 CT scan demonstrating the anatomical relations of the head, body, and tail of the pancreas (h,b,t). The antrum (a) and body (s) of the stomach are shown as anterior relations of the head and body, while the duodenal loop (d) and the gall bladder are anterolateral relations of the head. The inferior vena cava (c) forms a posterior relationship to the head of the pancreas. The position of the superior mesenteric artery (*white arrowhead*) and of the left renal vein (*black arrowheads*) in relationship to the neck and body of the pancreas are well shown. The relationship of the tail of the pancreas to the left kidney (lk) and the spleen (s) is illustrated. Incidentally, there is dilatation of the common bile duct in the head of the pancreas.

separately from the major ducts (pancreas divisum) (Sugawa *et al.*, 1987).

Blood supply (Figs 24.9, 24.10; Reuter & Redman, 1972)

The pancreas is fed by branches of the coeliac axis and superior mesenteric arteries. The coeliac trunk arises just cephalad to the pancreas. The common hepatic artery courses to the right in close relation to the neck and subsequently the head of the pancreas, here dividing to give rise to the gastro-duodenal artery and the proper hepatic artery. The gastroduodenal artery courses inferiorly, lying ventral to the head of the pancreas, giving rise to anterior and posterior superior pancreatico-duodenal arteries, which supply the head of the pancreas and join the anterior and posterior inferior pancreaticoduodenal arteries, which derive from the superior mesenteric artery,

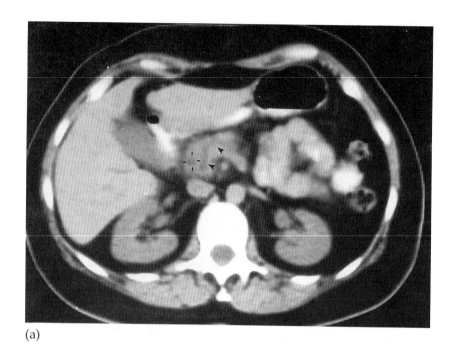

(a)

Fig. 24.6 (a) CT scan showing the relative positions of the common bile duct (as marked) and the pancreatic duct (*arrowheads*) in the head of the pancreas. Both of these are dilated, allowing easier recognition.

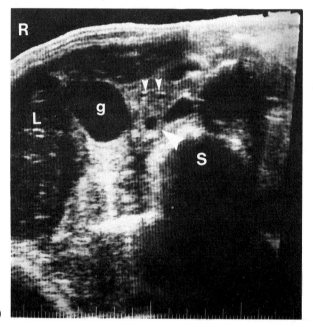

(b)

Fig 24.6 (b) Ultrasound scan demonstrating anatomical relations of the head of the pancreas, illustrating the common bile duct (*large arrowhead*) and branches of the pancreatic arcade (*small arrowheads*). The gall bladder (g) is an anteromedial relation of the head of the pancreas. L = liver; LS = spine.

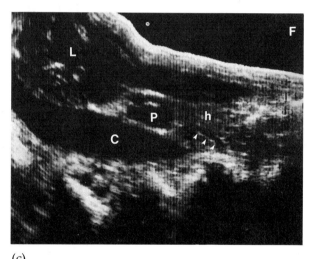

(c)

Fig. 24.6 (c) Longitudinal, oblique ultrasound scan showing the head of the pancreas (h) and its relationship to the inferior vena cava (C) and portal vein (P). L = liver. The *small arrowheads* indicate the course of the common bile duct within the pancreatic head. F = feet.

producing the pancreatic arcades. The splenic artery arises from the coeliac trunk and follows an undulating course along the superior aspect of the body of the pancreas, occasionally becoming embedded within the pancreatic parenchyma and giving supply to the dorsal pancreatic artery, which also takes origin from the coeliac axis and superior mesenteric arteries following a longitudinal course within the body and tail. Occasionally one of the vessels of supply from the splenic artery to the pancreas is larger than the others and is then termed the pancreatica magna. The superior mesenteric artery arises from the anterior surface of the aorta, coursing caudally and emerging from

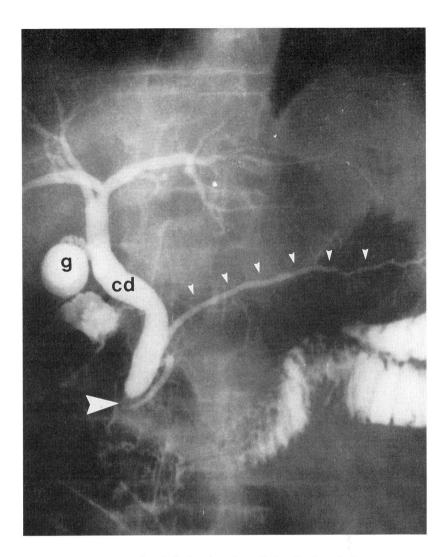

Fig. 24.7 ERCP demonstrating the anatomical relations of the pancreatic duct (*small arrowheads*) and the common bile duct (cd). The *large arrowhead* points to the ampulla of Vater and its relationship to contrast in the duodenum. The gall bladder (g) is also shown. The common bile duct is slightly dilated.

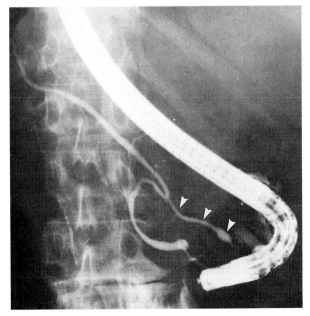

Fig. 24.8 ERCP demonstrating freely patent accessory duct of Santorini (*arrowheads*). (Patient in prone position).

the inferior border of the body of the pancreas, passing anterior to the uncinate process where it forms a landmark for sectional imaging. Venous drainage is via small veins from the body and tail of the pancreas directly into the splenic vein, which lies adjacent to the posterior superior aspect and runs to the right to join the superior mesenteric vein posterior to the neck of the pancreas, thus forming the portal vein. The inferior pancreatico-duodenal veins drain the head of the pancreas into the superior mesenteric vein, while the posterior superior pancreaticoduodenal veins join the portal vein directly.

Anatomical variations

These include variations in pancreatic position and variation in arterial branches. Although the pancreas and duodenal loop are retroperitoneal structures and therefore theoretically fixed, the pancreas may lie as low as the sacral promontory

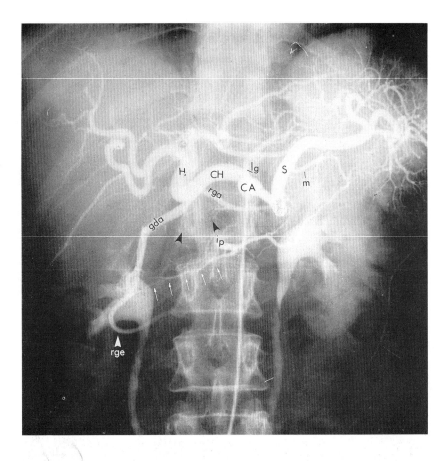

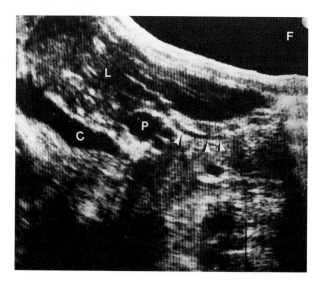

Fig. 24.9 Coeliac axis angiogram showing the origin of the common hepatic (CH), the left gastric (lg) and the splenic (S) arteries. The right gastric artery (rga) and the gastroduodenal artery (gda) are also shown; there is retrograde filling of the inferior pancreatic artery (ip). The blood supply to the pancreas in terms of the posterior pancreatic arcade (*arrowheads*), taking origin from the gastroduodenal artery proximally and the right gastric artery and anterior pancreatic arcade (*white arrows*) is shown. The pancreatica magna artery arising from the splenic trunk (m) should be noted. rge = right gastroepiploic artery.

(Fig. 24.11) or may even lie totally to the left of the mid-line (Fig. 24.12). Although changes in the position of the pancreas may be caused by surgery (a left nephrectomy causing displacement of pancreas to the left, for example), such displacement may occur in the absence of operative procedures (Dunn & Gibson, 1986).

The peripancreatic vascular anatomy is of vital importance to the imager, providing landmarks for the demonstration of the pancreas. However, there are multiple and frequent variations in vascular origin and course (Michels, 1955). Indeed, the so-called normal arrangement of hepatic and splenic arteries arising from the coeliac axis, with superior mesenteric artery supplying only pancreas and small and large gut, is present only in just over one-half of cases. The most common anatomical variant seen in pancreatic imaging is where the right lobe of the liver is partially or completely supplied by an artery arising from the superior mesenteric trunk (Figs 24.13, 24.14). In this case the aberrant hepatic artery will pass posterior to the head of the pancreas and then may lie either anterior or posterior to the portal vein in the porta hepatis.

24.10 Longitudinal oblique ultrasound scan just to the right of the mid-line, demonstrating the gastroduodenal artery (*arrowheads*), coursing through the head of the pancreas, and related the portal vein (P). L = liver; C = inferior vena cava; F = front.

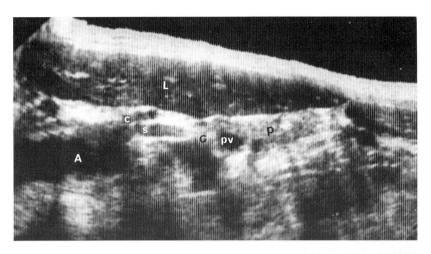

Fig. 24.11 Longitudinal ultrasound scan of the upper abdomen showing the origin of the coeliac axis and superior mesenteric artery (c,s) from the anterior surface of the aorta (A). The relationship of the pancreas (p) to the portal vein (pv) should be noted. G = gas in the pyloric antrum; L = Liver. In this patient the unusually caudal position of the pancreas should be noted.

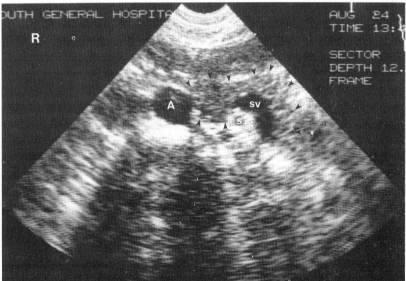

Fig. 24.12 Transverse ultrasound scan in the region of the transpyloric plane. In this patient the pancreas (*arrowheads*) lies completely to the left of the aorta (A) but retains a constant relationship to the superior mesenteric artery (s) and the splenic vein (sv).

Age-related change

Even in the absence of disease the pancreas gradually decreases in size with increasing age. Pancreatic tissue becomes gradually replaced by fat and fibrous tissue, and the organ often assumes a more lobular outline. This natural ageing process has implications for the interpretation of pancreatic images (May & Gardiner, 1987). (see Figs 24.3, 24.38, 24.45).

Methods of pancreatic imaging

Introduction

There are many different indications for imaging the pancreas. Patients may present with relatively non-specific symptoms such as epigastric pain, diarrhoea, or collapse. Although pancreatic pain is classically described as epigastric radiating to the back, this is not invariable and may also be seen in other conditions such as leaking aortic aneurysms. Frequently in conditions such as acute pancreatitis, pain will be accompanied by symptoms, signs, and biochemical features that limit the validity of imaging techniques for primary diagnosis, which should then be reserved for the diagnosis of complications.

Pancreatic imaging forms an integral part of the investigation of jaundice when it has been established that the jaundice is obstructive in nature. A pancreatic carcinoma may present in this way, but similarly may present with distant metastases, an epigastric mass, pain, or non-metastatic complications of malignant disease such as thrombophlebitis migrans. Other tumours may present as

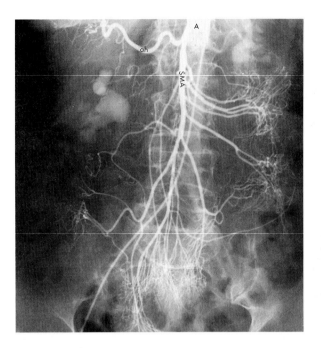

Fig. 24.13 Selective superior mesenteric arteriogram (SMA). There is in this case an accessory hepatic artery (ah) serving the right lobe of the liver. A = aorta.

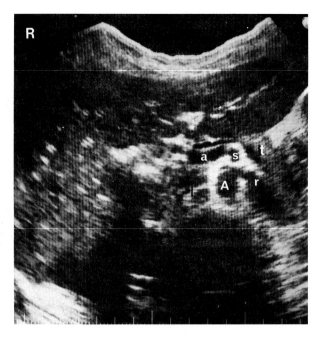

Fig. 24.14 Transverse ultrasound scan just below the transpyloric plane, demonstrating an aberrant origin of an accessory hepatic artery (a) from the superior mesenteric artery (s). The tail of the pancreas (t), the aorta (A), and left renal vein (r) are also shown.

a result of endocrine activity, in which case pancreatic imaging is required to localize rather than to diagnose the tumour.

Finally, the patient may present with symptoms of pancreatic insufficiency, in which not only functional but morphological tests may prove of value in the demonstration, for instance, of occult carcinoma and chronic pancreatitis.

Because of the multiple modes of presentation of pancreatic disease there is no clear-cut algorithm for the investigation of the pancreas. The author has therefore considered different imaging modalities separately; in each case attempting to stress those areas in which the technique has particular application.

Plain radiography

CHEST FILMS

Features suggestive of pancreatic disease seen on a plain chest X-ray include pleural effusions (usually left-sided) and basal atelectasis in association with diaphragmatic elevation in acute pancreatitis and its complications (Fig. 24.15). Occasionally pancreatic pseudocysts may extend into the mediastinum where they may present as smooth, rounded masses in either anterior or posterior mediastinum. Pulmonary metastases, particularly small multiple nodules and the linear and nodular shadowing of lymphangitis carcinomatosa, may represent the first feature of a pancreatic carcinoma. There are features on the chest X-ray characteristic of cystic fibrosis of the pancreas and these features may be used to indicate the severity of the disease, but they will not be considered here.

ABDOMINAL FILMS (Geokas *et al.*, 1985)

The supine abdominal film will usually suffice but occasionally erect lateral decubitus, oblique, and lateral films will facilitate the detection of pancreatic disease. Punctate calcification in the pancreatic bed is indicative of chronic pancreatitis (Fig. 24.16). The degree of calcification varies in extent and density but does not bear any relation to endocrine deficiency (Lankisch *et al.*, 1986). Frequently the calcification may overlie the vertebral bodies, and oblique or lateral views of the abdomen may be necessary for adequate demonstration (Fig. 24.17). Pancreatic calcification may occur in cystadenocarcinoma of the pancreas but this is extremely rare.

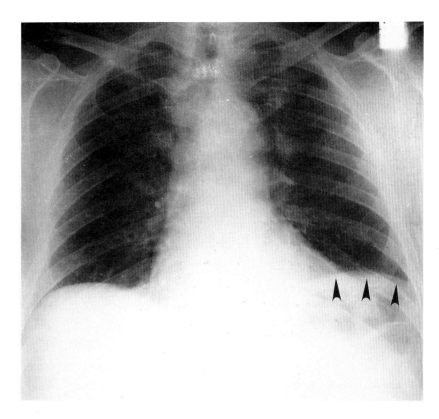

Fig. 24.15 Chest X-ray demonstrating elevation of the left hemidiaphragm with some blunting of the left costophrenic recess in a patient with acute pancreatitis.

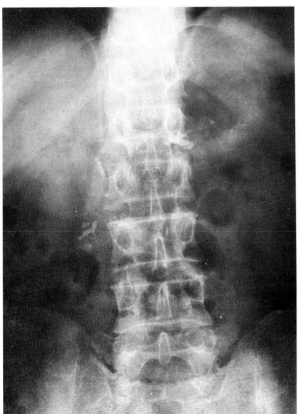

Fig. 24.16 Plain abdominal film showing punctate calcification in the bed of the pancreas in a patient with chronic pancreatitis.

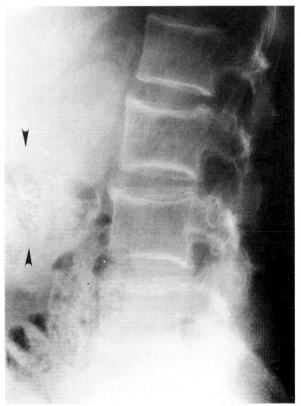

Fig. 24.17 Lateral film of the abdomen demonstrating pancreatic calcification (*arrowheads*) not visualized on the AP film because of superimposition upon the lumbar vertebrae.

In acute pancreatitis there may be paralytic ileus commonly affecting the duodenum, the transverse colon, or a loop of jejunum. Focal loop ileus is said to be characteristic of acute pancreatitis and is referred to as a 'sentinel loop' (Fig. 24.18). There may be blurring of the left renal outline and of the left psoas margin. Many of these signs while occurring frequently in acute pancreatitis occur also in other conditions and are therefore not specific (Field, 1984).

It is occasionally possible to identify soft-tissue mass lesions on plain radiography both by increase in density and by displacement of adjacent organs. (Fig. 24.18) The diagnosis of a pseudocyst may be suggested on this basis. Furthermore, in the right clinical setting, the demonstration of a mass containing gas bubbles is highly suggestive of a pancreatic abscess.

Contrast radiological studies

BARIUM STUDIES (Trenkner & Laufer, 1984)

The double-contrast barium meal utilizing smooth-muscle relaxant and gaseous distension has to a large extent supplanted the tubed hypotonic duodenogram, and produces satisfactory mucosal coating of the duodenum and distension of the duodenal lumen (Fig. 24.19). Widening of the duodenal loop may be seen in any process that causes pancreatic enlargement, but effacement of the medial duodenal folds (Fig. 24.20), and more particularly mucosal destruction, are features of carcinoma of the pancreatic head (Fig. 24.21). Acute pancreatitis may cause inflammatory thickening of the mucosal folds of the duodenum. Occasionally the barium study may reveal the cause of pancreatitis, such as annular pancreas or posterior perforating duodenal ulcer.

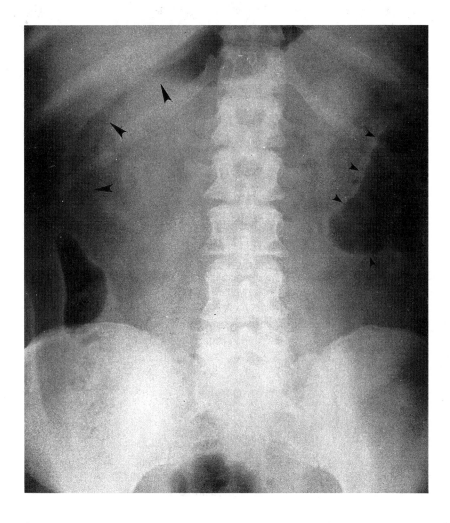

Fig. 24.18 Plain abdominal film in a patient with acute pancreatitis. There is distortion of the gas shadow of the antrum of the stomach and widening of the duodenal loop (*large arrowheads*) as well as dilated sentinel loops of small bowel (*small arrowheads*).

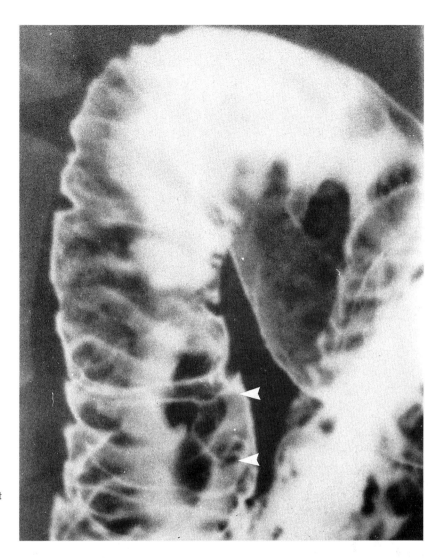

Fig. 24.19 Normal 'C' loop in a tubeless hypotonic duodenogram performed as part of a double-contrast barium meal. The normal appearance of the duodenal mucosa and the major papilla (*arrowheads*) is shown.

CHOLECYSTOGRAPHY

The use of modern contrast media during imaging of the gall bladder regularly allows the demonstration of the common bile duct. Dilatation of the duct may allow the inference of a pancreatic lesion but is not specific.

PERCUTANEOUS TRANS-HEPATIC CHOLANGIOGRAPHY

This is often used to evaluate a patient in whom the diagnosis of obstructive jaundice has been made by ultrasound (US) or computerized tomography (CT) by the demonstration of dilated ducts.

A 22 gauge (Chiba) needle is inserted into the liver from the right lateral approach. Dilute contrast medium (e.g. Hypaque 45) is slowly injected under fluoroscopic control as the needle is gradu-

ally withdrawn until contrast is seen to enter the duct system. Contrast is then continuously injected until all the intrahepatic ducts are filled (usually between 20 and 40 ml), when the needle is withdrawn. Changing the patient position to prone and erect will usually provide adequate filling of the common bile duct. Distal obstruction is characterized by one or more intraluminal filling defects in the presence of calculus obstruction. Pancreatitis may produce a long stricture. Pancreatic carcinoma may produce an abrupt or tapering obstruction (Fig. 24.22), or there may be an irregular stricture or occasionally nodular intraluminal filling defects. High duct obstruction may be seen with porta hepatis nodes secondary to a carcinoma in the body or tail of the pancreas.

The use of a fine needle carries only a low risk of biliary leak or significant haemorrhage. However,

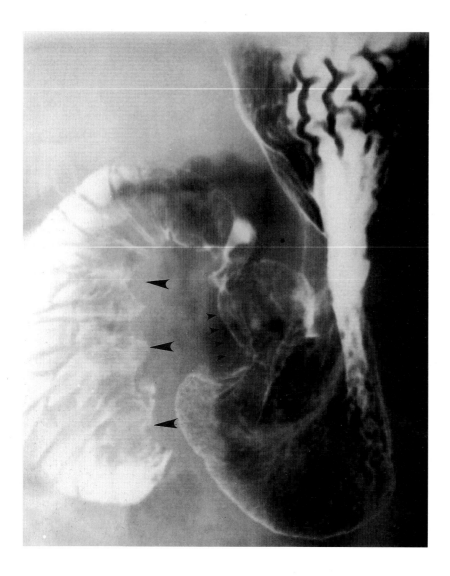

Fig. 24.20 Double-contrast barium meal showing widening of the duodenal loop, distortion and irregularity of the antrum of the stomach (*small arrowheads*), and effacement and some destruction of the mucosal folds of the duodenum (*large arrowheads*) in a patient with carcinoma of the head of the pancreas.

clotting factors should be corrected, if necessary, prior to the technique; the patient should be given antiobiotic cover (80 mg gentamicin with the premedication) and a surgeon should be involved in patient management prior to puncture (May & Gardiner, 1987).

ENDOSCOPIC RETROGRADE CHOLANGIOPANCREATOGRAPHY
(Classen & Phillip, 1984)

Endoscopic retrograde cannulation of the bile and pancreatic ducts allows opacification of these ducts with water-soluble contrast in approximately 80% of cases. The endoscopic technique has a further advantage, however, of allowing biopsy of peri-ampullary lesions, papillotomy, and interventional procedures such as the placement of a biliary stent.

Contrast injection into the pancreatic duct is performed under fluoroscopic control at a pressure insufficient to cause parenchymal filling (Fig. 24.23). Spot films are taken in prone, left posterior oblique, right posterior oblique, and occasionally lateral positions; the supine position is occasionally necessary to fill the pancreatic tail. In spite of care, infection or pancreatitis occurs in approximately 2% of cases and the complication rate is higher in the presence of pancreatic pseudocyst.

The duct tapers gently from its maximum diameter in the head to a minimum diameter in the tail (Fig. 24.24). The upper limits of normal for pancreatic duct diameter at ERCP are 6.5, 5.0 and 3.0 mm, respectively, for the head, body, and tail, although the diameter of the duct increases with age. There are between 20 and 30 side-branches, although the number of these that fill decreases

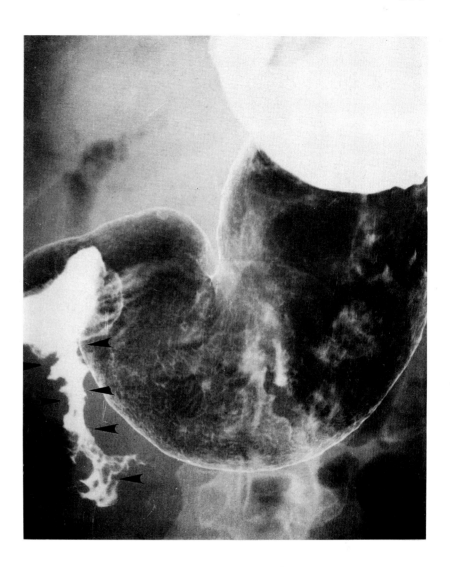

Fig. 24.21 Double-contrast barium meal in extensive pancreatic carcinoma demonstrating widespread mucosal destruction in the duodenal loop (*arrowheads*).

with advancing years (Fig. 24.25). Diagnostic criteria of ERCP are based on evaluation of the duct diameter, the degree of filling of side-branches, and the speed of drainage of the duct (Fig. 24.26). Duct dilatation and beading occurs in chronic pancreatitis, together with underfilling, truncation, and sometimes cystic dilatation of the branch ductules (Fig. 24.27). Duct strictures and occlusions occur in neoplastic disease although they may also occur particularly in focal acute pancreatitis (Fig. 24.28). The double-duct sign with dilatation of both the common bile duct and of the pancreatic duct is strongly suggestive of malignant disease of the pancreatic head (Fig. 24.29). It is possible to combine digital subtraction techniques to achieve greater parenchymal detail during ERCP but this technique appears to carry a greater risk of pancreatitis, presumably because of a tendency to attempt to achieve greater branch filling (Lavelle *et al.*, 1985).

ANGIOGRAPHY (Lunderquist, 1985, Reuter & Redman, 1972; see Figs 24.8, 24.9)

The role of angiography in the evaluation of pancreatic disease has undergone a period of re-evaluation since the advent of non-invasive imaging procedures such as computerized tomography and ultrasound. Indications for angiography have become much more limited. However, there remains a role occasionally in the determination of operability of pancreatic tumour as well as in the demonstration of small islet-cell tumours of the pancreas. (Even in these areas dynamic computerized tomography and high-resolution endoscopic ultrasound may eventually replace the angiogram.)

The technique involves the selective catheterization of both the coeliac axis and the superior mesenteric artery, normally by the Seldinger approach. It may be necessary to use subselective

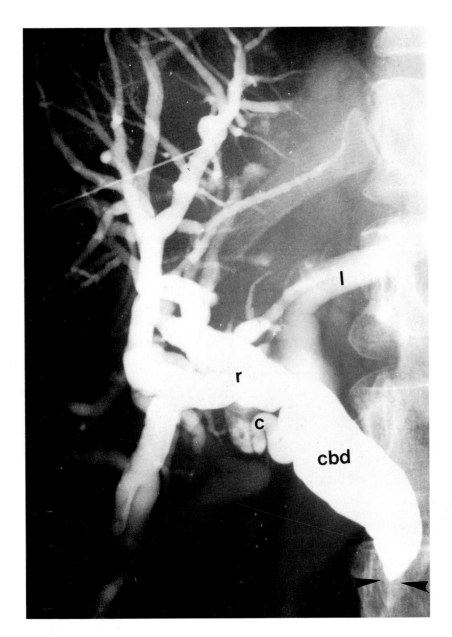

Fig. 24.22 Percutaneous trans-hepatic cholangiogram in a patient with pancreatic carcinoma showing the site of the needle puncture in a branch of the right hepatic duct (r). The left hepatic duct (l) is rather less well filled, although this is not unusual. All the ducts are markedly dilated. cbd = common bile duct; c = cystic duct. The site of the obstruction is identified by the *arrowheads*.

injections of the hepatic and splenic arteries or even superselective gastroduodenal and dorsal pancreatic catheterization to improve pancreatic arterial filling, although clearly the more selective the catheterization the more difficult the technique (Fig. 24.30). Adrenaline may be given prior to injection to augment pancreatic filling, as the pancreatic vessels tend to constrict less in response to intra-arterial adrenaline than do the hepatic vessels. Films are taken throughout the arterial phase, but the procedure also includes delayed films to evaluate the venous phase. Film subtraction, magnification, and digital subtraction all may improve diagnostic accuracy (Fig. 24.31). Vessels in the body and tail of the pancreas are best

filled during splenic injection, while those in the head are best filled during injection of the hepatic and superior mesenteric arteries. Arterial filling is commonly followed by a parenchymal flush that continues into the early venous phase. The frequency of arterial variants has already been described and clearly these are often encountered during pancreatic angiography.

Angiography is rarely used in the inflammatory diseases of the pancreas although abnormalities of vessel calibre and course do occur. More importantly however is its use in the demonstration of vascular complications such as aneurysm and pseudoaneurysm formation consequent upon the inflammatory disease.

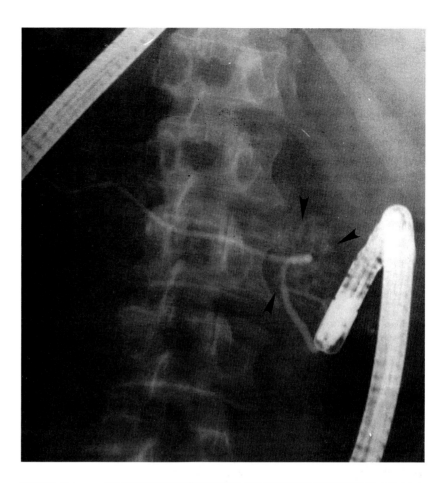

Fig. 24.23 Prone oblique film in an ERCP in which can be seen some parenchymal filling (*arrowheads*) in the region of the pancreatic head.

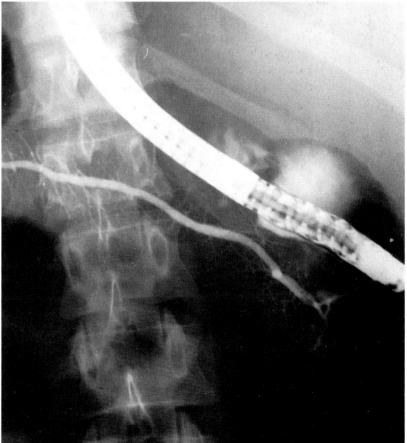

Fig. 24.24 Normal ERCP (prone) in a 24-year-old woman. The calibre of the duct and the side-branch filling is well shown.

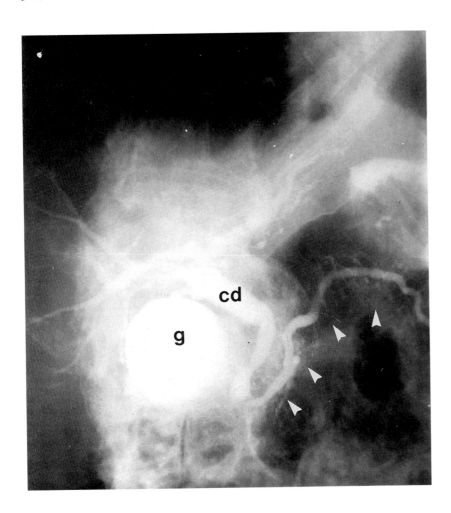

Fig. 24.25 Normal pancreatogram in an 84-year-old man. The duct calibre on this supine oblique view is rather greater, as is the calibre of the common bile duct (cd). There is rather less filling of the side-branches (*arrowheads*). g = gall bladder.

In the evaluation of pancreatic carcinoma, angiography has to a large part been replaced by other imaging techniques. Angiographic changes that occur are subtle and difficult to interpret, but encasement and distortion of vessels are predictive signs of inoperability (Fig. 24.32). However, in the localization of functioning islet-cell tumours, angiography is extremely accurate, up to 80% of insulinomas being correctly identified by this means. Most tumours are identified by a dense tumour blush (Fig. 24.33), but there is also frequently vessel displacement. Angiography is less reliable in the demonstration of gastrinomas, partly because the tumours are smaller as a general rule, but also because they are frequently less vascular. Digital subtraction angiography (DSA) appears to offer little advantage because of reduced spatial resolution, and small tumours are therefore difficult to identify (Ariyama *et al.*, 1986).

PERCUTANEOUS TRANS-HEPATIC PORTOGRAPHY AND SPLENIC VENOGRAPHY

This procedure is the direct catheterization of the portal venous system by trans-hepatic needle and subsequent catheter placement. The procedure allows not only the opacification of the venous system draining the pancreas, but also direct portal venous sampling for the accurate localization of hormonally active pancreatic tumours.

SCINTIGRAPHY (Gross *et al.*, 1984)

The role of isotope imaging has to a large extent been supplanted by the sectional imaging techniques and ERCP. [75]Selenomethionine had been the most widely used radiopharmaceutical, but even with the use of differential subtraction studies using colloid liver scans, the sensitivity

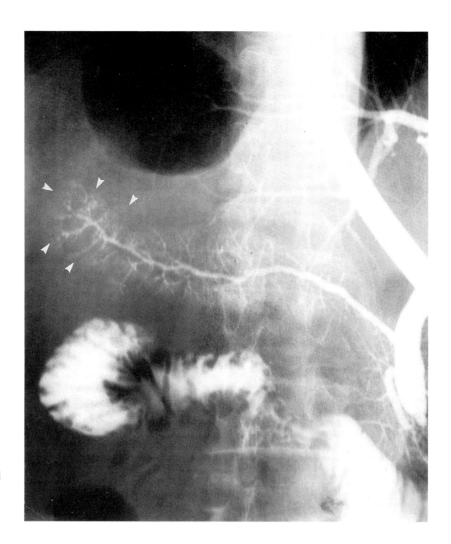

Fig. 24.26 Prone oblique view of the pancreatic duct in a patient with mild chronic pancreatitis with some duct ectasia, particularly notable in the region of the tail (*arrowheads*).

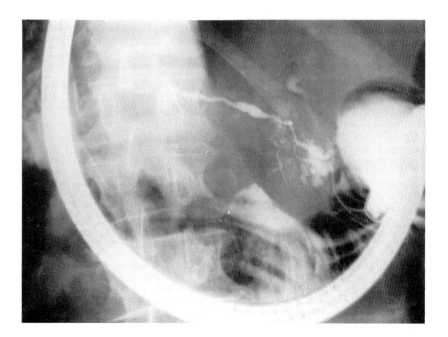

Fig. 24.27 ERCP in a patient with severe chronic pancreatitis. Prone oblique view. There is marked duct ectasia in the region of the head of the pancreas, together with multiple focal stenoses and dilatations.

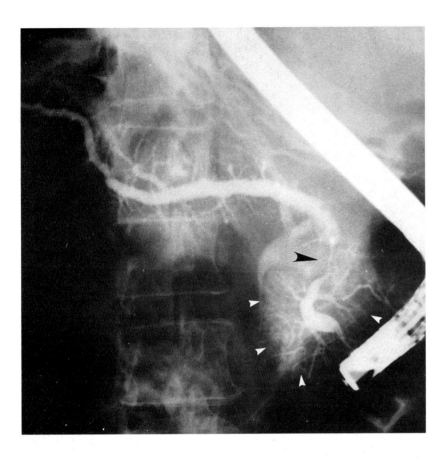

Fig. 24.28 Prone oblique ERCP in a patient with a focal stricture (*large black arrowhead*) caused by a pancreatic carcinoma. There is significant side-duct and parenchymal filling in the region of the head of the pancreas (*small white arrowheads*) because of the pressure required to fill the more proximal pancreatic duct, which is significantly dilated.

and more particularly the specificity of the technique has remained poor. Tomographic techniques such as longitudinal multiplane emission tomography (LMET) or positron emission tomography (PET) have improved specificity, but these improvements have not been sufficient to supplant CT and ultrasound using current techniques, and therefore there is little place for isotope imaging of the pancreas. Although some studies suggest that [111]Indium-labelled leukocyte imaging in pancreatitis may be a useful predictor of complication rate, this seems unlikely to better that predicted by CT (Anderson *et al.*, 1986).

New pancreas-seeking radiopharmaceuticals are currently being evaluated. Of these several isotopes of zinc may hold some promise, although perhaps the most exciting possibility is the use of labelled monoclonal antibodies for the demonstration of pancreatic tumours and metastases. These techniques are, however, currently only experimental (Montz *et al.*, 1986, Fujibayashi *et al.*, 1986 a,b).

ULTRASOUND IMAGING (Kurtz & Goldberg, 1984, Meire, 1984)

Ultrasound imaging in pancreatic disease remains one of the mainstays for diagnosis in spite of imaging difficulties. CT more reliably demonstrates the entire gland, and certain diseases of the pancreas, specifically acute pancreatitis, by producing focal ileus, give rise to conditions that interfere markedly with adequate imaging of the pancreas by ultrasound (Fig. 24.34). However, the diagnosis of acute pancreatitis is unlikely to depend on imaging techniques, but is made on the basis of clinical presentation and biochemical findings. Ultrasound is thus used for the assessment of complications, and while CT may be superior in the diagnosis of pancreatic abscess, the demonstration of pancreatic pseudocyst by ultrasound is reliable, and pseudocyst follow-up is probably best performed by this technique.

Two generalizations are, however, perhaps worth making. These are that in general the obese

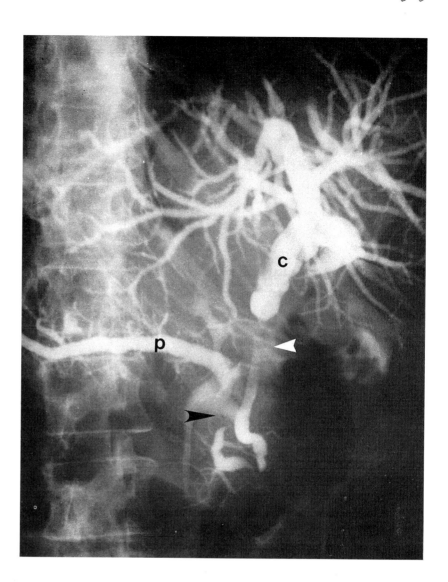

Fig. 24.29 ERCP demonstrating the double-duct sign of pancreatic tumour, with strictures in the common bile duct (c) and the pancreatic duct (p) identified by the *arrowheads*.

patient is better examined by CT, the thin patient by ultrasound, and while CT is better for visualization of the whole pancreas, ultrasound better demonstrates parenchymal abnormalities of the pancreatic head. The spatial resolution of endoscopic and operative ultrasound appears to be better than CT.

Advances in transducer design and electronic focusing have improved pancreatic resolution. Furthermore, the advent of real-time ultrasound has improved the flexibility of the technique and consequently improved the visualization of the pancreas. Ultrasound frequencies of between 3.5 and 7.5 MHz are used, depending upon the proximity of the pancreas to the anterior abdominal wall. The patient is examined in the supine, both posterior oblique positions, and in the erect position (Figs 24.35, 24.36). Changes in patient pos-

ition alters the relative position of adjacent organs. Specifically, in the erect position the liver descends into the abdomen rather more than the pancreas, and the left lobe may then be used as an acoustic window to visualize the pancreatic body and head. The right posterior oblique position will displace gas from the duodenal cap and may allow small amounts of fluid to enter the duodenal loop, thus allowing better identification of the head of the pancreas and of the distal common bile duct. The tail of the pancreas may be demonstrated in the prone position but is more reliably identified on coronal scans using the spleen as an acoustic window (Paivansalo & Suramo, 1986). All these changes in patient position may be augmented by the ingestion of water. (Although other fluids may be used, this is the simplest and cheapest, and is also extremely effective!) (Fig. 24.37). Water will dis-

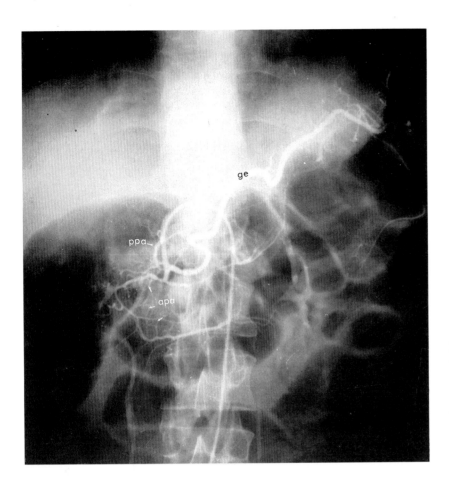

Fig. 24.30 Selective catheterization of the gastroduodenal artery showing the proximal origin of the posterior pancreatic arcade (ppa) and the vascular supply from the terminal branch, the anterior pancreatic arcade (apa). The other terminal branch, the gastroepiploic artery (ge) can also be seen.

place gas from the body and antrum of the stomach and will frequently displace other bowel loops and allow the stomach to be used as an acoustic window for more complete pancreatic visualization. However, in spite of these technical improvements the pancreas is inadequately visualized in up to 15% of cases, and possibly more in patients with a diagnosis of acute pancreatitis. The pancreatic tail is least reliably demonstrated by ultrasound.

Prior to improvements in ultrasound imaging the location of the pancreas was inferred by the position of various marker vessels. Although pancreatic parenchyma can now be clearly visualized these marker vessels remain important for the delineation of anatomy, the recognition of anatomical variants, the determination of scan planes, and most particularly for the identification of the small atrophic pancreas. The position of the pancreas relative to these vessels may, however, vary as has been stated (see Fig. 24.10). Similarly there may be dynamic changes in position of the pancreas in individual patients, depending upon whether the patient is erect or supine or in one or

other of the oblique or decubitus positions. Such changes in position may also alter the shape of the pancreas, the more dependent portion appearing more bulky.

The parenchymal texture of the pancreas varies with increasing age. In childhood the reflectivity of the pancreas is slightly less than, or equal to, that of the liver: the reflectivity of the pancreas gradually increases with advancing age so that in the elderly pancreatic tissue is sufficiently reflective to be indistinguishable from the surrounding peripancreatic fat (Fig. 24.38a,d). These changes in reflectivity are probably related to the gradual fatty replacement of the pancreas with age, and this postulate is supported by correlation with CT appearances. The changes are furthermore important, since changes in pancreatic reflectivity have been correlated with pancreatic disease. Where such changes are focal, such as the decreased reflectivity that occurs in most pancreatic carcinomata, interpretation is relatively easy, but when the changes are diffuse, the reporting of either increased or decreased reflectivity would really

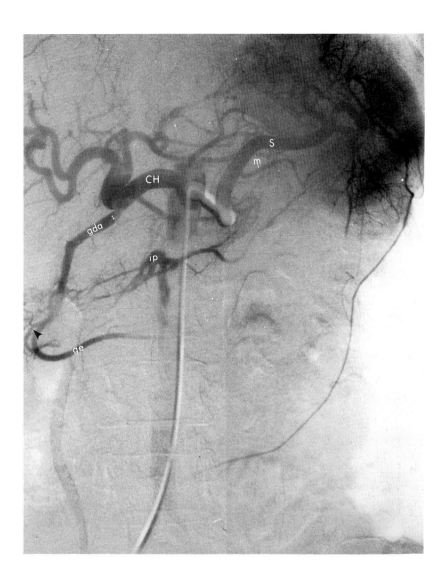

Fig. 24.31 Film subtraction angiogram of the coeliac axis with retrograde filling of the inferior pancreatic artery (ip). gda = gastroduodenal artery; ge = gastroepiploic artery; m = pancreatica magna artery; CH = common hepatic; S = splenic artery. *Arrowhead* identifies the origin from the gastroduodenal artery of the anterior pancreatic arcade.

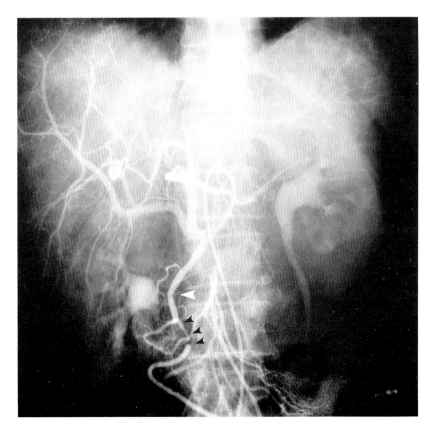

Fig. 24.32 Coeliac axis angiogram in a patient with a carcinoma of the pancreatic head. Abnormal angulation and splinting of the gastroduodenal artery are identified at the *large white arrowhead*. There is narrowing and encasement of the vessels in the region of the anterior pancreatic arcade (*arrowheads*).

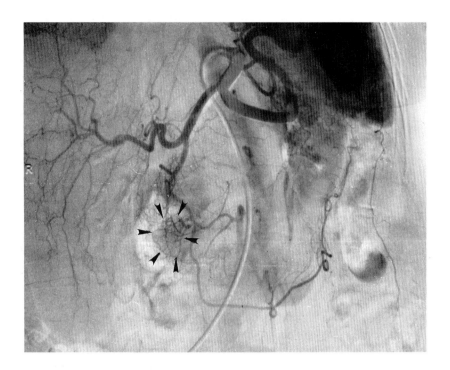

Fig. 24.33 Film subtraction angiogram of a coeliac axis injection showing neovascularity and a tumour blush in a patient with an insulinoma (*arrowheads*).

demand a knowledge of the appearance of the organ prior to the onset of pancreatic disease, since changes in pancreatic reflectivity do not occur at predetermined ages. Thus in a patient of 40 years a normal pancreas may be occasionally equally reflective to the liver, most commonly slightly more reflective than the liver, and occasionally very much more reflective than the liver.

The pancreatic duct may be seen in up to 90% of normal ultrasound examinations. It is uncommon, however, to demonstrate more than short segments of the duct, and these are most commonly seen in the region of the neck and body when the duct is at right angles to the ultrasound beam (Figs 24.38a, 24.39b). The most frequent appearance is that of a single or double linear reflection without a demonstrable lumen, although luminal diameters of up to 2 mm are normal and in some cases a luminal diameter of 3 mm has been seen in an apparently normal pancreas.

Morphological changes indicative of disease

Ultrasound may demonstrate enlargement, either focal or diffuse, alterations in echo texture, and alterations in duct calibre (Fig. 24.39). If tumours are insufficiently large to cause enlargement of the gland, these may be missed on CT but identified on ultrasound on a basis of reduced reflectivity (Fig. 24.40). Acute pancreatitis may produce enlargement of the gland with diffuse decrease in reflectivity (Fig. 24.41). Extrapancreatic involvement may be demonstrated and used as a prognostic sign in similar fashion to CT for the development of complications, *vide infra* (Jeffrey *et al.*, 1986). Chronic pancreatitis may display inhomogeneous increase in reflectivity, duct dilatation, and calcification (Fig. 24.42). The 'bright pancreas' of chronic pancreatitis is, however, of-ten indistinguishable from the normal elderly pancreas.

Pancreatic pseudocysts either in the pancreatic bed or elsewhere in the abdomen are reliably identified by ultrasound and this represents the technique of choice for follow-up (Fig. 24.43).

Ancillary findings of pancreatic disease can be demonstrated by ultrasound. Gall stones may be demonstrated within the gall bladder, and biliary obstruction can be identified. Increased reflectivity of the liver with effacement of portal vein walls and rounding of the inferior margins is a non-specific sign, but may identify cirrhosis secondary to alcohol excess and may also be seen in children with cystic fibrosis, in addition to the reduction in size of the gland and increased reflectivity seen in this condition (Swobodnik *et al.*, 1985, McHugo *et al.* 1987). Occasionally even fluid-filled loops of bowel are identified as paralytic ileus in response to pancreatitis. Although ultrasound is a reliable method for demonstration of pancreatic pseudocysts, the presence of ileus and of gas actually

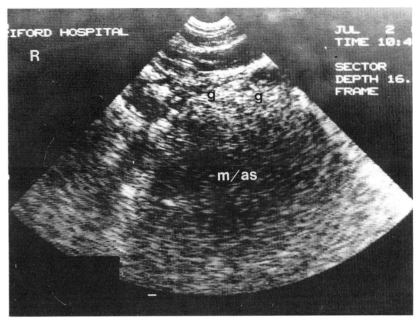

(a)

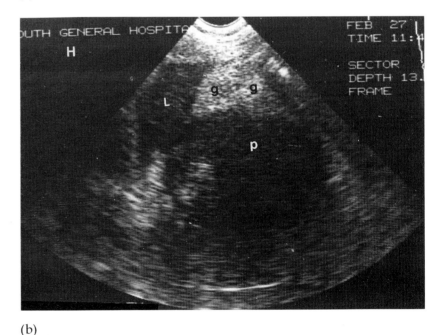

(b)

Fig. 24.34 (a) Transverse ultrasound scan in the region of the transpyloric plane, demonstrating a mass in the pancreas (m) obscured by the acoustic shadow (as) produced by abdominal bowel gas (g).
(b) Longitudinal ultrasound scan in the region of the head of the pancreas. Here acoustic shadowing from bowel gas (g) produced the false impression of a large mass in the head of the pancreas (p). H = head; L = liver.

within the lesions makes it less suitable than CT for the investigation of pancreatic abscess or pancreatic phlegmon.

Operative ultrasound (Smith *et al.*, 1985, Bowerman *et al.*, 1985)

It is now possible to use sterilizable high-frequency transducers at operation. The transducer is placed directly on the pancreas or within 'a water delay' achieved by forming a sump of saline within the wound. Direct application of the high-frequency transducer to the pancreas at the time of surgery allows accurate localization of certain smaller tumours, particularly those of islet-cell origin. It may also be used to guide open biopsy and aspiration.

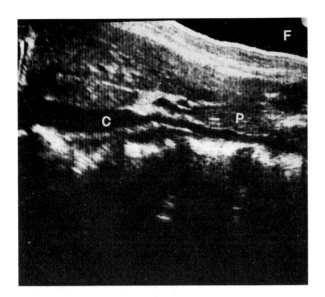

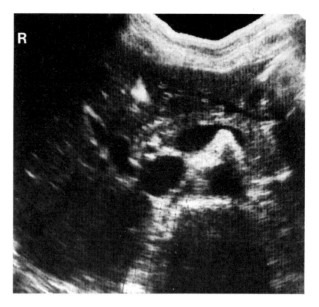

Fig. 24.35 Longitudinal scan demonstrating the normal pancreas. The head of the pancreas (P) forms a slight impression on the anterior surface of the inferior vena cava (C). F = foot.

Fig. 24.36 Transverse scan demonstrating the normal pancreas.

Endoscopic ultrasound (Lux & Heyder, 1986, Sivak & Kaufman, 1986)

It has recently become possible to combine a modified flexible endoscope with small real-time ultrasound transducers incorporated into the tip of the endoscope. Although this technique has inherent difficulties related to some loss of flexibility of the endoscope, some loss of optical field of view, a limited ultrasound field of view, and limited ultrasound tissue penetration, it has the advantage of allowing higher-frequency and therefore higher-resolution ultrasound to be used

without recourse to operation. Several reports attest to its value in the diagnosis of small pancreatic tumours and also in the demonstration of subtle or mild chronic pancreatitis. The technique is currently limited by the inherent inflexibilities and equipment cost, but certainly appears to have a role in the investigation of obscure pancreatic pain and in the preoperative evaluation of islet-cell tumours (Lees, 1986).

Doppler

Doppler techniques have a limited role. It is poss-

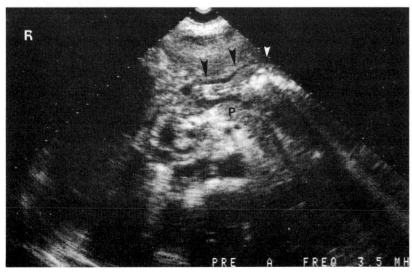

(a)

Fig. 24.37 (a) Transverse scan in the transpyloric plane of the pancreas (P) partially obscured by gas in the stomach (*arrowheads*).

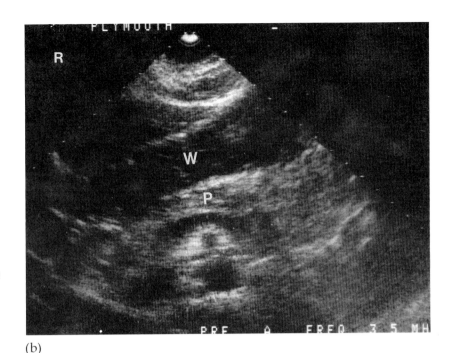

Fig. 24.37 (b) Following the ingestion of water the pancreas (P) is more clearly seen through the water (W) within the body of the stomach. The water is used as an acoustic window.

(b)

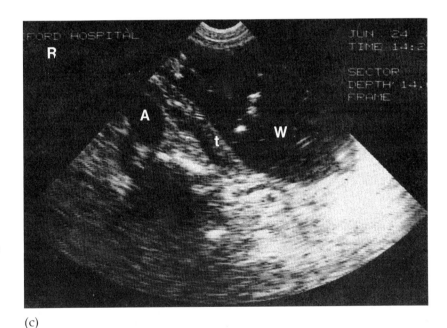

Fig. 24.37 (c) The tail of the pancreas (t) is more clearly seen with the patient in the left decubitus position, when water collects in the body of the stomach (W). A = aorta.

(c)

ible to demonstrate blood flow when there is difficulty in differentiating ducts from vessels. Aneurysms and pseudoaneurysms may be confirmed by the demonstration of blood flow. It may be possible to identify tumour encasement by alterations of flow characteristics within pancreatic vessels, but this is currently experimental.

Computerized tomography (May & Gardiner, 1987, Donovan, 1983)

Demonstration of the pancreas with CT has always been reliable, but reduction of scanning times below 5 s and the achievement of slice thicknesses of between 2 and 5 mm has resulted in improved resolution. The examination is performed after the administration of oral contrast medium: approximately 300 ml of dilute contrast (either water-soluble or barium sulphate, e.g. Ezcat) are given

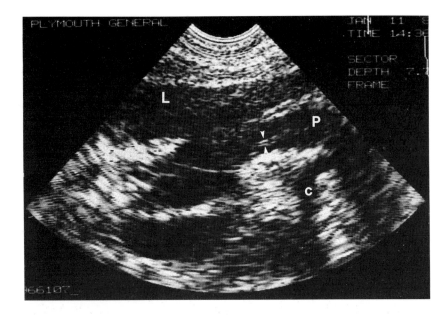

Fig. 24.38 Different pancreatic reflectivity with increasing age. L = liver; P = pancreas; sv = splenic vein; s = superior mesenteric artery; A = aorta. (a) The *small arrowheads* show a portion of pancreatic duct. The pancreas is somewhat cephalad in its position, being related to the coeliac axis (C). The pancreas is less reflective than the liver.

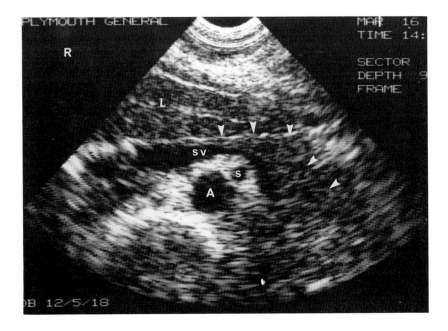

Fig. 24.38 (b) The *large arrowheads* identify the outline of the pancreas. A = aorta; sv = splenic vein; s = superior mesenteric artery. The pancreas is of equal reflectivity to the liver.

between 30 min and 1 h prior to the examination, and a further 300 ml immediately prior to the scan. Intravenous contrast enhancement is usually employed either by bolus or slow infusion. Although either technique will allow the demonstration of marker vessels such as the coeliac axis, the superior mesenteric arteries, and splenic and superior mesenteric veins, a separate rapid bolus injection immediately prior to dynamic scanning may allow the demonstration of the pancreatic vessels, and indeed a tumour blush. A scout film or digitized radiograph is usually obtained prior to commencing sequential slices to determine the upper limit (the dome of the right hemidiaphragm) and lower limit (the tip of the right lobe of the liver) of the examination. Section intervals are usually between 5 and 10 mm with contiguous slicing. The patient is usually examined supine, although the right lateral decubitus position may allow contrast to enter the duodenal loop.

Factors that contribute to suboptimal imaging include metallic surgical clip artefact, and a similar

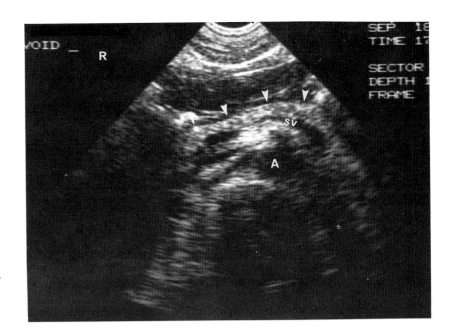

Fig. 24.38 (c) Note the outline of the pancreas, the aorta (A) and splenic vein (sv). Pancreatic reflectivity is greater than that of fat.

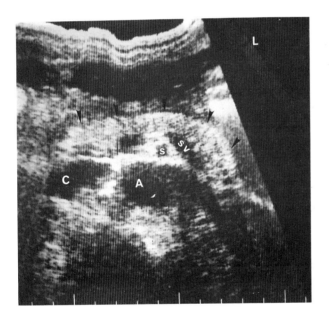

Fig. 24.38 (d) C = IUC. A = aorta. Pancreatic reflectivity is greater than that of fat.

artefact from non-dilute barium and motion. The contribution of retroperitoneal fat to optimum CT imaging is paramount and those patients with reduced amounts of fat are often best examined by ultrasound. Although it is possible for computer reconstruction of images in both coronal and sagittal planes, resolution in these planes is usually poorer than in the original axial form. The entire pancreas is not seen on a single axial slice as a

general rule because of its oblique lie within the abdomen, therefore appearing in parts on several sequential slices (Fig. 24.44).

Dynamic computerized tomography (Berland *et al.*, 1983) (Fig. 24.45)

The evaluation of certain pancreatic lesions is augmented by rapid scanning following a bolus of intravenous contrast. This has the facility of demonstrating small vessels and of identifying capillary, parenchymal, and venous phases of contrast enhancement.

The technique demands rapid scan times as well as short interscan periods for its adequate performance, but is limited not only by these factors but also by tube performance, heating, etc. which will govern the number of contiguous and sequential slices that may be performed at certain power levels. If rapidity of image acquisition is achieved at the expense of the use of ideal exposure factors, then quantum mottle and poor signal: noise ratio will obviate the advantages of the technique. Such factors limit usually the review of the entire pancreas by this technique, and a single level or several sequential levels are predetermined for special study by the digitized 'scout' film or on precontrast scans.

Intravenous contrast (150 ml Urografin 370) is given by rapid injection. Scanning is commenced 15s after commencement and completed within 2 min of the end of the injection.

Added information achieved by this technique

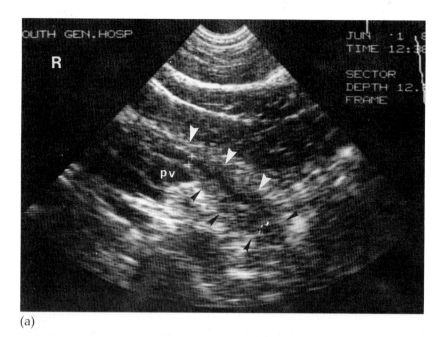

(a)

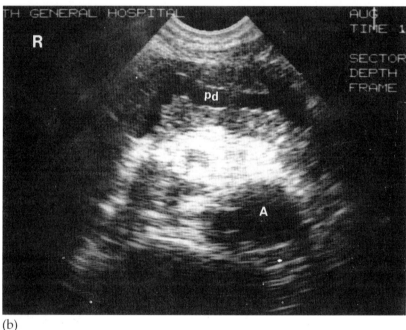

(b)

Fig. 24.39 Pancreatic duct dilatation.
(a) The echo-poor pancreatic duct runs a tortuous course through the centre of the pancreatic body and tail, identified by the *arrowheads*, and is measured by the on-screen cursors at 4 mm. pv = portal vein;
(b) There is even more marked dilatation of the pancreatic duct (pd). A = aorta.

includes the demonstration of vascular encasement by tumour. The better definition of pseudocyst walls contributing to the assessment of pseudocyst 'maturity', and the demonstration of hyper-vascularity and tumour blush.

The pancreas is of uniform soft-tissue density. It may be smooth or lobular in outline although it is generally more smooth in the young patient, becoming more lobular with age as a result of fatty replacement (Fig. 24.46a, b). With advancing age this fatty replacement may become very extensive and these changes parallel the increased reflectivity

seen on ultrasound (Heuck *et al.*, 1987). Also with advancing age and commensurate with the fatty replacement there is a reduction in size of the pancreas. While measurements of the head of the pancreas may be as high as 3 cm and the body and tail as high as 2.5 cm each in the younger age groups, this has reduced to 2.5, 1.7 and 1.5 cm, respectively, by the 70s. Although the entire pancreas is seen in most cases, visualization of the pancreatic duct is very much less reliable, probably being identified in 50% of cases or less (Fig. 24.47a, b).

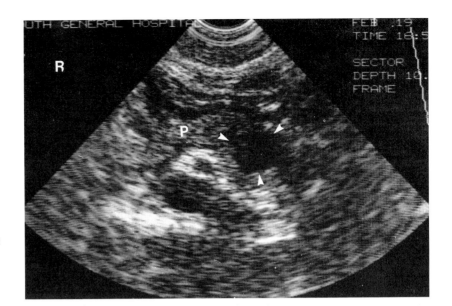

Fig. 24.40 Tumour of the pancreatic tail. A small tumour identified by the *arrowheads* is detected by decreased reflectivity rather than by significant distortion of the pancreatic outline. P = body of pancreas.

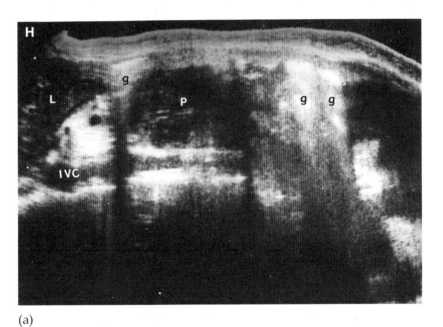

(a)

Fig. 24.41 Ultrasound in acute pancreatitis. (a) Long-axis scan demonstrating a large echo-poor pancreatic head (p). There is widespread bowel gas (g). L = liver; IVC = inferior vena cava; H = head. (b) Transverse scan in transpyloric plane. A large inhomogeneous echo-poor pancreas is identified by the *arrowheads*. s = superior mesenteric artery; A = aorta.

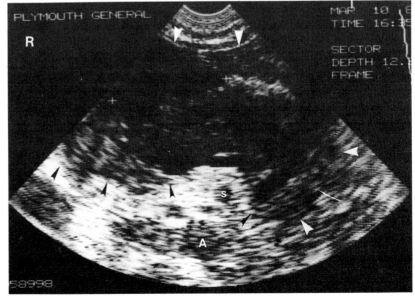

(b)

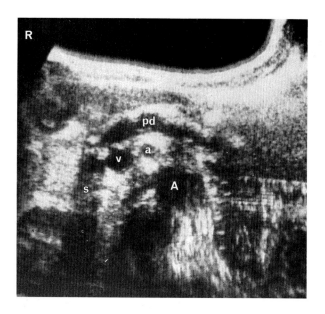

Fig. 24.42 Transverse ultrasound scan in a patient with chronic pancreatitis. The pancreatic duct (pd) within the centre of a highly reflective pancreas produces acoustic shadowing where there is calcification (s). A = aorta; a = superior mesenteric artery; v = superior mesenteric vein.

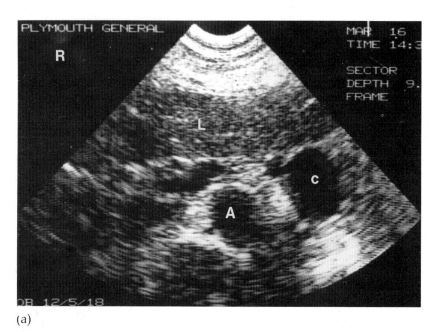

(a)

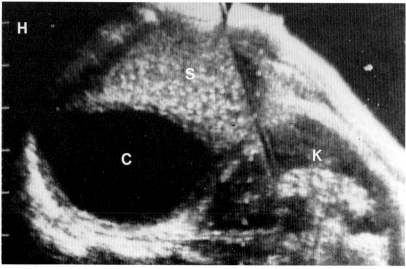

(b)

Fig. 24.43(a) Small pancreatic pseudocyst (c) in the region of the tail of the pancreas in this transverse ultrasound scan. A = aorta; L = liver. (b) Coronal ultrasound scan in the left upper quadrant demonstrating an intrasplenic pancreatic pseudocyst (C). S = spleen; K = left kidney; H = head.

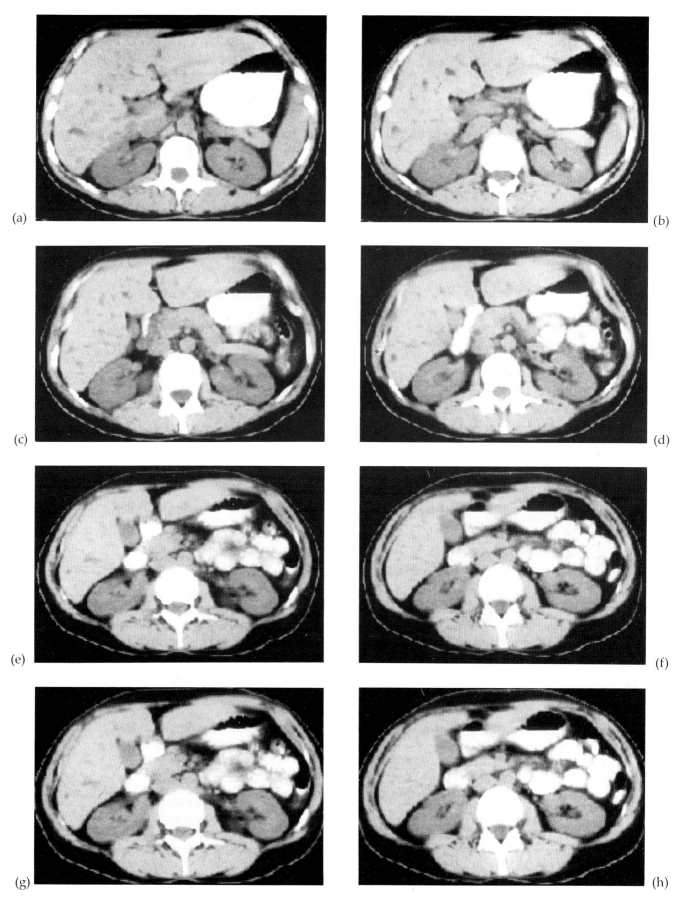

Fig. 24.44 Sequential CT scan through the pancreas showing the visualization of different sections at different levels. Incidentally, this patient has Caroli's disease, identified by the multiple low-attenuation, focally dilated ducts within the liver.

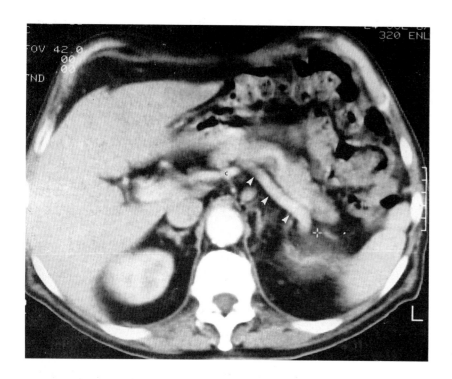

Fig. 24.45 Dynamic CT scan of the body of the pancreas demonstrating contrast in the coeliac trunk and its branches (c), and in the splenic vein (*arrowheads*). There is a parenchymal blush within the pancreas itself.

Features suggestive of pathology

Diffuse or focal enlargement of the pancreas can be seen in inflammatory or neoplastic disease (Figs 24.48, 24.49). It remains impossible to differentiate on the basis of morphology between focal pancreatitis and pancreatic neoplastic disease. Tumours are generally of similar density to normal pancreatic parenchyma except when necrotic, or in the case of cystic tumours. CT can reliably demonstrate invasion of the retropancreatic fat, although this is occasionally confused by coexistent or consequent pancreatitis. Pancreatic calcification can be more clearly demonstrated on CT than on plain radiography or ultrasound, but calcification within the splenic artery should not be confused with this (Fig. 24.50). CT is however, currently the most sensitive technique for the evaluation of pancreatic complications, particularly pancreatic abscess and phlegmon (Jeffrey *et al.*, 1987). The use of CT early in the course of acute pancreatitis may allow the prediction of significant intra-abdominal complications based on whether or not the disease is confined to the pancreas alone. Such predictions are, however, anatomic and are not useful in prognostication about renal and pulmonary complications (Nordestagaard *et al.*, 1986).

Magnetic resonance imaging (May & Gardiner, 1987)

Magnetic resonance imaging is not currently widely available. Although satisfactory sectional images of the pancreas may be produced in axial coronal and sagittal planes by manipulation of the magnetic field, image resolution is limited by image construction time and the associated artefact related to breathing and motion. Morphological information therefore is inferior to that of computerized tomography, and probably also to ultrasound. It has been suggested that improved resolution may be achieved with some reduction of artefact by improvement of coil design, and the use of surface coils appears to be one way of improving image quality (Simeone *et al.*, 1985). Although it is possible with modern magnets to achieve good or excellent images of the pancreas using both T_1 and T_2 weighted images, it does not seem that T_1 and T_2 relaxation times and MR signal intensities will produce specific and reproducable patterns allowing differentiation between normal and diseased pancreatic tissue or the distinction between tumour and inflammation. It may be that in certain selected cases MRI may provide additional information to other imaging

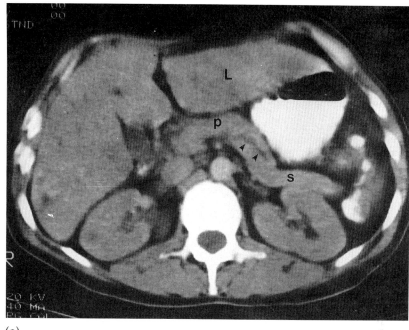

(a)

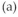

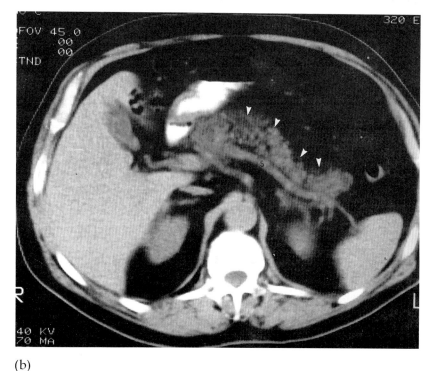

Fig. 24.46 (a) Ct scans through the head and body of the pancreas (p) showing a smooth outline to the pancreas. The *arrowheads* identify the marginations between the splenic vein (s) and the pancreas. L = liver. (b) CT scan through the upper abdomen in a patient with a pancreas partially replaced by fat and with an irregular outline. S = splenic vein.

(b)

techniques, for instance improving staging of pancreatic carcinoma, but the technique has yet to be found a definite role in the evaluation of the pancreas (Tscholakoff *et al.*, 1987).

Interventional techniques

Both ultrasound and CT may be used for the accurate localization of pancreatic pathology for needle placement.

The selection of imaging technique depends on local availability of equipment and expertise. We

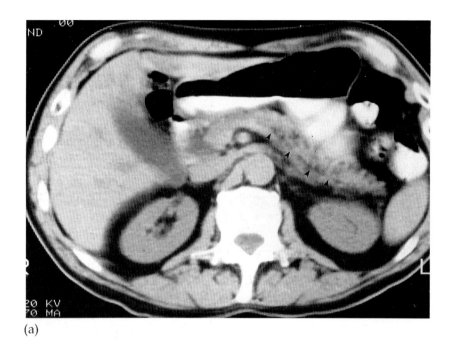

(a)

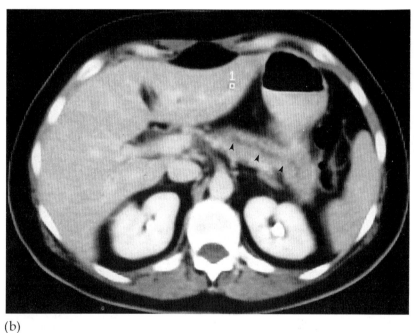

(b)

Fig. 24.47 (a) CT scan through the body and tail of the pancreas. A pseudopancreatic duct is suggested by the fat plane between the splenic vein and the body and tail of the pancreas (*arrowheads*). (b) CT scan through the body and tail of the pancreas in a patient with a slightly dilated pancreatic duct (*arrowheads*).

use a combination of CT to evaluate the relative position of gut (when relevant) and ultrasound for the continuous (real-time) monitoring of the needle tip during placement.

PANCREATIC BIOPSY

Much of the literature reports the use of fine (19–23 gauge) needles for aspiration biopsy. While some of these claim to have a cutting edge and therefore produce a core biopsy, in our experience the yield of such a core from pancreatic lesions is unreliable, and usually only samples sufficient for cytology are achieved, although with a good cytology laboratory overall accuracy rates of 88% can be achieved (Phillips *et al.*, 1985). There is, however, the suggestion that the vigorous motion of the needle within the pancreas, which is required to yield adequate tissue fluid, is as likely to result in complications such as pancreatitis, haemorrhage

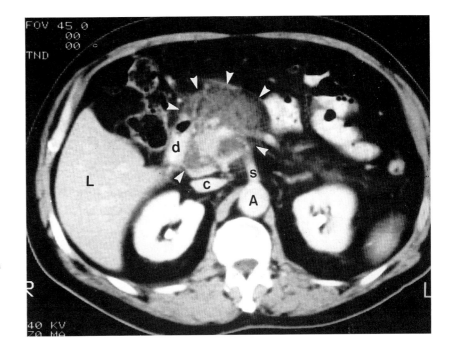

Fig. 24.48 CT scan of acute pancreatitis. Focal ill-defined mass in the region of the pancreas identified by the *arrowheads*. d = duodenum; L = liver; c = inferior vena cava; s = superior mesenteric artery; A = aorta.

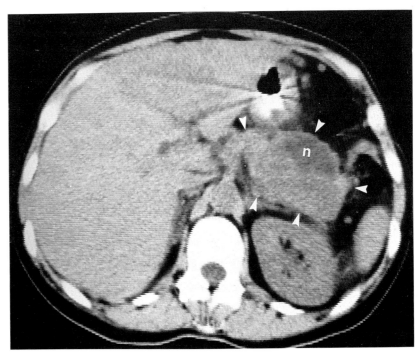

Fig. 24.49 Large mass in the region of the tail of the pancreas on CT scan (*arrowheads*). There is some necrosis (n) in the periphery of this pancreatic tail neoplasm.

and tumour seeding as it is using fine-needle core biopsy needles such as 'Biopty Cut' (Radiplast). It is now our practice routinely to use these core biopsy needles for pancreatic biopsy. Diagnostic yield is higher and incidence of side-effects does not appear to be increased.

The use of CT and ultrasound to guide needle placement may also be extended for the insertion percutaneously of needles and catheters for aspiration and/or drainage of pancreatic abscesses and pseudocysts. While many would advocate catheter drainage for pancreatic pseudocyst, the results are variable, with some authors suggesting that drainage procedures do not alter the natural history of the cyst. In our practice therapeutic aspiration of pseudocysts is performed using ultrasound

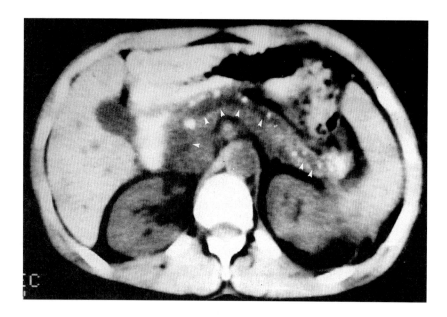

Fig. 24.50 CT scan of a patient with chronic pancreatitis, showing pancreatic duct dilatation (*arrowheads*) together with multiple areas of calcification.

guidance usually through the gastric wall with a 14–16 gauge needle/cannula combination (Long-dwel) as a 'holding procedure' in the severly ill patient. Such a technique, repeated when necessary, usually allows sufficient patient resuscitation to allow the definitive marsupialization of the pseudocyst by surgical techniques.

However, it is possible to combine endoscopic and ultrasound guidance for the placement of a double pigtail catheter draining the pseudocyst into the stomach. The long-term survival of these catheters has not been established, nor has the time for removal.

Percutaneous drainage of pancreatic abscesses is probably best performed using CT for planning an optimum route (often through the flank) for catheter placement, although the initial needle pass may then be guided by ultrasound. The catheter is usually placed using the Seldinger catheter ex-change technique after dilatation of the track, although in situations where the abscess has a superficial component a trochar and cannula technique may be used.

Recent work suggests that transcutaneous needle placement within the pancreas under ultra-sound or CT guidance may be used for intra-tumoral chemotherapy (Livraghi *et al.*, 1986).

Summary

Ultrasound and CT represent the mainstays for diagnostic imaging of the pancreas. ERCP provides further information about duct course and calibre, while in addition allowing collection of pancreatic juice for laboratory analysis and the performance of papillotomy and biopsy. Ultrasound and CT provide imaging for the guidance of diagnostic and therapeutic procedures such as biopsy and drainage.

Other techniques have a lesser role in the evaluation of the pancreas, and for many indications a simple algorithm of ultrasound followed by CT and/or ERCP provides detailed information of the anatomy and pathology of the pancreas. In some cases ultrasound or CT in isolation, perhaps augmented by guided biopsy techniques, may be all that is required.

Although there are limited indications for other techniques, presentation of pancreatic disease is far from characteristic in all cases and therefore features that are characteristic or suggestive of pancreatic disease on plain radiographs and con-trast studies are important to recognize if the correct diagnostic pathway is to be followed.

References

Anderson, J.R., Spence, R.A., Laird, J.D., Ferguson, W.R. & Kennedy, T.L. (1986) Indium-111 autologous leukocyte imaging in pancreatitis. *Journal of Nuclear Medicine*, **27(3)**, 345–352.

Ariyama, J., Shimaguchi, S., Suyama, M. & Shirakabe, H. (1986) Intra-arterial digital subtraction angiography in the diagnosis and treatment of gastrointestinal disorders. *Gastrointestinal Radiology*, **11**, 177–182.

Berland, L.L., Lawson, T.L. & Foley, W.D. (1983) Dynamic pancreatic scanning. In Siegelman, S.S. (ed) *Computed*

Tomography of the Pancreas, pp. 33—60. Churchill Livingstone, New York.

Bowerman, R.A., McCracken, S., Silver, T.M. & Knake, J.E. (1985) Abdominal and miscellaneous applications of intraoperative ultrasound. *Radiologic Clinics of North America*, **23(1)**, 107—113.

Classen, M. & Phillip, J. (1984) Endoscopic retrograde cholangiopancreatography (ERCP) and endoscopic therapy in pancreatic disease. *Clinics in Gastroenterology*, **13(3)**, 819—842.

Donovan, P.J. (1983) Technique of examination and normal pancreatic anatomy. In Siegelman, S.S. (ed) *Computed Tomography of the Pancreas*, pp. 1—32. Churchill Livingstone, New York.

Dunn, G.D. & Gibson, R.N. (1986) The left sided pancreas. *Radiology*, **159(3)**, 713—4.

Field, S. (1984) Plain films: The acute abdomen. *Gastroenterology*, **13(1)**, 3—40.

Fujibayashi, Y., Saji, H., Yomoda, I., Suzuki, K.H., Torizuka, K. & Yokoyama, A. (1986a) A new approach toward a pancreas-seeking zinc radiopharmaceutical. II. 62Zn-EDDA (ethylenediamine-n, n′-diacetic acid) for pancreas PCT imaging. *European Journal of Nuclear Medicine*, **11(12)**, 488—493.

Fujibayashi, T., Saji, H., Yomoda, I., Suzuki, K.H., Torizuka, K. & Yokoyama, A. (1986b) A new approach toward a pancreas-seeking zinc radiopharmaceutical. I. Accumulation of 65Zn-amino acid and aminopolycarboxylic acid complexes in pancreatic tissue slices. *European Journal of Nuclear Medicine*, **11(12)**, 484—487.

Geokas, M.C., Baltaxe, H.A., Banks, P.A., Silva, J. & Frey, C.F. (1985) Acute pancreatitis. *Annals of Internal Medicine*, **103**, 86—100.

Gross, M.D., Shapiro, B., Thralls, J.H., Freitas, J.E. & Beierwaltes, W.H. (1984) The scintigraphic imaging of endocrine organs. *Endocrine Reviews*. **5(2)**, 221—281.

Heuck, A, Maubach, P.A., Reiser, M., Fuerbach, S., Allgayer, B., Lukas, P., Kahn, T. (1987) Age related morphology of the normal pancreas on computed tomography. *Gastrointestinal Radiology*, **12**, 18—22.

Jeffrey, R.B. Jr., Grendell, J.H., Federle, M.P., Meyer, A.A., Wing, V.W., Wall, S.D. & Shea, W.J. (1987) Improved survival with early C.T. diagnosis of pancreatic abscess. *Gastrointestinal Radiology*, **12(1)**, 26—30.

Kurtz, A. & Goldberg, B.B. (1984) Pancreas. In Goldberg, B.B. (ed) *Abdominal Ultrasonography*, 2nd edn, pp. 163—207. John Wiley, New York.

Lankisch, P.G., Otto, J., Erkelenz, I. & Lembcke, B. (1986) Pancreatic calcifications: No indicator of severe exocrine pancreatic insufficiency. *Gastroenterology*, **90(3)**, 617—621.

Lavelle, M.I., Tait, N.P., Walsh, T., Alderson, D. & Record, C.O. (1985) Demonstration of pancreatic parenchyma by digital subtraction techniques during endoscopic retrograde cholangiopancreatography. *Clinical Radiology*, **36(4)**, 405—407.

Lees, W.R. (1986) Endoscopic ultrasound of chronic pancreatitis and pancreatic pseudocysts. *Scandinavian Journal of Gastroenterology*, (Suppl), **123**, 123—129.

Livraghi, T., Bajetta, E., Matricardi, L., Villa, E., Lovati, R. & Vettori, C. (1986) Fine needle percutaneous intratumoral chemotherapy under ultrasound guidance: A feasibility study. *Tumori*, **72(1)**, 81—87.

Lunderquist, A. (1985) The pancreas. *Clinics in Gastroenterology*, **14(2)**, 355—369.

Lux, G. & Heyder, N. (1986) Endoscopic ultrasonography of the pancreas; technical aspects. *Scandinavian Journal of Gastroenterology*, (Suppl), **123**, 112—118.

McHugo, J.M., McKeown, C., Brown, M.T., Weller, P. & Shah, K.J. (1987) Ultrasound findings in children with cystic fibrosis. *British Journal of Radiology*, **60**, 137—141.

May, G. & Gardiner, R. (1987) *Techniques of Imaging. Clinical Imaging of the Pancreas*, pp. 16—49. Raven Press, New York.

Meire, H. (1984) Ultrasound in gastroenterology. *Clinics in Gastroenterology*, **13(1)**, 183—204.

Michels, N.A. (1955) *Blood Supply and Anatomy of the Upper Abdominal Organs*. Lippincott, Philadelphia.

Montz, R., Klapdor, R., Rothe, B. & Heller, M. (1986) Immunoscintigraphy and radioimmunity in patients with pancreatic carcinoma. *Nuklearmedizin*, **25(6)**, 239—244.

Nordestagaard, A.G., Wilson, S.E. & Williams, R.A. (1986) Early C.T. as a predictor of outcome in acute pancreatitis. *American Journal of Surgery*, **152**, 127—132.

Paivansalo, M. & Suramo, I. (1986) Ultrasonography of the pancreatic tail through spleen and through fluid filled stomach. *European Journal of Radiology*, **6**, 113—115.

Phillips, V.M., Hersh, T., Erwin, B.C. *et al.*, (1985) Percutaneous biopsy of pancreatic masses. *Journal of Clinical Gastroenterology*, **7(6)**, 506—510.

Reuter, S.R. & Redman, H.C. (1972) Vascular anatomy. In *Gastrointestinal Angiography*, pp. 20—54. W.B. Saunders, Philadelphia.

Simeone, J.F., Edelman, R.R., Stark, D.D. *et al.*, (1985) Surface M.R. imaging of the abdominal viscera, Part III, The pancreas. *Radiology*, **157(2)**, 437—41.

Sivak, M.V. & Kaufman, A. (1986) Endoscopic ultrasonography in the differential diagnosis of pancreatic disease. A preliminary report. *Scandinavian Journal of Gastroenterology* (Suppl), **123**, 130—134.

Smith, S.J., Vogelzang, R.L., Donovan, J., Atlas, S.W., Gore, R.M. & Neiman, H.L. (1985) Intraoperative sonography of the pancreas. *American Journal of Roentgenology*, **144(33)**, 557—562.

Sugawa, C., Walt, A.J., Nunel, D.C. & Masuyama, H. (1987) Pancreas divisum: Is it normal anatomic variant? *American Journal of Surgery*, **153(1)**, 62—7.

Swobodnik, W., Wolf, A., Wechsler, J.G., Kleihauer, E. & Ditschunett, H. (1985) Ultrasound characteristics of the pancreas in children with cystic fibrosis. *Journal of Clinical Ultrasound*, **13(7)**, 469—474.

Trenkner, S.W. & Laufer, I. (1984) Double contrast examination oesophagus, stomach and duodenum. *Clinics in Gastroenterology*, **13(1)**, 41—73.

Tscholakoff, D., Hricak, H., Thoeni, R., Winkler, M.L. & Margulis, A.R. (1987) M.R. imaging in the diagnosis of pancreatic disease. *American Journal of Roentgenology*, **148(4)**, 703—709.

Wyburn, G.M. (1964) Anatomy of the Pancreas. In G.J. Romanes (ed) *Cunningham's Anatomy*, 10th edn, pp. 440—443, Oxford Medical Publications, London.

25: Pancreatic Inflammatory Disease

W.R. LEES

Acute pancreatitis

Aetiology

In most countries of the Western world the incidence of alcoholic pancreatitis is increasing. Despite this over 60% of cases of acute pancreatitis in the United Kingdom are still caused by gall stones which is more likely to result in a fatal outcome. This is probably due to bacterial contamination of necrotic pancreatic tissue at a much earlier stage (Trapnell & Duncan, 1975, Imrie & White, 1975).

The mumps virus, hyperlipidaemia and hypercalcaemia can all cause acute pancreatitis, and although many other aetiologies are listed in the medical literature these are relatively unimportant and are largely based on anecdotal case reports.

Many different experimental models of acute pancreatitis have been constructed but only three features of relevance to the disease in man can be derived from animal work; reflux of bile or duodenal contents into the pancreatic duct system, an increase in intraduct pressure, and bacterial contamination of the interstitial space of the pancreatic parenchyma.

The most consistent experimental cause is elevation of the pressure in the pancreatic duct system. Above 60 cm of water the basement membranes of the alveoli rupture and duct contents escape into the interstitium. This alone is enough to cause acute pancreatitis, but the presence of bile or duodenal content, particularly enterokinase, leads to more rapid enzyme activation. Bacterial contamination leads to early infection of necrotic material.

The mechanism of alcohol in inducing pancreatitis is unclear.

Definition

An accepted international definition of acute pancreatitis is 'an acute condition typically presenting with abdominal pain and usually associated with raised pancreatic enzymes in blood or urine, due to inflammatory disease of the pancreas.' The general nature of this definition shows how poor is our understanding of the underlying pathology (Sarner & Cotton, 1984).

Most of our knowledge of the progress of acute pancreatitis is based on radiological studies, and the separation of acute pancreatitis into acute interstitial and necrotizing pancreatitis is a useful one. Acute interstitial pancreatitis (AIP) is mild, with rapid recovery and complete restitution of the pancreas to normal. Necrotizing pancreatitis may be subclassified as mild or severe, depending on the extent of necrosis. If more than 50% of the pancreas is necrosed then the pancreatitis is severe, and the risk of death increases considerably (Banks et al., 1983).

Pathomorphology

Histopathological studies of acute pancreatitis are difficult to perform because of the rapid autodigestion that occurs in pancreatic tissue after death. Despite this, all cases of severe and long-standing pancreatitis show a common feature, which is large and confluent foci of peripancreatic fat necrosis. These foci extend along the interstitial septae into the parenchyma and are associated with necrosis of contiguous acini.

Venous thrombosis, haemorrhage, and infarction characterize advanced parenchymal damage, and involvement of the parenchyma is irregular with necrosis often very localized. Gyr has concluded from these observations that acute pancreatitis advances mainly through progression of fat necrosis to confluent necrosis on the surface of the gland, with subsequent patchy vascular damage leading to infarction (Gyr et al., 1984).

This theory does not conflict with the available imaging evidence, where glandular tissue can appear well perfused with normal architecture in the first 24 h, with patchy or confluent necrosis only becoming evident at 48 h or more.

Clinical grading

There are two commonly used clinical methods for early assessment of the severity of acute pancreatitis. The original scheme was proposed by Ranson *et al.*, in 1974 and consists of a cumulative score of clinical features. On admission the key factors are; age > 55 years, a white blood cell count > 16 000, a blood glucose > 10 mmol/1, serum LDH > 700 iu, and an AST > 250 units. Other important prognostic factors within the first 48 h of admission are a rise in blood urea and nitrogen (BUN) > 5 mg%, a Pao_2 < 60 mm/mg, and a serum calcium < 2 mmol/1.

Prognostic factor analysis provides a reliable method of identifying patients at risk of severe disease early in the course of the illness and has an accuracy of approximately 80% (Ranson *et al.*, 1974, Imrie & White, 1975).

McMahon has proposed a simple method of peritoneal lavage and analysis of the returned fluid. This can be performed at the bedside and has similar accuracy in discriminating severe from mild pancreatitis. If the returned lavage fluid has the appearance of prune juice, then this is a good indication of pancreatic necrosis with extension of the inflammatory process into the peritoneal cavity (McMahon *et al.*, 1980).

Radiological grading methods based on morphological criteria have also been developed (*vide infra*).

Despite the increasing incidence of acute pancreatitis, mortality rates have been steadily reducing over the past 10 years. There are three reasons for this reduction:
1 Improved metabolic maintenance, particularly total parenteral nutrition.
2 Better management of patients in respiratory failure.
3 Active radiological monitoring of acute pancreatitis and its complications, with detection of pancreatic necrosis or abscess leading to earlier intervention.

Acute interstitial pancreatitis (AIP)

Mild acute pancreatitis causes swelling of the parenchyma of the gland, which may be focal or lobular in scale. There is attenuation of the duct system. Oedema and fluid accumulate in the peripancreatic fat spaces and there may also be a small transudate into the lesser sac or close peritoneal recesses.

A definite diagnosis of acute pancreatitis is made when the serum amylase is elevated above 1000 iu. Even in severe pancreatitis the elevation in serum amylase may be transitory and unrecorded, and the diagnosis may be unclear.

Both ultrasound and CT scanning are highly specific in the diagnosis of AIP. Ultrasound typically demonstrates pancreatic enlargement, a generalized reduction in parenchymal echogenicity, and a relative increase in echogenicity of the walls of a normal or diminished calibre duct system. Small fluid accumulations are easy to recognize with ultrasound, but oedema in the surrounding fat may obscure pancreatic boundaries (Fig. 25.1). It is important to note that the changes in mild AIP may be focal, and patchy oedema or necrosis can be confined to one or more individual pancreatic lobules. These are 7–8 mm in diameter and are divided from one another by fine fibrous septae.

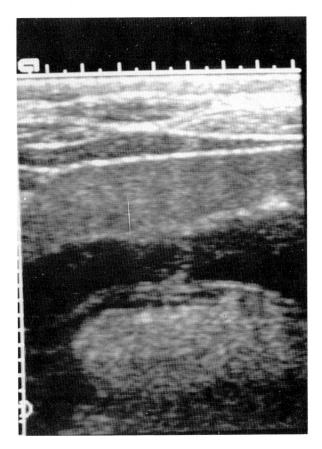

Fig. 25.1 Transverse ultrasound scan of acute interstitial pancreatitis. Fluid is seen to outline the peritoneum of the posterior border of the lesser sac. The butterfly sign described by Weill.

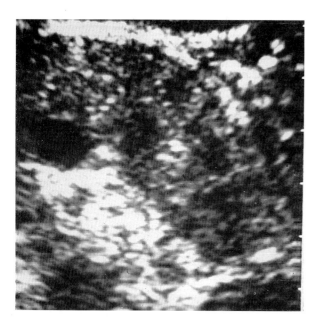

Fig. 25.2 Acute interstitial pancreatitis. There is a reduction in echogenicity of individual pancreatic lobules with prominence of the interlobular septa.

Intrapancreatic oedema may render the septae visible as thin, bright lines radiating from the centre to the periphery of the gland (Fig. 25.2).

CT is less sensitive in showing intrapancreatic changes in mild AIP but is more sensitive than ultrasound in showing the effects on the surrounding tissues. Oedema in peripancreatic fat will result in a density midway between fat and fluid, and small fluid collections are easily recognized. Thickening of the peritoneum and Gerota's fascia yield specific evidence of retroperitoneal inflammation, but if these are the sole features on CT, they do not necessarily indicate the presence of active disease (Freeny, 1984).

The diagnosis of acute pancreatitis is usually made on clinical grounds and the majority of patients will recover without the need for any imaging. For these patients, the most important examination is an ultrasound scan of the gall bladder and biliary tree. Over 30% of patients with gall stone pancreatitis will have further attacks of pancreatitis within 6 months of the initial episode, and the subsequent attacks are often more severe than the first. Virtually all of these can be prevented by interval cholecystectomy. The ultrasound scan is best performed immediately prior to discharge, when visualization will be almost certainly better than at the diagnostic scan performed at admission.

Complications are uncommon following AIP,

but significant pseudocysts can follow even mild attacks and should be excluded by ultrasound or CT scanning prior to discharge (Siegelman *et al.*, 1980).

Necrotizing pancreatitis (NP)

For patients with clinically severe acute pancreatitis the initial diagnostic ultrasound examination should concentrate on the biliary tree, when evidence of significant dilation (CBD > 6 mm) is considered by many to be an indication for urgent endoscopy and biliary sphincterotomy with removal of any choledochal stones (Safrani & Cotton, 1981).

An ultrasound scan performed too early in the disease process may well be misleading, as the pancreas can look remarkably normal in the first 24 h. Meteorism, abdominal tenderness, and other problems of the acute abdomen often preclude satisfactory ultrasound visualization, although views of the head and tail of the pancreas can usually be obtained through the flanks (Fig. 25.3a,b).

CT scanning is best performed 48 h after admission, using the dynamic bolus technique with large volumes of contrast to assess perfusion of the pancreatic parenchyma. Pancreatic necrosis cannot be diagnosed by ultrasonography or magnetic resonance scanning and can only be inferred from secondary signs (Fig. 25.4).

The Ulm Pancreas Group have performed dynamic enhanced CT scanning on 41 patients selected for surgery by clinical criteria. Scans were performed after a prolonged bolus injection of 150 ml of contrast medium. There were 35 patients with operatively proven necrotizing pancreatitis. CT without contrast gave evidence of pancreatic necrosis in 39% by showing low-density regions within the parenchyma. After contrast enhancement, 26 patients with 20–50% necrosis demonstrated a low-enhancement area of corresponding size. The size of pancreatic necrosis was overestimated in one patient and there was failure to demonstrate an enhancement defect in five. In nine patients with total or subtotal pancreatic necrosis, a corresponding area of poor enhancement was demonstrated in five (56%). In two cases pancreatic necrosis was underestimated. In two further patients the dimensions of the necrosis were significantly underestimated (Buchler *et al.*, 1986, Maier, 1986).

Overall the scale of partial necrosis was determined correctly in 77% of cases and total or sub-

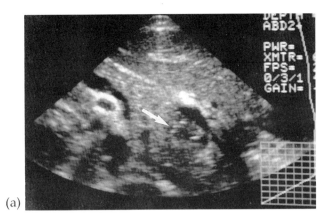

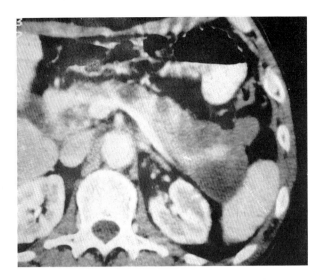

Fig. 25.4 Thirty per cent pancreatitic necrosis on a dynamic CT scan taken at 48 h.

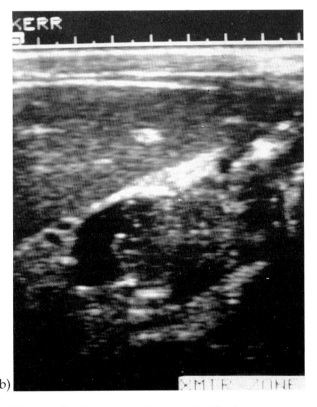

Fig. 25.3 Focal necrosis with associated fluid.

total pancreatic necrosis was diagnosed in 78%. Some of the discrepancies can be explained by the interval between CT and subsequent surgery, which was up to 24 h in some cases, by technical problems of CT scanning in patients with respiratory distress or by difficulty in assessing true volume of necrosis at surgery. The conclusion, however, is clear. Enhanced CT using high volumes of contrast is able to exclude necrosis if a normal enhancement pattern is demonstrated. Patients with less than 50% necrosis will probably be managed successfully with supportive therapy

alone. More than 50% necrosis requires surgery to pre-empt the development of complications (Beger & Buchler, 1986).

In the early stages of total or subtotal pancreatic necrosis there may be only minimal phlegmonous change, with gross extrapancreatic involvement only becoming apparent after several days (Fig. 25.5). The approximate natural history of necrotizing pancreatitis is given in Figs 25.6 and 25.7.

Most other schemes for radiological grading of acute pancreatitis have evaluated the distribution of disease within the pancreas and surrounding fat spaces (see Table 25.1). The success of these methods is very dependent on the time course of necrotizing pancreatitis, and progressive involvement of contiguous fat spaces is an indication of severe necrosis. The lesser sac and those fat spaces close to the body and tail of the pancreas tend to be involved first, with spread into more distant retroperitoneal or peritoneal compartments if activated pancreatic enzymes continue to be discharged from necrotic areas of pancreatic tissue (White et al., 1986) (Figs 25.8, 25.9).

Initial results based on an early grading CT scan yielded a predictive value in high grades of over 60% for severe complications such as pancreatic abscess. However, a more recent prospective study by Vernacchia, using his own previously successful criteria, showed abscess formation in only 30% of those in grades D and E. He now no longer recommends the routine use of CT and concludes that it should be selectively performed only in patients who fail to respond to clinical supportive therapy or in whom complications are suspected.

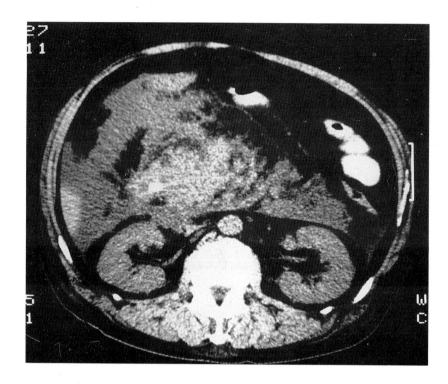

Fig. 25.5 Extensive oedema and fluid accumulation in the peripancreatic spaces.

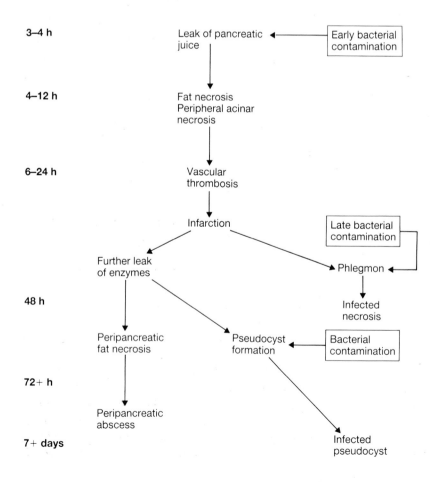

3–4 h	Leak of pancreatic juice ← Early bacterial contamination
4–12 h	Fat necrosis Peripheral acinar necrosis
6–24 h	Vascular thrombosis
	Infarction
	Further leak of enzymes → Phlegmon ← Late bacterial contamination
48 h	Infected necrosis
	Peripancreatic fat necrosis → Pseudocyst formation ← Bacterial contamination
72+ h	Peripancreatic abscess
7+ days	Infected pseudocyst

Fig. 25.6 Necrotizing pancreatitis.

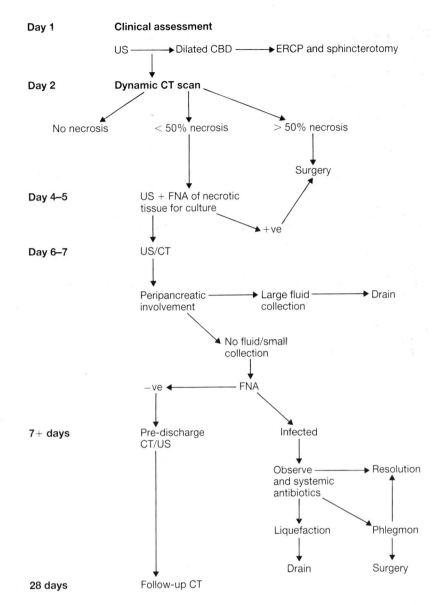

Fig. 25.7 Radiological landmarks in severe acute pancreatitis.

The great majority of surgeons would agree with this less aggressive approach (Vernacchia *et al.*, 1987) (Fig. 25.10).

Lethal pancreatitis

There are three main causes of death in acute pancreatitis. Respiratory failure from respiratory distress syndrome is the most common cause of death early in the disease process, particularly in patients with fulminant necrosis. This is potentially reversible by modern ventilation therapy. Impairment of renal function and renal failure is particularly prevalent in severe necrotizing pancreatitis and in older patients. Neither renal nor respiratory failure indicate the presence of pancreatic sepsis, but respiratory failure is usually easier to manage after resection of the phlegmon.

The other major cause of death is from septic complications of pancreatitis. These are: cholangitis, infected pancreatic necrosis, and infection of the peripancreatic spaces (Ranson, 1984).

Cholangitis can be rapidly lethal in the presence of continuing biliary obstruction, but in the absence of complete obstruction it is unlikely to be life-threatening. Infected pancreatic necrosis still carries a mortality of over 90% and the only effective treatment is resection of the necrotic area. Neither CT nor ultrasound scanning is able to diagnose infection in the absence of gas formation,

Grade	1	2	3
Each fat space	< 25%	25–50%	> 50%
Non-fat spaces (e.g. lesser sac)	< 3 cm	3–5 cm	> 5 cm
Intrapancreatic	Focal or diffuse enlargement	Mass or fluid < 5 cm	Mass or fluid > 5 cm
Ascites/pleural fluid	< 100 ml	100–300 ml	> 300 ml

Table 25.1 CT grading of acute pancreatitis (Vernacchia *et al.*, 1987)

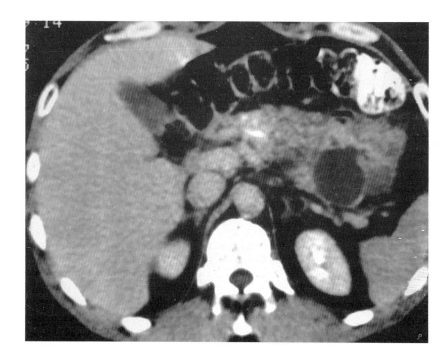

Fig. 25.8 Lesser sac phlegmon with cystic changes. Dynamic CT.

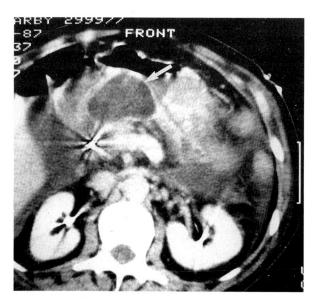

Fig. 25.9 Pancreatic ascites.

which Vernacchia and colleagues found in only 2 out of 15 patients with surgically proven abscess (Vernacchia *et al.*, 1987). The only effective method of diagnosing infection is biopsy.

Gerzhof recently reported a series of 67 fine-needle aspirations in 57 cases of suspected pancreatic sepsis. There were 18 phlegmons, 33 pseudocysts, and 16 peripancreatic collections. Forty-one were sterile and 26 infected. There were no complications and only two deaths occurred from sepsis in this series. His group concluded that demonstration of infected necrosis on immediate Gram stain should be an indication for urgent surgery (Gerzhof *et al.*, 1986).

Infected pancreatic necrosis can rarely be drained by catheter, although percutaneous lavage techniques may have some value. Infection of a pseudocyst or a peripancreatic space is a less

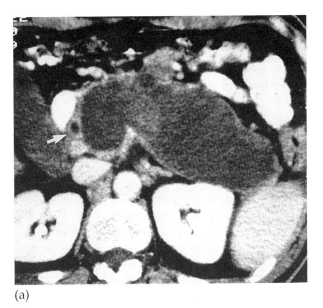
(a)

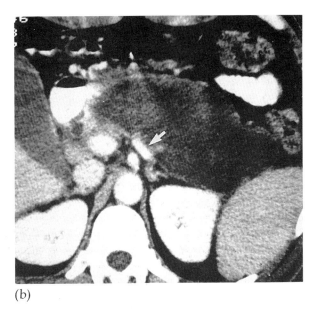
(b)

Fig. 25.10 Sterile phlegmon the pancreas in 95% destroyed. (a) The bile duct is displaced. (b) The splenic artery is incorporated in the wall of the phlegmon.

urgent complication which does not necessarily require surgical intervention and may be managed solely by catheter drainage. Freeny has recently reported percutaneous catheter drainage of 18 patients with pancreatic abscesses. Sixteen were successfully drained and only two required subsequent surgery. There were three complications in the series, two cases of self-limiting haemorrhage and one empyema of the pleural cavity. Several important points were raised by this study. The time to resolution was up to 6 months and the majority of patients required very prolonged drainage. Four of the 18 patients had communications with the main pancreatic duct system, and seven had pancreatoenteric fistulae (Freeny *et al.*, 1986) (Fig. 25.11).

The important long-term complications of acute pancreatitis are:
- Biliary obstruction.
- Obstruction to the gastrointestinal tract.
- Splenic vein thrombosis.
- Pancreatic acites.
- Renal obstruction.
- Pseudoaneurysm formation.
- Pseudocysts formation.

Most of these are minor and require no active intervention (Fig. 25.12).

A pseudoaneurysm is potentially lethal and should be searched for by dynamic CT scanning in any case of severe necrotizing pancreatitis. It is important to note that this is a long-term complication, pseudoaneurysms are rarely detected before 2–3 weeks after the initial onset (Freeny, 1984).

Virtually all patients with clinically significant acute pancreatitis will have peripancreatic fluid collections in the 1st week of the disease (Hill *et al.*, 1982; Sarti, 1977). Bradley has shown that the majority resolve within 6 weeks, but that less than 20% of fluid collections seen after this time resolve spontaneously (Bradley & Clements, 1976). Only a few peripancreatic fluid collections progress to true pseudocyst formation, but all pseudocysts are preceded by a collection in the early phase.

The pathologist defines a true pseudocyst as a collection of pancreatic fluid with a high amylase content surrounded by a fibrous wall. The thickness of the wall depends on the duration of the cyst, and most well-established pseudocysts will show significant rim enhancement on dynamic CT (Fig. 25.13).

Spillage of large quantities of pancreatic juice indicates disruption of the pancreatic duct system. If this involves a small branch duct, than healing of the fistula may occur and no communication will be apparent between the cyst and the pancreatic duct. Disruption of the main pancreatic duct leads to loss of larger volumes of pancreatic juice, although oedema and fibrosis in the cyst wall may temporarily occlude the communication.

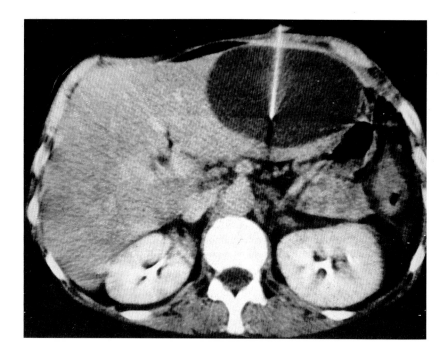

Fig. 25.11 CT guided drainage of an infected pseudocyst.

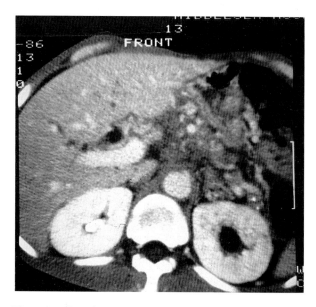

Fig. 25.12 Portal vein thrombosis with compensating collateral veins seen on a dynamic CT.

Percutaneous drainage of the cyst may well reveal the underlying communication once the pressure within the cyst falls below the secretion pressure of the drained segment of pancreas.

The surgical and radiological literature are replete with descriptions of bizarre pseudocysts which have dissected through various tissue planes to unusual locations (Sankaran & Walt, 1975). This phenomenon is largely a function of chronicity, and with prompt diagnosis and early treatment few cysts should be allowed to develop thick walls or to dissect into remote locations. The vast majority are now to be found in close contiguity with the pancreas (Vernacchia et al., 1987). In the early stages considerable regression and healing may occur with total parenteral nutrition. If response does not occur within a few weeks, early percutaneous drainage may be curative.

The organs most vulnerable to a pseudocyst are the spleen and splenic pedicle, and splenic vein thrombosis and splenic infarction are commonly found in association with untreated cysts at the splenic hilum. Damage to the splenic artery by a pseudocyst is the most common cause of pseudoaneurysm formation.

Peripancreatic fluid collections can be seen in up to 50% of patients 2–3 weeks after a severe attack of acute pancreatitis and may still be present after the 6-week time limit described by Bradley (Sarti, 1977). At this point management decisions are needed. Catheter drainage under ultrasound or CT control is a simple, well tolerated procedure, and pseudocysts can be adequately drained for prolonged periods of time through catheters as small as 5.5 Fr. It is rarely necessary to use catheters of larger then 7.5 Fr. Once the pseudocyst is decompressed and evacuated, an improvement in

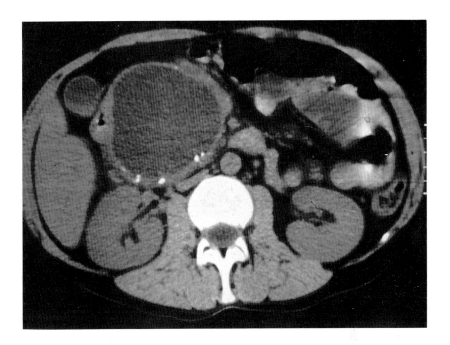

Fig. 25.13 Chronic pseudocyst with a calcified thick wall.

the patient's general condition can be expected and the radiologist and surgeon are then left to chose between early surgery or prolonged catheter drainage.

With non-communicating cysts, drainage ceases promptly after evacuation of the cyst contents and the catheter can be safely removed after a few days following a check ultrasound or CT scan. If there is any communication with the underlying duct system, this is revealed as a constant flow of 30−200 ml of pancreatic juice daily. An antegrade tubogram may fail to reveal the fistula in the 1st week of drainage and this may not become apparent for 3−4 weeks until healing has occurred. If no communication develops and if drainage continues, endoscopic retrograde pancreatography should demonstrate the site of disruption of the pancreatic duct. Although this procedure is contraindicated in the presence of an undrained pseudocyst, the available evidence suggests that this risk is minimal with a catheter *in situ* (Fig. 25.14).

The reported success rates for curative percutaneous drainage for pseudocysts following acute pancreatitis vary between 16 and 60%, with most authors reporting less than 30% success (Barlin *et al.*, 1981). Recent evidence suggests that these results can be significantly improved by maintaining percutaneous drainage for up to 6 months (Freeny *et al.*, 1986). Our own policy is to manage the pseudocyst initially with percutaneous drainage

for 2−3 weeks to improve the general condition of the patient and promote local healing. If drainage persists after this time then a definitive resection of the pancreas distal to the duct disruption is performed following mapping pancreatography by the endoscopic or antegrade route. Our present algorithm for pseudocyst management is given in Fig. 25.15.

Surgical cyst-gastrostomy is the traditional method of dealing with pseudocysts but has also had very variable success. Results are best in long-standing pseudocysts which have a thick and fibrous wall to which a suitable enterostomy can be made. Its success in the acute phase with underlying duct disruption is very low, whereas a simple distal pancreatectomy is almost always successful. Virtually all cyst-gastrostomies will have closed after 6−8 weeks, and the advantage of this procedure over catheter drainage is unproven.

Traumatic pancreatitis

Severe pancreatic trauma almost always results in duct disruption and spillage of pancreatic juice into the peripancreatic spaces. Some of the largest pseudocysts have their origin in transection of the main pancreatic duct. With blunt trauma this usually occurs in mid-body at the point where the pancreas crosses the aorta. With penetrating injury, the disruption can occur at any point within

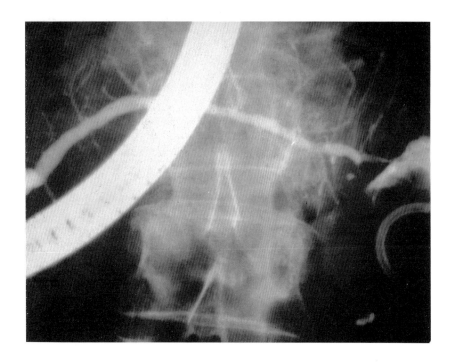

Fig. 25.14 ERCP showing communication with a pseudocyst previously drained by catheter.

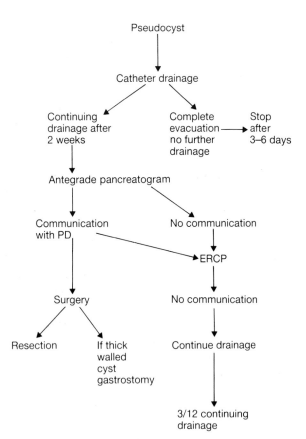

Fig. 25.15 Algorithm for pseudocyst management.

the pancreas and is usually associated with traumatic necrosis (Vallon *et al.*, 1979).

Even complete transection of the pancreas can be clinically silent and go unnoticed until the development of pancreatic ascites or a large pseudocyst. Distal pancreatectomy is essential if there has been complete disruption of the main pancreatic duct. This can only be adequately planned after obtaining a pancreatogram. This may be performed as an immediate preoperative procedure and will show either a block in the main pancreatic duct at the point of disruption or spillage of contrast medium and juice into the retroperitoneum.

As with communicating pseudocysts, decompression of the fluid collection by a percutaneous catheter will improve the general condition of the patient, and if performed in conjunction with a contrast study will usually show the condition of the distal pancreas (Fig. 25.16).

Relapsing pancreatitis

The concept of a relapsing form of acute pancreatitis was originally proposed in Marseilles in 1960, but this is no longer recognized as a distinct entity (Singer *et al.*, 1985). Repeated attacks of acute pancreatitis are certainly common in patients with gall stones and in cases of untreated hypercalcaemia and hyperlipidaemia. Acute pancreatitis can also occur as a complication of chronic pancreatitis. It is this latter group of patients that has caused most of the confusion. Recurrent attacks of acute pancreatitis in patients with underlying

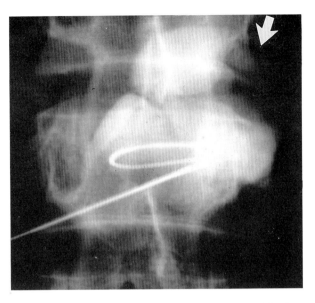

Fig. 25.16 Complete disruption of the MPD in mid body. The resulting pseudocyst is drained by catheter. The distal duct is faintly outline (*arrow*). Treatment is distal pancreatectomy.

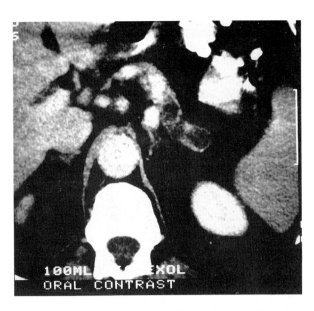

Fig. 25.17 The duct in the tail of the pancreas is distended by mucus and the parenchyma is atrophic. The underlying papillary carcinoma was only seen on endoscopic ultrasonography.

chronic pancreatitis may vary from bouts of abdominal pain to full-blown attacks of pancreatitis. Careful ultrasonography will usually reveal a focus of reduced echogenicity confined to a single segment of pancreas, occasionally even to a single lobule. This may also be associated with small localized peripancreatic effusions or intrapancreatic collections. Similar bouts of focal acute pancreatitis may follow percutaneous biopsy procedures and ERCP if the injection pressure has been too high.

Obstructive pancreatopathy

Pancreatic fibrosis and atrophy of parenchyma follow from partial or complete obstruction of the main pancreatic duct. This is commonly seen as a desmoplastic reaction surrounding infiltrating pancreatic carcinomas, but is also recognized in conjunction with any intraduct lesion producing obstruction to free flow of pancreatic juice (Sahel & Sarles, 1984). Obstruction may be by small tumours, neurofibromata, smooth-muscle tumours, and even by heterotopic pancreatic tissue infiltrating the major or minor papilla. The obstructing lesion may be hidden by the surrounding fibrosis, and can be hard to find even in resected specimens. (Fig. 25.17). (Lowes *et al.*, 1989)

Many cases of pancreatitis secondary to con-

genital abnormalities of the pancreas have their origin in incomplete drainage.

The pancreas divisum anomaly is found in approximately 6% of the Western population. It is seen in a higher proportion of patients with acute pancreatitis or obstructive pancreatopathy but whether it is a genuine aetiological factor or simply reflects selection bias of patients for ERCP has never been satisfactorily resolved.

The pancreas divisum anomaly can modify the distribution of disease in pancreatitis, and an acute attack of gall stone pancreatitis may result in a pure ventral pancreatitis with drainage of the dorsal segment unaffected. Drainage via the minor papilla is more precarious and a pure dorsal obstructive pancreatopathy is a well-recognized disorder.

Other congenital anomalies of pancreatic drainage are rare and, with the exception of the annular pancreas, usually asymptomatic. Drainage of the annular pancreas may be so poor that it results in pancreatic fibrosis with subsequent duodenal stenosis (Fig. 25.18).

Chronic pancreatitis

Aetiology and pathomorphology

Chronic pancreatitis is a relatively uncommon disease varying in incidence from 0.2% to 3% in

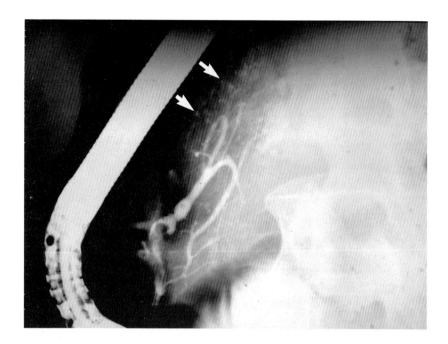

Fig. 25.18 Congenital short pancreas with acinar calcification.

autopsy series. The incidence has been increasing in the past 20 years and this almost certainly reflects a genuine increase rather than more effective means of diagnosis. This rise has mainly been caused by an increase in alcohol consumption.

The pathogenesis of chronic pancreatitis is still unclear and it is even uncertain whether chronic pancreatitis is a discrete entity within the pancreatic inflammatory disease or is related to acute pancreatitis. Evidence for this concept is based on the fact that acute and chronic pancreatitis are both related to alcohol abuse and thus there may be some common direct effect of alcohol on the pancreas.

The morphological features of advanced chronic pancreatitis are irregular scarring of the pancreatic parenchyma, typically on a lobular scale, strictures of the main pancreatic duct, and stenosis of the side-branches usually at the junction with the main duct. Intraductal protein plugs are a common finding and are frequently calcified in severe disease. Many cases show evidence of focal tissue necrosis with intrapancreatic pseudocyst formation.

Sarles has suggested that the initial lesion in alcoholic chronic pancreatitis is formation of an abnormal juice, leading to precipitation of protein plugs that give rise to secondary duct lesions by obstruction, initially of the main branches and subsequently with calcification within the main pancreatic duct system itself. Duct obstruction then leads to a focal obstructive pancreatitis with degeneration and fibrosis of the pancreatic parenchyma (Sahel & Sarles, 1984).

An alternative theory proposed by Klöppel suggests that alcohol damages the pancreatic parenchyma directly, leading to focal necrosis with healing by fibrosis that subsequently causes strictures of the duct system. This reduces the flow of pancreatic secretions, leading to precipitation of protein plugs upstream from the stenoses. At this point the mechanism of obstructive pancreatopathy becomes the dominant process. It is probable that both mechanisms operate in the majority of patients with alcoholic pancreatitis.

The theory of Sarles explains the phenomenon of idiopathic calcific chronic pancreatitis; that of Klöppel explains the predominantly parenchymal changes in the alcoholic with severe pancreatic pain but minimal duct changes on pancreatography (Klöppel, 1986).

It is important for the radiologist to understand the evolution of chronic pancreatitis in the individual patient in order to understand the morphology as demonstrated by radiological techniques (Nagata *et al.*, 1981, Amman *et al.*, 1984).

Early chronic pancreatitis

The morphological features of early chronic pancreatitis are:

1 Parenchymal damage with focal fibrosis.

2 Periductal fibrosis predominantly at bifurcations of the duct system

3 Irregularities of the main pancreatic duct.

4 Increase in bulk in pancreatic parenchyma.

5 Intraduct protein plugs.

No single imaging technique is capable of demonstrating all of these features. Pancreatography is undoubtedly the most sensitive method for demonstrating duct changes and is generally regarded as the most specific method of diagnosis (Cotton *et al.*, 1980; Kasugai *et al.*, 1984).

In non-calcific chronic pancreatitis CT scanning has a sensitivity of no better than 50% and may be very misleading unless there is significant duct dilatation or cyst formation (Malfertheiner *et al.*, 1984) (Table 25.2).

Modern ultrasonography is capable of demonstrating parenchymal changes involving the main pancreatic duct, and under good conditions of visualization can demonstrate the side-branches, but ultrasonography is notorious for being operator and patient-dependent and has a lower success rate than CT scanning in visualizing the entire pancreas (Fig. 25.19).

Severe chronic pancreatitis is easy to diagnose by ultrasound, CT, or even plain film radiography (Fig. 25.20).

The morphological features are:

1 Strictures of the main pancreatic duct with upstream dilatation.

2 Calculi within the duct system.

3 Confluent parenchymal fibrosis.

4 Cavities.

5 Involvement by inflammation of surrounding strictures.

CT scanning will give the most complete information, but the only pathognomonic feature is calcification, and this if present will be seen in at least 85% of cases by good conventional radiography (Kolmannskog *et al.*, 1981). To obtain adequate images in non-calcific chronic pancreatitis, good technique is important whichever imaging method is used.

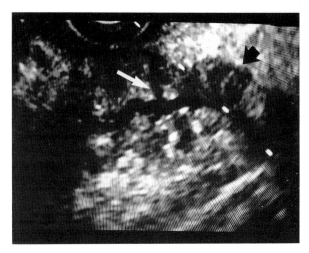

Fig. 25.19 Endoscopic ultrasound scan of mild chronic pancreatitis showing side-branch duct ectasia (*white arrow*) and lobular inflammation (*dark arrow*).

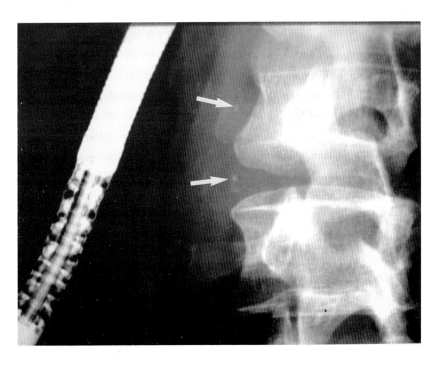

Fig. 25.20 Typical calcification of chronic pancreatitis.

Table 25.2 Sensitivity and specificity of CT in chronic pancreatitis

	Sensitivity (%)	Specificity (%)
Ferrucci *et al.*, 1979	84	56
Savarino, 1980	90	59
Kolmannskog *et al.*, 1981	80	—
Freeny, 1982	—	85
Malfertheiner, 1983	50 (mild CP)	

Technical factors

ENDOSCOPIC RETROGRADE CHOLANGIOPANCREATOGRAPHY (ERCP)

An adequate quality pancreatogram requires filling of the entire main pancreatic duct system and side-branches without causing acinar opacification. Overinjection is likely to lead to acute pancreatitis or duct 'blowout'. Another factor known to induce acute pancreatitis is repeated cannulation with trauma to the papilla of Vater (Axon *et al.*, 1984). A mild elevation of serum amylase up to 2000 iu is found in the majority of uncomplicated ERCPs. To obtain consistently good quality pancreatograms, scrupulous attention to detail is required, and even in a specialist centre, many of the films obtained may be unsuitable for retrospective analysis.

CT SCANNING

There are three requirements for a good pancreatic CT scan:
1 Adequate magnification of the area of interest and thin contiguous sections (4–5 mm) to identify the pancreatic duct system.
2 Adequate opacification of the duodenal loop with oral contrast. This may require duodenal paralysis and scanning in the left anterior oblique position.
3 Infusion of a slow bolus of intravenous contrast medium in adequate quantity; at least 100 ml of 35% non-ionic agent for a man of 70–80 kg body weight. This can be given just prior to rapid scanning through the pancreas, but best opacification and demonstration of the portal veins requires slow infusion throughout the scan (Fig. 25.21).

Identification of vascular lesions or small areas of infarction may also require true dynamic scanning after a rapid injection of a bolus of contrast.

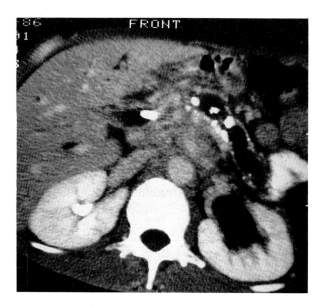

Fig. 25.21 Severe calcific chronic pancreatitis with ectasia of the MPD with intraduct calculi.

ULTRASONOGRAPHY

An adequate ultrasound study of the pancreas must include a description of the main pancreatic duct and of the volume of pancreas adequately studied. It is only possible to visualize the entire pancreas in the supine position in 30–40% of patients. The remainder require ingestion of 300–400 ml of degassed water, and careful positioning to displace gas from the gastric antrum and duodenal loop and to distend them with fluid. Some authors even propose the routine use of duodenal paralysis to maintain this acoustic window. Scanning in the right lateral or erect position after a fluid load provides a good acoustic window to the entire pancreas in at least 90% of patients.

Grading of chronic pancreatitis

All the various imaging techniques view the same morphological features in slightly different ways.

In order to establish a common descriptive base, a grading scheme for the morphology of chronic pancreatitis was proposed at the Classification Meeting in Cambridge in 1983 (Axon *et al.*, 1984, Sarner & Cotton, 1984). This is summarized in Table 25.3.

Except where there is definite evidence of strictures of the main pancreatic duct or calculi, it is difficult to make a definitive diagnosis of chronic pancreatitis on the basis of a single morphological

Table 25.3 Grading of chronic pancreatitis by imaging methods

Grade	US/CT	ERCP
1 Normal	Criteria for a normal study are fulfilled	
2 Equivocal	1 Abnormal sign only	< 3 abnormal branches
3 Mild	2+ Abnormal signs MPD 2–4 mm Gland 1–2 × normal Cavities < 10 mm Duct irregularity	> 3 abnormal branches
4 Moderate	Focal acute pancreatitis Parenchymal heterogeneity Increased echogenicity of duct wall Contour irregularity head/body	Above + MPD changes
5 Marked	All the above + 1 more: Cavity > 10 mm Intraduct filling defects Calculi Duct obstruction (stricture) Severe duct irregularity Contiguous organ invasion	

characteristic. If two features are present the diagnosis can be made, but with limited confidence; if three or more are present the diagnosis is highly specific. From pancreatography it is possible to classify non-calcific chronic pancreatitis into mild and moderate forms, depending on whether there is involvement of the main pancreatic duct system. Demonstration of at least three abnormal side-branches is required for diagnosis of mild chronic pancreatitis, and evidence of definite narrowing or irregularity of the main pancreatic duct for a diagnosis of moderate disease (Figs 25.22, 25.23).

Small cavities are frequently seen. These are pancreatic or peripancreatic collections which fill with contrast medium on pancreatography. They represent cysts, pseudocysts, or even abscesses and it is impossible to infer their true nature from the pancreatogram. Cavities may be large, but if smaller than 10 mm in diameter are rarely of major significance and are considered a feature of mild or moderate disease.

Common bile duct narrowing may be caused by fibrosis in the head of the pancreas. This is uncommonly seen in mild or moderate pancreatitis but is seen in up to 25% of patients with severe disease.

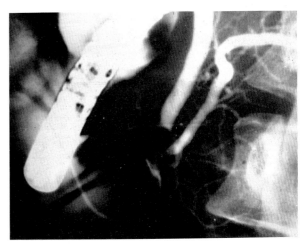

Fig. 25.22 ERCP of early chronic pancreatitis. There is good filling of all the side-branches with acinar opacification.

The features of severe chronic pancreatitis are intraduct calculi, strictures of the main pancreatic duct with upstream dilatation, cavities of greater than 10 mm in diameter, and evidence of extension of the inflammatory process to involve contiguous structures. Any one of these signs is sufficient to

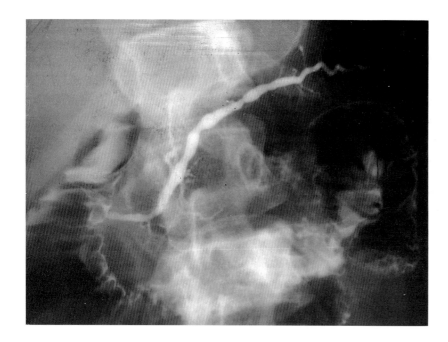

Fig. 25.23 Moderate chronic pancreatitis on ERCP.

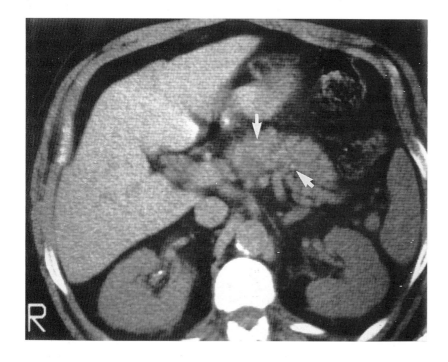

Fig. 25.24 Faint calcification on an unenhanced CT scan.

alter the grade from moderate to severe, provided that there is also involvement of the main pancreatic duct and its side-branches (Fig. 25.24).

Chronic pancreatitis may be a focal disease involving small segments of pancreatic tissue. The entity of 'groove' pancreatitis has recently been proposed by several German authors to explain the most common type of focal pancreatitis, which occurs in the segment of pancreas lying between the common bile duct and the duodenum. This may result in dense and focal fibrosis indistinguishable from a desmoplastic tumour (Nix & Schmitz, 1981) (Fig. 25.25).

The value of a grading system is that the underlying morphology can be described in the same precise terms by different imaging techniques, each of which shows only some of the features. This leads to repeatable description that allows populations to be compared and individual patients to be systematically followed up (Axon

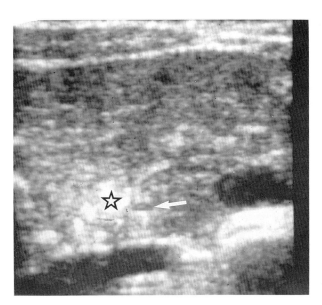

Fig. 25.25 The *star* indicates calcifications lying between the bile duct (*arrow*) and the duodenum.

et al., 1984.) A good correlation was recently shown between ERCP and ultrasonography when this scheme was tested (Jones *et al.*, 1988).

The natural history of chronic pancreatitis is still not adequately understood. In patients with alcoholic chronic pancreatitis who continue to drink, the disease appears to progress inexorably to calcific chronic pancreatitis with duct obstruction, fibrosis and atrophy of functioning pancreatic tissue (Amman *et al.*, 1984, Kalthoff *et al.*, 1984). The majority of patients with calcific chronic pancreatitis will have an impaired glucose tolerance test but only 5–10% will be frankly diabetic. Paradoxically the pain of chronic pancreatitis may be relieved when all functioning pancreatic tissue has been destroyed and hence chronic pancreatitis may 'burn out' in its end stages (Bornman *et al.*, 1980, 1984, Reimer *et al.*, 1984).

Complications of chronic pancreatitis

The principle complications of chronic pancreatitis are pseudocyst formation, biliary obstruction, portal vein thrombosis, and duodenal obstruction. Pseudocysts in this condition are almost always secondary to complete duct obstruction by a calculus and will rarely respond to conservative measures or percutaneous drainage (Freeny, 1986).

The peribiliary fibrosis of chronic pancreatitis classically leads to the 'rat tail' stricture in the distal common bile duct, but short strictures indistinguishable from their malignant equivalent are frequently seen. Evidence of previous portal-vein fibrosis is commonly seen on ultrasound or CT scanning, with visualization of varices or portal venous collaterals after obliteration of the main portal veins. The portal-vein thrombosis has usually been clinically silent with full physiological compensation via the collateral circuit (Ferrucci *et al.*, 1979).

Duodenal obstruction is uncommon even in severe calcific chronic pancreatitis, but some degree of duodenal narrowing is seen in up to 20% of patients with calcific chronic pancreatitis.

Surgery and chronic pancreatitis

Our indications for pancreatic surgery are intractable pain with duct dilatation or focal fibrosis, recurrent pseudocyst formation, or biliary or duodenal obstruction.

Focal pancreatitis with fibrosis can be impossible to distinguish from pancreatic cancer with a desmoplastic reaction, and biopsy is essential to establish a diagnosis prior to surgical intervention. Guided fine-needle aspiration cytology has traditionally been used but has a sensitivity of no better than 82% in large series (Hall-Craggs & Lees, 1986). More recently cutting biopsy needles of 1.2 mm diameter have been employed to give true histology. These have a higher complication rate but are more sensitive in the diagnosis of cancer; they can give a specific histological diagnosis of chronic pancreatitis (Figs 25.26a,b; 25.27a,b).

New imaging techniques in pancreatic inflammatory diseases

Magnetic resonance imaging

The spatial resolution of magnetic resonance imaging is now sufficient to demonstrate the common bile duct, portal venal system, and even the dilated main pancreatic duct, and the contrast resolution of the technique is as capable as CT scanning in showing oedematous changes of the peripancreatic fat or surrounding fascia. To date, no clinical advantage has been demonstrated over CT scanning where dynamic contrast enhancement techniques have been used, even in a group with over 450 cases (Engleholm, 1987, personal communication) (Fig. 25.28a,b).

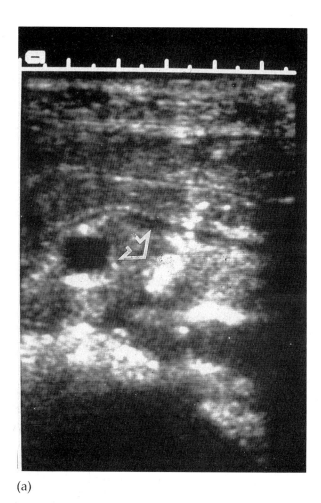

(a)

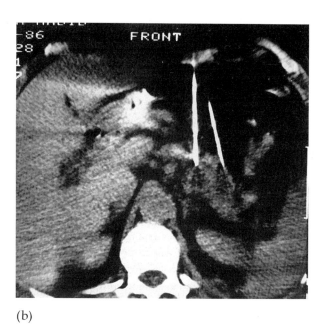

(b)

Fig. 25.26 (a) Ultrasound guided biopsy of the mid body of the pancreas. (b) CT guided biopsy of the tail of the pancreas.

Percutaneous pancreatography

Where there is clear ultrasonographic visualization of even a slightly dilated pancreatic duct, puncture of the duct with a fine needle under ultrasound control is relatively simple and a pancreatogram can be obtained by contrast instillation down the needle. The technique appears safe and we have experienced no significant complications in over 120 percutaneous punctures. The technique is extremely useful in the 10−20% of cases of chronic pancreatitis where the pancreatogram provides inadequate information as to the complete anatomy of the duct system, either through failure to cannulate or from a complete block in the main pancreatic duct (Fig. 25.29).

A complete map of the pancreatic duct system is essential to adequate surgical planning, and the success rate of this technique is over 90% where the duct exceeds 3 mm in diameter.

Endoscopic ultrasonography

Commercial devices are now available that incorporate high-resolution, high-frequency ultrasound probes mounted on the end of conventional side-viewing duodenoscopes. These operate at frequencies of 7.5 or 10 MHz and are capable of resolution of the order of 0.2 mm. By placing a tip-mounted ultrasound probe into the second part of the duodenum using endoscopic techniques, the probe can be withdrawn past the ampulla of Vater, around the duodenal loop into the gastric antrum, and then along the greater curve of the stomach. The technique can visualize the entire pancreas in over 70% of patients, and over 75% of the pancreas in 90%. The soft-tissue resolution obtainable by this technique is very much higher than that obtained by conventional ultrasonography or CT scanning and it is capable of routinely showing the anatomy of the side-branches of the pancreatic

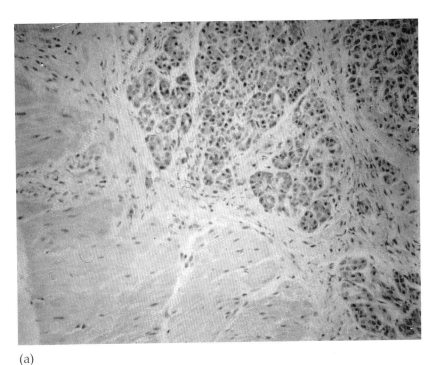

(a)

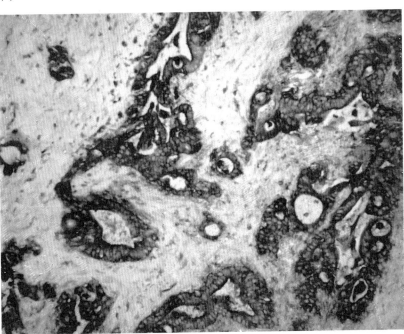

Fig. 25.27 (a) H&E stain of infiltrating pancreatic cancer. (b) Higher magnification showing strong surface staining for CEA.

(b)

duct system together with high-contrast resolution of the surrounding parenchyma. This technique is useful in discriminating the normal from the abnormal pancreas in patients with pain of suspected pancreatic origin, and for differentiating focal pancreatitis from pancreatic carcinoma. Of patients with pancreatic disease, 10–15% cannot be adequately evaluated with conventional imaging methods, and in our experience this technique is, next to biopsy, the most specific diagnostic method currently available.

Pancreatic endosonograhy is as well tolerated as any simple upper gastrointestinal endoscopy, carries no significant hazard, and can be performed as an out-patient procedure.

The very small field of view obtained by the

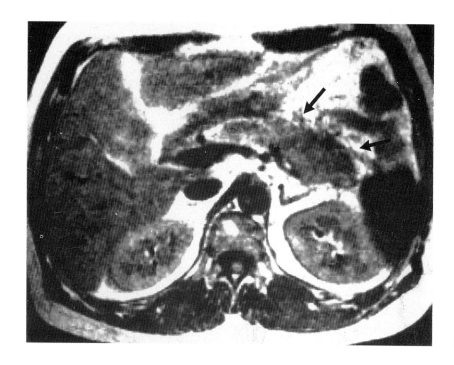

Fig. 25.28 (a) Horizontal MR section of mild acute pancreatitis.

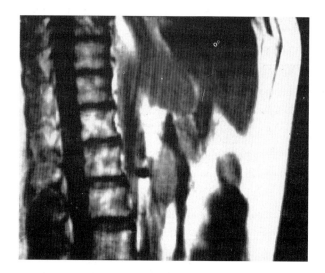

Fig. 25.28 (b) Sagittal MR section of mild acute pancreatitis.

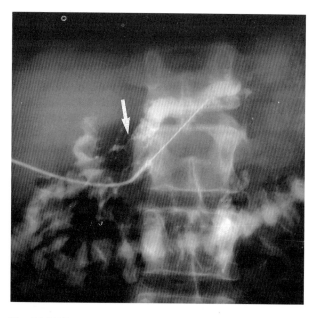

Fig. 25.29 Percutaneous pancreatogram showing a stricture in the MPD.

instrument and the invasive nature of the technique will limit its application in the early stages of evaluation of pancreatic disease, but it is finding increasing acceptance in specialist pancreatic centres for the investigation of difficult pancreatic problems.

References

Ammann, R.W., Akovbiantz, A., Largiader, F. & Schueler, G. (1984) Course and outcome of chronic pancreatitis. Longitudinal study of a mixed medical−surgical series of 245 patients. *Gastroenterology*, **86**, 820−828.

Axon, A.T.R., Classen, M., Cotton, P.B. *et al.* Pancreatography in chronic pancreatitis: international definitions. *Gut*, **36**, 517—520.

Balthazar, E.J., Ranson, J.H., Naidich, D.P. *et al.* (1985) Acute pancreatitis: prognostic value of CT. *Radiology*, **156(3)**, 767—772.

Banks, S., Wie, L. & Gersten, M. (1983) Risk factors in acute pancreatitis. *American Journal of Gastroenterology*, **78**, 637—640.

Barlin, J.S., Smith, F.R., Pereiras, R. *et al.* (1981) Therapeutic percutaneous aspiration of pancreatic pseudocysts. *Digestive Diseases and Sciences*, **26**, 585—586.

Beger, H.G. & Buchler, M. (1986) Outcome of necrotizing pancreatitis in relation to morphological parameters. In Malfertheiner, P. & Ditschuneit, H. (eds) *Diagnostic Procedures in Pancreatic Disease*, pp. 135—139. Springer Verlag, Berlin.

Bornman, P.C., Marks, I.N., Girdwood, A.H., Clain, J.E., Narusnky, L., Clain, D. J. & Wright, J.P. (1980) Is pancreatic duct obstruction or stricture a major cause of pain in calcific pancreatitis? *British Journal of Surgery*, **67**, 425—428.

Bornman, P.C., Marks, I.N. & Girdwood, A.H. (1984) Mechanism of pain in chronic alcohol-induced pancreatitis (CAIP). In Gyr, K., Singer, M.V. & Sarles, H. (eds), *Pancreatitis; Concepts and Classification*, pp. 193—195, Elsevier, Amsterdam.

Bradley, E.L. & Clements, L.J. (1976) Spontaneous resolution of pancreatic pseudocyst: implications for timing operative intervention. *American Journal of Surgery*, **129**, 23—28.

Buchler, M., Malfertheiner, P. & Beger, H.G. (1986) Correlation of imaging procedures, biochemical parameters, and clinical stage in acute pancreatitis. In Malfertheiner, P. & Ditschuneit, (eds). *Diagnostic Procedures in Pancreatic Disease*, pp. 123—129.

Cotton, P.B., Lees, W.R., Vallon, A.G. *et al.* (1980) Grayscale ultrasonography and endoscopic pancreatography in pancreatic diagnosis. *Radiology*, **134**, 453—459.

Ferrucci, J.T. Jr., Wittenberg, J. Mueller, P.R. *et al.* (1979) Computed body tomography in chronic pancreatitis. *Radiology*, **130**, 175—182.

Freeny, P.C. (1984) Computed tomography of the pancreas. *Clinical Gastroenterology*, **13**, 791—818.

Freeny, P.C., Marks, W.M. & Ball, T.J. (1983) Impact of high-resolution computed tomography of the pancreas on utilisation of ERCP and angiography. *Radiology*, **142**, 35—39.

Freeny, P.C., Lewis, G.P. & Marks, W. (1986) Percutaneous catheter drainage of infected pancreatic fluid collections and abscesses. *Radiology*, **161(P)**, 89.

Gerzhof, S.G., Banty, P.A., Robbins, A.H. *et al.* (1987) Percutaneous aspiration for diagnosis and management of suspected infection in complicated pancreatitis. *Radiology*, **165(P)** Suppl. **(55)**, 28.

Gyr, K., Heitz, P.U. & Beglinger, C. (1984) Pancreatitis. In Kloppel, G. & Heitz, P.V. (eds), *Pancreatic Pathology*, pp. 44—72. Churchill Livingstone, Edinburgh.

Hall-Craggs, M.A. & Lees, W.R. (1986) Fine needle aspiration biopsy: pancreatic and biliary tumours. *American Journal of Roentgenology*, **147**, 399—403.

Hill, M.C., Barkin, J., Isikoff, M.B. *et al.* (1982) Acute pancreatitis: clinical vs CT findings. *American Journal of Roentgenology*, **139**, 263—269.

Imrie, C.W. & White, S. (1975) A prospective study of acute pancreatitis. *British Journal of Surgery*, **62** 490—494.

Jensen, A.R., Matzen, P., Malchow-Moller, A., Christoffersen, I. and The Copenhagen Pancreatitis Study Group (1984) Pattern of pain, duct morphology, and pancreatic function in chronic pancreatitis. A comparative study. *Scandinavian Journal of Gastroenterology*, **19**, 334—338.

Jones, S.N., Frost, R.A. & Lees, W.R. (1988) Diagnosis and grading of chronic pancreatitis by morphological criteria derived by ultrasound and pancreatography. *Clinical Radiology*, **39(1)**, 43—48.

Kalthoff, L., Layer, P., Clain, J.E. & DiMagno, E.P. (1984) The course of alcoholic and nonalcoholic chronic pancreatitis. *Digestive Diseases and Sciences*, **29**, 953.

Kasugai, T., Kurimoto, K., Fujiwara, K., Tenehiro, K. & Kuno, N. (1984) Criteria for ERCP diagnosis of chronic pancreatitis based on histological evaluation. In Gyr, K.E., Singer, M.C. & Sarles, H. (eds) *Pancreatitis, Concepts and Classification*, pp. 225—229. Elsevier, Amsterdam.

Klöppel, G., Adler, G. & Kern, H.F. (1986) Pathomorphology of acute pancreatitis in relation to its clinical course and pathogenesis. In Malfertheiner, P. & Ditschuneit, H. (eds) *Diagnostic Procedures in Pancreatic Disease*, pp. 135—139. Springer Verlag, Berlin.

Kolmannskog F., Schrumpf, E., Bergan, A. & Larsen, S. (1981) Diagnostic value of computer tomography in chronic pancreatitis. A comparison with current diagnostic tests. *Acta Radiologica*, **22(6)**, 649—55.

Lowes, J.R., Lees, W.R. & Cotton, P.B. (1989) Pancreatic duct dilatation after secretin stimulation in pancreas divisum. *Pancreas*, **4(3)**, 371—374.

McMahon, M.J., Playforth, M.J. & Pickard, I.R. (1980) A comparative study of methods for the prediction of severity of attacks of acute pancreatitis. *British Journal of Surgery*, **67**, 22—25.

Maier, W. (1986) Grading of acute pancreatitis by computed tomography morphology. In Malfertheiner, P. & Dischuneit, H. (eds) *Diagnostic Procedures in Pancreatic Disease*, pp. 44—48. Springer Verlag, Berlin.

Malfertheiner, P., Buchler, M., Beger, H.G. & Ditschuneit, H. (1984) Exocrine pancreatic function in correlation to morphological findings (assessed by different imaging procedures) in chronic pancreatitis. In Gyr, K.E., Singer, M.V. & Sarles, H. (eds), *Pancreatitis: Concepts and Classification*, pp. 231—234. Elsevier, Amsterdam.

Nagata, A., Homma, T., Tamai, K. *et al.* (1981) A study of chronic pancreatitis by serial endoscopic pancreatography. *Gastroenterology*, **81**, 884—891.

Nix. G.A., & Schmitz, P.I. (1981) Diagnostic features of chronic pancreatitis distal to benign and to malignant pancreatic duct obstruction. *Diagnostic Imaging*, **50 (3)**, 130—137.

Ranson, J.H.C. (1984) Acute pancreatitis: pathogenesis, outcome and treatment. *Clinical Gastroenterology*, **13**, 843—863.

Ranson, J.H.C., Rifkind, K.M., Roses, D.F., Fink, S.D., Eng, K. & Spencer, F.C. (1974) Prognostic signs and the role of operative management in acute pancreatitis. *Surgery, Gynecology and Obstetrics*, **139**, 69—81.

Safrany, L. & Cotton, P.B. (1981) A preliminary report: urgent duodenoscopic schincterotomy for acute gallstone pancreatitis. *Surgery*, **89**, 424—428.

Sahel, J. & Sarles, H. (1984) Chronic calcifying pancreatitis and obstructive pancreatitis. Two entities. In Gyr, K.E., Singer, M.V. & Sarles, H. (eds), *Pancreatitis: Concepts and Classification*, pp. 47–49. Elsevier, Amsterdam.

Sankaran, S. & Walt, A.J. (1975) The natural and unnatural history of pancreatic pseudocysts. *British Journal of Surgery*, **62**, 37–44.

Sarner, M. & Cotton, P.B. (1984) Classification of pancreatitis. *Gut*, **25**, 756–759.

Sarti, D.A. (1977) Rapid development and spontaneous regression of pancreatic pseudocysts documented by ultrasound. *Radiology*, **125**, 789–793.

Siegelman, S.S., Copeland, B.E., Saba, G.P. *et al.* (1980) CT of fluid collections associated with pancreatitis. *American Journal of Roentgenology*, **134**, 1121–1132.

Singer, M.V., Gyr, K.E. & Sarles, H. (1985) Revised classi-fication of pancreatitis. Report on the Second Inter-national Symposium on the Classification of Pancreatitis in Marseille, France, 28–30 March, 1984. *Gastroenterology*, **89**, 683–690.

Trapnell, J.E. & Duncan, E.H.L. (1975) Patterns of incidence in acute pancreatitis. *British Medical Journal*, **2**, 179–83.

Vallon, A.G., Lees, W.R. & Cotton, P.B. (1979) Gray-scale ultrasonography and endoscopic pancreatography after pancreatic trauma. *British Journal of Surgery*, **66**, 169–172.

Vernacchia, F.S., Jeffrey, R.B. Jr., Federle, M.P. *et al.* (1987) Pancreatic abscess: predictive value of early abdominal CT. *Radiology*, **162(2)**, 435–438.

White, E.M., Wittenberg, J., Mueller, P.R., *et al.* (1986) Pancreatic necrosis: CT manifestations. *Radiology*, **158(2)**, 343–346.

26: Non-Endocrine Pancreatic Neoplasms

R.A. WILKINS AND D.E. KATZ

Introduction

The last decade has seen a marked increase in the incidence of pancreatic cancer throughout the world. It now accounts for about 3% of all cancers and is the 5th most common cause of cancer deaths after lung, bowel, breast and prostate (Silverbeg & Lubera, 1986). Pancreatic cancer can affect people of any age but there is a rapidly increasing incidence after the age of 50. The tumours are more common in males with a male : female ratio of 2 : 1. The highest incidence is in Polynesians such as the Maori's of New Zealand and in native Hawaiians. There is also an unduly high incidence in Blacks in the USA (Fraumeni, 1975). An increased incidence is seen in smokers (Liu & Kessler, 1981) and there is controversial evidence to suggest an increased risk in coffee drinkers (McMahon et al., 1981), even if they drink decaffeinated coffee (Wynder et al., 1986). The causal relationship between diabetes and pancreatitis is at best speculative (Beazley & Cohn, 1981).

Pathology

Most cancers are adenocarcinomata (95%) Cubella & Fitzgerald (1979). The large majority of non-endocrine pancreatic neoplasms arise from ductal elements (89%). In only 1% of cases do tumours arise from the acini, but in almost 10% of cases the site of origin is unknown (Shorten et al., 1986). Mucinous adenocarcinomata form a small subgroup of adenocarcinomata that produce a mucinous material within the tumour. The treatment and prognosis is identical to the other adenocarcinomata. Cystic neoplasms are rare tumours and are of three distinct types (i) mucinous cystic tumours (cystadenocarcinomata), which have a malignant potential, (ii) microcystic adenomata (cystadenomata), which are benign (Wynder et al., 1973), and (iii) papillary cystic neoplasms (solid and papillary). This latter group occurs predominantly in young women and is malignant, though it may be cured by radical resection (Kaufman et al., 1986). Very rare tumours that may affect the pancreas but account for less than 1% of all pancreatic neoplasms are sarcomata, haemangiomata, lymphangiomata, lymphomata, and metastases. Tumours arise in the head of the pancreas in more than half the cases, and in the body and tail in the remainder.

Clinical manifestations

Pain, weight loss and unremitting jaundice are the three outstanding symptoms. Pain is the most common symptom of pancreatic cancer, and is usually vague and poorly defined initially, but becomes more intense with growth; it frequently radiates to the back and is often relieved by sitting forward (Gambill, 1970).

Weight loss is invariably present and is probably due to a combination of the tumour per se and associated symptoms of early satiety and anorexia, and consequent poor nutrition.

Jaundice is the initial symptom in almost half the patients with tumours of the head, and occurs as a later manifestation in about a quarter of patients with tumours of the body and tail. Painless jaundice which is firmly entrenched as a classic finding of pancreatic cancer occurs in only about 25% of cases (Braganza & Howat, 1972).

Malabsorption and steatorrhoea may occur as late manifestations following pancreatic-duct obstruction and subsequent lack of secretion of pancreatic enzymes.

Diabetes mellitus is frequently associated with pancreatic cancer (25–50%) (Melnyk, 1973). The relationship is unclear but it seems likely that the diabetes occurs secondary to duct obstruction rather than inducing the cancer. The combination of abdominal pain with acute onset to diabetes mellitus must arouse the suspicion of pancreatic cancer (Cohen, 1965).

Spontaneous venous thrombosis is a common but non-specific finding in pancreatic cancer and would appear to bear no relationship to the size or extent of the tumour (Lieberman *et al.*, 1961).

Diagnosis

Pancreatic carcinoma remains one of the most difficult tumours to detect early in its course. The search for accurate tumour marker continues and some success has been reported with CA 19−9 and carcinoembryonic antigen (CEA) (Del Favero *et al.*, 1986). The combination of tumour marker assays and diagnostic imaging methods is potentially more accurate than either of these methods alone.

Imaging investigations

Plain X-rays

Abdomen

The plain abdominal X-ray is often the first radiological investigation performed on patients with pancreatic cancer who present with pain and/or jaundice, and may provide valuable clues to the diagnosis. Large tumours may cause displacement of the gastric air bubble or a grossly distended gall bladder may be recognized. Non-specific signs such as congestive splenomegaly secondary to splenic vein invasion or ascites may also be seen.

Pancreatic calcification is readily recognized on plain films. There is some evidence to suggest an increased incidence of carcinomata in chronic calcific pancreatitis, but it should be remembered that pancreatic calcification is indicative of benign disease in over 95% of patients (Eaton & Ferruci, 1973).

Primary ductal carcinomata virtually never calcify, but tumoral calcification is occasionally seen in benign cystic neoplasms of the pancreas (Becker *et al.*, 1965). Calcification in phleboliths has also been described in cavernous lymphangiomata (Dodds *et al.*, 1969).

Chest

Lung metastases occur late and are seen more frequently with tumours of the body and tail. Spread may occur either haematogenously, or rarely from direct extension from mediastinal lymph nodes.

Spine

Bony metastases may be seen either from haematogenous spread or from direct extension of tumour into contiguous vertebrae. Bony involvement is rare, however, and occurs in only 1% of cases. The metastases are typically osteolytic but osteoblastic metastases have been described (Freeny & Lawson, 1982).

Barium examinations

The widespread use of more direct imaging modalities had led to a dramatic reduction in the utilization of what, for many years, had been the primary imaging technique for the detection of pancreatic tumours. Barium examinations are, however, often requested as an early investigation in patients with persisting abdominal pain. The overall accuracy of this indirect method of visualizing masses is relatively low and only a positive finding is of diagnostic value. Diagnostic accuracy for tumours of the pancreatic head is much higher than for lesions of the body and tail, with a diagnostic accuracy of up to 95% reported in some series (Eaton & Ferruci, 1973). An impeccable technique using either direct intubation hypotonic duodenography or a careful double-contrast barium meal technique with gas distension and an anticholinergic drug is essential for accurate assessment.

The classical duodenal changes produced by pancreatic carcinoma include (i) extrinsic pressure, displacement or encasement of the duodenal loop; (ii) Frostberg's 'reversed-3' sign caused by traction on the medial wall of the duodenum by the pancreatic tumour (Fig. 26.1); (iii) mucosal irregularity; and (iv) barium reflux into the pancreatic or common bile duct. Displacement or direct invasion of the stomach and colon may also be recognized on barium examinations.

Ultrasound

Accurate ultrasound diagnosis requires a meticulous technique, and despite this the technical failure rate is often high. The presence of a dilated common duct or pancreatic duct should signal the need for careful assessment technique. It is often necessary to examine patients on several occasions and in varied positions and to use techniques such as filling the stomach with water to gain a better access window. Both high-resolution real-

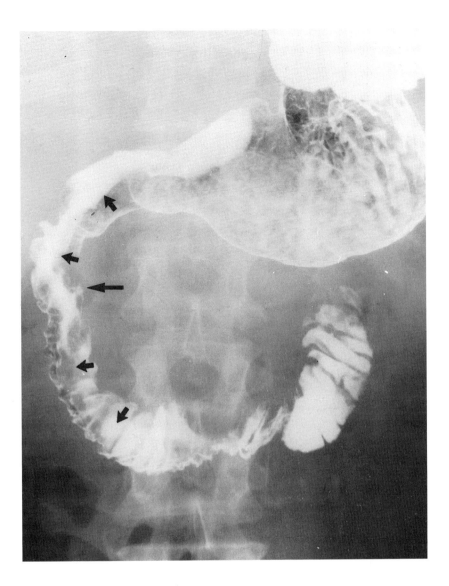

Fig. 26.1 Frostbergs' reversed-3' sign. The tumour of the pancreatic head has stretched and invaded the duodenal loop (*short arrows*) with relative fixity of the ampulla (*long arrow*).

time and B-scanners should be available for a complete examination. Tumours of the tail are the most difficult to detect because of air in the stomach or splenic flexure, and are often best seen through the left kidney in the prone position.

Tumours usually present as focal or diffuse masses and generally need to be more than 2 cm in diameter to be detected reliably (Doust, 1975). The margins of the pancreas are usually smooth but may be nodular or irregular with tumour enlargement (Cotton *et al.*, 1980).

Body and tail tumours are usually focal, but tumours of the head, while initially focal, often cause duct obstruction that causes distal pancreatitis and results in a diffusely enlarged gland with distal inflammatory swelling.

The texture pattern of pancreatic cancer is variable. The most common appearance is loss of the normal 'cobblestone' appearance and replacement by a less echogenic, coarser mass. Occasionally high-level echoes are superimposed on the background low-level tumour, and rarely the tumour may be of increased echogenicity (Weinstein *et al.*, 1979).

There is considerable variation in texture of the normal pancreas, and overlap between changes seen in inflammatory and neoplastic disease. None the less, carcinoma must be strongly considered when there is a focal or diffuse mass, a dilated pancreatic duct, or a focal alteration in texture, particularly a decrease in echogenicity. Pancreatic-duct dilatation is a feature of both pancreatitis and carcinoma. In general the duct in carcinoma tends to dilate more uniformly and to have parallel walls, whereas in chronic pancreatitis the duct may have a more irregular contour.

Carcinoma of the head of the pancreas causes obstructive jaundice in 80–90% of cases. Ultrasound allows distinction between medical and surgical jaundice in 95% of cases but the detection of the site of obstruction is much more difficult, with an accuracy range of between 55 and 85% (Neiman & Mintzer, 1977, Taylor & Rosenfeld, 1977).

Ultrasound allows the simultaneous evaluation of the liver, and metastases are present in almost half of patients with pancreatic tumours at the time of presentation (Freeny & Lawson, 1982).

Endoscopic ultrasound has recently become a talking point. The ultrasound probe is introduced into the stomach via an endoscope, and the pancreas scanned through the stomach wall. Theoretically this should be more accurate than conven-

tional ultrasound, though early results have yet to confirm this. Sivak detected 60% of carcinoma in a small series in this way (Sivak & Kaufman, 1986).

Computerized tomography

The most common finding in carcinoma is enlargement of the gland beyond the normal limits. There is a wide variation in the normal dimensions of the pancreas and one cannot rely on absolute measurements. Where the pancreas does not show the gradual normal tapering from head to tail, or where there is a discrepancy in this tapering, carcinoma of the pancreas should be suspected (Fig. 26.2). In about 13% of cases there is a diffuse

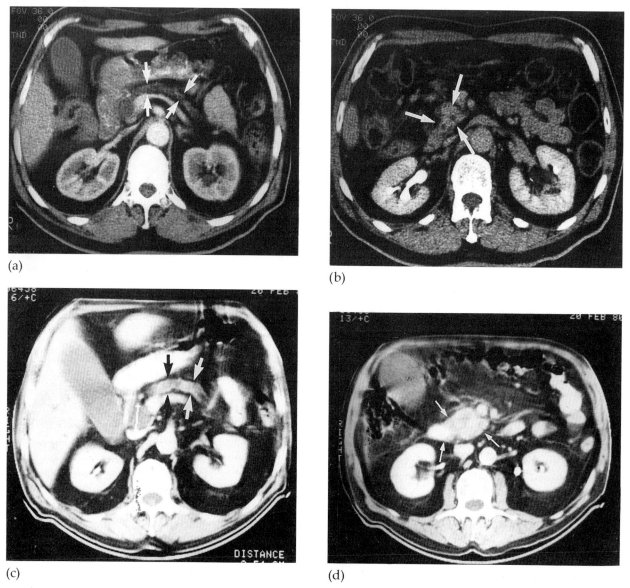

(a)

(b)

(c)

(d)

Fig. 26.2 Two cases of carcinoma showing a thin atrophic body and tail of pancreas (a and c) and a 'normal' sized head (b and d). This discrepancy in size is often an indication of tumour.

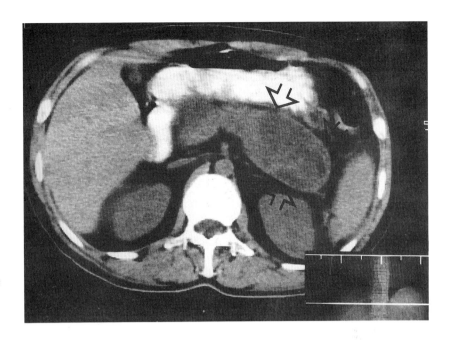

Fig. 26.3 Cystadenocarcinoma of the tail of the pancreas. The expanded tail (*arrows*) shows areas of low attenuation within.

enlargement of the gland. In these cases the pancreatic margins are often irregular and indistinct (Wittenburg *et al.*, 1982).

Tumour masses usually need to be 2–3 cm in diameter to produce a recognizable alteration in contour. Obviously the size and site of the tumour within the gland will to some extent determine the ease with which each tumour can be recognized (Ward *et al.*, 1983).

Tumours of the head or body of the pancreas often produce ductal obstruction and atrophy of the tail of the pancreas. The tail may merely look small, or the dilated duct may be seen as a tubular lucency in the centre of the atrophic tail. Obstruction may also cause retention cysts proximal to the mass.

Density differences can be recognized in about 50% of carcinomata of the pancreas. Tumours usually have slightly lower attenuation than the surrounding gland and this is often more evident with dynamic scanning after bolus injection of contrast (Haaga & Alfidi, 1983). Central necrosis within tumours may result in areas of fluid density and the appearance may closely resemble that of a pseudocyst. Mucinous adenocarcinomata, cystadenomata and cystadenocarcinomata may also produce low-density areas within the pancreas (Fig. 26.3). The cystic areas in mucinous adenocarcinomata tend to be smaller and slightly denser than their counterparts in cystadenomata and cystaenocarcinomata. Tumours may be difficult to distinguish from pseudocysts, and percutaneous needle aspiration may be needed for cytological evaluation.

Tumour spread is typically by direct lymphatic invasion, vascular invasion, and perineural extension. Metastases are frequent to liver, lymph nodes, peritoneum, and lung. Less frequently tumour spreads contiguously to adrenal glands, duodenum, kidneys, stomach, gall bladder, colon and spleen. Ascites is present in about 9% of cases (Freeny & Lawson, 1982). CT at a single examination will allow detection of spread as well as assessment of local tumour (Fig. 26.4).

Computerized tomography versus ultrasound

Freeny and Lawson (1982) compared the accuracy statistics of several large series of pancreatic ultrasound (total 908 patients), and pancreatic CT (1310 patients). Results showed that CT is more sensitive (92 vs. 78%), produces virtually no technically unsatisfactory results, (ultrasound failed to image the pancreas adequately in 14%), and has a high negative predictability (93 vs. 86% for ultrasound). Most important, however, is the ability of CT to provide a wider range of diagnostic information than ultrasound. Ancillary findings that are well shown on CT, such as regional lymph node involvement, local extension into the retroperitoneum, and invasion of contiguous organs, are often not accurately depicted on ultrasound and necessitate further examination for adequate evaluation. The

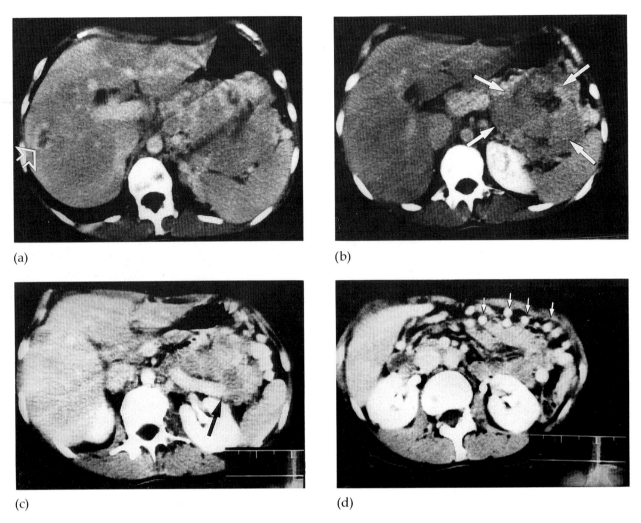

(a)   (b)

(c)   (d)

Fig. 26.4 CT shows the full extent of disease in a patient with weight loss and backache. (a) Liver metastases (*arrowed*); (b) Large tumour mass of mixed attenuation (*arrowed*) in tail of pancreas; (c) After bolus enhancement invasion of the splenic vein is seen (*arrow*); (d) Extensive collateral circulation (*arrows*).

current recommendation is that CT should be the examination of choice in suspected pancreatic cancer.

Magnetic resonance imaging

Despite advances in imaging techniques there has been little improvement in the mortality or morbidity in neoplastic disease of the pancreas. Magnetic resonance imaging (MRI) is a rapidly evolving technique with exciting potential for early diagnosis. At the time of writing, reported work has involved a variety of magnets, using different field strengths and with variable results. At present there do not appear to be any distinct advantages of MRI over CT. With MRI it is often difficult to

identify all the normal pancreas. The anatomy is usually clearly defined posteriorly owing to lack of signal because of the splenic and portal vein, but anteriorly lack of fat and the proximity of stomach and jejunum may make identification difficult. Overall, CT is superior to MRI for visualizing the normal pancreas because the margins are much more clearly delineated. The inability of MR to recognize calcification within the pancreas is a major pitfall, as calcification is often used as a differentiating point between benign and malignant pancreatic disease.

MRIs potential sensitivity and specificity for detection and differentiation of tumours provide hope that with refinement and experience there may be a large step forward in pancreatic imaging.

Percutaneous cholangiography

In most institutions ultrasound and/or CT are the front-line diagnostic tools in carcinoma of the pancreas. If the diagnosis is not made by either of these modalities, and in order to define precisely the location of an obstructing lesion, some form of direct cholangiography is necessary. This may be obtained by a percutaneous or an endoscopic approach.

Percutaneous cholangiography can be undertaken either by a trans-hepatic or a transjugular method. The transjugular is more complex and has largely been replaced by fine-needle direct percutaneous methods. Only in cases of severe coagulopathy would a transjugular approach be considered and even in such circumstances it may be preferable to do a percutaneous procedure with 'plugging' of the tract on removal of the needle with Gelfoam to prevent leak or bleeding.

Percutaneous trans-hepatic cholangiography (PTC) was first described by Huard & Do-Zuan-Hop in 1937. The procedure became established using an 18 gauge sheathed needle but there was a moderately high complication rate, particularly of bile leakage and bleeding. The acceptability of the technique was transformed by the introduction of the fine needle (Okuda et al., 1974). Success rate was raised from 87 to 98% and the complication rate overall dropped by a factor of nearly 4 (Harbin et al., 1980). Reported mortality rates of fine-needle technique range from 0 to 0.28% (Meyerovitz & Bettmann, 1987).

TECHNIQUE

Either a 22 or 23 gauge needle can be used. In most instances a right lateral approach is chosen, though occasionally if it is necessary to puncture the left duct an anterior epigastric approach may be employed. The only major contraindication to this alternative approach is the radiation hazard to the operator as the needle is in the direct beam.

Using the lateral approach the first step, having obtained informed consent, is to get the patient's co-operation for the study. This means explaining the procedure and practising breathing techniques. It is our normal practice to ask the patient to arrest respiration at a random point in the cycle and then to breathe gently when instructed.

The site for the puncture can be chosen either by fluoroscopy or percussion. The aim is to make the puncture in the mid-part of the right lobe, yet

avoiding the pleural reflection. A suitable site is planned in the anterior axillary line in an appropriate intercostal space. Care must be taken to avoid the intercostal artery, which runs along the inferior border or the rib.

Having chosen the correct location, local anaesthesia is applied and then with the respiration arrested as indicated the needle is introduced parallel to the table-top in a single pass to a point some 3–4 cm above the hilum of the liver. This point can either be marked fluoroscopically prior to the passage of the needle or judged by fluoroscopic control during its passage. The patient is then instructed to breathe gently.

The next step is to remove the obturator and connect, via a flexible connecting tube, a syringe filled with contrast medium. A suitable contrast medium would be a non-ionic compound of about 300 mg% iodine concentration or less. Under direct fluoroscopic vision a small amount of contrast medium is carefully infused through the needle as it is gradually withdrawn. A characteristic appearance indicates the location of the tip of the needle. If it is in the parenchyma, a diffuse blush occurs. If in a vessel, contrast will flow rapidly along the line of the vessel, the anatomical arrangement of which is detailed in Chapter 1. When the needle tip is in the bile duct the contrast will pool in the duct and gradually flow along the duct either in a caudal or cephalad direction. This appearance is very easily recognized after a limited experience. At this point the withdrawal of the needle is stopped and the contrast medium is infused until the duct system is well filled. Even in a dilated duct system it is seldom necessary to introduce more than 30 ml of contrast medium, which, by positioning, can be induced to opacify the entire system. If possible it is good practice to try to aspirate a few drops of bile for culture at this point prior to removing the needle. No further precautions are required and a simple dressing on the skin is all that is needed.

If on the first pass no bile ducts are entered, the passes can be repeated until such time as a bile duct is entered. It is good practice to terminate contrast medium injection and to repeat the pass prior to complete withdrawal of the needle, i.e. about 2–3 cm deep to the capsule. This has two advantages. Firstly, it tends to reduce the amount of contrast medium that finds its way beneath the capsule (this is important as it becomes painful), and secondly, it allows repeat passes to be made with only a single puncture of the capsule, hence minimizing leakage problems. The only need to terminate the procedure prior to successfully puncturing a bile duct is the development of a complication or some adverse reaction. Having filled the biliary tree with contrast medium the patient is rotated and/or tipped into appropriate positions so that the entire anatomy can be displayed and suitably documented on radiographs.

In patients with impaired clotting, prior to removal of the needle after filling the duct system, small pledgets of Gelfoam are injected into the liver parenchyma between the punctured duct and the capsule. These may be injected at more than one site as the needle is slowly removed.

INTERPRETATION

As ultrasound is now so accurate in distinguishing hepatocellular versus cholestatic jaundice, there is seldom a need to undertake cholangiography on an undilated system. In the great majority of circumstances therefore, the main purpose of the PTC will be to define the severity, location, and nature of an obstruction.

In carcinoma of the pancreas the biliary system may be narrowed or obstructed at several locations. The common bile duct lies within the substance of the head of the pancreas over its terminal portion, and clearly a carcinoma arising at this point can obstruct the duct by direct invasion. The duct may also be obstructed by direct invasion in a suprapancreatic location or less frequently by the involvement of metastatic nodes at the porta. An obstruction occurring in a peri-ampullary location may be due to a carcinoma of the pancreas or an ampullary carcinoma, but these cannot be distinguished radiographically (Freeny & Ball, 1981).

Other causes of bile-duct strictures include cholangiocarcinoma (Fig. 26.5), and benign conditions such as inflammatory disease related to stones and cholangitis, and previous surgery. Theoretically, the occlusion of the bile duct by a carcinoma of the pancreas has a smoothly tapered appearance, though this is not in any way diagnostic. Freeny and Lawson (1982) analysed the pattern of obstruction in 55 cases. More than half the cases (58%) had a smooth, rounded, or tapered appearance, one-third showed an irregular obstruction, and a small number (9%) a squared cut-off. Where the stenosis or obstruction is in the suprapancreatic portion of the common bile duct the bile duct is frequently and characteristically drawn medially at the site of obstruction. This is a characteristic

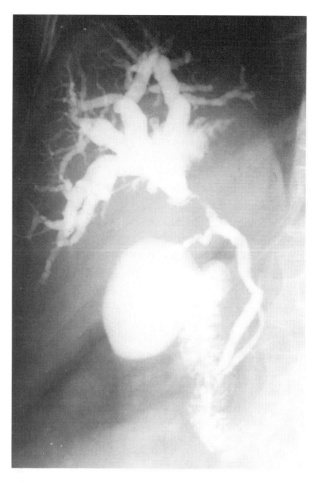

Fig. 26.5 PTC. A cholangiocarcinoma causing an irregular stricture of the common hepatic duct with proximal dilatation.

feature and is illustrated in Fig. 26.6. The severity of the stenosis together with the duration will determine whether the degree of proximal dilatation. The origin of the cystic duct in relationship to the stricture will determine whether the gall bladder is dilated or not.

PTC is very accurate in locating the site of block in obstructive jaundice. In a retrospective multicentre study from Japan (Tsuchiya *et al.*, 1986), PTC was said to be diagnostic in 34 of 49 patients with obstructive jaundice, and abnormal in all of them. PTC was also undertaken in the same study on 20 patients without jaundice, though the indications for this examination are not clear. In this group the PTC was diagnostic of carcinoma in 9 of the 20 patients, and again abnormal in all of them.

The choice between endoscopic retrograde cholangiopancreatography (ERCP) and PTC will be

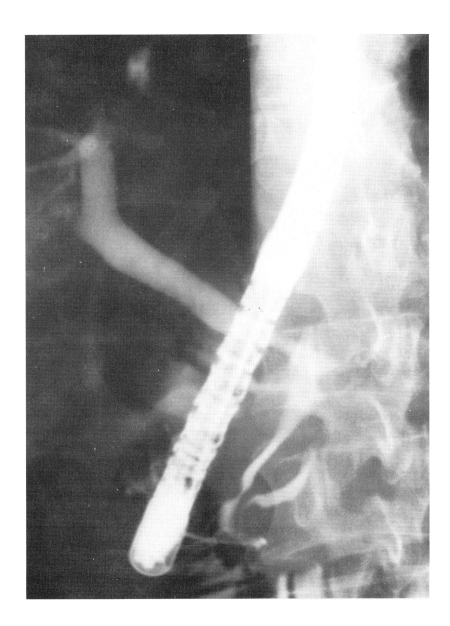

Fig. 26.6 ERCP. A carcinoma of the body of the pancreas obstructs the pancreatic duct and produces a characteristic deviation and narrowing of the common bile duct.

discussed below but one of the main indications for PTC is to progress at the same study or subsequently to drainage procedures. These procedures will be discussed in Chapter 10.

COMPLICATIONS

Using the fine-needle technique, leakage of blood or bile is unlikely (occurring in less than 1% of patients). The most serious complication developing with any frequency is sepsis. The incidence is higher in patients with cholelithiasis.

Some authors advocate the routine use of prophylactic antibiotics starting 12–24 h before PTC (Meyerovitz & Bettmann, 1987). If the operator is careful not to overdistend the biliary system and the outflow is not totally or subtotally obstructed, then it is probably safe to leave the patient without antibiotic cover. If the duct system is obstructed, prompt drainage either transcutaneously or surgically is the best way to avoid sepsis, though antibiotic cover is required.

The development of sepsis may be delayed, though release of endotoxins by the procedure can be very rapid and cause septicaemia and endotoxic shock actually during the examination. This requires management to maintain vital signs, the drawing of samples for culture, and the immediate infusion of intravenous antibiotics (Meyerovitz & Bettmann, 1987).

Endoscopic retrograde cholangiopancreatography (ERCP)

Whatever the pros and cons of ERCP versus PTC, there can be no doubt that if the working clinical diagnosis is of carcinoma of the pancreas or if a pancreatic mass is suspected from ultrasound or CT then ERCP should be the investigation of choice if available on site. This is simply because using ERCP the duct systems of both the pancreas and the biliary tree can be filled at the same examination. With skilled operators this is possible in the majority of patients and greatly enhances the diagnostic yield of the study. Gilinsky *et al.* (1986) found ERCP to be the most accurate of all diagnostic modalities. The findings in the biliary system in carcinoma of the pancreas are identical to those described above in the section on percutaneous cholangiography and the pitfalls of interpretation are much the same.

Just one word of warning, in practical terms when the contrast medium is introduced through a contaminated system (that is, via an endoscope passed through the mouth, oesophagus, etc.) there is a potential for the contrast media to contain bacteria. In a normally draining duct system this is probably of no great consequence, but in an obstructed system there is a potential for the induction of cholangitis or pancreatitis and septicaemia. The radiologist, if not actually performing the ERCP but assisting at it, has an important role to play in the acquisition of suitable radiographs and in aiding the endoscopist to obtain correct filling and positioning of the patient to obtain a diagnostic study. He may be able to obviate overfilling by his knowledge of the apperances of the biliary and pancreatic duct systems. In a multicentre survey by Cotton (1977) there was an 0.37% incidence of cholangitis with an 0.05% mortality. It is important to note that in 90% of the cases developing cholangitis the bile ducts were obstructed. Other studies (Vennes *et al.*, 1974) have found a much higher incidence of up to 15% of cholangitis developing after ERCP of an obstructed system.

Management is as described in the section on PTC. Similarly, pancreatitis may be a complication of ERCP, particularly in an obstructed system. In Bilbao's survey (Bilbao *et al.*, 1976) 80% of deaths were in obstructed ducts, yet the total incidence of pancreatitis was only 0.3%.

Prophylactic antibiotics are thought to be of benefit when stagnation is present. This is a recommendation of the British Society of Gastroenterologists (Cotton, 1977). Gentamicin and cephalosporin are commonly employed. Relief of the obstruction if at all possible is an important part of management.

A common ampulla for the bile duct and pancreatic duct is present in 60% of patients and the pancreatic duct can be filled by redirecting the ERCP cannula into the pancreatic duct. Alternatively if a second ampulla is present this will have to be cannulated independently. The pancreatic duct system is in normal patients of small volume and there is a real danger of overfilling the system. If the pancreatic duct system is overfilled, contrast will appear in the substance of the gland, the so-called acinar pattern. In the days of ionic contrast medium this often led to complications and in particular to pancreatitis, but with the newer nonionic contrast media this danger is reduced. Nevertheless, amylassaemia or occasionally pancreatitis can be precipitated by overfilling the duct system (Twomey & Wilkins, 1982).

RADIOGRAPHIC FINDINGS

The commonest radiographic finding in carcinoma of the pancreas is duct obstruction, and in the literature review by Freeny & Lawson (1982), totalling 530 cases, obstruction was present in 46%. The obstruction is usually smooth and tapered, but this is not diagnostic and identical appearances can be seen in inflammatory disease. Coexistent pancreatitis is not infrequently seen in carcinoma of the pancreas and in a review by Gambill (1971), 10% of 225 cases were seen to have these two diseases. Radiographically it may be very difficult to distinguish chronic pancreatitis with stricturing or occlusion of the duct from a carcinoma. Chronic pancreatitis traditionally causes multiple strictures and occlusions of the duct system (Chapter 25). If this is seen proximal to a stricture but not downstream of the stricture, then the diagnosis is likely to be carcinoma with coexistent pancreatitis (Fig. 26.7). If, on the other hand, the changes of chronic pancreatitis are seen both upstream and downstream of the stricture then the cause is likely to be an inflammatory stricture.

The second most common finding on ERCP is a stricture of the duct that has not progressed to a complete obstruction. In Freeny's review (Freeny & Lawson, 1982), this was present in 40%. The duct system proximal to the stricture is dilated and may show the changes of pancreatitis. There is no

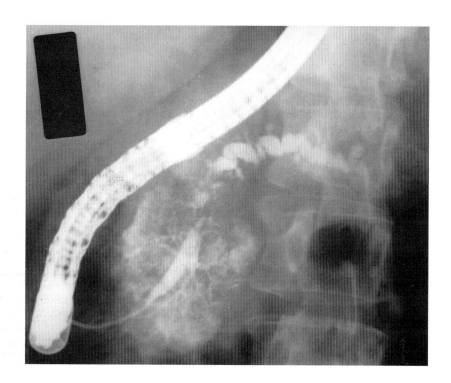

Fig. 26.7 ERCP. Proximal to the obstructing carcinoma the ducts are dilated and exhibit many strictures. Downstream the duct system is normal.

need, and in fact it is contraindicated, to introduce more than the very minimum amount of contrast medium beyond the stricture to identify the duct proximally.

Associated with the obstruction or stricture of the main duct there is frequently an associated acinar field defect (Fig. 26.8). When the carcinoma arises in a location remote from the principal ducts it is theoretically possible to have a field defect without any recognizable duct changes. This is not surprisingly a rare finding, and in Freeny's review of 530 cases occurred in just 2% (Freeny & Lawson, 1982).

Occasionally the tumour may undergo central necrosis which connects with the duct system, and cavitation may be detected as contrast medium enters the tumour. Even more rarely the carcinoma may be of a diffuse infiltrating type that narrows the duct system over a long length.

FURTHER MANAGEMENT

In equivocal cases pancreatic juice can be obtained by stimulating the pancreas with i.v. pancreozymin. This may be sent for cytology, which may then confirm the diagnosis (Hatfield *et al.* 1976).

Alternatively, percutaneous biopsy may be undertaken using the images obtained during ERCP as a guiding mechanism. This is an alterna-

tive to the use of ultrasound or CT for guided biopsies. Localization in two dimensions is clearly very easy using fluoroscopically directed biopsy techniques. Depth cannot be judged directly, but with practice the location of the needle tip can be judged by distortion and movement of the contrast-filled ducts adjacent to the proposed biopsy site. Avoiding other organ systems during the passage of the needle can to some extent be assessed at ERCP, in particular it is usually possible to identify and avoid the transverse colon. Other structures need not be avoided if a fine needle (22 gauge) is used.

Although it is correct medical practice to obtain histological or cytological proof of pancreatic carcinoma, the radiographic appearances are frequently highly characteristic. This is due to the regrettable fact that these tumours often present late. The typical presentation is of pain and obstructive jaundice, mass in the pancreas shown on ultrasound or CT and an ERCP showing obstruction or stricture of the pancreatic duct. The only management decision is based on size of tumour and potential for an attempt at curative resection. In a recent survey by Kalser *et al.* (1985), only 5% of patients had a small tumour (median size 9 cm^2) and were deemed suitable for radical surgery. This group survived, on average, 73 weeks: significantly longer than group 2 with larger tumours, where

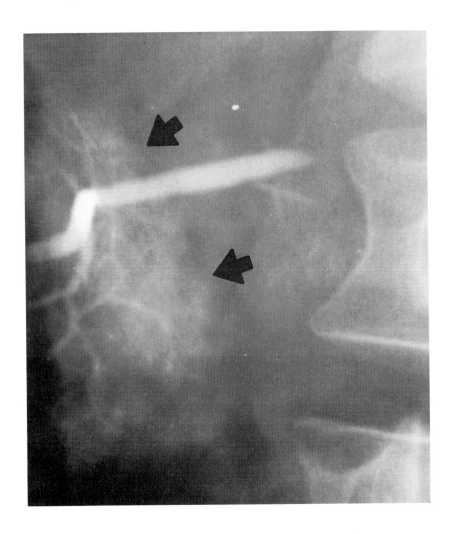

Fig. 26.8 ERCP. The carcinoma obstructs the main duct but infiltrates into the gland several centimetres distally. The 'acinar field defect'.

median survival was 33 weeks, and group 3, with advanced disease, who survived 10 weeks.

Tsuchiya *et al.* (1986) undertook a retrospective multicentre trial to assess diagnosis and management of small tumours. One hundred and six cases with carcinomata 2 cm or less in diameter were reviewed. It was possible to resect 99% of these. At surgery, however, less than half (44%) were stage I with no capsular or retroperitoneal invasion and no evidence of nodal spread. In this group survival rates were high (89.5% at 1 year and 37% at 10 years). Encouraging though these figures are it must be remembered that this group (stage I, 2 cm or less) represented just 45 patients from a review of 3315 in total.

Angiography

Pancreatic angiography for diagnostic purposes is no longer employed in the majority of centres due to advances in cross-sectional imaging. The only exception being in suspected cases of cystic tu-

mours. These lesions can be divided into mucinous cystadenomata or cystadenocarcinomata, microcystic adenomata, and papillary cystic tumours. In these tumours the characteristic angiographic pattern is of hypervascularity, though a range of vascularity is described (Freeny *et al.*, 1978). The principal difference is that the mucinous cystadenocarcinomata, which are highly malignant, show in addition characteristic angiographic signs of invasion, namely vessel encasement and obstruction. It is claimed that all cystadenomata will become cystadenocarcinomata in time (Compagno & Oertel, 1978).

In pancreatic carcinoma the place for angiography is now mainly in assessment of resectability and in definition of the vascular anatomy prior to resection. Selective catheterization of the gastroduodenal artery is required and in some cases further superselective studies are needed. The angiogram needs to be extended to cover the venous phase, and there may be a place for magnification to improve accuracy. In order to obtain good venous-phase information, digital subtraction is helpful. The use of vasodilators is recommended if good venous filling cannot be obtained without.

Angiography is undertaken in a standard manner using a transfemoral approach. Either Sidewinder or cobra-shaped catheters are most often suitable for selective gastroduodenal catheterization. In some cases, and when more selective studies are required, a range of specialized guidewires must be available, including movable tapered core, torque-control, and injectable. The volume of contrast medium injected depends mainly on the degree of selectively and size of vessel. In the gastroduodenal artery a typical volume may be 15–20 ml.

Pancreatic carcinomata are essentially avascular, though in some cases patchy hypervascularity has been seen (Reuter, 1975). The most important angiographic sign is of vessel encasement. In the largest series published, Tylen (1973) found arterial encasement in 103 of 116 cases, with 32 cases of venous encasement. Encasement, as the name implies, is direct involvement of the vessel by the scirrhous tumour, which partly compresses it but distorts it at the same time. This leads to a characteristic serpiginous or saw-tooth deformity.

In assessment of resectability the angiographer's aim is to look for evidence of extrapancreatic extension of the neoplasm. Thus, encasement of the extrapancreatic arteries including the gastroduodenal artery, and occlusion or encasement of veins such as the splenic vein, are clear evidence of unresectability.

Biopsy

Pancreatic tissue for cytological or histological purposes may be obtained percutaneously or endoscopically. On stimulation with i.v. pancreozymin, pancreatic secretions can be collected by aspiration through an endoscope, spun, and stained. A cytological specimen may also be obtained using a brushing device passed through the endoscope.

Transcutaneous biopsy of the pancreas was first reported by Oscarson et al. (1972). This development was one of a series of advances in diagnosis which were enabled by the introduction of the flexible 22 gauge 'Chiba' needle. The technique of aspiration is critical to the diagnostic yield. The needle is introduced attached to an empty 10-ml syringe, so that the tip lies at the point of interest. Suction is applied to the needle using the syringe and the needle is moved a short distance to and fro to help loosen the cells. The needle may also be rotated during this process for the same purpose. The vacuum is then released on the aspirating syringe and the needle withdrawn. Cytological slides are then prepared by ejecting the material collected with the needle onto a slide. The slide is prepared and fixed immediately. Ideally the material should be examined immediately by a cytologist so that adequacy of the specimen may be judged. Cytological material may also be obtained transcutaneously using the Rotex device (Vrsus Konsult AB, Sweden).

More recently it has been shown (Lees, personal communication) to be possible to obtain histological samples safely using an 18 gauge automatic biopsy device (Biopty, Henleys Medical Supplies, London). This needle is a variation of the Trucut design but the sample can be taken automatically and very quickly by a spring system that can be used one-handed. This is very useful when guiding the biopsy under ultrasound. Localization of the pancreatic mass other than by ultrasound can also be by CT guidance or under fluoroscopic control during an ERCP. Aspiration biopsy may also be obtained using angiography or PTC as a guiding mechanism, but accuracy rates are low and these methods cannot be recommended.

The ease and convenience of ultrasound localization for biopsy is to some extent offset by the slightly discouraging published accuracy figures. In a small and early series only 50% accuracy was noted (Clouse et al., 1977), though more recent studies (Mitty et al., 1981) record a sensitivity of 86% and a specifity of 100%. The major source of error is probably the accurate localization of the tip of the needle. Needle tips with a roughened surface (Cook Inc., Bloomington, USA) reflective to ultrasound may help to overcome this. Localization by CT is advocated as a highly accurate method by Freeny & Lawson (1982), who recorded 19 of 22 correct diagnoses, but the same author was also able to record a 96% accuracy rate using ERCP as a guidance method (Freeny et al., 1980). Whatever guidance is used, complication rates are low, with no deaths recorded and only a single case of tumour seeding along the tract (Ferrucci et al., 1979).

Other pancreatic neoplasms

The endocrine tumours are discussed in Chapter 15. Other than adenocarcinoma and the rare cystic neoplasms, other tumours may occasionally be seen in the pancreas. Lymphoma may frequently lie adjacent to the pancreas and at a late stage invade this organ directly. It is reported that 0.7% of extranodal non-Hodgkin's lymphoma originates in the pancreas (Freeman *et al.*, 1972). Extramedullary plasmacytoma in the pancreas has been described (Rice *et al.*, 1981) as have sarcomata, haemangiomata and lymphomata, but all are very rare.

Metastatic disease to the pancreas may be seen from various primaries including bronchus and melanoma. With all these rarities diagnosis is normally dependant on tissue sampling, though the lymphomata may be diagnosed by non-invasive methods.

Management

Surgical treatment of pancreatic carcinoma is traditional but the results are generally discouraging, as detailed above. Palliative non-surgical treatment for relief of jaundice includes the placement of stents through the obstructed biliary system by either an endoscopic or a percutaneous approach. Alternatively, the jaundice may be relieved by external drainage. These techniques are discussed in detail in Chapter 22.

References

Beazley, R.M. & Cohn, I. (1981) Pancreatic cancer. *Cancer*, **31**, 346–358.

Becker, W.F., Welsh, R.A. & Pratt, H.S. (1965) Cystadenoma and cystadenocarcinoma of the pancreas. *Annals of Surgery*, **161**, 845–863.

Bilbao, M.K., Dotter, C.T., Lee, T.G. & Katon, R.M. (1976) Complications of Endoscopic retrograde cholangiopancreatography (E.R.C.P.). A study of 10,000 cases. *Gastroenterology*, **70**, 314–320.

Braganza, J.M. & Howat, H.T. (1972) Cancer of the pancreas. *Clinical Gastroenterology*, **1**, 219–237.

Clouse, M.E., Greeg, J.A., McDonald, D.G. *et al.* (1977) Percutaneous fine needle aspiration biopsy of pancreatic carcinoma. *Gastrointestinal Radiology*, **21**, 67–69.

Compagno, J. & Oertel, J.E. (1978) Mucinous cystic neoplasms of the pancreas with overt and latent malignancy (cystadenocarcinoma and cystadenoma). A clinicopathologic study of 41 cases. *American Society of Clinical Pathologists*, **69(6)**, 573–580.

Cohen, G.F. (1965) Early diagnosis of pancreatic neoplasms in diabetics. *Lancet*, **ii**, 267–269.

Cotton, P.B. (1977) E.R.C.P. *Gut*, **18**, 316–341.

Cotton, P.B., Lees, W.R., Vallon, A.G. *et al.* (1980) Gray-scale ultrasonography and endoscopic pancreatography in pancreatic diagnosis. *Radiology*, **134**, 453–459.

Cubella, A.L. & Fitzgerald, P.J. (1979) Classification of pancreatic cancer (non endocrine). *Mayo Clinic Proceedings*, **54**, 449–458.

Del Favero, G., Fabris, C., Plebani, M. *et al.* (1986) CA 19–9 and carcinoembryonic antigen in pancreatic cancer diagnosis. *Cancer*, **57**, 1576–1579.

Dodds, W.J., Margolin F.R. & Goldberg, H.I. (1969) Cavernous lymphangioma of the pancreas. *Radiology Clinical Biology*, **38**, 267–270.

Doust, B.D. (1975) Ultrasonic examination of the pancreas. *Radiologic Clinics of North America*, **13**, 467–478.

Eaton, S.B. & Ferruci, J.T. (1973) *Radiology of the Pancreas and Duodenum*, p. 58. Saunders, Philadelphia.

Ferrucci, J.T. Jr., Wittenberg, J., Margolies, M.N. & Carey, R.W. (1979) Malignant seeding of the tract after thinneedle aspiration biopsy. *Radiology*, **130**, 345–346.

Fraumeni, J.F. (1975) Cancers of the pancreas and biliary tract: Epidemiological considerations. *Cancer Research*, **35**, 3437.

Freeman, C., Berg, J.W. & Cutler, S.J. (1972) Occurrence and prognosis of extranodal lymphomas. *Cancer*, **29**, 252–260.

Freeny, P.C. & Ball, T.J. (1981) Endoscopic retrograde cholangiopancreatography (ERCP) and percutaneous transhepatic cholangiography (PTC) in the evaluation of suspected pancreatic carcinoma: Diagnostic limitations and contemporary roles. *Cancer*, **47**, 1666–1678.

Freeny, P.C., Kidd, R. & Ball, T.J. (1980) ERCP-guided percutaneous fine-needle pancreatic biopsy. *Western Journal of Medicine*, **132**, 283–287.

Freeny, P.C. & Lawson, T.L. (1982) *Radiology of the Pancreas*. Springer-Verlag, New York, Heidelberg, Berlin. 397–496.

Freeny, P.C., Weinstein, C.J., Taft, D.A. *et al.* (1978) Cystic neoplasms of the pancreas: New angiographic and ultrasonographic findings. *American Journal of Roentgenology*, **131**, 798–802.

Gambill, E.C. (1970) Pancreatic and ampullary carcinoma: Diagnosis and prognosis in relationship to symptoms, physical findings and elapse of time in 255 patients. *Southern Medical Journal*, **63**, 1119–1122.

Gambill, E. (1971) Pancreatitis associated with pancreatic carcinoma: a study of 26 cases. *Mayo Clinic Proceedings*, **46**, 174–177.

Gilinsky, N.H., Bornman, P.C., Girdwood, A.H. & Marks, I.N. (1986) Diagnostic yield of endoscopic retrograde cholangiopancreatography in carcinoma of the pancreas. *British Journal of Surgery*, **73**, 539–543.

Haaga, J.R. Alfidi, R.J. (1983) *Computed Tomography of the Whole Body*, pp. 639–680. C.V. Mosby, St Louis, Toronto.

Harbin, W.P., Mueller, P.R. & Ferrucci, J.T. (1980) Transhepatic cholangiography: Complications and use patterns of the fine-needle technique. *Radiology*, **135**, 15–22.

Hatfield, A.R.W., Smithies, A., Wilkins, R. *et al.* (1976) Assessment of endoscopic retrograde cholangiopancreatography (ERCP) and pure pancreatic juice cytology in patients with pancreatic disease. *Gut*, **17**, 14–21.

Huard, P. & Do-Zuan-Hop. (1937) La ponction transhepatique des canaux biliares. *Bulletin de la Société de Médecine et Chirurgie L'Indochine*, **15**, 1909–1100.

Kalser, M.H., Barkin, J. & MacIntyre, J. M. (1985) Pancreatic carcinoma: Assessment of prognosis by clinical presentation. *Cancer*, **56**, 397–402.

Kaufman, S.L., Reddick, R.L., Stiegel, M., Wild, R.E. & Thomas, C.G. (1986) Papillary cystic neoplasm of the pancreas — a curable pancreatic tumor. *World Journal of Surgery*, **10**, 851—859.

Lieberman, J.R., Borrero, J., Urdaneta E. *et al.* (1961) Thrombophlebitis and cancer. *Journal of the American Medical Association*, **177**, 542—546.

Lin, R.S. & Kessler, L. (1981) A multifactorial model for pancreatic cancer in man. Epidemiological evidence. *Journal of the American Medical Association*, **245**, 147—152.

MacMahon, B., Yen, S., Trichopoulos, D., Warren, K. & Nardi, G. (1981) Coffee and cancer of the pancreas. *New England Journal of Medicine*, **304**, 630.

Melnyk, C.S. (1973) Carcinoma of the pancreas. In Sleisenger, M.H. & Fordtran, J.S. (eds), *Gastrointestinal Disease*, pp. 1198—1205. Saunders, Philadelphia.

Meyerovitz, M.F. & Bettman, M.A. (1987) Transhepatic biliary procedures. In *Complications in Diagnostic Imaging*, 2nd ed, pp. 171—185. Blackwell Scientific Publications, Oxford.

Mitty, H.A., Efremidis, S.C. & Yeh, H.C. (1981) Impact of fine-needle biopsy on management of patients with carcinoma of the pancreas. *American Journal of Roentgenology*, **137**, 1119.

Neiman, H.L. & Mintzer, R.A. (1977) Accuracy of biliary duct ultrasound: comparison with cholangiography. *American Journal of Roentgenology*, **129**, 979—982.

Okuda, K., Tanikawa, K., Emura, T. *et al.* (1974) Nonsurgical percutaneous transhepatic cholangiography — diagnostic significance in medical problems of the liver. *American Journal of Digestive Diseases*, **19**, 21—36.

Oscarson, J, Stormby, N. & Sundgren, R. (1972) Selective angiography in fine-needle aspiration cytodiagnosis of gastric and pancreatic tumours. *Acta Radiologica: Diagnosis*, **12**, 737—748.

Reuter, S.R. (1975) Superselective pancreatic angiography. In Anacker, H. (ed), *Efficiency and Limits of Radiologic Examination of the Pancreas*, pp. 149—158. Georg Thieme, Stuttgart.

Rice, N.T., Woodring, J.H., Mostowycz, L, & Purcell, M. (1981) Pancreatic plasmacytoma: Sonographic and computerized tomographic findings. *Journal of Clinical Ultrasound*, **9**, 46.

Shorten, S.D., Hart, W.R. & Petras, R.E. (1986) Microcystic adenomas (serous cystadenomas) of pancreas. *American Journal of Surgical Pathology*, **10(6)**, 365—372.

Silverberg, E. Lubera, J. (1986) Cancer statistics. *CA. A Cancer Journal for Clinicians*, **36**, 9—25.

Sivak, M.V Jr & Kaufman, A. (1986) Endoscopic ultrasonography in the differential diagnosis of pancreatic disease: a preliminary report. *Scandinavian Journal of Gastroenterology*, **21** [Suppl 123], 130—134.

Taylor, K.J.W. & Rosenfeld, A.T. (1977) Gray scale ultrasonography in the differential diagnosis of jaundice. *Archives of Surgery*, **112**, 820—825.

Tsuchiya, R., Noda, T., Harada N. *et al.* (1986) Collective review of small carcinomas of the pancreas. *Annals of Surgery*, **203(1)**, 77—81.

Twomey, B.P. & Wilkins, R.A. (1982) Pancreatic parenchymography using Metrizamide. *Gut*, **23**, A 432.

Tylen, U. (1973) Accuracy of angiography in the diagnosis of carcinoma of the pancreas. *Acta Radiologica*, **14**, 449—466.

Vennes, J.A., Jackson, J.R. & Silvis, S.E. (1974) Endoscopic cholangiography for biliary system diagnosis. *Annals of Internal Medicine*, **80**, 61—64.

Ward, E.M., Stephens, D.H & Sheedy, P.R. (1983) Computed tomographic characteristics of pancreatic carcinoma. An analysis of 100 cases. *Radiographics*, **3**, 547.

Weinstein, D.P., Wolfman, N.T. & Weinstein, B.J. (1979) Ultrasound characteristics of pancreatic tumours. *Gastrointestinal Radiology*, **4**, 245—251.

Wittenburg, J., Simeone, J.F., Ferruci, J.T. *et al.* (1982) Nonfocal enlargement in pancreatic carcinoma. *Radiology*, **144**, 131.

Wynder, E.L., Dieck, G.S. & Hall, N.E.L. (1986) Case-control study of decaffeinated coffee consumption and pancreatic cancer. *Cancer Research*, **46**, 5360—5363.

Wynder, E.L., Mabuchi, K., Maruchi, N. & Fortner, J.G. (1973) Epidemiology of cancer of the pancreas. *Journal of the National Cancer Institute*, **50**, 645.

Part 5
The Spleen

27: The Spleen

D.M. KING

Introduction

Historically the radiological assessment of the spleen has been limited to the plain abdominal radiograph. The information gained was rarely more than an approximation of splenic size and radiodensity together with the demonstration of abnormal calcification. Direct imaging techniques that were available in the past proved to be inaccurate and often hazardous.

With the advent of ultrasound, nuclear medicine studies, computerized tomography (CT) and magnetic resonance imaging (MRI) techniques, imaging is no longer confined to the crude morphology of the spleen; detailed evaluation of the internal structure, physiological function and even biochemical abnormalities is now possible. The spleen is rarely imaged in isolation with these newer techniques, and multiple organ demonstration often increases diagnostic precision.

Anatomy

The spleen is an intraperitoneal organ lying posteriorly and laterally in the left upper quadrant of the abdomen beneath the 9th, 10th and 11th ribs. It is the size of a fist and weighs between 75 and 100 g in the healthy adult. It is situated in the supramesocolic space together with the liver, stomach, duodenum and gall bladder.

Anteriorly the spleen is related to the greater curve of the stomach and the splenic flexure of the colon, whilst the lateral and superior surfaces are bordered by the diaphragm and lateral abdominal wall. Inferiorly, medially, and posteriorly the spleen abuts the upper pole of the left kidney and at its hilum it is impressed by the pancreatic tail. The visceral surface of the spleen thus shows several variable indentations caused by these adjacent organs, and conversely these organs show splenic impressions which may be mistakenly interpreted as abnormal. The spleen may as a result be responsible for a 'pseudotumour' indenting the

colon or the greater curve of the stomach. The prominence or 'hump' on the lateral aspect of the left kidney produced by the spleen may confuse the inexperienced observer and suggest the presence of an intrinsic renal mass.

The axis of the spleen is variable because its position is only maintained by pressure from adjacent organs. Most commonly its long axis is oblique, running along the line of the 10th rib, but rarely it adopts a transverse position lying between the gastric fundus and the left hemidiaphragm. Occasionally it is compressed by adjacent organs, becoming thinned and lying in a vertical plane along the lateral abdominal wall; it is in this situation that the splenic tip may be palpable and splenomegaly is incorrectly diagnosed. It is a mobile intra-abdominal organ and this mobility may be demonstrated during computerized tomography examination, particularly if the patient is examined both supine and prone, and ultrasound scanning in the erect position may show considerable descent of the spleen.

Two reflections of peritoneum, the gastrosplenic and the splenorenal ligaments, form the major supporting structures. The latter contains the splenic artery, splenic vein, and pancreatic tail, whilst the former contains the left gastroepiploic artery and short gastric arteries. Splenocolic and splenophrenic ligaments also provide the organ with further support. These ligaments together with the spleen itself form the lateral recess of the lesser sac. Occasionally these ligaments become elongated producing the 'wandering spleen', and this phenomenon may be demonstrated by CT, or more specifically by scintigraphy. These methods of imaging are also able to identify the site and number of accessory or multiple spleens. These have been reported at autopsy in between 10 and 30% of normal subjects and have been found in many different sites, most commonly around the splenic artery branches, pancreatic bed, and in gastroepiploic omentum. Foci of splenic tissue have also been reported in distant sites including the testes, peritoneum, and periureteric and presacral areas.

The splenic artery normally arises as a major branch of the coeliac axis at the level of the 12th dorsal vertebra. It traverses the left upper quadrant and passes behind the stomach above the splenic vein. It is closely related throughout its course to the superior border of the pancreas, to which it donates a supply via short pancreatic branches. Shortly before it enters the splenic hilum some branching occurs. Approximately six arterial branches enter the spleen itself and several short gastric branches are usually present, as well as the left gastroepiploic artery.

The venous drainage is predominantly by the splenic vein, which passes medially, uniting with the inferior mesenteric vein in the mid-line to form the portal vein. The splenic vein has a much greater calibre and a straighter course than the splenic artery and this, together with its ease of identification and constant position, make it an important and reliable landmark, particularly for the ultrasonographer.

The lymphatic vessels from the spleen drain into small nodes at the hilum and thence to a chain of glands along the pancreas. Finally they enter the superior mesenteric and coeliac axis glands.

The spleen is clothed by a thick double-layered capsule, the inner layer of which contains fibrous tissue and smooth muscle fibres. Trabeculae arise from the capsule and penetrate the splenic pulp, carrying with them the intrasplenic arteries. The spleen is thus divided into compartments which contain both red and white pulp. The white pulp lies centrally around the main arterial branch and is made up of lymphatic nodules and periarterial lymphatic sheaths forming a framework for lymphocytes and macrophages. Thin-walled sinuses are separated by cords within the red pulp and these form an intermediate system of spaces between capillaries of the arterial and venous systems. Approximately 90% of the blood entering via arterioles into the red pulp passes through an 'open' system initially into the cords and then into the sinuses. The remaining 10% flows directly through arteriovenous communications. Most of the red cells pass to the cords, having been separated from serum in the white pulp and it is this difficult and sluggish passage through the cords into the sinuses which requires the inherent deformability of red cells. Blood flow through a normal adult spleen averages 300 ml per minute.

Physiology

Haematology

In the fetus the spleen has an important role as an organ of haemopoiesis, but this activity normally ceases by the 7th month of intrauterine life. Haemopoiesis in the spleen may, however, be reactivated in adult life as a response to any severe anaemia or as a consequence of bone-marrow failure. This explains why extensive skeletal metastases and Albers-Schönberg disease may be accompanied by splenomegaly.

In the adult the major function of the spleen is in the identification and destruction of aged red blood cells and lymphocytes. This is probably performed by macrophages stored in the spleen, and thus haemolytic anaemias are frequently accompanied by enlargement of the spleen. Phagocytosis of platelets is also a normal function of the spleen and this process is often abnormally increased in splenomegaly as a result of increased platelet retention and destruction. Thrombocytopenia frequently, therefore, accompanies hypersplenism.

Although the spleen contains at any time a large quantity of red cells and their precursors it has no storage function. It does, however, act as a reservoir of platelets, storing up to 30% of the total platelet mass.

Defence

The spleen is a major source of macrophages and antibodies produced by plasma cells, and is thus of considerable importance in the mechanism of defence against infection. It plays a valuable rôle in the phagocytosis of bacteria, particularly encapsulated bacteria such as pneumococci. Many other bacterial infections are also accompanied by splenomegaly; these include typhoid, brucellosis, and subacute bacterial endocarditis. Indeed, septicaemia of any cause may produce a degree of splenomegaly, and enlargement also accompanies viral infections such as viral hepatitis and infectious mononucleosis. World-wide the commonest infections associated with splenomegaly are malaria, leishmaniasis, and schistosomiasis.

The importance of the spleen in the mechanism of defence is highlighted by the changes in immunological competence that may occur after splenectomy. When the spleen has been removed a state of diminished resistance to infection occurs, and children in particular may be susceptible to overwhelming pneumococcal infection (Likhite, 1976). There is also an increased incidence of sepsis in adults, and vaccination against pneumococcal infection is therefore recommended in children and adults following splenectomy. This should be supplemented in children by penicillin administration until the age of 18 years.

Plain radiography

Until relatively recently radiological examination of the spleen was indirect, relying on plain radiography and contrast studies of adjacent organs to identify and define changes in splenic size and contour.

Indirect methods of examination of the spleen were first described in 1912 by LePage, who described a method involving gaseous distension of the stomach. Direct imaging was achieved by Oka and his colleagues in 1929, using the technique of hepatolienography in which Thorotrast was used as the contrast agent. Thorotrast is a 20% colloidal suspension of thorium dioxide which, at that time, was used in cerebral angiography. It was found to

be radioactive, being an alpha-particle emitter, and its use was rapidly abandoned when its toxic effects became apparent. The technique of hepatolienography depended on the function of the reticuloendothelial tissue within the spleen in removing injected particulate radio-opaque material from the circulation. Numerous contrast media were assessed, without success, but the functional aspects of this technique formed the basis for later nuclear medicine studies. The advent of splenoportography and selective arteriography in the early 1950s allowed, for the first time, an assessment of parenchymal architecture and the detection of focal abnormalities.

The abdominal radiograph remains a most useful indicator of significant splenomegaly, whether as a plain study or as part of an intravenous urogram or barium examination (Fig. 27.1). Attention should also be paid to the chest film, in either posteroanterior or a lateral projection, as this may also allow identification of splenomegaly (Fig. 27.2). Fortunately, precise demonstration of splenic size is rarely required in practice, as only marked and therefore obvious splenomegaly is of clinical relevance. The normal spleen reaches its

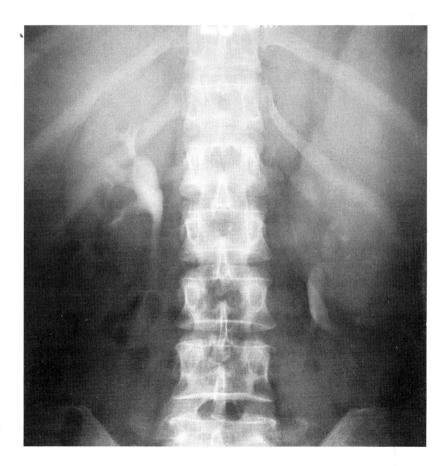

Fig. 27.1 Intravenous urogram demonstrating enlargement of the spleen compressing the upper pole of the left kidney.

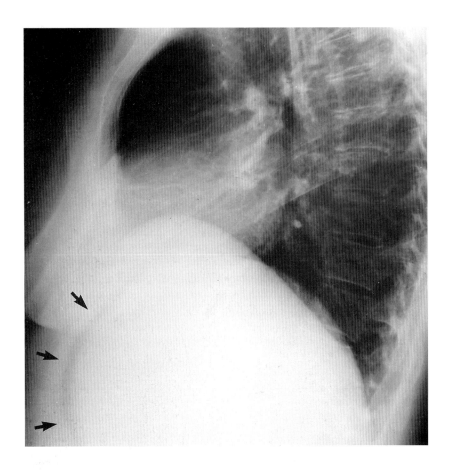

Fig. 27.2 Marked enlargement of the spleen seen on a lateral chest radiograph. The anterior splenic margin is well demonstrated by adjacent fat (*arrows*).

maximum size in young adults and with increasing age a degree of atrophy occurs.

As a result of the posterior and subcostal position of the spleen, the clinical recognition of enlargement is often delayed and its volume is generally assumed to be at least twice that of normal when it becomes palpable. The plain radiograph assessment of splenic size is aided by the situation of the low-density fat deposits that lie against it. This fat, which is variable in quantity, normally outlines the lateral and inferior margins. Fat within the greater omentum may also abut the inferior and medial surface, thus occasionally delineating the splenic hilum, but this is not dependable, as perisplenic fat varies markedly from patient to patient and insufficient fat in a thin patient may render the spleen invisible.

Quantitative assessment of the normal size of such an irregular and variably shaped organ is particularly difficult, as reproducible end-points for measurement are almost impossible to standardize. Generally the spleen is between 10 and 13 cm in length, 6–8 cm in width and 3–4 cm in thickness. Papers have been published describing normal splenic dimensions and methods of measurement (Blendis *et al.*, 1969, Asher *et al.*,

1976), but these methods are of little practical value and determination of splenic size is largely subjective. Clinically suspected splenomegaly may now readily be confirmed or refuted by ultrasonography, CT, or nuclear medicine studies. Not infrequently the spleen whose inferior tip is readily palpable is shown on these examinations to be a long, thin, or anomalously positioned organ of normal volume.

Splenomegaly is frequently a dominant feature of blood dyscrasias and myelofibrosis as well as leukaemia and lymphoma (Fig. 27.3). Patients with 'storage' disease such as Gauchers or a mucopolysaccharidosis will also usually show significant enlargement of the spleen. Haemolytic anaemias are usually accompanied by splenomegaly, but massive enlargement is particularly associated with thalassaemia major. In contrast the splenomegaly which accompanies childhood sickle-cell disease usually diminishes in the young adult as a result of repeated infarctions and the end-stage spleen is often shrunken.

The numerous infective causes of splenomegaly have already been described but non-infective inflammatory conditions such as rheumatoid arthritis, systemic lupus erythematosus, and

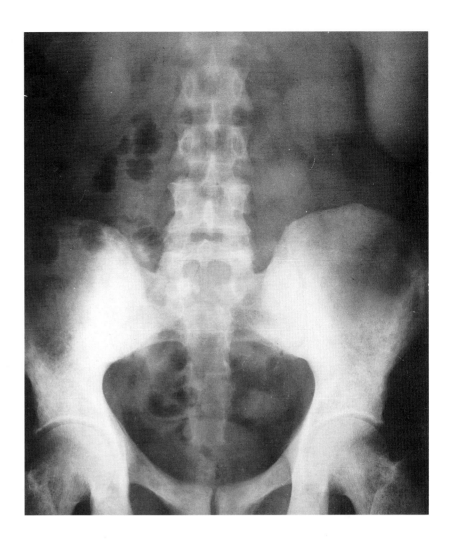

Fig. 27.3 Myelofibrosis. Splenomegaly and diffuse, symmetrical bony sclerosis affecting the pelvis.

sarcoidosis may be associated with splenic enlargement. Significant enlargement often occurs in liver failure or cirrhosis as a result of portal hypertension.

Closed abdominal injury may result in intracapsular rupture of the spleen, and the presence of an enlarged splenic shadow on a radiograph after trauma should alert the radiologist to the possibility of this dangerous condition. Associated rib or vertebral fractures or signs of pulmonary contusion should increase the index of suspicion.

Calcification overlying or adjacent to the spleen is usually easily detectable on the plain abdominal or chest radiograph. Punctate, irregular calcification is seen following tuberculous or histoplasma infection and occasionally in cysticercosis (Fig. 27.4). Tuberculous calcification of the spleen is usually associated with hepatic and nodal calcification and a similar type of coarse, irregular or punctate calcification may be seen in splenic venous phleboliths. As elsewhere in the body, phleboliths are seldom clinically significant and

they appear as oval or irregular foci between 2 and 5 mm in diameter. Larger phleboliths may show evidence of layering and they may have a low density centre. They are particularly common in the pathologically enlarged spleen and in splenic angiomas. Diffuse or granular calcification may be associated with previous infarction and is particularly seen in patients with sickle-cell disease. In this condition the abnormal crescentic erythrocytes are unable to deform and as they pass through the splenic cords they are trapped within the spleen. In conditions of reduced oxygen tension and stasis, sickling of red cells occurs and numerous micro-infarctions may follow. Subsequently the infarctions may calcify.

Occasionally diffuse granular calcification develops in intrasplenic metastases but this is almost always part of disseminated abdominal disease, usually adenocarcinoma from ovary or bowel. Rarely, intrasplenic deposits from breast carcinoma show calcification.

Tortuous parallel-line or curvilinear calcification

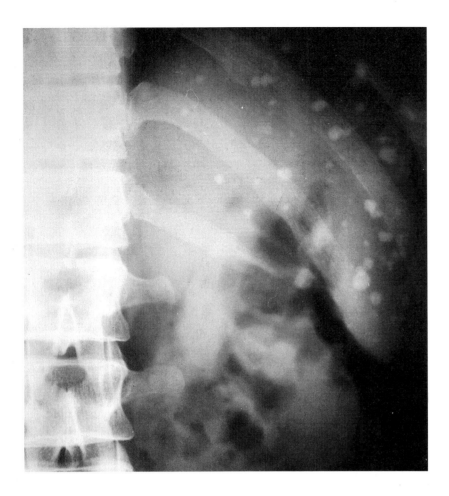

Fig. 27.4 Calcification in tuberculous granulomata in the spleen. Note the focus at the splenic hilum indicating calcification in an adjacent lymph node.

outside the spleen is not infrequently present in association with atheromatous disease and represents calcification of the splenic artery. A single large radius ring calcification in the region of the spleen often denotes the presence of a splenic artery aneurysm. Aneurysms at this site are second only to the aorta in frequency and are more common in women than men, particularly in the premenopausal age group (Sherlock & Learmonth, 1952). Most commonly they are between 1 and 3 cm in diameter but occasionally reach 15 cm. Typically, their presence produces no symptoms at all and they are found incidentally during unrelated urographic or barium studies. Ring calcification is present on the abdominal radiograph in 70% of cases. Occasionally the aneurysm ruptures; this is most commonly seen in young women, often during pregnancy, and an acute intraperitoneal haemorrhage results.

Fine or linear calcification, noted at or near the splenic hilum, may indicate a previous thrombosis of the splenic vein. However in this condition, which may complicate pancreatic or gastric carcinoma, features of oesophageal or gastric varices will usually be found. Ring calcification overlying the splenic shadow may delineate the wall of a hydatid cyst (Fig. 27.5). Hydatid cysts of the spleen are usually solitary but they may reach considerable size, sometimes containing several litres of fluid. Hydatid disease is not, however, usually confined to the spleen, being more commonly part of widespread infestation. World-wide, two-thirds of all splenic cysts are due to echinococcal infection. They are particularly common in southern Europe, South America, Australia, and Alaska.

Curvilinear calcification around the margin of the splenic shadow may be found after a subcapsular or perisplenic haemorrhage, and further imaging may be required for confirmation (Fig. 27.6). Trauma is also an aetiological factor in the development of most pseudocysts found in the spleen, which are a consequence of resorption and liquefaction in the haematoma. Approximately 20% show some amorphous or punctate calcification, and pseudocysts comprise 70–80% of all non-parasitic cysts found in the spleen. So-called 'simple' cysts are rare but their ease of detection on CT and ultrasound examination has resulted in

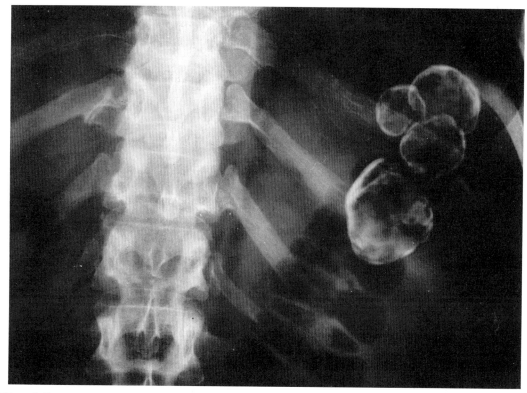

Fig. 27.5 Rim calcification in the walls of splenic hydatic cysts. The extent of calcification and number of cysts is unusual.

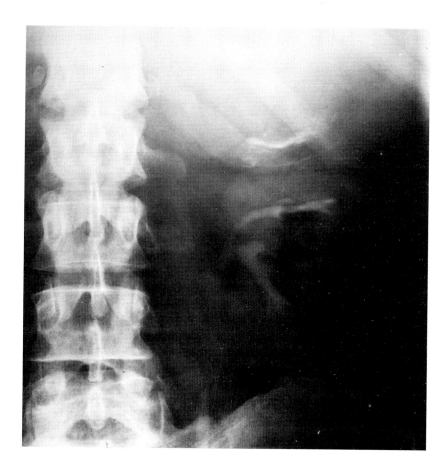

Fig. 27.6 Splenic haematoma. Rounded enlargement of the lower pole of the spleen compresses and distorts the upper pole of the left kidney. Curvilinear calcification lies in the margin of the haematoma.

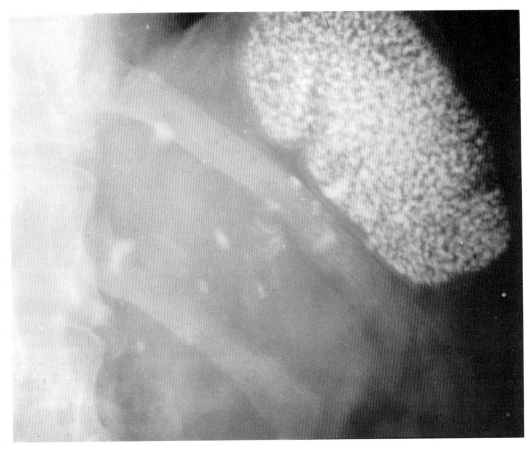

Fig. 27.7 Thorotrast. Accumulation of high-density material within the spleen. Note the low-density deposition in the capsule, the atrophy, and the lymph node opacification.

increased awareness of their existence. Simple cysts are usually silent and are lined by flattened or cuboidal cells originating from infolding of peritoneal mesothelium during splenic development. Epidermoid cysts may occur in the spleen, most commonly in children and young adults, and cystic dermoids have been reported.

Calcification should not, however, be confused with the presence of Thorotrast which can mimic true splenic calcification (Fig. 27.7). Following its intra-arterial injection many years previously this contrast medium remains permanently in the spleen, regional lymph nodes, and liver. It forms dense granular shadowing in the spleen and its retention is usually associated with significant splenic atrophy.

Evidence of excessive haemosiderin deposition in the spleen as a consequence of severe haemolytic anaemia or haemachromatosis may be found on the plain abdominal radiograph. Deposition within the spleen produces a diffuse increase in radiodensity, but focal deposition may also occur in which case multiple dense nodules up to 3 mm in diameter may be seen.

Nuclear medicine

Until recently radionuclide imaging was the only available technique capable of evaluating the size, shape and homogeneity of the spleen. Although sensitivity and specificity of splenic scintigraphy are lower than computerized tomography and ultrasound, it remains an easy-to-perform, cost-effective, and painless method of splenic imaging. It requires the intravenous injection of a radio-pharmaceutical and a few minutes in front of a gamma camera to produce images of the spleen. These images are reproducible, easy to interpret and require comparatively little observer experience.

Most requests for splenic imaging follow from a clinical observation of splenomegaly, and scintigraphy remains a useful method of clarifying this problem. Ectopic, aberrant, or regenerating splenic tissue can only be identified with confidence by scintigraphic techniques because this test is the only method of splenic imaging that is specifically dependent upon the presence of functioning splenic tissue.

The liver contains 80% of the body's reticuloendothelial tissue, the spleen contains 15% and bone marrow the remaining 5%. The tissue macrophages of the reticuloendothelial system are able to ingest foreign particles from the blood stream, and this property forms the basis of scintigraphic studies of the liver and spleen.

In 1965 the use of ^{99m}technetium sulphur colloid was first described for hepatic and splenic scintigraphy (Harper *et al.*, 1965). This still remains the most widely used radiopharmaceutical in splenic scintigraphy, and images may be obtained approximately 15 min after an injection of between 2 and 5 mCi of labelled colloid. The colloid is prepared in the form of particles approximately 0.01 μm in diameter, which after intravenous injection are rapidly cleared by the reticuloendothelial system. The efficiency of this extraction is dependent only on the functioning state of the reticuloendothelial cells and an adequate blood flow to the organ. The use of other radiocolloids such as ^{99m}technetium microaggregated albumin, ^{113m}indium colloid, and ^{198}gold has largely been abandoned because their use involves the exposure of the patient to much higher doses of radiation.

By this method the spleen is imaged as part of a liver scan, and routine projections consist of anterior and posterior views together with both lateral projections. If splenic images alone are required then anterior and posterior projections of the left upper quadrant of the abdomen will suffice. Investigation of suspected ectopia, polysplenia, or asplenia will require views of the whole abdomen.

In the normal subject the uptake of the colloid by the spleen occurs at approximately the same rate per unit volume as that of the liver, and thus maximum count densities are usually similar. Hepatic parenchymal disease, however, almost always affects the function of the Kupffer cells as well as the blood flow to the liver, and consequently there is diminished liver concentration and relatively increased splenic retention of the colloid. The splenic image is therefore of correspondingly increased activity and the organ is usually enlarged. If the liver disorder is severe,

then reticuloendothelial tissue is the bone marrow will take up the colloid and activity in the bones will be detected.

The demonstration of focal space-occupying lesions within the spleen depends upon the replacement of splenic reticuloendothelial tissue by tumour. Unfortunately, the sensitivity of this method varies according to the position within the spleen of the abnormality. Contrast between areas of activity and areas of photon deficiency at or near the surface will be marked, hence lesions as small as 2 cm in diameter in this area may be detectable. However, quite large masses situated deep within the spleen may go undetected.

Focal defects in the scintigraphic image may be seen as the result of any intrasplenic mass, and this method of examination is unable to discriminate between benign masses such as cysts and soft-tissue masses. Malignant infiltration may produce clearly marginated discrete defects (Fig. 27.8). but not infrequently a patchy image of reduced overall activity is seen. This is particularly common in association with lymphomatous infiltration and chronic lymphocytic leukaemia.

Defects resulting from infarction may be apparent as wedge-shaped areas of reduced activity. This finding is seen in patients with subacute bacterial endocarditis and is also known to occur in sarcoidosis. Splenic infarctions are also not uncommon in the enlarged spleen of myelofibrosis. Ultimately, after multiple infarctions, the spleen will show reduced or even absent activity. Localized intrasplenic haematomata may produce large, sometimes irregular defects within the image which occasionally transect the spleen. Subcapsular collections characteristically result in the medial displacement of the spleen away from the abdominal wall. A crescentic lateral margin produced by the haematoma impressing the parenchyma is virtually pathognomonic. Further useful scintigraphic information may be obtained by combining colloid studies of the spleen together with lung scanning, in order to emphasize the defect produced by the haematoma.

The diagnosis of splenic rupture will usually be aided by a history of abdominal trauma. However, splenic rupture is not always preceded by severe injury and may occur spontaneously in association with diffuse parenchymal disease. Patients with scintigraphic suspicion of this dangerous condition should be promptly referred for more specfic CT or ultrasound examination. Nuclear medicine studies may be particularly valuable in monitoring

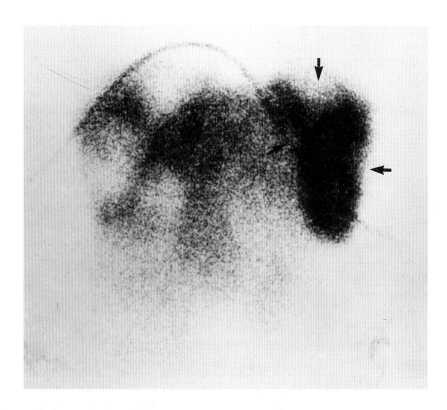

Fig. 27.8 Liver/spleen scintigram. The anterior projection demonstrates multiple rounded photon-deficient areas in both liver and spleen (*arrows*) in a patient with malignant melanoma.

those patients who are being managed conservatively, as serial examinations can be performed at minimal cost, risk or discomfort.

Isolated splenic uptake without associated hepatic uptake may be particularly appropriate when an enlarged liver abuts or obscures the splenic margin. Selective splenic uptake is also preferable when ectopic position or regeneration after splenectomy is suspected, and in order to resolve this problem it is necessary to utilize the spleen's unique ability to sequester damaged red blood cells from the circulation. Heating has been found to be the most satisfactory method of damaging the red cells and the exposure of a suitably anticoagulated sample of the patient's blood to a temperature of 49.5°C for 20–30 min will produce a satisfactory sample of pyrospherocytes. The pyrospherocytes are labelled with ^{99m}technetium and returned by intravenous injection to the patient. These labelled cells are cleared by the spleen within 5–15 min, and specific scintigraphic images of the spleen alone may then be obtained. The use of ^{51}chromium as the label has been superseded by ^{99m}technetium, which although more difficult to prepare, involves a lower absorbed dose by the patient.

It is interesting that successful trapping by the spleen depends upon the degree of damage suffered by the cells, and they require heating at a specific temperature for a precise time (Hamilton *et al.*, 1976). Erythrocyte damage using antibodies, and chemical damage, have been shown to be either blood-group dependent or too imprecise for clinical use.

The utilization of the physiological function of the spleen enables the identification of the pathological state of 'functional asplenia'. This condition is characterized by the presence of Howell–Jolly bodies in the peripheral blood even though the spleen is present. In this situation the spleen is unable to trap colloid or labelled pyrospherocytes. Reversible forms of this condition may be seen in neonates or following haemolysis, but it is particularly found in sickle-cell disease. Occasional cases have also been noted in adults with coeliac disease as well as ulcerative colitis (Pearson *et al.*, 1969). The inclusion of the spleen in a therapeutic irradiation field may also result in functional asplenia and these patients have been shown to have an increased incidence of pneumococcal sepsis (Coleman *et al.*, 1982.)

Computerized tomography

Computerized tomography (CT) undoubtedly provides the most sensitive and thorough assessment of the spleen. The ability of CT to display not only the internal anatomy of the spleen but also all the adjacent structures increases its value in the investigation of abnormalities in the left upper quadrant of the abdomen. As well as morphology, functional CT studies may be performed, involving dynamic scanning during intravenous injection of contrast, thus facilitating the diagnosis of vascular abnormalities and reducing the need for angiography.

The clear presentation of detailed anatomy by CT ensures its popularity with clinicians and radiologists alike. Its limitations are high cost, limited availability, and lengthy procedure time. It is inflexible in its use and requires a patient fit enough to endure and co-operate in what is frequently a time-consuming and uncomfortable procedure. It may be impossible or impractical to perform a CT examination on the very ill patient. In addition, although most machines are now able to achieve very short scan times, the patient must still be able to arrest respiratory movement for a few seconds.

Although CT, unlike magnetic resonance imaging and ultrasound, produces high-quality images only in a fixed transverse axial plane, this is not, in the examination of the spleen, a practical problem. Indeed, it might be argued that the rigid presentation of images of CT allows the reproducible and comparable examination techniques to be performed.

The majority of diagnoses of splenic abnormalities made during any imaging procedure are incidental and unrelated to the presenting clinical problem. This fact simply reflects the absence of symptoms that accompanies splenic pathology of either focal or diffuse nature. As all CT examinations of the abdomen and most examinations of the thorax include sections of the spleen it should not be surprising that it is this technique, above all others, which has increased awareness of splenic pathology.

CT studies performed without intravenous contrast enhancement demonstrate a homogeneous parenchymal pattern within the spleen with a density, depending on machine and operating technique, of between 40 and 45 Hounsfield units. The normal liver is almost always of greater density than the spleen and the constancy of the numerical relationship of the densities has been stressed by several workers (Piekarski et al., 1980). This characteristic may be of practical value, being particularly applicable to the identification of diffuse hepatic parenchymal infiltrations, most commonly fat.

Rarely, an objective increase in the attenuation of the spleen may be seen in conditions which require treatment by multiple blood transfusions. This increased density is the result of excessive haemosiderin deposition (Long et al., 1980).

Vascular studies

After a rapid intravenous bolus of contrast medium the splenic artery will usually be visualized on CT after 10–15 s, and the splenic vein to 10–15 s later. This vascular enhancement may be particularly valuable in confirming the presence of splenic artery aneurysms or varices. Characteristic time–density curves allow separation of aneurysms from venous malformations. Sequential scans after intravenous injection of contrast also allow assessment of patency in the splenic and portal venous systems, which may be particularly important in the presurgical work-up of patients with hepatic disease. As a consequence, angiographic demonstration may be unnecessary.

Splenic parenchymal texture after injection of intravenous contrast medium is typically patchy, unlike the uniform increase in density seen in the the liver. Unlike the liver, therefore, where contrast enhancement may increase the detection of focal disease, enhancement of the spleen does not significantly increase the chance of detecting focal abnormalities. Indeed the unwary may easily fall into the trap of misdiagnosing the uneven parenchymal density as evidence of malignant infiltration within the spleen. The splenic inhomogeneity after contrast enhancement occurs as a result of the unique structure of the splenic pulp, and in particular in the two different modes of blood flow through the organ. Most of the blood passing via arterioles into the red pulp passes through the 'open' system initially into the cords and then into the sinuses. Transit of blood by this route is sluggish and flow rates uneven. The direct passage through the remaining 'closed' system of arteriovenous communication is much more rapid, and thus differing concentrations of contrast may be found at different times in different compartments of the spleen (Fig. 27.9). An even parenchymal density is rarely achieved until approximately 120 s after intravenous injection, and at this point the density usually increases by 60–70 Hounsfield units (Claussen & Lochner, 1985).

Characteristic enhancement of splenic tissue following intravenous contrast is, however, of practical help in identifying accessory spleens which

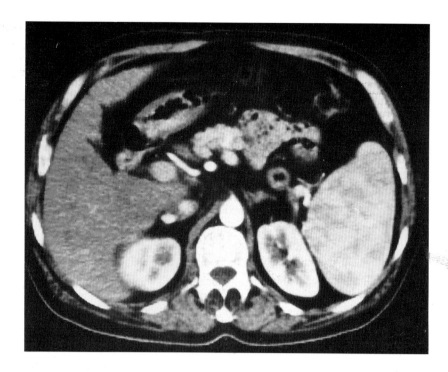

Fig. 27.9 CT demonstration of marked inhomogeneity of the spleen after rapid intravenous injection of contrast. Note the opacified splenic and hepatic arteries.

may, in the unenhanced scan, have the appearances of enlarged lymph nodes. This discrimination is particularly important in patients with non-Hodgkin's lymphoma, as over 50% will show adenopathy at the splenic hilum (Breiman *et al.*, 1978). After splenectomy any unresected accessory spleen may enlarge (Fig. 27.10). and subsequently the patient may re-present with a mass in the left upper quadrant and the return of features of hypersplenism. Implantation of splenic tissue in anomalous sites may occur after trauma or abdominal surgery, and intrathoracic splenosis is a particular complication that may be first noted on a chest radiograph or CT examination. The combination of CT with splenic scintigraphy will localize the splenic tissue, confirming the diagnosis and thus preventing unjustified surgical intervention. CT is also a useful non-invasive aid in the clarification of the asplenia or polysplenia syndromes, in which there may be a congenital absence or multiplicity of spleens. Multiple spleens are usually right-sided but may be bilateral. The varying manifestations of these syndromes include anomalies of the vena cava and heart, together with intestinal tract malrotation, situs inversus, symmetrical hepatic lobes, or absence of the gall bladder.

Encouraging results demonstrating increased sensitivity for the detection of focal intrasplenic lesions have been reported following intravenous injection of iodinated lipoid emulsions such as ethiodol oil emulsion 13 (EOE−13). This is a selective imaging agent for liver and spleen prepared by emulsifying iodized poppy seed oil (ethiodol, lipiodol) in water. It is administered by intravenous infusion over 1 h at a dose of 0.25 ml per kg body weight. Currently its availability is generally restricted to research institutions, but it has been clearly shown to increase the sensitivity for the detection of hepatic and splenic metastases by CT (Miller *et al.*, 1984). Similar studies of the spleen using this agent have also shown greatly increased sensitivity for the detection of lymphoma, and detection rates of 8% before EOE−13 have been increased to 92% after its administration (Thomas *et al.*, 1982).

Pathology

CYSTS

The aetiology and incidence of cysts within the spleen has already been described. Simple cysts exhibit anticipated water-density readings but parasitic cysts may be non-homogeneous masses of low-density material. Calcification within the cyst or its wall is particularly well demonstrated by CT, and enhancement after intravenous contrast may be seen in the wall, particularly in hydatid cysts. These may also have a multiloculated appearance when daughter cysts have developed within them. (Fig. 27.11) The wall of a non-parasitic

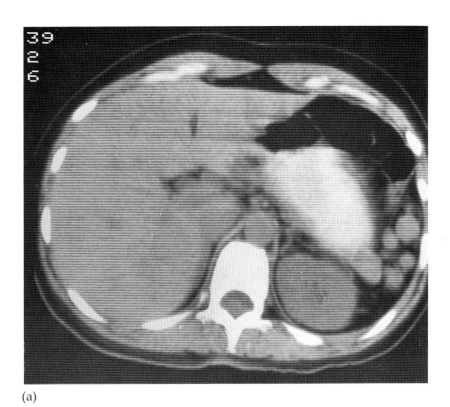

(a)

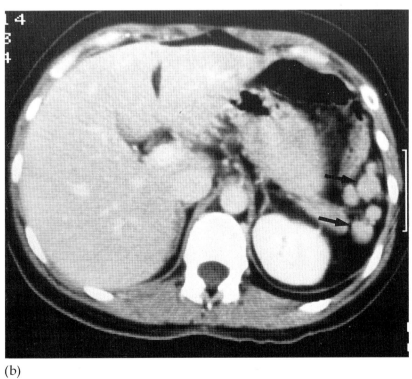

Fig. 27.10 (a) and (b) Pre and post-intravenous contrast CT sections showing four enhancing splenunculi 1 year after splenectomy.

(b)

cyst is usually thinner and more clearly defined than that of a hydatid cyst and no enhancement will be evident. Simple or post-traumatic cysts are usually unilocular, producing characteristic 'beaking' of the compressed adjacent normal spleen.

NEOPLASMS

Benign neoplasms of the spleen are extremely rare. Haemangiomata, cystic lymphangiomata, hamartomata and myxomata have all been described but

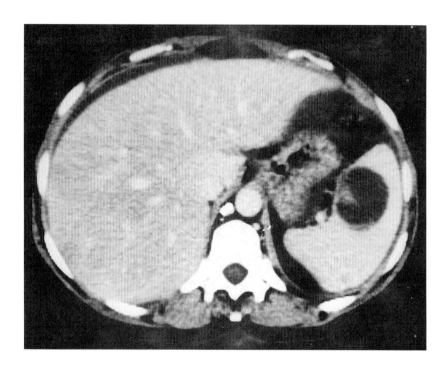

Fig. 27.11 Hydatid disease. Note the clearly defined margin and the loculation within the cyst.

they have no particular characteristics on CT and appear as focal low-density or cystic masses. Haemangiomata, of which there have been at least 100 reported cases, are probably the most common benign lesion and are of the cavernous type. Enhancement after intravenous contrast is a variable and unreliable feature. Massive splenomegaly may occur and a splenic weight of 1.3 kg has been reported. These patients usually remain asymptomatic but spontaneous rupture has been recorded in 25% of cases (Husni, 1961).

Primary splenic neoplasms are also extremely rare and are always angiosarcomata. Only 58 cases have been described and characteristically they present a rapidly progressive course culminating in death within 6 months of diagnosis. They metastasize early in the course of the disease of liver, lung, lymph nodes, and bone, and approximately 33% are complicated by spontaneous rupture. Unlike hepatic angiosarcomata there is no known association with a chemical carcinogen. There are no characteristic CT features, and they normally appear as non-homogeneous low-density focal areas within an enlarged spleen. Occasionally rim enhancement may be apparent after contrast administration but this feature is frequently absent. This is all the more surprising considering the underlying vascular nature of the tumour, and in this disease angiographic examination has been found to be more specific.

The reported incidence of secondary malignant involvement of the spleen varies widely, ranging from 4% in some series up to 36% in others (Das Gupta & Brasfield, 1961). Post-mortem studies reveal a 9% overall incidence of splenic metastases in cases of epithelial malignancies (Abrams & Spiro, 1950), but when present, splenic deposits have been identifiable macroscopically in only 67% of cases, and microscopic examination has been required for identification of the remaining 37% (Marymont & Gross, 1963). This latter group would clearly be undiagnosable on CT, and a negative CT examination should not, therefore, be assumed to exclude the presence of metastatic disease. The tumour with the greatest propensity for dissemination to the spleen is probably malignant melanoma, but splenic deposits are also regularly detected by CT in cases of ovarian carcinoma. Splenic deposits are also occasionally detected in patients with carcinoma of the pancreas, colon, and breast. In most carcinomata, splenic metastases are associated with known metastases elsewhere, most commonly in the liver or lungs. (Fig. 27.12) Consequently the demonstration of deposits within the spleen seldom alters therapy or prognosis. Isolated splenic metastases have been reported (Piekarski *et al.*, 1980), and their detection may have a major impact on management. Splenectomy may be justified in these cases, but more commonly surgical intervention in cases of splenic

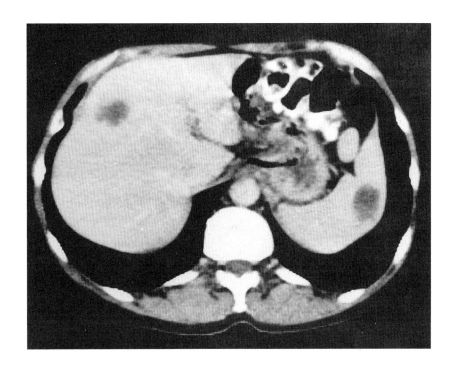

Fig. 27.12 Metastases from carcinoma of the ovary involving liver and spleen. This post-enhancement study emphasizes the low-density content.

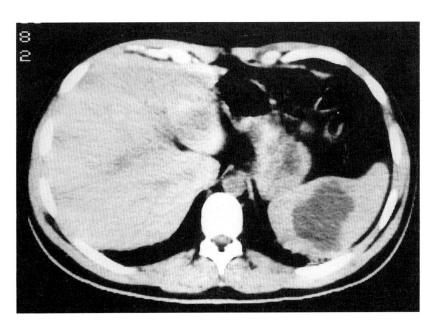

Fig. 27.13 A large low-density metastasis in a patient with teratoma of the testis. There were no other signs of dissemination.

metastases results from the sudden development of intraperitoneal haemorrhage following the spontaneous rupture of a deposit.

Splenic metastases have a variable, non-characteristic appearance on CT but are most commonly fairly well-marginated focal lesions of low density (Fig. 27.13). They may occasionally appear cystic, and their differentiation from benign cysts on CT criteria alone may prove impossible. In this instance fine-needle aspiration under CT or ultrasound guidance may obtain sufficient material for cytological diagnosis. Reported series involving this technique stress its high degree of safety (Soderstrom, 1976 Solbiati *et al.*, 1983).

It might be expected that CT of the spleen would play an important role in the management of lymphoma, since the spleen may well be the first or only organ involved. Unfortunately, most lymphomatous spleens are involved by micronodular disease, which is undetectable by CT. Consequently the only demonstrable abnormality by CT in most cases of lymphoma is generalized enlarge-

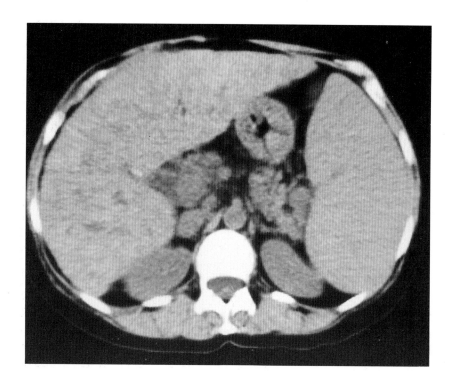

Fig. 27.14 Diffuse splenomegaly in a patient with lymphoma. Following resection the histological examination demonstrated diffuse splenic involvement.

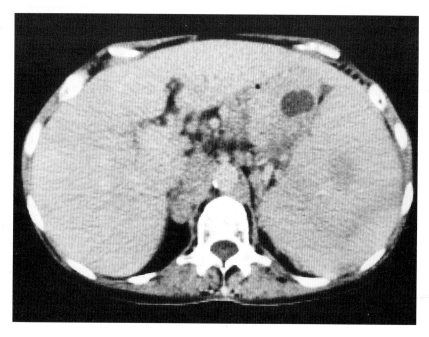

Fig. 27.15 Disseminated intra-abdominal lymphoma. The enlarged spleen shows the presence of a typical central low-attenuation area.

ment (Fig. 27.14). If massive splenomegaly is demonstrated in a patient with lymphoma then involvement is very likely, but conversely the demonstration of a normal sized spleen does not exclude involvement because at least one-third of spleens involved by lymphoma will show no detectable enlargement (Vermess *et al.*, 1981). Occasionally, lymphomatous nodules within the spleen are large enough to be detectable,

when they usually appear as low-density, non-enhancing focal areas (Fig. 27.15).

INFECTION

Most splenic abscess result from haematogenous spread of bacteria and are most common in patients who are immunosuppressed or have pre-existing splenic disease. Splenic infarctions, which may be

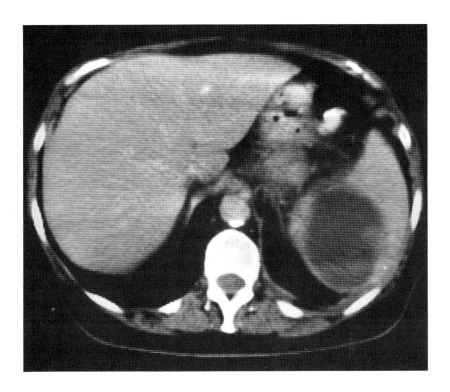

Fig. 27.16 A large splenic abscess in an immunosuppressed patient.

seen in intravenous drug addicts, are often complicated by abscess formation and they are also occasionally seen in cases of subacute bacterial endocarditis. Only rarely will the spleen be secondarily involved in an inflammatory process originating in an adjacent organ, but direct extension does sometimes complicate a left subphrenic abscess or a pancreatic pseudocyst.

Splenic abscesses usually appear as small, multiple, poorly marginated low-density foci, some of which may possess a fluid component (Fig. 27.16). Larger solitary masses do, occasionally develop, but enhancement after intravenous contrast does not generally occur in splenic abscesses. CT scanning may facilitate percutaneous fine-needle aspiration for diagnosis or therapeutic catheter drainage of larger localized lesions. CT has been shown to be particularly valuable in the search for sites of infection in immunocompromised patients when sepsis may insidiously develop within the spleen.

TRAUMA

Following closed abdominal injury the spleen is the most frequently damaged organ (Fitzgerald *et al.*, 1960). It has a large blood supply and rupture may very rapidly result in death from intra-abdominal haemorrhage and shock. Clinical evaluation is often difficult because of the protected positioned of the spleen, and rupture may at first result in few or no symptoms or signs, particularly if the haemorrhage is contained within the capsule. In consequence the condition may initially go undetected, only for the patient to present later in severe shock. Hitherto scintigraphy and arteriography provided the only useful information, but now CT and ultrasound provide the most sensitive methods of diagnosis.

Unfortunately the patient with multiple injuries may be unsuitable for CT due to the need for urgent resuscitation. In the immediate casualty room assessment ultrasound is a more appropriate abdominal imaging tool, and CT studies are usually delayed until the resuscitation is complete. Major trauma is not always required to produce rupture of the spleen, and haemorrhage may occasionally follow minimal insult when there is pre-existing parenchymal damage; the most common predisposing cause for this is infectious mononucleosis.

Immdiately after trauma an intrasplenic or subcapsular haematoma may appear isodense or even hyperdense on an unenhanced CT examination. More often the haematoma becomes apparent only after contrast enhancement of the adjacent normal splenic tissue (Fig. 27.17 a,b). Subcapsular collections usually produce elliptical filling defects in

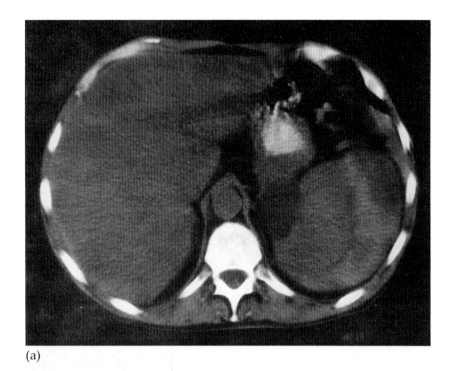

(a)

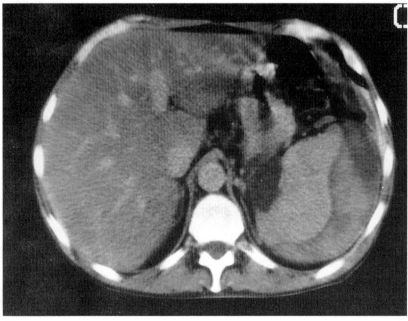

(b)

Fig. 27.17 (a) Unenhanced CT examination of the spleen following blunt trauma to the abdomen. The fresh perisplenic haematoma (*arrows*) shows a density slightly above that of the adjacent spleen. (b) Following intravenous contrast enhancement of normal spleen, the laterally situated haematoma becomes more clearly visible.

the splenic margin, but laceration may be evident as a low-density cleft through the full thickness of the spleen (Fig. 27.18). Subsequent scanning of patients managed conservatively demonstrates reducing density of the haematoma as it ages and liquefaction of the contents may occur, resulting in a post-traumatic pseudocyst.

CT examination when properly performed has been shown to have an accuracy of 95% in the diagnosis of splenic injury, and it has justifiably replaced scintigraphy and arteriography in most instances (Jeffrey *et al.*, 1981).

THROMBOSIS AND INFARCTION

Thromboembolic occlusion of splenic arteries produces segmental wedge-shaped areas of reduced attenuation. Not surprisingly these are highlighted by post-contrast studies and later, following involution, they may be evident as seg-

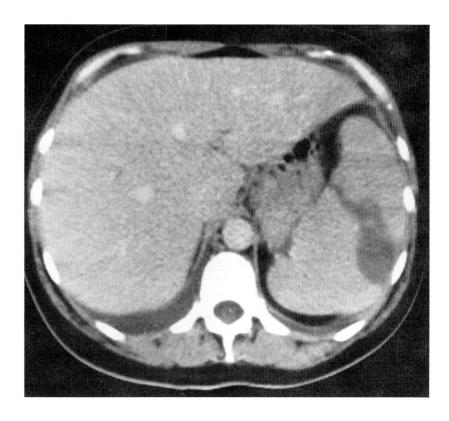

Fig .27.18 Abdominal CT examination. Two weeks after road-traffic accident showing complete transection of the spleen. Note the enhancement in the remaining normal parenchyma.

ments of retraction near the capsule of the spleen.

Dynamic CT studies employing rapid injections of large volumes of contrast may very clearly demonstrate thrombosis of the splenic vein, together with the consequent collateral venous drainage. This condition is usually accompanied by splenomegaly and it typically occurs as a complication of intra-abdominal sepsis or pancreatic carcinoma. Varices and splenomegaly with splenic or portal-vein thrombosis will commonly be seen in patients with portal hypertension. A single CT study may quickly, thoroughly, and non-invasively demonstrate conditions which previously required assessment by time-consuming, invasive, and inaccurate radiological studies.

Ultrasound

Ultrasound examination of the spleen is painless, non-invasive, widely available, and cost-effective. The recent development of high-resolution real-time machines has increased the usefulness of ultrasonography in the evaluation of the spleen by reducing the technical difficulty involved in obtaining high-quality images. Ultrasound imaging by static 'B' scanning alone is time-consuming, difficult, and often unsatisfactory because of poor sonographic access to an organ which often obs-

cured by rib or bowel gas. A thorough examination of the spleen and splenic bed by this method is rarely possible. Real-time transducers of the mechanical or phased array type employ small contact 'footprints' to produce wide sector images and they are thus able to take advantage of narrow intercostal acoustic windows. Although subcostal access is only feasible in cases of splenomegaly, most of the normal-sized spleen should be accessible through acoustic windows in the 10th and 11th intercostal spaces where the longest axis will be found. Attention should be paid to the superior and lateral margins of the spleen, which may be particularly difficult to image due to the interposed costophrenic recess. By taking advantage of all the available acoustic windows, no part of the spleen need be excluded from examination. Fortunately, although the normal spleen may prove awkward to examine, requests for splenic ultrasound normally result from clinical suspicion of enlargement, and in this situation the target organ is easily imaged.

Although ultrasound examination is less time-consuming than previously it remains a skill which depends heavily on the operator's experience. The wider use of real-time equipment increases rather than decreases the subjective nature of the examination and encourages a survey-type attitude to the procedure where little importance is attached to the production of 'hard copy' images. In consequence, ultrasonography remains a method of imaging where retrospective review is unreliable and clinical confidence in the technique difficult to generate. By contrast this is not a problem in scintigraphy and computerized tomography, where the images are reproducible irrespective of the skill of the radiologist.

Despite the interpretative problems involved in its use, the favourable physical characteristics of ultrasound have ensured that it has become the initial splenic imaging method. Clinical suspicion of splenomegaly requires confirmation by sonographic examination, and underlying focal abnormalities within the spleen are usually easily identified. Reproducible quantitative measurements of splenic size and volume are particularly difficult to obtain by this method of imaging, and generally the various rules and formulae derived in order to produce such measurements by ultrasound have been found to be inaccurate. In practice, therefore, estimation of splenic volume by ultrasound depends largely on subjective assessment by the ultrasonographer.

Normal splenic parenchyma is usually slightly less reflective than liver and it returns a homogeneous echo pattern with a greater concentration of finer echoes than the liver. It contains virtually no recognizable internal anatomical structure and vessels are only usually seen at the hilum. The parenchyma is surrounded by a thin, poorly reflective capsule, which is scarcely visible as it is closely applied to the splenic pulp. Separation of the two by an echo-poor or echo-free rim suggests the presence of a subcapsular fluid collection. The calibre of the splenic and portal veins should be noted during the examination, particularly when cirrhosis and portal hypertension are clinically suspected, and by using the spleen itself as an acoustic window reasonable access to the hilum and splenic bed is usually possible. Varices and splenic-artery aneurysms may thus be imaged (Fig. 27.19), and if equipment is available Doppler studies of these vessels may allow valuable assessment of blood flow.

Pathology

SPLENOMEGALY

Malignant infiltrations produce variable and inconstant change in parenchymal reflectivity. Lymphoma and chronic leukaemia may be associated with marked enlargement, and typically the splenic tissue returns a pattern of diminished echo level. Occasionally, however, strongly reflective spleens may be encountered in these diseases. Focal disease within the spleen may result in almost echo-free areas but through-transmission of sound is minimal or absent. These conditions may also be associated with enlarged lymph nodes at the

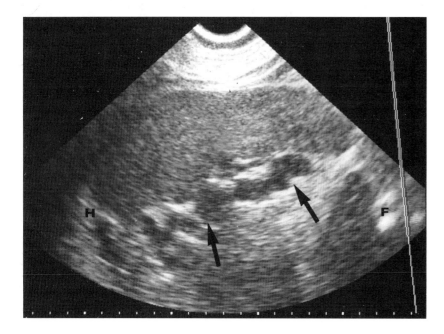

Fig. 27.19 An oblique longitudinal ultrasound section through the spleen showing varices (*arrows*) extending from the hilum.

splenic hilum, and the ultrasonographer should therefore pay particular attention to this area when lymphoma or leukaemia is suspected.

Splenomegaly resulting from congestion or haematological disorders usually produces little change from the normal echo pattern. Only when the spleen subsequently becomes scarred and shrunken, as in sickle-cell disease, will there be a pattern of increased reflectivity. In acute infections mild splenomegaly may be noted and ultrasound examination will display a parenchymal pattern of reduced echo level. As the disease progresses enlargement may increase and the echo pattern may return towards normal. Finally the parenchymal pattern may show generalized increased in reflectivity. Attempts have been made to characterize pathological processes within the spleen (Mittelstaedt & Partain, 1980, King *et al.*, 1985). Whilst good correlation between clinical and sonographic estimations of splenic size have been obtained, the correlation between parenchymal pattern and pathological process is poor.

FOCAL ABNORMALITY

Cysts within the spleen, as elsewhere, are characteristically echo free, showing through-transmission of sound. Many may be classed as simple and innocent although a large number of these will actually be post-traumatic pseudocysts (Fig. 27.20). They are usually detected as incidental observations during a general abdominal examin-

ation, but it is important to avoid mistakenly interpreting a cyst in the left upper quadrant as arising within the spleen when it actually represents an unrelated renal cyst or pancreatic pseudocyst. Hydatid cysts (*Echinococcus granulosus*), in addition to anticipated sonographic features, may contain calcium in their walls, thus resulting in echogenic foci within the cyst. Calcification, suspected on ultrasound examination, may be confirmed by plain radiography.

Malignant cystic masses within the spleen are occasionally seen in patients with disseminated ovarian carcinoma or teratoma of the testis, but cysts of this type are usually less clearly marginated than those of a benign aetiology and are frequently accompanied by other focal areas of parenchymal abnormality.

Non-homogeneous, echo-poor masses will exhibit only minimal or no through-transmission of sound; abscesses or intrasplenic haematomata may exhibit these characteristics (Fig. 27.21). Focal metastases, which may be of the characteristic 'target' appearance, are not uncommonly seen in disseminated malignant melanoma, and less frequently in metastatic carcinoma (Fig. 27.22). Echo-rich metastases occur, as they do in the liver, most frequently in patients with disseminated colorectal carcinoma. Echo-poor lesions are not infrequently seen in the terminal stages of disseminated breast carcinoma. Localized lesions showing virtual absence of echoes but with little through transmission are classically found in lymphoma.

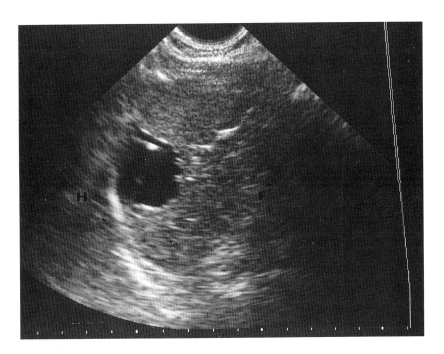

Fig. 27.20 Splenic cyst. The echo-free content and clearly defined but irregular margin should be noted.

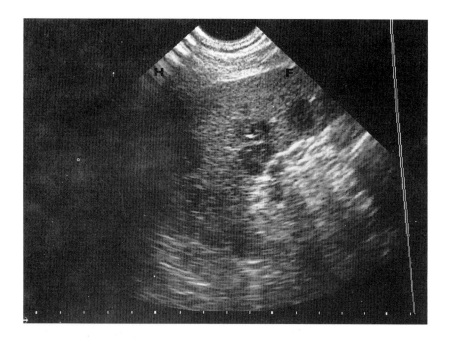

Fig. 27.21 Multiple intrasplenic abscesses showing varying size, poor marginal definition, and irregular echo-poor content.

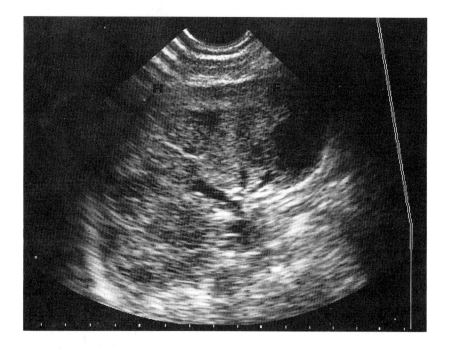

Fig. 27.22 Multiple intrahepatic metastases in a patient with malignant melanoma.

TRAUMA

Previously the ruptured spleen was promptly removed but there is now good evidence to suggest that resection should be avoided where possible and the patient managed conservatively (Buntain & Lynn, 1979). This change in surgical practice stems from an increasing awareness of the reduction in immunological competence that follows splenectomy. In this situation it is vital to be able to monitor the condition of the spleen closely and regular splenic imaging is therefore necessary so that any deterioration in the condition of the patient can be detected promptly. Whilst there remains a place for angiography in the initial assessment of splenic trauma and CT elegantly displays the full extent of damage, both these methods are unsuitable for regular follow-up. Ultrasound has the favourable physical characteristics together with flexibility and mobility that make it eminently suitable for this role and it is also important in the initial assessment of damage to the spleen.

In examining a patient with suspected splenic injury the ultrasonographer should be alert to evidence of intrasplenic haematoma, which is usually echo-poor, ill-defined, and frequently only slightly different from normal parenchyma (Fig. 27.23). Large intrasplenic haemorrhages will be associated with considerable parenchymal damage and should be correspondingly easier to detect (Fig. 27.24). Bleeding contained within the spleen is frequently accompanied by a subcapsular fluid collection that will present as an echo-free rim around the parenchyma (Fig. 27.25). Fortunately the smallest collections of fluid are readily detectable and their presence should alert the radiologist to the possibility of significant intrasplenic damage. In severe trauma the capsule will often tear and blood will collect in the left upper quadrant (Fig. 27.26). The observation of such a collection should alert the ultrasonographer to the serious nature of the condition, and collapse of the patient may be imminent.

Angiography

The vasculature of the spleen may be displayed by several different routes.

The arterial supply is most easily demonstrated by selective cannulation by a retrograde approach

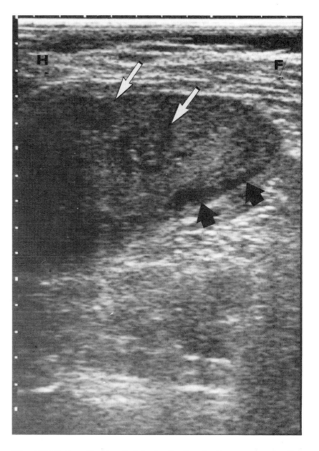

Fig. 27.23 Small rounded foci of mixed echo pattern in the inferior tip of the spleen (*short arrows*). An echo-free subcapsular collection can be identified medially (*long arrows*).

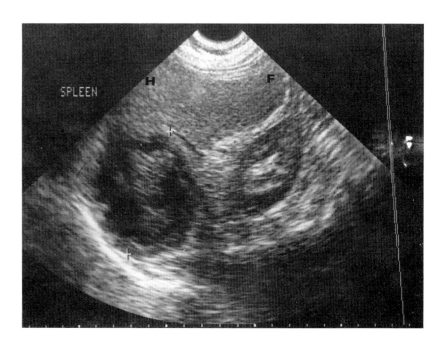

Fig. 27.24 A large irregular intrasplenic haematoma demonstrated on oblique longitudinal sonography.

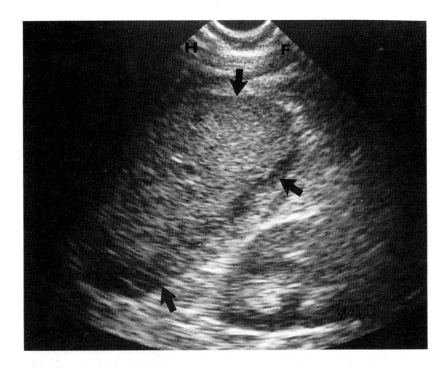

Fig. 27.25 Intracapsular rupture of the spleen. Echo-poor fluid encircles the splenic parenchyma (*arrows*).

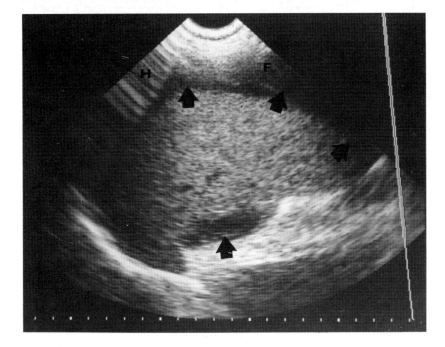

Fig. 27.26 An oblique longitudinal ultrasound section showing the spleen 'floating' in echo-free fluid (*arrows*) after a tear of the splenic artery.

from the femoral artery. Occasionally an antegrade route from above my be required when there is severe peripheral arterial disease. Usually a catheter introduced from below into the coeliac axis readily and indeed preferentially enters the splenic artery and this may be a source of frustration to the radiologist wishing to catheterize the hepatic artery (Fig. 27.27).

The splenic artery is the largest of the three branches of the coeliac axis; the others being the hepatic and left gastric arteries. A flush injection into the abdominal aorta is traditionally advocated in order to provide a 'roadmap' of the major branches of the aorta prior to their selective catheterization. In practice, the origin of the coeliac axis will usually be found easily at or just below the left pedicle of the 12th dorsal vertebra. The splenic artery is a high-flow vessel and image

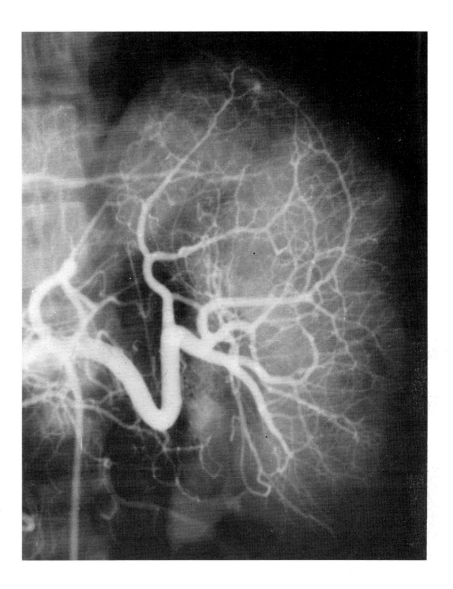

Fig. 27.27 Normal splenic arteriogram following injection into the coeliac axis.

quality is enhanced by the use of generous volumes of contrast given by pressure injection.

Splenic angiography is now increasingly rarely performed. It is insensitive at detecting parenchymal abnormalities and this invasive technique is now seldom indicated in the investigation of a patient with splenomegaly. From time to time the preoperative assessment of splenic artery aneurysms and venous malformations will justify an angiogram, and the course and appearance of varices can easily be demonstrated by this technique. However, the most important role for angiography of the spleen remains in the diagnosis of rupture and haemorhage. Features of splenic trauma range from disruption of the vascular tree and transection of major arteries when damage is gross, to localized areas of avascularity and extravasation when less severe. Extrasplenic and subcapsular haematomata are also usually well shown,

compressing the normal parenchyma (Fig. 27.28). In 1981 Fisher and his colleagues stressed the value of arteriography in defining the therapeutic options in the management of splenic trauma. In so doing they described a detailed angiographic classification of damage to the spleen which allows selection of those patients who may safely be managed conservatively.

It is also possible to display the venous drainage of the spleen adequately via the arterial route by taking delayed films after selective arterial injection, as the spleen has only one major vein and very few tributaries (Fig. 27.29). In recent years the increased use of improved arteriographic techniques has been responsible for the decline in the practice of the more direct but traumatic procedure of splenoportography.

This technique involves the direct puncture of the splenic pulp by a large-calibre needle, 12–15

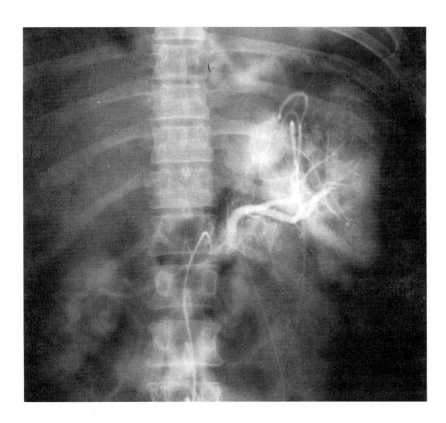

Fig. 27.28 Rupture of the spleen. Note the uneven parenchymal opacification, the loss of splenic outline, intrasplenic vascular displacement, and extrinsic compression along the lateral margin of the spleen by the haematoma.

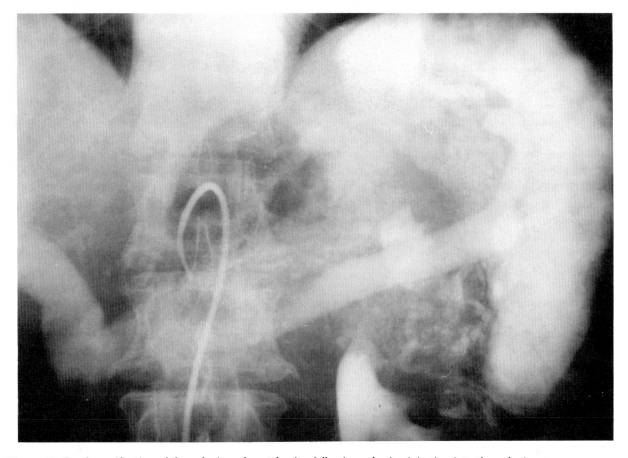

Fig. 27.29 Good opacification of the splenic and portal veins following selective injection into the splenic artery.

cm long, and it requires an accurate assessment of the position and size of the spleen. The puncture of a normal sized spleen is usually via an approach between the 9th and 10th ribs, but obviously the examination is easier when the spleen is enlarged. Unfortunately splenic enlargement is often a reflection of parenchymal disease and although splenomegaly increases the chance of successful puncture, intrasplenic pathology correspondingly increases the complication rate. The needle should be introduced under direct screening and should be angled so that it lies parallel with the long axis of the organ, with its tip aimed at the hilum.

After a test dose has confirmed a satisfactory position, 20–30 ml of contrast is injected over 3–5 s. Serial radiographs, taken over the succeeding 20 s, allow maximal visualization of the splenic and portal veins. The needle is removed immediately after the injection and the patient should be confined to bed for 8 h. The most serious complication is bleeding from the splenic puncture site after withdrawal of the needle, and in an attempt to reduce this risk a plug of Gelfoam may be left in the needle track (Probst et al., 1978.)

A clear demonstration of the anatomy of the splenic and portal veins is possible by this technique. The calibre of the normal splenic vein, by splenoportography, varies between 7 and 16 mm and its length on average is 13 cm. However, the aim of this technique is rarely to delineate the splenic vein itself, and more commonly the requirement is to display the portal vein and venous collaterals in a patient with cirrhosis.

Techniques using digital radiography have more recently been described which allow the administration of lower volumes of contrast and the use of smaller-calibre needles. Using this equipment, satisfactory examinations have been performed with a total of only 16 ml of contrast, injected through a 21 gauge needle (Braun et al., 1985). Despite these technical improvements, the procedure of splenoportography has largely been rendered obsolete by the development of ultrasound, CT, and improved splenic angiography.

A third route to the portal and splenic venous system is via a percutaneous trans-hepatic route for which a catheter, selectively introduced into an intra-hepatic portal venous branch, is guided under direct screening control into the portal vein and thence into the splenic vein. This technique allows not only the acquisition of high-quality diagnostic images but also makes possible the therapeutic occlusion of varices. There are only a small number of selected patients, however, in whom this technique is appropriate and arguably it should be performed only in specialized centres.

Interventional radiology

Therapeutic arterial embolization of the spleen was first described in 1973 by Maddison as a method of non-operative ablation of splenic function. This technique is particularly useful because many patients with hypersplenism have disordered haematology and are poor surgical risks. Schwartz et al. (1970) reported an overall mortality rate of 7.1% and a major complication rate of 18% following splenectomy in this high-risk group. Infarction of the spleen by the radiologist will usually improve the haematological picture sufficiently to permit a safer subsequent splenectomy.

Autologous clot was the material chosen as the embolic agent in the first hypersplenic patient to undergo therapeutic infarction. Subsequently many other methods and materials have been described. These include absorbable gelatin sponge (Sterispon), polyvinyl alcohol sponge, silicone spheres, lyophilized human dura (Lyodura), stainless steel coils, and absolute ethanol.

Complete splenic embolization as a one-stage procedure results in a high incidence of complications, particularly splenic abscess, splenic rupture, pneumonia, and septicaemia (Wallace et al., 1976, Lunderquist et al., 1980). It is therefore prudent to embolize the spleen in two or three stages over several weeks. Distal, partial, and segmental embolization will also reduce any possibility of including gastric or short pancreatic branches in the embolization.

Allison et al. (1981) have particularly recommended that embolization should only be considered when it can be followed, if necessary, by splenectomy. The same workers reported the development in some patients of free intraperitoneal gas several hours after splenic infarction. They suggested that the gas might have been released by the large amount of blood contained in the spleen at the moment of embolization, but this alarming phenomenon did not in itself appear hazardous.

Despite the possibility of major complications, this relatively simple procedure can be vital in the management of patients suffering from severe hypersplenism. Following successful embolization, the hyperdynamic state that may complicate hypersplenism is usually diminished, and platelet counts have been shown to increase in nearly all patients within 1 month. The beneficial effects are usually maintained and long-term increase in platelet levels has been recorded following embolization of the spleen (Yoshioka *et al.*, 1985).

References

Abrams, H.L. & Spiro, R. (1950) Metastases in carcinoma. *Cancer*, **3**, 74.

Allison, D.J., Fletcher, D.R. & Gordon-Smith, E.C. (1981) Therapeutic arterial embolisation of the spleen: a new cause of free intraperitoneal gas. *Clinical Radiology*, **32**, 617–621.

Asher, W.M., Parvin, S. & Virgillo, R.W. (1976) Echographic evaluation of splenic injury after blunt trauma. *Radiology* **118(2)**, 411–415.

Blendis, L.M., Williams, R. & Kreel, L. (1969) Radiological determination of spleen size. *Gut*, **10**, 433–435.

Braun, S.D., Newman, G.E. & Reed Dunnick, N. (1985) Digital splenoportography. *American Journal of Roentgenology*, **144**, 1003–1004.

Breiman, R., Castellino, R., Harrell, G., Marshall, W., Glatstein, E. & Kaplan, H. (1978) CT — pathologic correlations in Hodgkin's disease and non-Hodgkin's lymphoma. *Radiology*, **126**, 159–166.

Buntain, W.L. & Lynn, H.B. (1979) Splenorrhaphy: Changing concepts for the traumatised spleen. *Surgery*, **86**, 748.

Coleman, C.N., McDougall, I.R., Dailey, M.O., Ager P., Bush S. & Kaplan, H.S. (1982) *Annals of Internal Medicine*, **96**, 44–47.

Claussen, C. & Lochner, B. (1985) *Dynamic Computed Tomography*, pp 98–102. Springer-Verlag, Berlin.

Das Gupta, T. & Brasfield, R. (1961) Metastatic melanoma. A clinico-pathological study. *Cancer*, **17**, 1323.

Fisher, R.G., Foucar, K., Estrada, R. & Ben-Menachem, Y. (1981) Splenic rupture in blunt trauma. Correlation of angiographic and pathologic records. *Radiologic Clinics of North America*, **19(1)**, 141–165.

Fitzgerald, J.B., Crawford, E.S. & DeBakey, M.E. (1960) Surgical considerations of nonpenetrating abdominal injuries; An analysis of 200 cases. *American Journal of Surgery*, **100**, 22–29.

Hamilton, R.G., Alderson, P.O., Harwig, J.F. & Siegel, B.A. (1976) Splenic imaging with technetium 99 m labeled erythrocytes: a comparative study of cell damaging methods. *Journal of Nuclear Medicine*, **17**, 1038–1043.

Harper, P.V., Lathrop, K.A. & McCardle, J. (1965) Technetium 99 m as a scanning agent. *Radiology*, **85**, 101–105.

Husni, E.A. (1961) The clinical course of splenic hemangioma. *Archives of Surgery*, **83**, 681.

Jeffrey, R.B., Laing, F.C., Federle, M.P. & Goodman, P.C. (1981) Computed tomography of splenic trauma. *Radiology*, **141**, 729–734.

King, D.J., Dawson, A.A. & Bayliss, A.P. (1985) The value of ultrasonic scanning of the spleen in lymphoma. *Clinical Radiology*, **36**, 473–474.

LePage, R. (1912) *La radioscope et la radiographie de la rate*. Theses, Facultie Medicine, Paris

Likhite, V.V. (1976) Immunological impairment and susceptibility to infection after splenectomy. *Journal of the American Medical Association*, **236**, 1376.

Long, J.A., Doppman, J.L., Nienhus, A.W. & Mills, S.R. (1980) Computed tomographic analysis of beta-thalassemic syndromes with hemochromatosis: Pathologic findings with clinical and laboratory correlation. *Journal of Computer Assisted Tomography*, **4**, 159–164.

Lunderquist, A., Owman, T. & Alwmark, A. (1980) *Intervention Radiology*, pp 258–261. Excerpta Medica, Amsterdam, Oxford, Princeton.

Maddison, F.E. (1973) Embolic therapy for hypersplenism. *Investigative Radiology*, **8**, 280–283.

Marymont, J.H. Jr & Gross, S. (1963) Patterns of metastatic cancer in the spleen. *American Journal of Clinical Pathology*, **40**, 58–66.

Miller, D.L., Vermess, M., Doppman, J.L. *et al.* (1984) CT of the liver and spleen with EOE-13. *American Journal of Roentgenology*, **144**, 235–243.

Mittelstaedt, C.A. & Partain, C.L. (1980) Ultrasonic–pathologic classification of splenic abnormalities: gray scale patterns. *Radiology*, **134(3)**, 697–705.

Oka, M. (1929) Eine neue Methode zur Röntgenologischen Darstellung der Milz (Lienographie). *Fortschritte au de Gebiete der Röntgenstrahlen und der Nuklearmedizin*, **40**, 497.

Pearson, H.A., Spencer, R.P. & Cornelius, E.A. (1969) Functional asplenia in sickle cell anemia. *New England Journal of Medicine*, **281**, 923–926.

Piekarski, J., Goldberg, H.I., Royal, S.A., Axel, L. & Moss, A.A. (1980) Difference between liver and spleen numbers in the normal adult: Its usefulness in predicting liver disease. *Radiology*, **137**, 727–729.

Probst, P., Rysavy, J.A. & Amplatz, K. (1978) Improved safety of splenoportography by plugging of the needle tract. *American Journal of Roentgenology*, **131**, 445–449.

Schwartz, S.I, Bernard, R.P., Adams, J.T. & Bauman, A.W. (1970) Splenectomy for hematological disorders. *Archives of Surgery*, **101**, 338–347.

Sherlock, P.V. & Learmonth, R. (1952) Aneurysm of the splenic artery: with an account of an example complicating Gaucher's disease. *British Journal of Surgery*, **30**, 151.

Soderstrom, N. (1976) How to use cytodiagnostic spleen puncture. *Acta Medica Scandinavica*, **199**, 1–5.

Solbiati, L., Chiara Bossi, M., Bellott, E., Ravetto, C. & Montal, G. (1983) Focal lesions in the spleen. Sonographic patterns and guided biopsy. *American Journal of Roentgenology*, **140**, 59–65.

Thomas, J.L., Bernardino, M.E., Vermess, M. *et al.*, (1982) EOE-13 in the detection of hepatosplenic lymphoma. *Radiology*, **145**, 629–634.

Wallace, S., Gianturco, C., Anderson, J.H., Goldstein, H.M., Davies, L.J. & Bree, R.L. (1979) Therapeutic vascular occlusion utilising steel coil techniques: clinical applications. *American Journal Roentgenology*, **127**, 381–387.

Vermess, M., Bernardino, M.E., Doppman, J.L., Thomas, J.L., Velasquez, W.S., Fuller, L.M. & Russo, A. (1981) The use of intravenous liposoluble contrast material for the examination of the liver and spleen in lymphoma. Preliminary report. *Journal of Computer Assisted Tomography*, **5**, 709–713.

Yoshioka, H., Kuroda, C., Hori, S. *et al.*, (1985) Splenic embolization for hypersplenism using steel coils. *American Journal of Roentgenology*, **144**, 1269–1274.

Part 6
The Abdomen

28: Magnetic Resonance Imaging of the Pancreas and Spleen

F.W. SMITH

Introduction

The accurate diagnosis of pancreatic disease by radiological methods remains difficult and the full potential of all the available techniques has not been investigated. Pancreatitis commonly produces diffuse glandular enlargement which may be well demonstrated both with ultrasound and X-ray CT, but both may have difficulty in differentiating it from cancer. Whilst the usefulness of magnetic resonance imaging (MRI) is well established for the investigation of the central nervous system, especially the cerebellum, brainstem, cranial nerves and spinal cord, its role in imaging the abdomen is not well documented. Early work examining the liver has illustrated the potential of MRI for hepatobiliary imaging, but as yet it has not been shown to be better than any of the established radiological techniques (Smith *et al.*, 1981, Alfidi *et al.*, 1982, Doyle *et al.*, 1982, Moss *et al.*, 1984, Stark *et al.*, 1984, Vermess *et al.*, 1985). Very little work has been published using MRI for the investigation of the pancreas and spleen. Again, only its potential for diagnosis has been presented, with no indication as to its place in diagnosis (Smith *et al.*, 1982, Stark *et al.*, 1984.)

Magnetic resonance imaging of the abdomen has been restricted because normal body motion — cardiovascular, respiratory, and intestinal peristalsis — cause image degradation and artefact production during the relatively long imaging times required for data acquisition. The problem of cardiac and respiratory motion may be overcome by the use of cardiac and respiratory gating, which incurs the penalty of increasing the already lengthy image acquisition time. Peristalsis may be abolished by the use of a spasmolytic. Before describing the magnetic resonance appearances of the upper abdomen, we should first consider the methods used to produce MR images to better understand their appearance.

Imaging method

Image production depends upon the detection of two types of signal emitted from the patient in the collection phase of imaging, immediately following the radiofrequency pulse. The two types of signal contribute to both the spatial and contrast resolution of the final image. The origin of contrast in the image is due to the differing concentrations of hydrogen protons within the molecules which make up the different tissues in each section, and also their different relaxation times. The contribution of proton concentration or density is obvious. The greater the concentration of protons, the stronger the signal, so soft tissue will appear white or grey and air and bone, with fewer protons, will appear black. The difference in proton density in soft tissues is not very large ($\pm$ 20%) and this component does not contribute greatly to soft-tissue contrast. The relaxation times of different tissues have a much larger range ($\pm$ 200%) and dominate image contrast.

Relaxation time is the term given to the process by which the protons release the energy they absorbed during the irradiating radiofrequency pulse, and is measured in milliseconds (ms). Most MR images contain signals due to two relaxation time processes, which occur simultaneously and are associated with the environment of the protons, the intensity of the emitted radiation falling exponentially at a rate characteristic for the environment of which they are part.

The first of these relaxation time processes is the proton spin-lattice relaxation time or T_1, and is the length of time required for the proton to realign with the magnetic field following irradiation. The T_1 varies, depending upon the rate at which it takes for the radiation to pass to the surrounding lattice of molecules in the tissue. The easier it is for protons to pass energy to neighbouring molecules, the more quickly they can relax to their original state and the faster is the fall of intensity of the emitted signal. Thus, tissues with a large amount of bound water, with protons closely bound to proteins, such as muscle, liver, and pancreas, have a short T_1. If the protons are more closely bound together as they are in hydrocarbons found in fat, then their T_1 is very short, whereas fluids with free water such as urine, cerebrospinal fluid, and ascitic fluid have a long T_1.

The second relaxation process is called the spin-spin relaxation time or T_2 and is more difficult to describe. The irradiating or excitation pulse not only causes protons to absorb energy, but it also generates an order or coherence in those protons it excites. The detectable signal emitted by the protons is only the coherent part. Thus, following an irradiating pulse, the signal that is detected, amplified, digitized, and stored in a computer, decays in two ways. Firstly the total signal decays to zero (T_1), and secondly the detectable component of the signal decays (T_2). The T_2 of tissue is about 10 times faster than the T_1.

Different tissues have different relaxation times often by an order of magnitude or more. It is this phenomenon which gives MR images improved soft-tissue contrast over X-ray CT. Furthermore, the T_1/T_2 ratio varies for different tissues. Malignant tissues have a longer T_1 than the equivalent normal tissue, but unfortunately this observation alone is not reliable for making a diagnosis of malignancy, because other conditions such as inflammation and oedema also have longer than normal T_1 values.

Imaging sequences

Magnetic resonance images are reconstructed from signals obtained using a series of different intervals and combinations between pulses of radiofrequency radiation. These combinations and intervals between the pulses are known as the pulse sequence. A particular pulse sequence can be chosen to make the resultant image more or less dependent on a particular source of contrast. If for example tissue oedema is of interest, a sequence which is T_2-dominated may be chosen.

Before constructing a pulse sequence it is important to understand the terminology and components of such a sequence. The time between successive excitation pulses initiating each pulse sequence is known as T_R. The time between the excitation pulse and collection of the re-radiated or emitted signal is known as the echo delay or T_E.

Spin-echo imaging using differing T_R and T_E values is the most commonly used imaging technique. This is because by choosing suitable T_R and T_E values, images dependent on proton density, T_1 and T_2 can be made. When images are wanted that are more dependent on T_1 then specific 180° pulses are used at a time interval T_I after T_R to produce inversion recovery images that have high spatial resolution but less contrast than spin-echo images, and are less sensitive to pathological changes in tissue.

Using spin-echo pulse sequences a series of different images can be made in any of three planes, sagittal, coronal or axial, which display both the anatomy of the region under examination and its T_1 and T_2 characteristics. Whenever MR imaging is being performed, images in at least two planes should be made using at least two different pulse sequences, thus ensuring the maximum amount of information from the examination.

Partial saturation images using a short T_E interval of < 10 ms and varying T_R intervals can be made. These images are composed of predominantly proton density information, especially when a very long, > 10 s, T_R is used. Medium, approximately 1 s, and short, < 100 ms, T_R intervals add T_1 weighting to the relatively contrast-free partial saturation images. The spin-echo sequences used most often are made using T_E intervals of between 50 and 200 ms at different T_R values. Short T_R intervals of less than 1000 ms with T_E values of between 50 and 200 ms yield T_1-weighted images. When the T_R is increased to between 2000 and 5000 ms they become T_2 weighted, and above 10 s they are predominantly proton density.

An ideal method for examining the upper abdomen is to perform a multisection acquisition in the coronal plane using a T_R of 500 ms and a T_E of between 35 and 50 ms. This yields a series of images in a short-time, which are a mixture of T_1 and T_2 data, but predominantly T_1. This should be followed by a multisection acquisition in the axial plane using a T_R of between 2000 and 3000 ms and T_E values of 50 and 100 ms. This so-called multi-echo sequence will give two sets of images with progressively more T_2 weighting. The longer the T_E that is employed, the stronger the signal that is gained from tissues and substances with a long T_2. The use of more than two echoes is also possible and a multi-echo sequence with up to eight echoes can be obtained without increasing the imaging time. Echoes in multiples of the first T_E are used, i.e. 45, 90, 135. The image quality of the later echoes is often significantly worse than if a single-echo sequence of long T_E were used. If high spatial resolution is wanted as well as contrast then two separate acquisitions using different T_E values is advisable.

Inversion recovery sequences can be constructed that will give both high tissue contrast and help to differentiate tumours from oedema where both have long T_I values.

The use of short T_I sequences, such as T_R 1000 T_I 100 T_E 40, give good resolution images because they are less vulnerable to body motion. This is partly due to the short T_R used and partly because of the weak signal obtained from fat using this sequence. Subcutaneous fat is a major source of motion artefact when imaging the abdomen, and a reduction in the fat signal minimizes this. Longer T_I intervals will provide good contrast between tissues of different T_1 value when a T_I value intermediate between the values is used. A further use of the long T_I sequence is to suppress the signal from long T_1 fluids such as ascites and bowel contents by using values of between 800 and 1200 ms. In the same way that it is possible to use a multi-echo sequence when employing a spin-echo sequence, so it is possible to construct a double-inversion recovery sequence that will suppress both the fat signal and the signal from fluids. These double sequences take a significantly longer time to acquire and may show some reduction in lesion contrast. A suitable double sequence for abdominal imaging is T_R 3000 ms T_I 1200 ms T_I 00 ms T_E 44 ms (Bydder & Young, 1985).

Imaging time

One of the drawbacks of MRI is the comparatively long data acquisition time for each pulse sequence as compared with CT and conventional radiological techniques. This results in image degradation due to patient movement and means that fewer patients can be examined in a given time as compared with CT. Image quality is dependent upon the pulse sequence, imaging matrix, and the signal strength. The contribution that pulse sequence length makes is self-evident, the longer the interval between pulse sequences the longer it will take to acquire the data; sequences using long T_R intervals take longer to acquire than those using short T_R values. Similarly the use of a 256 × 256 matrix to produce high spatial resolution will take

longer to acquire than a lower-resolution 128 × 128 matrix acquisition. Signal strength increases with increasing magnetic field strength, but even at relatively high fields (0.5–2.0 Tesla) the signal is not particularly strong and a number of acquisitions from each section under examination must be acquired and added together before being averaged (number of buffers). It is therefore important to understand how to calculate the acquisition time when planning each patient investigation. The acquisition time for each sequence is equal to the T_R × matrix size × number of buffers, i.e. a fast, low-resolution sequence suitable for use in positioning a patient, which takes just 1 min to acquire, would use a T_R of 500 ms, a 128 matrix, and only one buffer. A more diagnostically useful sequence using a T_R of 2000 ms, a 256 matrix, and collecting four buffers will take 34 min. This sequence may be shortened to 25.6 min by reducing the matrix size to 192 without significant loss in spatial resolution. Acquisition time is independent of T_E and T_I and largely independent of the number of sections acquired in a multi-slice acquisition. The number of sections that can be obtained from any given sequence is dependent upon the T_R used. Using a T_R of 500 ms, only 3–5 sections can be obtained but using a T_R of 2000 ms, up to 17 or 19 sections may be acquired.

The effects of cardiac, respiratory, and peristaltic motion on image quality have already been mentioned as one of the main causes of image degradation due to 'ghosting'. These causes of artefact can be removed by a number of different means. Cardiac gating, where the pulse sequence is initiated 1 ms after the occurrence of the cardiac R wave, results in slight improvement to abdominal images and does not significantly add to imaging time when T_R values of less than 1000 ms are used. Respiratory gating abolishes the major 'ghosting' artefact caused by subcutaneous fat and considerably improves image quality, but adds significantly to imaging time. Using a rubber bellows fastened around the chest it is possible to monitor the respiratory excursion and to choose either end-inspiration or end-expiration as the trigger for pulse sequence initiation. Because the normal respiratory rate is about 15–18 cycles per minute imaging time may be up to four times that of non-gated imaging. A suitable compromise that does not add significantly to imaging time is to set the gate to exclude only those breaths which fall outside the normal regular breathing cycle. This excludes the occasional deep inspiration that may be made by a bored or restless patient and which tends to spoil the image.

Unlike X-ray CT, bowel gas and fluid do not cause artefact on MR images, but peristaltic movement will. Peristalsis may be reduced by administering a spasmolytic agent such as glucagon 1–2 mg intravenously immediately prior to imaging. It has been suggested that fasting for 6 h prior to imaging may be beneficial in emptying the stomach and small intestine. This is useful when examining the lower abdomen and pelvis because fluid-filled small bowel may be mistaken for pelvic pathology. However, when examining the upper abdomen it is better to have some fluid in the stomach and duodenum to outline them accurately, since the relaxation time of stomach, duodenum pancreas, and liver are very similar. Any oral fluid is suitable as an upper gastrointestinal contrast agent, milk being particularly suitable, and it seems unlikely that a specialized, paramagnetic oral contrast agent will be necessary.

The presence of barium in either the upper or lower gastrointestinal tract is not a contraindication to MR imaging, since it does not cause any artefact and appears as an area of either low or absent signal in the bowel. Metallic surgical clips may cause artefact on the image, depending upon their constituents. If the clip is ferromagnetic it will cause an area of no signal on the image, but will not cause any line artefact as is seen on CT images. Imaging of patients with ferromagnetic clips may be hazardous to the patient when high-field MR imagers are used, because the clips may be moved by the strong magnetic forces employed. Non-ferrous clips are not a problem; they will not move in the magnetic field and do not cause any artefact, appearing as small areas of no signal. Patients with ferromagnetic clips and implants should therefore be excluded from MRI as should those with cardiac pacemakers, which may be damaged by the rapidly changing electromagnetic gradients.

The pancreas

Magnetic resonance images of the pancreas are similar in many respects to CT images. Changes in morphology are easily recognized but changes in relaxation time signal, which may increase contrast between lesion and organ, are not specific enough to allow for more accurate tissue diagnosis.

The normal pancreas may be identified in most patients using either spin-echo or inversion re-covery sequences. The pancreas, which in adults measures between 12 and 15 cm runs almost horizontally but obliquely from the splenic hilum over the abdominal aorta and inferior vena cava to the right side of the abdomen where its head is bordered by the duodenal loop. It may be best demonstrated with MR by axial and coronal sections through the upper abdomen. The course taken by the pancreas varies from patient to patient and determines the number of sections required in any plane to completely visualize the organ. The boundaries of the normal pancreas appear smooth and slightly lobulated (Figs 28.1–28.6). The presence of retroperitoneal fat is important for the clear demonstration of the organ. In thin patients and children, sparse retroperitoneal fat makes if difficult to distinguish the pancreas from bowel. MRI can best identify bowel when it contains fluid or gas but occasionally the presence of fluid-filled small bowel may be confused with an enlarged pancreas (Fig. 28.2). The shape of the pancreas is variable, its diameter usually decreasing from the head towards the tail. Minor variations in diameter are normal and may be simulated in axial sections by the intersection of a curved organ at different levels (Fig. 28.3).

The main pancreatic duct runs centrally through the body and tail. Its diameter of between 2 and 4 mm is too narrow to be readily demonstrated in normal sections, which are usually 8–10 mm thick.

The intensity of signal from the normal pancreas is similar to that of normal liver and bowel. The contrast between two tissues is governed by a number of properties of the tissues, the T_1 and T_2 relaxation times, the spin density, and blood flow in the tissues all contributing. The T_1 and T_2 relaxation times for different tissues may be calculated, but because there is considerable overlap in these values between liver and pancreas and between different pathological states, they are not a useful measurement for either tissue localization or diagnosis. The range of T_1 measurement for liver is 275–425 ms and for pancreas 275–725 ms. The T_2 measurements are 37–55 ms and 55–85 ms, respectively, when measured at 0.8 T. When the ratio spin densities between the organs and that of skeletal muscle are studied there is again overlap. For liver the ratio is 0.84 ± 25 and for pancreas it is 0.77 ± 10 (Schmidt et al., 1985.)

Reliable diagnosis using MRI rests not only upon an understanding of the relationships of image brightness and contrast and the corresponding properties of tissue, but also on the ability to

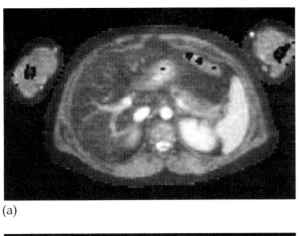

(a)

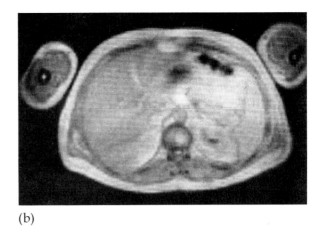

(b)

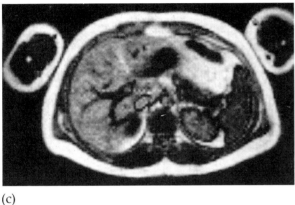

(c)

Fig. 28.1 (a) Calculated T_1. (b) Proton density. (c) Inversion recovery. Normal liver, spleen and pancreatic tail. Blood vessels seen as white in the T_1 image, splenic vein demonstrated running along pancreas.

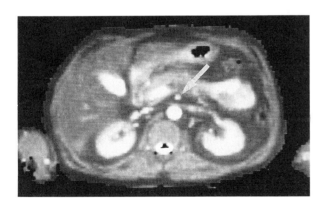

Fig. 28.2 Normal pancreas. Stomach and duodenum contain fluid and duodenum appears white. Loops of small bowel adjacent to pancreatic tail mimic tumour. Superior mesenteric artery (*arrow*).

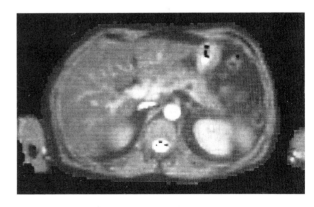

Fig. 28.3 Normal pancreas demonstrating the irregular appearance of this organ when sectioned through different thicknesses of tissue.

recognize the organ being examined and its adjacent structures. This is especially true of the pancreas, where recognition of the surrounding blood vessels is of paramount importance (see Fig. 28.4). Both veins and arteries are easily seen without the use of intravenous contrast material on all MR images whatever pulse sequence is used. Using the spin-echo technique the blood in all vessels appears as a 'void'. The blood is black and the vessel wall is visible as a grey structure. Similar appearances are seen using inversion recovery sequences (Fig. 28.1). When T_1-calculated images are viewed, blood appears as a strong signal and is displayed as white (Figs 28.1–28.6).

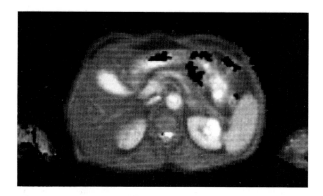

Fig. 28.4 Normal pancreas. The strong intensity signal from the region of the pancreatic head is due to the partial volume effect of the portal vein and duodenum and must not be mistaken for a pancreatic tumour.

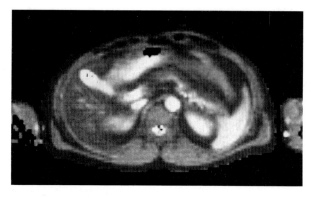

Fig. 28.5 Tortuous splenic vein lying along the posterior border of the pancreas.

The superior mesenteric artery serves as an important landmark for localizing the body of the pancreas, which lies in front of this artery (Figs 28.5, 28.6).

The splenic vein runs along the posterior border of the pancreas (Figs 28.1, 28.5, 28.6) and may sometimes run within the organ. Its recognition is important because posterior displacement is indicative of an intrapancreatic lesion and anterior displacement is a sign of a retropancreatic lesion.

The splenic artery runs a more tortuous course than the vein and is situated along the upper surface of the pancreas (Fig. 28.7).

The superior mesenteric vein and portal vein, which are not easily seen on the non-enhanced CT scan, are often recognized. The superior mesenteric vein lies to the right of the superior mesenteric artery and the portal vein is behind the body of the pancreas. The duodenum that surrounds the lateral and inferior margins of the head of the pancreas is best demonstrated when filled with fluid. The fourth part of the duodenum can then be differentiated from the uncinate process, both of which lie behind the superior mesenteric vein and artery.

The common bile duct runs a short part of its course vertically through the pancreatic head. It is recognizable because of the strong signal, both T_1 and T_2, from bile making it appear white in T_1 and T_2-weighted images, and the relatively low proton density of bile making it appear dark grey in proton-density and partial-saturation images.

The intrahepatic ducts are not visualized unless they are dilated, at which time they are easily differentiated from the portal vein by their strong

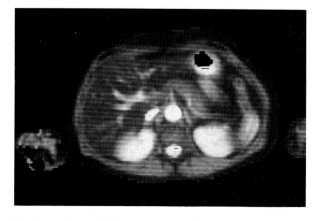

Fig. 28.6 Normal abdomen sectioned at the level of the origin of the superior mesenteric artery.

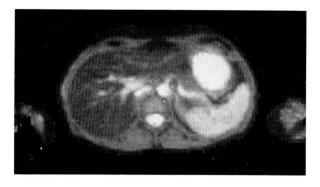

Fig. 28.7 Normal abdomen at level of splenic artery. Fluid in stomach appears white.

intensity T_1 and T_2 signals and low proton density (Fig. 28.8).

Tumours of the pancreas

The diagnostic criteria for tumours of the pancreas are similar to those applied to CT examination, the

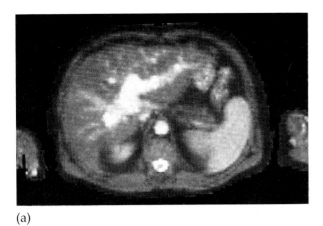

(a)

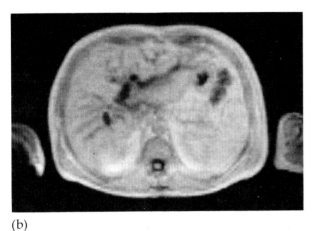

(b)

Fig. 28.8 (a) T_1. (b) Proton density. Dilated intrahepatic bile ducts due to a carcinoma in the head of the pancreas (*not visible*). The strong T_1 relaxation time signal makes bile appear white, whilst the low proton density of bile shows as black in (b) and clearly delineates the dilated bile ducts.

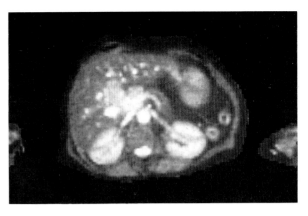

Fig. 28.9 Carcinoma of head of pancreas extending into the porta hepatis and causing biliary obstruction.

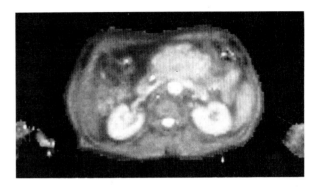

Fig. 28.10 Carcinoma of body of pancreas.

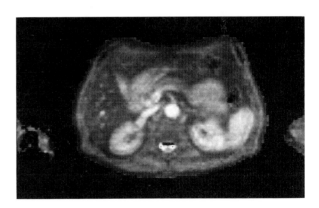

Fig. 28.11 Carcinoma of tail of pancreas.

localized solid mass within the pancreas being the most important diagnostic feature. Care has to be taken when assessing a pancreas which has an irregular configuration with abrupt changes in thickness, to differentiate a normal variant from early tumour.

The most common benign tumour of the pancreas, the cystadenoma will appear as a well demarcated mass containing a number of cysts of long T_1 and T_2. The signal from these mucinous cysts will not be as strong as from the exudate in retention cysts and pseudocysts.

In most cases of adenocarcinoma the signal intensity from the tumour is similar to that of normal pancreas (Figs 28.9–28.11) when both T_1 and T_2-weighted images are viewed. In some cases, however, the relaxation times are longer than in the normal pancreas (Figs 28.12, 28.13) and the tumour is easily recognized. Obliteration of the adjacent fat planes surrounding the retroperitoneal structures by tumour infiltration is a useful sign easily seen in MR images. Involvement of any major blood vessel is also clearly seen (Fig. 28.14). Areas of necrosis within large tumours will have a low proton density and strong T_1 and T_2 signal, the strengths of the relaxation signals being dependent on the constituents of the necrotic tissue. Long

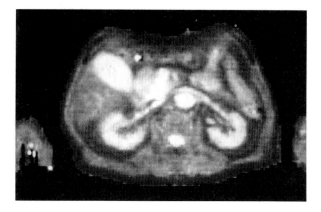

Fig. 28.12 Carcinoma of head of pancreas showing strong (*white*) signal from tumour.

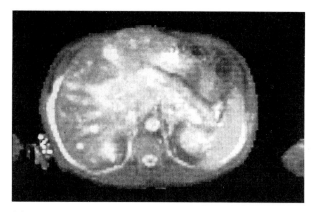

(a)

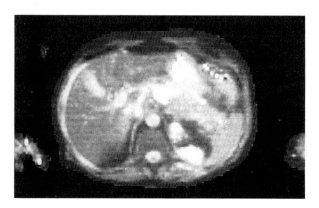

Fig. 28.13 Carcinoma of body of pancreas. Strong (*white*) signal necrotic area within tumour.

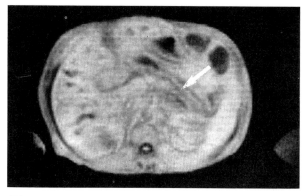

(b)

Fig. 28.14 (a) T$_1$. (b) Proton density. Infiltrating carcinoma of the pancreas causing biliary obstruction and ascites. Bile, ascites, and oedema of tumour appear *white* in(a). In (b) the proton-density image, the ascites and bile ducts appear *black* as does the dilated pancreatic duct (*arrow*).

relaxation times are due to the presence of fluid and may be mistaken for a pseudocyst. The presence of blood or other protein-rich material within the necrotic area will shorten the relaxation time and therefore decrease the signal strength. Biliary obstruction may occur when the tumour is situated in the head of the pancreas. The pancreatic duct may also become obstructed and dilated, but this is not a reliable sign of carcinoma since it may also occur in pancreatitis (Neff *et al.*, 1984).

Regional lymph node enlargement occurs in approximately 65% of cases of adenocarcinoma and large nodes are easily recognized. Large nodes in the porta hepatis may be difficult to differentiate from primary tumour in the head of the pancreas because of the similarity in signal intensity. Ascites is more commonly seen in acute pancreatitis but occurs in between 10 and 15% of cases of carcinoma. It may be demonstrated when very small amounts are present in the peritoneal space

because of its very long relaxation time and resultant strong signal (Fig. 28.14). Metastases within the liver are generally of stronger signal intensity than normal liver and easily differentiated (Fig. 28.15).

Islet-cell carcinomata, although often very small, may be recognizable as space-occupying masses which do have significantly increased signal intensity as compared with normal pancreas. This increased signal intensity is predominantly due to T$_2$ and is best demonstrated with T$_E$ values greater than 50 ms.

Sarcoma also gives a strong intensity signal and may be difficult to differentiate from islet-cell carcinoma.

Similarly gastrin-secreting adenomata have been demonstrated which have a long relaxation time (Smith, 1983). Little experience with secondary tumours is available but it is likely that the MRI appearances will be non-specific, and the

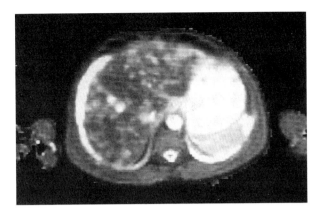

Fig. 28.15 Metastatic deposits in liver appear *grey*, dilated bile ducts white from a carcinoma of pancreas (*not shown*), which is also obstructing the duodenum, resulting in gastric dilatation and retention of fluid (*white*). Ascites is also present.

diagnosis of pancreatic tumour dependent upon morphological changes in the pancreas and secondary signs such as duct obstruction, regional metastases, liver metastases, and malignant ascites.

Pancreatitis

Acute pancreatitis is usually characterized by excessive enlargement of the pancreas, with an increase in relaxation time resulting in a stronger intensity signal from the organ (Fig. 28.16). However, this is not invariably the case and the gland may appear to be enlarged and have a normal signal intensity, in which case it is only the presence of exudate which enables the diagnosis to be made (Fig. 28.17). This exudate has a very long relaxation time, both T_1 and T_2, and is easily recognizable. Large and small amounts of malignant ascites are likewise easily differentiated because of their strong signal intensity, but are difficult to distinguish from exudate or pus in the peritoneal cavity. No specific signs have been recorded that will differentiate oedematous pancreatitis, which has a good prognosis, from haemorrhagic pancreatitis. Difficulty may also be experienced in differentiating diffuse carcinoma of the pancreas from pancreatitis (Fig. 28.18). Abscess formation is a serious complication of acute pancreatitis and will be demonstrable as encapsulated, cystic structures in the region of the pancreas and perirenal areas. No reliable distinction between a pseudocyst and an abscess can be made, since both give strong T_1 and T_2 signals that

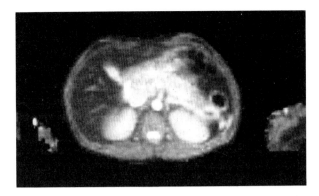

Fig. 28.16 Acute pancreatitis.

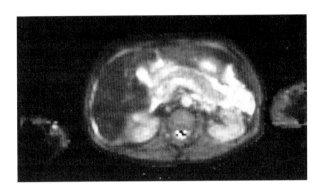

Fig. 28.17 Acute pancreatitis with surrounding exudate and pseudocyst formation in relation to the pancreatic tail.

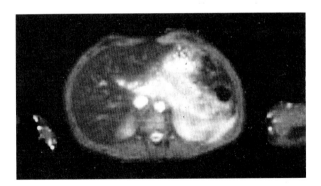

Fig. 28.18 Acute pancreatitis demonstrating similarity to infiltrating tumour.

vary depending upon the amount and type of protein present. The presence of gas within the mass is characteristic of infection.

In chronic pancreatitis the pancreas may be diffusely enlarged or atrophic and diagnosis may be difficult (Fig. 28.19). The presence of calcification, seen in about 30% of cases, is an important sign in X-ray CT but one which is not applicable

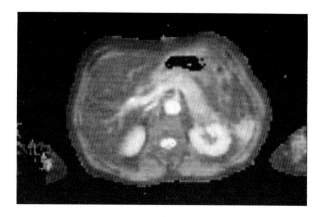

Fig. 28.19 Chronic pancreatitis.

to MRI. Calcification will be demonstrable as ill-defined low-signal-intensity areas when the calcification is larger than 1 cm. Smaller areas of calcification will not be detected. Changes in pulse sequence are unlikely to be helpful in the detection of calcification because no signal is obtained from calcium. Dilatation of the pancreatic duct may be seen in chronic pancreatitis but it must be remembered that pancreatitis may be secondary to carcinoma obstructing the ducts.

Metabolic disease

Pancreatic lipomatosis may occur in generalized adiposity and in the late stage of chronic pancreatitis. The presence of fat will result in a shortening of relaxation time, with resultant weakening of signal in T_1- and T_2-weighted images. The proton density will be increased and the appearances of the pancreas may approach those of abdominal fat. In patients with iron overload and haemochromatosis the paramagnetic effect of the iron results in a shortening of relaxation time and the pancreas may appear similar to one infiltrated with fat. Viewing of the proton-density-weighted images will differentiate the two, since in haemochromatosis the proton density is unchanged from normal.

Trauma

Blunt abdominal trauma tends to involve the body of the pancreas. It may cause contusion, incomplete or complete rupture of the capsule and duct, and is frequently associated with pseudocyst formation. MRI will demonstrate changes in the pancreas consistent with contusion and similar to those seen with CT. Haematoma will be recognizable, having a shorter relaxation time than the fluid seen in a traumatic pseudocyst (Fig. 28.20). As the haematoma ages so the relaxation time will decrease, and MRI can be used to assess its size and expansion in the retroperitoneal space. In common with CT, MRI cannot differentiate between a traumatic pseudocyst and an inflammatory one.

Intra-abdominal infection

Because of the ability of MRI to acquire data from any plane and its ability to demonstrate small fluid collections, it is ideally suited to the demonstration of perihepatic, pancreatic, and splenic abscess. The strong signal intensity in T_1- and T_2-weighted images, whilst not always able to give an accurate diagnosis of the fluid, will give a very accurate display of the size and extent of any collection (Fig. 28.21). When the history is one of abscess formation MRI will be particularly helpful for assessing its site and size.

Spleen

The shape of the spleen is variable, depending upon the site and size of adjacent organs. The stomach, left kidney, splenic flexure of the colon, and the diaphragm lie against the spleen and may influence its shape. The proton density of the spleen is similar to that of the adjacent kidney and stomach and also to that of the pancreas and liver. Its relaxation times, both T_1 and T_2, are longer than pancreas, liver, and stomach but very similar to those of kidney. The spleen therefore appears as an organ of stronger signal intensity than liver and

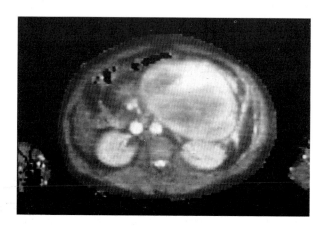

Fig. 28.20 Traumatic pancreatic pseudocyst.

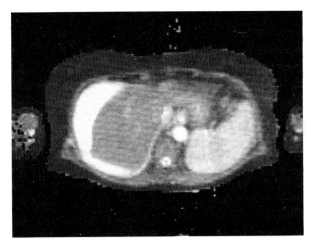

(a)

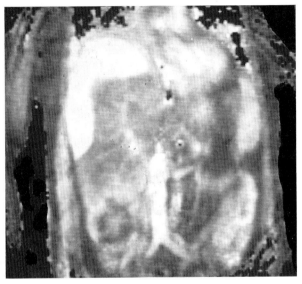

(b)

Fig. 28.21 (a) Axial. (b) Coronal T_1 images of large, right-side subphrenic abscess (*white*).

pancreas and is easily recognizable (Fig. 28.22). Anatomical variants such as polysplenia and accessory spleen appear as homogeneous, smooth encapsulated masses similar to the normal spleen.

Cysts of the spleen are rare, but when present appear as well circumscribed fluid collections of low proton density and long T_1 and T_2. Solid tumours of the spleen are uncommon, malignant lymphoma and plasmacytoma being the most common. Difficulty is experienced in demonstrating splenic tumours deep in the spleen because they very often have proton density and relaxation characteristics similar to normal spleen. Tumours that infiltrate through the capsule are more readily appreciated (Fig. 28.23).

Splenomegaly occurs in cirrhosis of the liver, acute and chronic infection, and in a number of haematological conditions. Apart from enlargement of the organ, no specific changes are seen in the homogeneity of the spleen or in the proton density or relaxation time signals. In cirrhosis of the liver, the appearances of the shrunken cirrhotic liver are diagnostic (Fig. 28.22) as are those of hepatic regeneration (Fig. 28.24) but the appearances in acute and chronic infection and haematological conditions such as thrombocytopenia are indistinguishable (Fig. 28.25). In common with abscesses elsewhere in the abdomen, abscesses in the spleen have long relaxation time signals and low proton density, but in the absence of a suitable history cannot be differentiated from cysts. The presence of gas within the lesion is pathognomonic of infection (Fig. 28.26).

Splenic trauma

The presence of fresh haemorrhage either within the spleen or under its capsule appears with a slightly lower proton density and stronger signal intensity than normal spleen on T_1- and T_2-weighted images (Figs 28.27, 28.28). With increasing age, the magnetic resonance properties of haemoglobin change, resulting in a shortening of relaxation time that may cause the haematoma to become isointense with normal spleen and thus not be visualized. For haemoglobin to bind oxygen, the iron in haem is in the reduced ferrous (Fe^{2+}) state. When it is removed from the circulation this ferrous iron becomes oxidized to the ferric (Fe^{3+}) state with the formation of methaemoglobin, which is paramagnetic and causes a reduction in relaxation time. This alteration in relaxation time of haematomata is well demonstrated in Fig. 28.28 where two large subcapsular haematomata of different ages are seen, the more recent, medial haemorrhage giving a much stronger signal than the older more peripheral one.

Contrast agents

The use of paramagnetic elements to alter the relaxation time of protons and thereby 'enhance' MR images has been developed for the study of the central nervous system. Their application to the investigation of abdominal organs has been slower, due to the limitations to abdominal imaging which have been discussed above. Both oral

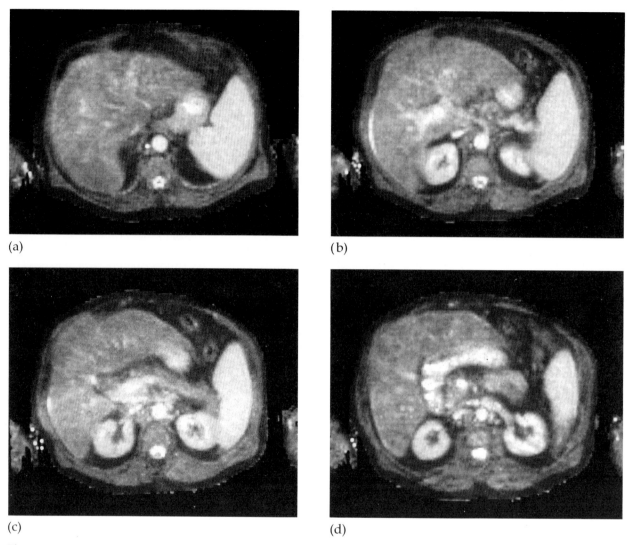

(a)

(b)

(c)

(d)

Fig. 28.22 (a,b) T_1 images of cirrohosis of the liver with splenomegaly and a large amount of intra-abdominal fat (*dark grey*). Small subcapsular, hepatic haematoma secondary to liver biopsy seen in (b) and (c). Splenic and hepatic arteries seen in (b). Left renal vein seen in (d).

and intravenous agents are available for altering the appearances of the gastrointestinal tract and solid organs of the abdomen, respectively.

Fluids such as normal gastrointestinal secretion, milk and other beverages have long T_1 and T_2 relaxation times and give a characteristic appearance. In most situations the presence of one or more of these fluids in the stomach, duodenum, or small bowel acts as a very suitable contrast agent.

There are situations, however, where the ability to change the MR signal from such structures may clarify the anatomy in the area being examined. A most suitable agent for this is ferric ammonium chloride, a safe compound used as an oral iron supplement. The paramagnetic property of the ferric ion to shorten relaxation time is the reason for its use (Wesbey *et al.*, 1985).

A number of other paramagnetic agents have been studied as potential intravenous contrast agents; they include chromium, copper, fluorine, nitroxide-stable free radicals, and a number of rare earth metal such as gadolinium. Unfortunately the majority of these potential contrast agents are toxic and have to be incorporated or chelated into a non-toxic molecule. The most useful element for intravenous use is gadolinium, a rare earth metal that can be rendered non-toxic by chelation into dimethyl penta-acetic acid (DTPA). When injected intravenously it is rapidly excreted by the kidneys, but while in the blood compartment it shortens

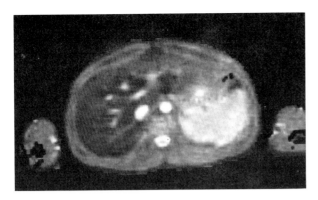

Fig. 28.23 Hodgkin's lymphoma of spleen, infiltrating through capsule.

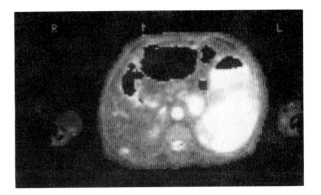

Fig. 28.26 Large splenic abscess. Pus has strong (*white*) signal and it contains a gas—fluid level. Stomach is displaced medially and is distended with gas. (T₁ image made at 0.04 Tesla.)

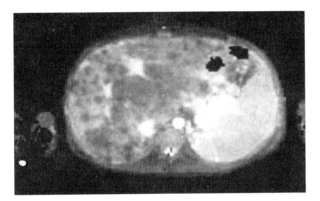

Fig. 28.24 Cirrhosis of the liver with dark-grey nodules of regenerating liver. Large spleen surrounded by a rim of ascites.

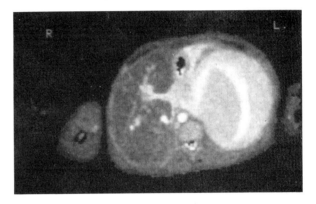

Fig. 28.27 Large splenic haematoma. Spleen is displaced medially by large haematoma exhibiting two distinct relaxation times. The outer *grey* mass is old haematoma, the *white* crescentic mass is recent haemorrhage. (T₁ image made at 0.04 Tesla.)

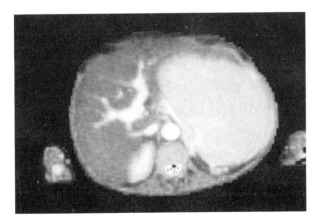

Fig. 28.25 Splenomegaly in a case of thrombocytopenia.

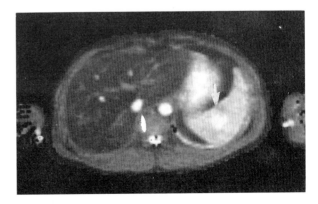

Fig. 28.28 Small intrasplenic haematoma (*arrow*).

the relaxation time and may be used to enhance the MR image. The use of gadolinium DTPA is to alter the T_1 and T_2 signal from vascular organs such as the liver, spleen, and pancreas, and enhance the contrast ratio between the organ under examination and any suspected lesion (Runge *et al.*, 1984).

Images

The images used to illustrate this chapter were made using a 0.08 Tesla (800 Gauss) resistive instrument. The instrument was designed and built at the University of Aberdeen and employs the spin-warp method of imaging. The pulse sequence used in all cases was T_R = 1000 ms, T_I = 200 ms, where the readout pulses occur every 1000 ms with alternate readout pulses preceded by inversion. The inversion is accomplished by adiabatic fast passage with a continuous delay of 200 ms. In other words the pulse sequence consists of interleaved saturation recovery (S_1) and inversion recovery (S_2) pulses from which proton density and inversion recovery images may be displayed. Calculated T_1 images are established from the formula T_1 = 200/In (2 × S_1/(S_1−S_2)).

The calculated T_1 image demonstrates short relaxation time structures as dark grey, intermediate relaxation time organs as shades of grey, and long relaxation time structures as white. The proton density image shows most soft tissue structures as grey with high-proton-density tissues such as fat appearing light grey and low-proton-density structures such as cortical bone and fluids as black. The inversion recovery image gives a strong (white) signal from very short relaxation time tissues such as fat, and also from very long relaxation time organs such as kidney and liver. Organs such as spleen and pancreas appear darker grey and fluids and some blood vessels appear black.

Whilst these images do not have the high spatial resolution available from instruments using powerful, high field strength (>0.5 Tesla) magnets, they accurately demonstrate the differences in relaxation time between different organs and in different disease states.

References

Alfidi, R.J., Haaga, J.R., Yousef, S.J. *et al* (1982) Preliminary experimental results in humans and animals with a super-conducting, whole body, nuclear magnetic resonance scanner. *Radiology*, **143**, 175−181.

Bydder, G.M. & Young, I.R. (1985) MR imaging: clinical use of the inversion recovery sequence. *Journal of Computer Assisted Tomography*, **9(4)**, 659−675.

Doyle, F.H., Pennock, J.M., Banks, L.M. *et al*. (1982) Nuclear magnetic resonance imaging of the liver: initial experience. *American Journal of Roentgenology*, **138**, 193−200.

Moss, A.A., Goldberg, H.I., Stark, D.B., Davis, P.L., Margulis, A.E., Kaufman, L & Crooks, L.E. (1984) Hepatic tumours: magnetic resonance and CT appearance. *Radiology*, **150**, 141−147.

Neff, C.C., Simeone, J.F., Wittenberg, J., Mueller, P.R. & Ferrucci, J.T. (1984) Inflammatory pancreatic masses. *Radiology*, **150**, 35−38.

Runge, V.M., Clanton, J.A., Herzer, W.A., Gibb, S.J., Price, A.C., Partain, C.C., & James, A.E. (1984) Intravascular contrast agents suitable for magnetic resonance imaging. *Radiology*, **153**, 171−176.

Schmidt, H.C., Tscolakoff, D., Hricak, H. & Higgins, C.B. (1985) MR contrast and relaxation times of solid tumours in the chest, abdomen and pelvis. *Journal of Computer Assisted Tomography*, **9(4)**, 738−748.

Smith, F.W. (1983) The value of NMR imaging in pediatric practice: a preliminary report. *Pediatric Radiology*, **13**, 141−147.

Smith, F.W., Mallard, J.R., Reid, A. & Hutchison, J.M.S. (1981) Nuclear magnetic resonance tomographic imaging in liver disease. *Lancet*, **i**, 963−966.

Smith, F.W., Reid, A., Hutchison, J.M.S. & Mallard, J.R. (1982) Nuclear magnetic resonance imaging of the pancreas. *Radiology*, **142**, 677−680.

Stark, D.D., Goldberg, H.I., Moss, A.A. & Bass, N.M. (1984a) Chronic liver disease: evaluation by magnetic resonance. *Radiology*, **150**, 149−151.

Stark, D.D., Moss, A.A., Goldberg, H.I., Davis, P.L. & Federle, M.P. (1984b) Magnetic resonance and CT of the normal and diseased pancreas: a comparative study. *Radiology*, **150**, 153−162.

Vermess, M, Leang, W.-L., Bydder, G.M., Steiner, R.E., Blumgart, L.H. & Young, I.R. (1985) MR Imaging of the liver in primary hepatocellular carcinoma. *Journal of Computer Assisted Tomography*, **9(4)**, 749−754.

Wesbey, G.E., Brasch, R.C., Goldberg, H.I., Engelstad, B.C., & Moss, A.A. (1985) Dilute oral iron solutions as gastro-intestinal contrast agents for magnetic resonance imaging; initial clinical experience. *Magnetic Resonance Imaging*, **3**, 57−64.

29: Trauma of the Upper Abdomen

E.M. McILRATH AND P.S. THOMAS

Introduction

The role of the radiologist in the investigation of upper abdominal trauma is secondary to that of the resuscitation team and the surgeon. The major cause of initial mortality in these patients is haemorrhage. Significant mortality and morbidity can be attributed to sepsis later in the course of the event. Any investigation, including plain films, must await attempts by the resuscitation team to produce a stable or controlled clinical situation (American College of Surgeons, 1976). It must be recognized that associated injuries, particularly to the cranial and respiratory systems may take precedence. They may not only increase morbidity and mortality directly but also distract attention from the abdominal injury.

It has been stated that imaging procedures provide decisive information regarding the necessity for emergency laparotomy in only 6% of patients, and this must be a major consideration at the early stage of assessment when time is of the essence (Strauch, 1973).

Isolated solid-organ injury within the upper abdomen is less common than presentation with associated injuries to the cranium, thorax, skeleton, hollow intra-abdominal viscera, mesentery, and retroperitoneal organs (Davis et al., 1976). A study of the incidence of isolated abdominal injury reveals that the spleen is the most commonly affected organ involved in blunt abdominal trauma.

The liver is only involved half as frequently in blunt trauma but is the most common organ involved in penetrating injury. Hepatic injury has the highest mortality (De Vincenti et al., 1968). Trauma to the pancreas is uncommon but is associated with a 20% mortality and complications is one-third of surviving patients (Jones, 1978).

While the incidence of visceral injury varies between blunt and penetrating trauma, this has a negligible effect on the radiological management, as the majority of surgeons consider exploration to be mandatory in all penetrating injuries, particularly missile wounds.

The overriding consideration at presentation is the clinical condition of the patient (Fig. 29.1). An understanding of the mechanism of injury will assist in the assessment of the consequences of trauma (Ben Menachem, 1981).

Blunt trauma. Localized impact such as that found in sports injuries associated with collision with the fist, foot, knee, or elbow will normally produce injury limited to structures adjacent to the impact. Diffuse impact is most frequently the result of a road traffic accident and is characterized by both

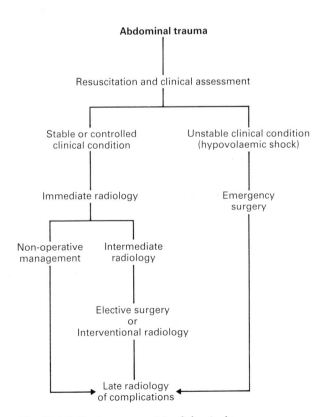

Fig. 29.1 Patient assessment in abdominal trauma.

489

widespread impact and deceleration components, causing injury at the points of impact and also remote from these areas.

Penetrating injuries

1 *Stab wounds*. These cause direct injury to organs in the line of assault. The depth of injury and possible deflection by bone are frequently difficult to assess.

2 *Flying fragments of metal or glass*. The extent of injury depends on the velocity of the fragments. The size of the entry wounds bears no relationship to the extent of visceral damage.

3 *Gunshot wounds*. Single projectiles can be divided into low- and high-velocity groups, the kinetic energy varying according to the formula $Ek = mv^2$, where Ek = kinetic energy, m = mass, v = velocity.

Low-velocity missiles have muzzle velocities of less than 0.75 km/s whereas high-velocity bullets can exceed 1.0 km/s. The importance of this observation to the radiologist is that the extent of temporary cavitation caused by a high velocity missile is large and therefore vascular damage and tissue necrosis will extend far beyond the track of the missile.

It is also worth noting that certain bullets are designed to yaw or tumble and thus the track will considerably exceed the calibre of the projectile.

Multiple projectile injuries will most commonly be caused by shotgun discharge. Penetration will be related to the distance from discharge. As with other low-velocity injuries deflection may occur from bony structures but it can also result from pellets striking shot already embedded within the tissues. The distance of deflection may be considerable and makes assessment of the track virtually impossible.

Iatrogenic trauma

The organs of the upper abdomen are not immune to trauma inflicted by both clinicians and radiologists. During surgery and notably in the emergency situation damage to both spleen, pancreas and bile ducts can go unrecognized. Percutaneous biopsy, image controlled or otherwise, can cause fistulae or vascular damage leading to intraperitoneal haemorrhage, or arteriovenous or biliary fistula.

Pre-existing pathology

It has long been recognized that a pathological organ is more vulnerable to the effects of trauma than its normal counterpart. This may be associated with an increase in the size of the organ but also appears to be related to alteration in the homogenecity of the parenchyma.

Clinical examination

While detailed clinical examination is outside the remit of this work it is necessary that the radiologist has access to and is aware of those parameters other than diagnostic imaging that will influence management.

History. The type of injury will be reflected in the number of organs or systems involved. Previous abdominal surgery is of obvious relevance.

Examination. Inspection for the external manifestations of trauma, evidence of peritoneal irritation, measurement of abdominal girth, auscultation for bowel signs, and pulse and blood pressure should be the mandatory minimum information available.

Laboratory investigations. Urinalysis, haematocrit, SGOT, SGPT and serum amylase will all assist both the surgeon and the radiologist in localizing and estimating the effect of trauma.

Peritoneal lavage. This technique is used in many centres. Warm saline, 500—1000 ml, is infused into the peritoneum and gentle movement of the patient is undertaken. Five minutes later as much of the fluid as can be siphoned off is removed for examination. The presence of bile, faecal staining, or a haemoglobin in excess of 1 g/l represent absolute criteria for laparotomy. Finally the amylase level is estimated as an indication of potential pancreatic damage (Odling-Smee & Crockard, 1981).

The residual fluid after siphoning can be visualized on ultrasound and CT examinations, and may cause displacement of either the liver and spleen evidenced during scintigraphy and arteriography.

Immediate radiological investigation

Conventional studies

The initial examination of the patient will normally

take place in the accident and emergency department and it is unlikely that sophisticated equipment will be available in the associated X-ray rooms.

The provision of trolleys designed to permit good-quality radiographs with minimum movement of the patient is essential. A cassette tray that moves through the whole length of the trolley and at the same time is designed to reduce object–film distance to a minimum is essential. The trolley should be flat-topped and free of accessories that would interfere with cross-table projections. A thin radiolucent fabric mattress provided with multiple handles aids transfer of the patient to a floating top bucky table, which will be more convenient if of elevator design. A ceiling-mounted tube crane and vertical bucky of either fixed or pedestal design must be adjacent to the bucky table.

In all cases a chest radiograph is indicated to exclude concomitant thoracic injury (Fig. 29.2), to provide information regarding pre-existing cardiopulmonary disease, and also to act as a baseline should the patient develop postoperative chest complications (Mindelzon & McCort, 1984).

The abdominal series should include supine and horizontal beam studies. The latter will most frequently be a left lateral decubitus because of the problems obtaining erect views in a patient who has suffered multiple injuries. Views at 90° are mandatory in projectile injuries, and interpretation is aided if the entry and exit wounds are identified by dressings with radio-opaque marked swabs. Despite the urgency of the situation and the frequently manifest impatience of the clinical staff, any temptation to accept suboptimal radiographs must be resisted.

Film density should be satisfactory in the flanks and the radiograph should visualize the area from the diaphragm to the symphysis pubis.

Radiographic signs

Intraperitoneal haemorrhage

Blood in the paracolic gutter may be seen as a band of homogenous density lying within the extraperitoneal fat line, displacing the colonic haustra medially and thus effacing the normal indentations that the haustra produce within the extraperitoneal fat (Fig. 29.3). As large amounts of blood within the peritoneum remain liquid, these signs will be optimized in the lateral decubitus position. Similarly the erect film will assist gravitation of blood into the cavity of the true pelvis, producing homogenous shadowing around the bladder with displacement of bowel loops upwards.

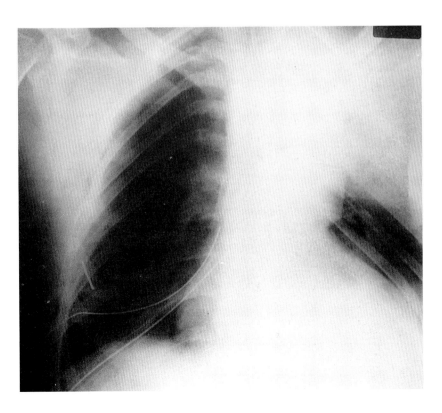

Fig. 29.2 Rupture of the aortic isthmus in a patient with liver trauma.

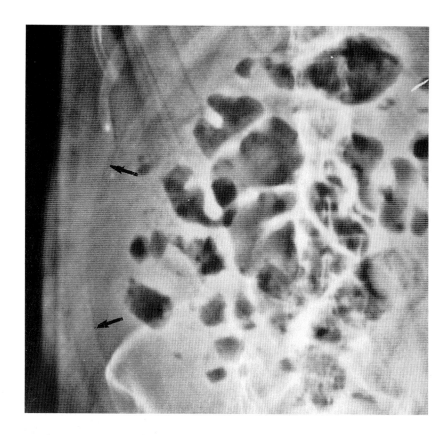

Fig. 29.3 Digital radiogram obtained prior to abdominal CT study showing evidence of blood in the right paracolic gutter.

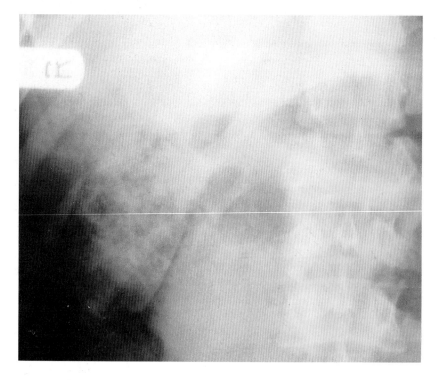

Fig. 29.4 Loss of the hepatic angle is associated with a blood-filled, distended gall bladder.

Blood collections around the inferior edge of the liver and spleen may efface the normal contours of these organs and be seen as a dense homogeneous mass (Fig. 29.4). Separations of the liver or spleen from the lower ribs may occasionally be noted and displacement of the gastric fundus, duodenal air bubble, or hepatic splenic flexures are also occasional features.

Retroperitoneal haemorrhage

Rupture of the pancreas can cause bleeding into the anterior pararenal space with loss of visualization of the upper renal poles and obliteration of the upper lateral aspect of the psoas muscles (Fig. 29.5). Pancreatic rupture may also be associated with duodenal ileus, suspected from the presence of persistent gas within a dilated duodenum, mucosal oedema, and enlargement of the duodenal loop (Fig. 29.6). Pancreatic injury can also be associated with the other signs of acute pancreatitis — sentinel loop, evidence of local ileus, colonic 'cut off' and left basal collapse, and pleural effusion.

Diaphragm

Elevation of the diaphragm if unilateral and associated with rib fractures may indicate specific injury to the liver or spleen (Fig. 29.7). Limited excursion of the diaphragm may be indicative of subphrenic haematoma, but more frequently will be a reflection of the clinical status of the patient from the pain produced by deep inspiration.

There must be continuing awareness, however, that patients with major upper abdominal trauma present a spectrum of associated injuries including thoracic injury (27%) and rupture of the diaphragm.

The preceding examinations should be concluded within 10–15 min, at which stage haematological and biochemical results will be becoming available. Consideration of these results together with the haemodynamic stability of the patient will enable a decision to be made regarding management, which will broadly fall into three:

1 Non-operative.
2 Emergency surgery.
3 Further imaging.

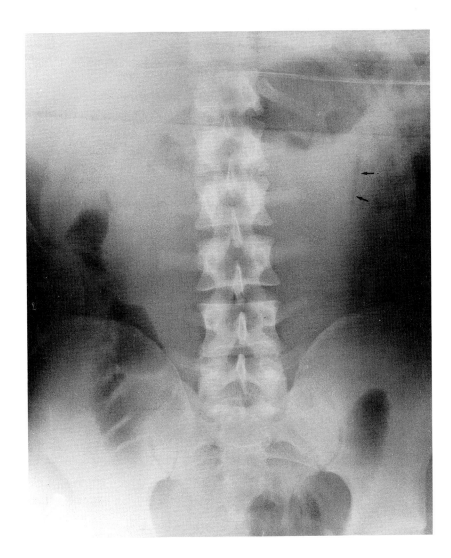

Fig. 29.5 Rupture of the pancreas with blood in the anterior pararenal space on the left side.

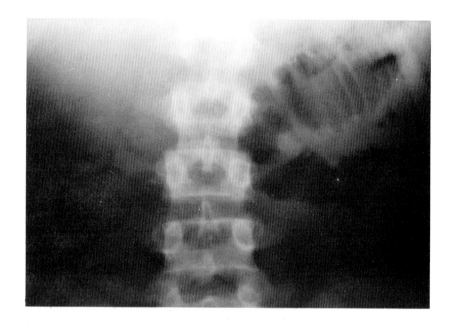

Fig. 29.6 Duodenal ileus associated with pancreatic rupture. (Seat-belt injury.)

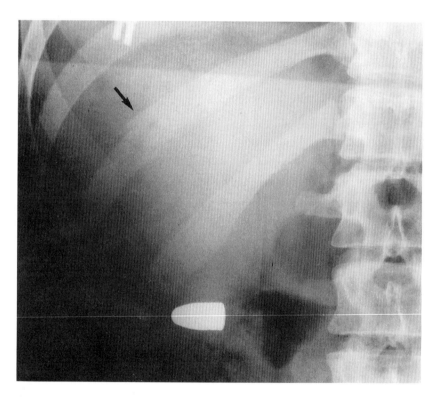

Fig. 29.7 Fracture of the right 11th rib with blood lying bilateral to the liver. The missile which entered through the right chest wall lies opposite L2.

Contrast studies

The use of contrast radiography has diminished with the increased availability of ultrasound, scintigraphy, and computerized tomography, and the recognition that contrast studies can produce only indirect evidence of solid-organ injury.

Oral contrast

The use of Gastrografin is limited firstly to the identification of the gastric fundus and its relationship to the spleen and the diaphragm, and secondly the size, shape, mucosal integrity, and motility of the stomach, duodenum, and upper jejunum.

Thus, while indirect evidence of solid-organ injury may be gained the main value will be in determining the integrity of the hollow organs directly visualized.

Intravenous contrast

The major indication for the use of i.v. contrast remains urinary tract trauma. The use of an adequate volume (300 ml, 21%) of contrast medium combined with films during the parenchymal phase has been stressed previously, and the concept of 'total body opacification' has been shown to demonstrate the size, shape, and position of both the liver and spleen.

It is difficult, however, to conceive that this method would be used except in the case of lack of availability of more modern diagnositic techniques.

Sinogram

The use of sinography in the assessment of stab wounds has, in the past, been advocated. However, more recent experience has revealed that this technique has been associated with an unnecessary laparotomy rate of 38% and enthusiasm has waned. The preferred method of evaluation is by local wound exploration and peritoneal lavage (Thompson et al., 1980).

Intermediate radiology

The objective of intermediate investigation is to produce further information as to the extent and severity of the abdominal injury. This is to enable the clinical team to define priorities of treatment. The investigations require that the patient should be haemodynamically stable and the subject's condition must continue to be monitored during investigation.

The radiologist should be aware of the opportunity to further elucidate injuries remote from the abdomen. For example, computerized tomography may be gainfully employed in combined cranial, spinal, pelvic, chest, and abdominal injuries. Similarly angiographic equipment based on an isocentric C or U arm can be utilized to produce satisfactory skeletal and spinal radiographs.

In abdominal trauma specific indications include:
1 Significant clinical findings within the abdomen.
2 Positive peritoneal lavage.

3 Falling haematocrit.
4 Continuing hypotension.
5 Clinical suspicion of abdominal injury in the presence of multisystem injuries.
6 Positive immediate radiology.

Choice of techniques

Straightforward contrast studies will be required only rarely and while the value of the intravenous urogram in renal trauma is not disputed this examination is unnecessary if there are indications for abdominal angiography. Four main investigations are of value:
1 Radionuclide imaging.
2 Ultrasound.
3 CT scanning.
4 Angiography.

In many centres the choice of technique will be dictated by the availability of equipment and expertise.

Both CT scanning and vascular studies *always* require the removal of the patient from the intensive care environment to the respective areas of the radiology department. Ultrasound equipment and gamma cameras may be available in mobile form but frequently this equipment is less suitable and less sophisticated than static units and the difficulty of performing a comprehensive examination in the alien atmosphere of an intensive care cubicle should not be underestimated.

Transport of the patient requires the support of adequate members of medical, nursing and ancillary staff. The use of a specially designed trolley enabling both vertical and lateral movement of the patient is invaluable in patients with multiple injuries.

CT and ultrasound scanning. These have been proven to provide information about the parenchymal pattern of organs, vascular structures, and the tissue planes within the abdominal cavity. Contrast-enhanced CT scanning may also provide information regarding perfusion of tissue and vascular extravasation.

Radionuclide scanning. While lacking the spatial resolution of other investigations, this provides parenchymal information about the liver and spleen. This feature is dependent on perfusion, and with dynamic 'first pass' scans extravasation may be seen. It is, however, specific to the targeted organ or organs.

Angiography. Prior to the availability of other methods, arteriography was widely utilized to provide information regarding the parenchymal pattern and integrity of organs. It offers few, if any, advantages in these spheres of imaging today and should be reserved for those patients who have symptoms related to vascular damage.

Finally, the overall condition of the patient will influence the choice of imaging technique (Ulthoff *et al.*, 1983). Patients who are disorientated or unmanageable or those who have external fixation applied to skeletal injuries may be more suitable for scintigraphy.

Those patients who have combined cranial–thoracoabdominal trauma, however, will frequently be examined by CT (Berg, 1983). The advice of a surgeon or anaesthetist can be invaluable if analgesia or sedation are required to produce a satisfactory examination.

Scintigraphy

The value of scintigraphy in trauma to the liver and spleen has been recognized for many years (Nebesar *et al.*, 1974) and several large series have been reported (Gelfand, 1984).

While many recent reports have concentrated on the use of newer techniques, including real-time ultrasound and CT, it should not be forgotten that the availability of gamma cameras with dynamic aquisition facilities have improved the accuracy of liver and spleen scanning while at the same time reducing the duration of the examination. Total examination time including preparation of the radionuclide should not exceed an hour.

Other advantages of scintigraphy include the aquisition of accurate information in subjects who would be unsuitable for other methods of assessment due to dressings, external fixation devices, or limited patient compliance. The indications for examination include:

1 Confirmation of a clinical diagnosis of liver or splenic trauma.
2 The assessment of the extent of such trauma.
3 The assessment of splenic viability.
4 The provision of comparative data on a follow-up basis to assess the course of injury.

TECHNIQUES

The examination should, wherever possible, take the form of a radionuclide angiogram using a wide field of view gamma camera with dynamic computer aquisition, followed by static organ scans in both anteroposterior and oblique projections.

A bolus of 185 MBq of ^{99m}technetium sulphur colloid is normally employed.

Assessment of the images

The general morphology of the organs should be examined, commencing with the external contours of the liver and spleen. Clefts or breaks in contour may represent lacerations particularly along the convex borders of both organs (Fig. 29.8), but care must be taken not to assume that the normally irregular areas around the splenic and liver hila represent pathology. Alterations in the position of the organ may be caused by extracapsular haematoma or fluid.

Contusion within the liver or spleen will be represented by multiple 'cold' areas of diminished uptake (Fig. 29.9) frequently irregular. Multiple lacerations and contusions of the spleen will produce the classical appearance of the 'fractured' spleen.

Extravasation of the isotope may be initially found during the dynamic phase of the examination (Bronfman *et al.*, 1981). Increasing accumulation of the isotope may occur during recirculation, which is aided by the reduced perfusion of the reticuloendothelial cells related to hypovolaemic shock. A similar aetiology may cause bone marrow uptake (Smith *et al.*, 1981).

Accumulation of extravasated isotope therefore represents active intraperitoneal bleeding. The presence of accessory splenic tissue should be sought and noted (Fig. 29.10).

Follow-up studies frequently reveal a rapid return to normal perfusion (Morayati *et al.*, 1983) in the absence of surgical intervention, and confirm the presence of functioning splenic tissue after surgery to preserve the spleen. The concept of splenic salvage has placed even greater importance on establishing accurate diagnosis of suspected splenic injuries. Scintigraphy offers a rapid reproducible method of assessment in hepatosplenic trauma. The technique has been recorded as producing less than 2% false negative and 7% false positive results (Gilday & Alderson, 1974).

Ultrasound

TECHNIQUE

The adoption of real-time scanning, particularly

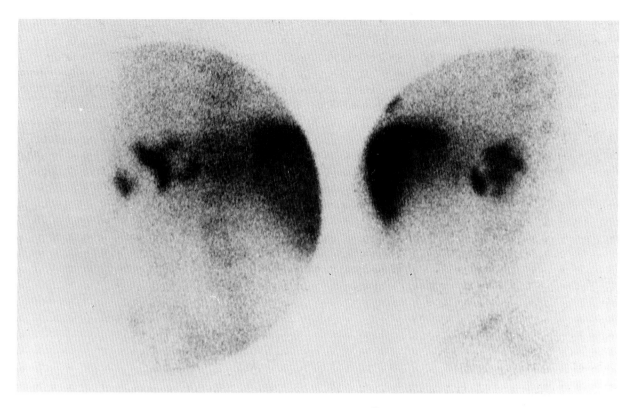

Fig. 29.8 Fragmentation of the spleen following a road-traffic accident. (^{99m}technetium sulphur colloid scan.)

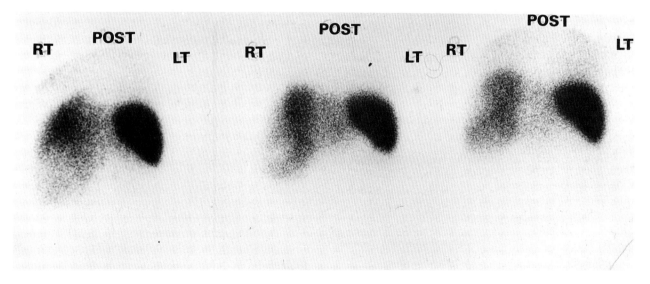

Fig. 29.9 A contusion of the right lobe of liver with development of a subcapsular haematoma followed by radionuclide scans over a period of 3 months. (Courtesy of Dr H. Carty.)

utilizing instruments with sector capability +3.5 + 5 MHz transducers has improved the role of ultrasound in trauma.

Examination time is reduced and the number of projections is unlimited, thus allowing better visualization of the abdominal organs with elimination of artefact. It may be necessary to obtain views through the lower intercostal spaces if the diaphragm is elevated and its excursion reduced by pain and associated thoracic injuries.

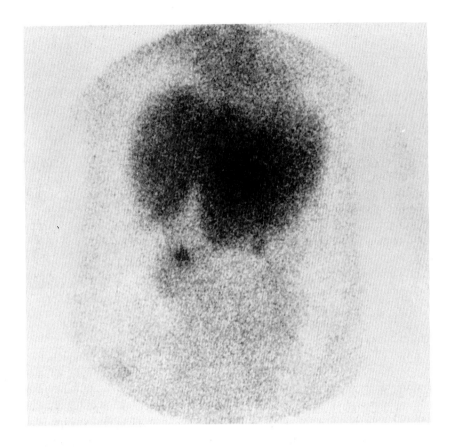

Fig. 29.10 Extrahepatic accumulation of isotope due to traumatic haemorrhage into the duodenum. (^{99m}technetiun sulphur colloid scan.)

Minimal elevation of the left side for splenic visualization or right side for the posterolateral liver segments is often necessary and can be achieved with care even in the severely traumatized patient.

A planned approach commencing from the subphrenic space, passing into the paracolic recesses, and thence into the pelvis will demonstrate the dependent peritoneal areas into which blood or fluid will gravitate. Artefact can be encountered if the transducer overlies the posterior costophrenic recess. (Foley *et al.* 1979).

Total visualization of the spleen is more difficult to achieve than that of the liver. This is solely due to the limited accessibility of the smaller, posteriorly placed spleen. Following the studies of the liver and spleen the central abdomen should be examined but this may prove difficult due to central displacement of bowel by intraperitoneal fluid and concomitant ileus.

Abdominal radiographs should be available and assessed for:
1 The position of the diaphragm.
2 The presence of rib fractures.
3 The distribution of visceral gas.

If peritoneal lavage has been undertaken this should be noted. The ultrasound images should be assessed as follows:
1 General quality of the image
2 The amount of each organ that has been adequately imaged.
3 The presence of fluid within the peritoneum.
4 The size, shape and position of liver, spleen, and pancreas.
5 The uniformity of parenchymal pattern.
6 The presence of intraperitoneal or retroperitoneal mass.

Spleen

The spleen is frequently enlarged by the effects of trauma, presumably due to the volume of intrasplenic haematoma. Serial examinations may demonstrate progressive enlargement. It must be recognized, however, that the splenomegaly may have preceded the episode of trauma, and be unassociated other than in increasing the vulnerability of the organ.

Irregularity of the splenic border must be interpreted with care, specifically on the medial border,

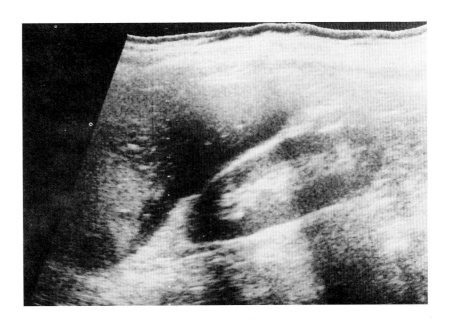

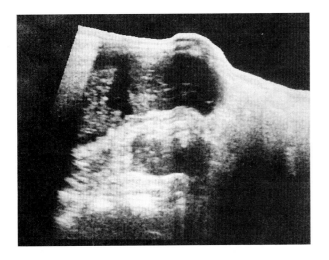

Fig. 29.11 Splenic rupture with subcapsular haematoma on the medial surface of the spleen. (Courtesy of Dr K.C. Dewbury.)

Fig. 29.12 Subscapular haematoma of the liver following RTA. (Courtesy of Dr. K.C. Dewbury.)

which is normally irregular (Asher *et al.*, 1976). Failure to image a segment of the border may also be due to gas or base of lung, or bone-induced artefact (Babcock & Kaufman, 1983).

The clinicopathological correlative study (Sonneburg *et al.*, 1983) suggests that traumatic changes in the splenic pulp should be diagnosed with considerable certainty. However, many other authors have advised caution in interpretation (Asher *et al.*, 1976, Kaufman *et al.*, 1984).

Subcapsular haematoma is normally visualized in profile as crescentic or spindle-shaped hypo-echoic areas paralleling or displacing the splenic pulp (Fig. 29.11).

Perisplenic haematoma has a similar echo pattern but will only be well-defined as it abuts on the spleen or diaphragm. Left paracolic haemorrhage should always be sought. Frank fractures through the splenic pulp are occasionally defined as an irregular anechoic line through the organ (Fig. 29.12). Contusions may be multiple and are most commonly of a hypoechoic nature. Difficulty in assessment arises because of lack of total visualization of the organ, artefacts from ribs and air-containing viscera, and the relatively sonolucent pattern of the splenic pulp. Thus, in his recent study, Kaufman states that sonography should not be the screening method of choice in paediatric patients, because of a prospective false-negative diagnostic rate of 50%.

While it is in the paediatric patient particularly that preservation of splenic function is important (Strauch, 1979), the evidence of an overall increase in morbidity and mortality is now irrefutable (Roy, 1984). Ultrasound offers neither the certainty of initial diagnosis nor reproducible parameters necessary for conservative management of splenic trauma.

Liver

The pathological changes demonstrable by ultrasound in hepatic trauma are similar to those in the spleen.

The size of the organ may vary with pre-existing disease and the contours may be difficult to determine over the spine. Irregularity of contour in the area of the porta hepatis and gall bladder fossa is a normal finding.

Accumulations of fluid above, lateral to, and in the Rutherford Morison pouch may be indicative of free intraperitoneal blood with the necessary reservations if peritoneal lavage has been undertaken.

Subcapsular haematoma (Figs 29.13, 29.14) and localized perihepatic haematoma in character similar to those around the spleen may be identified, and the right paracolic gutter examined for free blood. Parenchymal abnormalities can be assessed more definitely than in the spleen. Contusion is normally hypoechoic (Figs 29.15, 29.16). at initial presentation, becoming hyperechoic for a short time before reverting to hypoechoic characteristics and diminishing in size.

Fibrous septa may be demonstrated during the healing phase (Fig. 29.17). Occasionally an irregular area of hyperechoic character may be demonstrated at initial examination. Lesions high and posteriorly placed within the right lobe and over the spine within the left lobe may not be demonstrable.

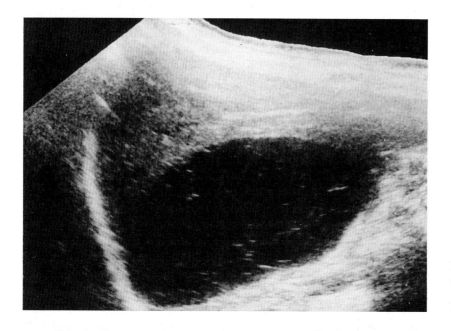

Fig. 29.13 Subcapsular haematoma of the liver following a road-traffic accident. (Courtesy of Dr K.C. Dewbury.)

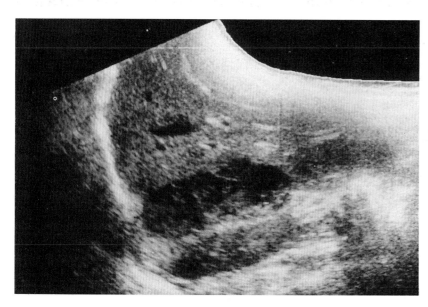

Fig. 29.14 Same patient as in Fig. 29.13. This illustration shows resolution of the haematoma 2 months after injury. (Courtesy of Dr K.C. Dewbury.)

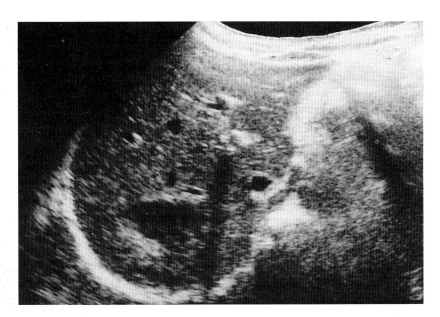

Fig. 29.15 Traumatic contusion of the right lobe of liver appearing as a hypoechoic area. (Courtesy of Dr K.C. Dewbury.)

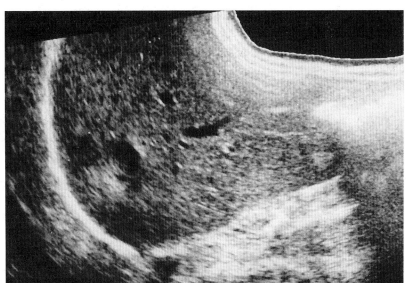

Fig. 29.16 Increasing echogenicity 2 weeks after the episode of trauma. (Courtesy of Dr K.C. Dewbury.)

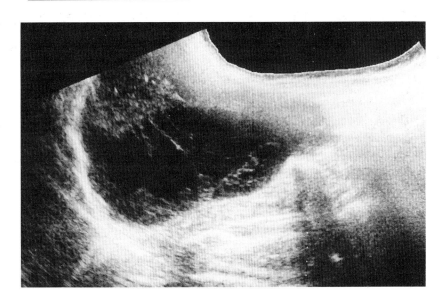

Fig. 29.17 Development of fibrinous septa during the course of traumatic hepatic haematoma. (Courtesy of Dr K.C. Dewbury.)

Pancreas

The signs of pancreatic trauma are limited to peripancreatic and retroperitoneal fluid collections evidenced by focal hypoechoic areas related to the gland, which may itself show generalized swelling (Figs 29.18, 29.19; Foley & Teele, 1979.)

Considerable difficulty, however, is encountered in consistently imaging the organ due to concomitant ileus. The fact that pancreatic injury is commonly associated with other severe visceral and retroperitoneal injuries complicates analysis of the findings.

CT scanning

In recent years the value of CT scanning in abdominal trauma has been reported by many authors. Case reports in the mid-1970s have been replaced by large, comprehensive series (Federle, 1983a). The fact that the vast majority of recent reports emanate from North America reflects economic circumstances rather than a differing clinical awareness.

TECHNIQUE

Contrast medium is given either orally or by a nasogastric tube, which should be withdrawn into the oesophagus during scanning. Five hundred

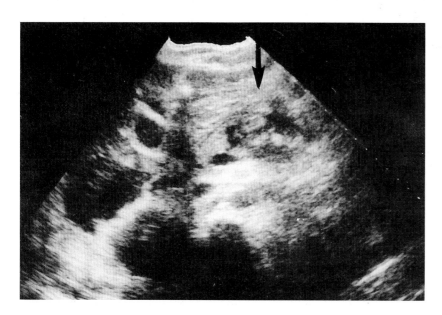

Fig. 29.18 Swelling of the pancreas with a small layer of fluid lying anterior to the gland, immediately after injury. (Courtesy of Dr K.C. Dewbury.)

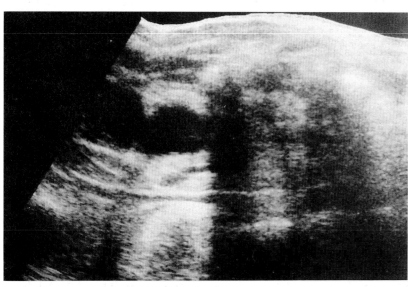

Fig. 29.19 Same patient as in Fig. 29.17. Development of a small pancreatic pseudocyst 1 week after injury. (Courtesy of Dr K.C. Dewbury.)

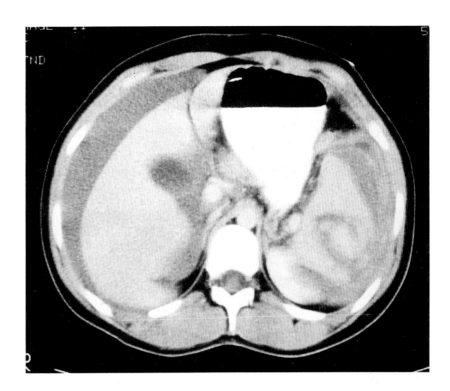

Fig. 29.20 Traumatic rupture of the spleen with widespread haemoperitoneum. (Courtesy of Dr B. Williamson.)

millilitres of 3% Gastrografin (Schering) is given as soon as the decision to proceed to CT is made. A further 200 ml is then administered on arrival at the CT unit. It has been suggested that further dilution of 1–2% would eliminate artefact (Federle, 1983b).

Intravenous administration of a 50 ml bolus of 300 mg % contrast medium, preferably non-ionic, should be followed by infusion of 100 ml of similar 300 mg % contrast medium diluted in 200 ml of normal saline.

Scanning speeds will vary with the equipment available, but should not exceed 5 s. The scanning protocol calls for contiguous scanning from just above the diaphragm to the lower poles of the kidneys, continuing at 1.5 cm intervals to the symphysis. The objectives are to produce a comprehensive abdominal examination with minimum artefact (Federle, 1984).

The images should be assessed as follows:
1 General quality, particularly identification of artefact.
2 Peritoneal cavity — presence of fluid or blood.
3 Retroperitoneum — presence of haematoma and renal morphology.
4 Size, shape and position of liver, spleen, and pancreas.
5 Parenchymal homogeneity of these organs.
6 Integrity of other organs.
7 Abnormal collections of contrast medium.

Fluid within the peritoneal cavity

The tendency is for blood or residual lavage fluid to accumulate in dependent peritoneal recesses. Thus, in the upper abdomen, inspection of the Rutherford Morisons pouch — the posterior subhepatic space — is mandatory.

In the mid-abdomen, the most definitive areas requiring inspection are the paracolic gutters. The pelvis is the most dependent area within the peritoneal cavity and the scanning sequence should continue to permit visualization of the rectouterine, rectovesical and paravesical fossae (Fig. 29.20).

Localized collections in relationship to the traumatized organs should be carefully sought and excluded. The attenuation value of every fluid collection identified should be assessed, taking care to avoid partial volume artefact.

A value greater than 30 HU differentiates blood from ascites. Organized thrombus tends to be an unusual feature within the peritoneum, but when focal aggregate occurs the attenuation value is always high, frequently exceeding 75 HU. More commonly, early thrombolysis occurs and attenuation values around 30–40 HU are then found. In the liver, spleen, and pancreas care must be taken not to confuse the linear artefact accentuated by ileus and poor control of respiration as representing contusion or laceration of the parenchyma.

Spleen

Crescentic or spindle-shaped low-attenuation fluid collections flattening the parenchyma represent a subcapsular haematoma (Figs 29.21, 29.22), more commonly identified on the convex edge; this may spread to the medial border (Korobkin *et al*. 1978). Irregular low-attenuation defects in the pulp, representing contusions, may be identified.

Well-defined linear defects representing laceration or fracture present little diagnostic difficulty (Fig. 29.23, 29.24). Peculiar mottled enhancement patterns may be analogous to the snow-storm appearance described on angiography (Fisher *et al.*, 1981). The presence of perisplenic and intraperitoneal blood is important in confirmation of splenic injury and in the interpretation of congenital splenic clefts and liver–spleen interface.

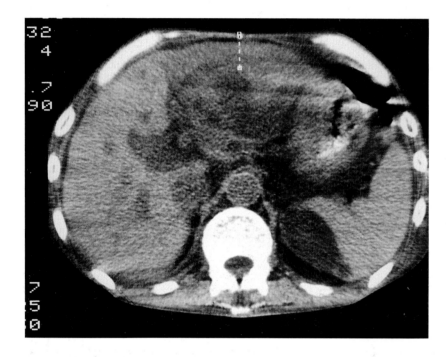

Fig. 29.21 Subcapsular haematoma on the posterior aspect of the spleen with rupture of the left lobe of liver.

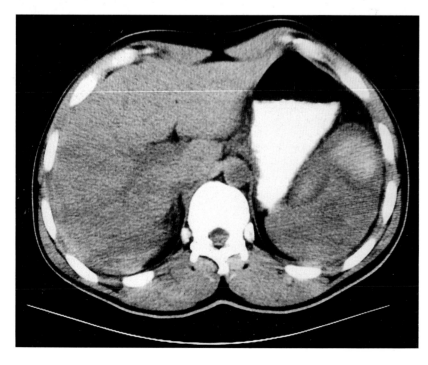

Fig. 29.22 Resolving splenic subcapsular haematoma. The increasing attenuation of the haematoma is well-demonstrated. (See Fig. 29.15.)

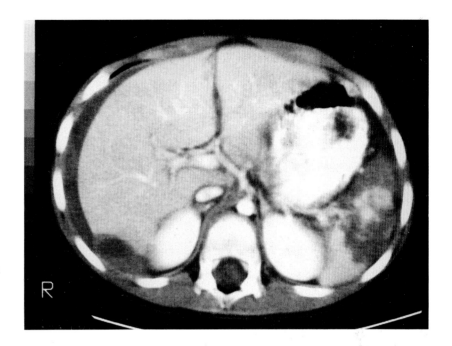

Fig. 29.23 Fracture of the spleen in the arterial phase of bolus infusion. There is a subcapsular haematoma on the posterior aspect of the right lobe of the liver and haemoperitoneum is present. (Courtesy of Dr B. Williamson.)

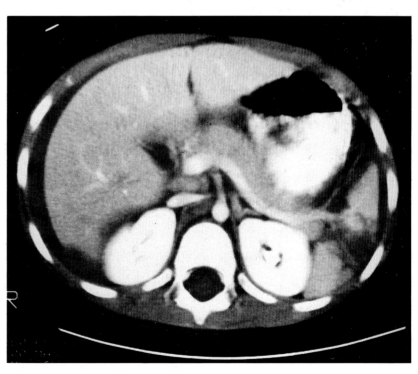

Fig. 29.24 Same patient as in Fig. 29.21 showing integrity of the pancreas and the splenic vein. (Courtesy of Dr B. Williamson.)

Liver

A subcapsular haematoma has appearances similar to those seen in the spleen (Fig. 29.25). Injuries to other organ systems may be present (Fig. 29.26). The most common finding is irregular linear or rounded areas of diminished attenuation representing contusion or laceration (Fig. 29.27) (Toombs *et al.*, 1982). Further reduction in attenuation represents lysis of the haematoma. Only occasionally are small areas of dense haematoma encountered whose attenuation is close to the enhanced hepatic parenchyma. Haemobilia may be represented by high-attenuation blood clot within the gall bladder (Fig. 29.28).

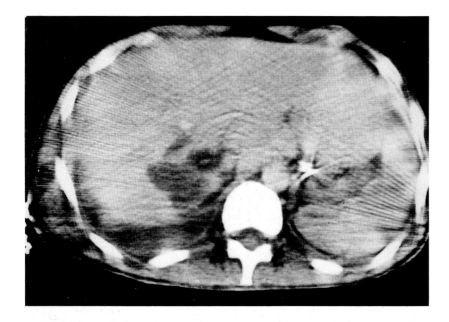

Fig. 29.25 A contusion of the right lobe of the liver related to the hepatic veins and associated with subcapsular and extracapsular haematoma.

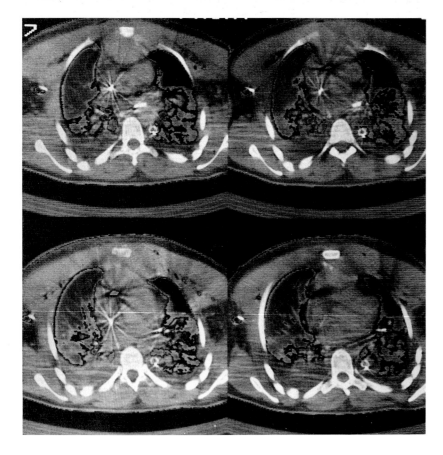

Fig. 29.26 Extensive mediastinal haematoma with haemothorax in the patient whose liver injury is demonstrated in Fig. 29.25.

Pancreas

Changes in the pancreas at the intermediate phase of investigation are limited to swelling of the gland of either focal or generalized type, and peri-pancreatic fluid collections (Figs 29.29, 29.30).

However, significant pancreatic injury is associated in up to 75% of patients with serious injury to other viscera, retroperitoneal structures, or the spine further complicating diagnosis.

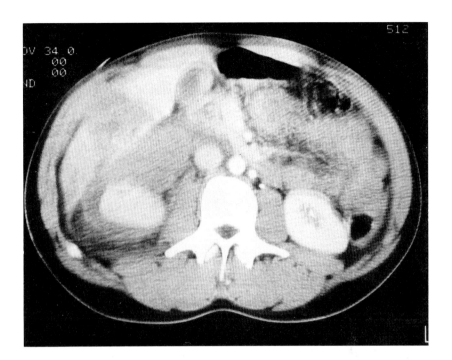

Fig. 29.27 Laceration of the right lobe of the liver following bolus enhancement. Laceration is represented as a low attenuation avascular area. (Courtesy of Dr B. Williamson.)

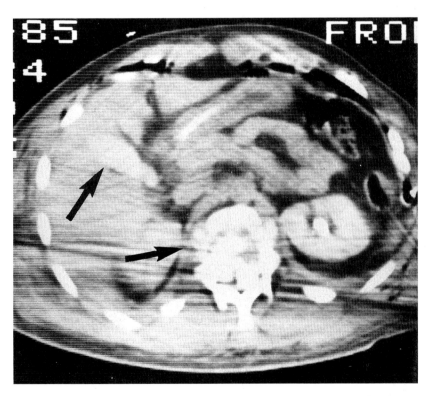

Fig. 29.28 The high attenuation in the gall bladder is due to haemobilia. A major vertebral injury is also demonstrated. (See Fig. 29.3.)

Diaphragm

While the diagnosis of rupture of the diaphragm is difficult on CT, the protocol requires the series of tomograms to commence above the diaphragm. This excludes pneumothorax, which may not be evident on chest radiographs (Wall *et al.*, 1983).

Angiography

The indications of arteriography are now almost totally restricted to the investigation of severe haemorrhage, to which may be added the possibility of interventional management of the cause of bleeding. The requirements for this form of

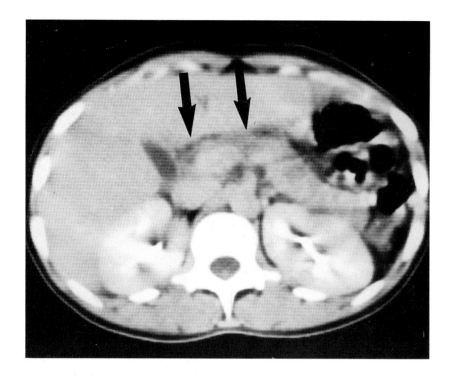

Fig. 29.29 A small amount of fluid outlines the anterior surface of the head and neck of the pancreas following trauma. (See Fig. 29.17.) (Courtesy of Dr B. Williamson.)

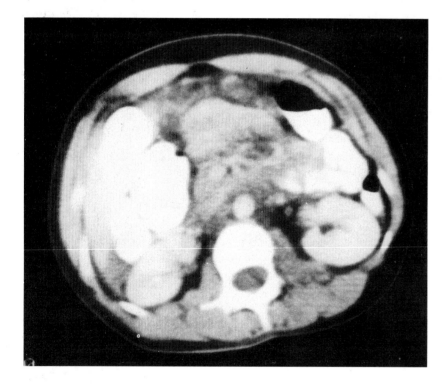

Fig. 29.30 Diffuse swelling of the pancreas 10 days following injury. (Courtesy of Dr B. Williamson.)

investigation are that the hospital offers full-time facilities for vascular investigation.

A dedicated multidirectional vascular X-ray unit is virtually essential and the availability of digital vascular imaging (DVI) is a considerable ad-vantage. Apparatus for anaesthesia and patient monitoring must be available, and a comprehen-sive stock of catheters, guide-wires and embolic materials are required.

TECHNIQUE

It must be appreciated that the time factor remains important and the assistance of qualified clinical, nursing, radiographic, and darkroom staff is mandatory.

All film programmes should include masks for future photographic subtraction. Frequently the film programme can be extended with benefit on the basis that the cardiac output is reduced in hypovolaemic states and that extravascular accumulation is delayed. Any tendency to reduce the dose of contrast medium should be resisted as inadequate visualization will lead to equivocal results and repeat examinations.

Only rarely will superselective injections be required, and the insertion of a 'pig-tail' catheter for flush aortography followed by a selective visceral catheter via the femoral artery will provide fast and adequate access. Occasionally the trans-axillary route will be necessary. Injections of 60–80 ml of non-ionic contrast medium of not less than 350 mg % at 15–20 ml/s will adequately outline the adult coeliac axis or superior mesenteric circulations.

The assessment of films include:
1 General quality including the adequacy of vascular filling in all phases.
2 The spatial arrangement and integrity of the arterial branches.
3 The homogeneity of the capillary phase.
4 The identification of venous filling and the uniformity of the rate of venous filling.
5 Identification of abnormal contrast accumulations.

Liver

Traumatic occlusion of arteries will possibly be evident but is rarely a significant indication for angiography, as necrosis of liver tissue is unlikely in the presence of normal portal venous supply.

Of more particular interest is damage to the arteries producing free haemorrhage, traumatic aneurysm, and arteriobiliary fistula or arterio-venous fistula (Figs 29.31, 29.32). (Clark *et al.*, 1983) Fistula is also a recognized complication of per-cutaneous liver biopsy (Figs 29.33, 29.34).

These latter conditions are amenable to trans-arterial embolization utilizing either Gianturco coils or detachable balloons (Fig. 29.35).

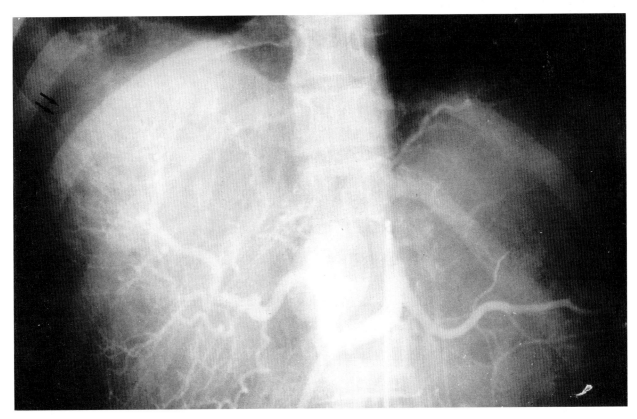

Fig. 29.31 Post-traumatic aneurysm of the hepatic artery following a road-traffic accident. Separation of the superolateral surface of the liver from the diaphragm is demonstrated. (Courtesy of Dr V. Cope.)

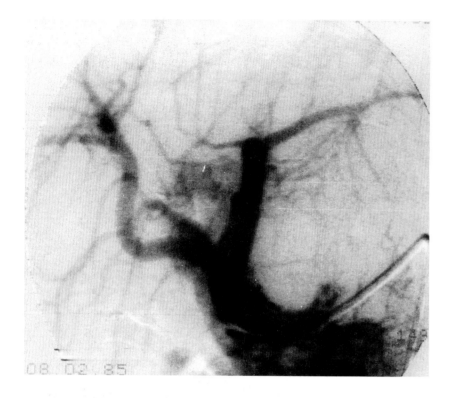

Fig. 29.32 Hepatic artery—portal vein fistula associated with rupture of the left lobe of the liver. (Intra-arterial digital study.)

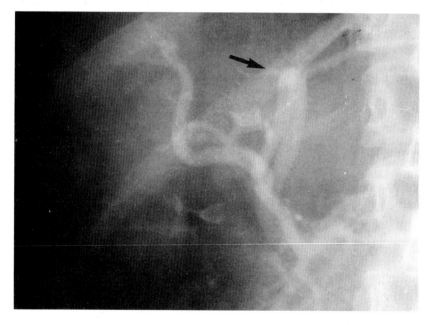

Fig. 29.33 Angiogram demonstrating hepatic artery—portal venous fistula following biopsy of the liver demonstrated on conventional angiography.

Therapeutic embolization may require the use of catheters suitable for superselective studies and the ability of the department to fabricate specifically shaped catheters is an advantage.

The recent development of guide-wires capable of carrying coils beyond the catheter tip, and of percutaneous needles which can be inserted under fluoroscopic control into lesions which cannot be reached by the intra-arterial route, have reduced the necessity for the placement of coils proximally in major hepatic arteries.

Experience indicates that use of materials such as Gelfoam and Ivalon, tend only to produce transient haemostasis in patients who have undergone massive blood transfusion. There appears to be little advantage in utilizing more permanent occlusive devices. The use of cyanocerylate has been limited to a few centres, and if

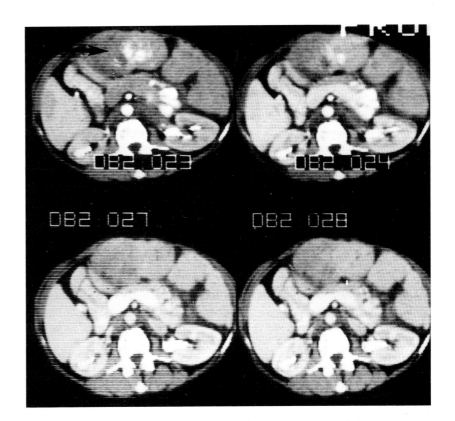

Fig. 29.34 CT angiogram demonstrating hepatic artery–portal venous fistula following biopsy of the liver demonstrated on angiocomputerized tomography.

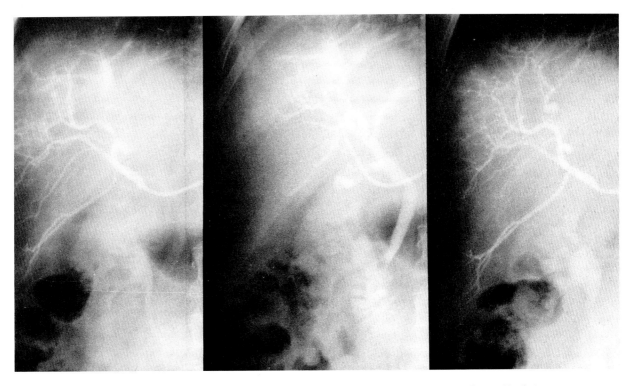

Fig. 29.35 Traumatic haemobilia following liver biopsy treated by embolization. (Courtesy of Dr J. Reidy.)

care is exercised in placement, this substance produces permanent occlusion.

Some workers have used a combination of particulate material such as Gelfoam and Ivalon with absolute alcohol to produce potentially more permanent occlusion than that produced by particulate matter alone. (Jander *et al.*, 1977).

Comprehensive experience in embolization in acute abdominal trauma is limited to a few centres. Patients will tend to be managed in relation to the individual problem and the experience of the radiologist involved.

It must be recognized that a recurrence of a haemorrhage, either from a site which has been embolized or from a separate point of trauma, may occur. This is more likely if a material such as Gelfoam has been used. There is, therefore, an advantage in leaving the arterial catheter in the lower aorta following embolization. The catheter can be infused with heparinized saline at a dose rate that maintains catheter patency but has no parenteral effect. The external portion of the catheter can be placed in a sterile polythene container within a sterile groin dressing. This technique expedites further embolization therapy or angiography to re-evaluate the situation.

Other arteriographic findings include disruption of the capillary—parenchymal pattern, separation of the liver from ribs or diaphragm, subcapsular indentation due to haematoma, slow filling, and displacement of venous radicles. The majority of these signs can now be elicited by other methods, particularly CT.

Spleen

Prior to the introduction of non-invasive methods for the diagnosis of splenic trauma, angiography had been utilized in some centres. Angiographic pathological correlative studies had demonstrated that excellent concurrence could be achieved and the technique was used to grade the degree of splenic injury and define the therapeutic approach (Fisher *et al.*, 1981). Subcapsular or perisplenic haematoma, fragmentation, laceration, and contusion of the splenic pulp can be identified and to a certain extent quantified (Figs 29.36, 29.37, 29.38).

Today it appears that angiography offers no advantage over non-invasive methods, particularly in the estimation of residual viable splenic tissue for conservation. Therapeutic embolization has only rarely been reported in splenic trauma (Wallace *et al.*, 1976). Similar technical considerations apply as in the case of the liver.

Pancreas

The angiographic signs of acute pancreatic rupture are subtle (Haertel & Fuchs, 1974). Dramatic bleeding from the pancreas due to trauma is

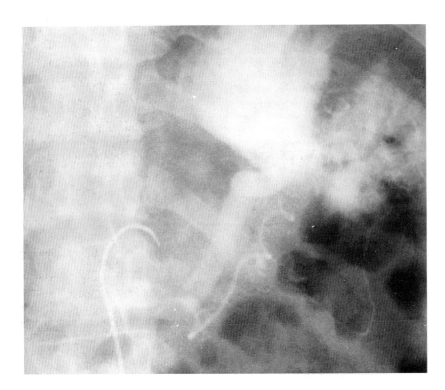

Fig. 29.36 Rupture of the spleen involving the mid and lower pole areas demonstrated on the venous phase of the coeliac axis angiography.

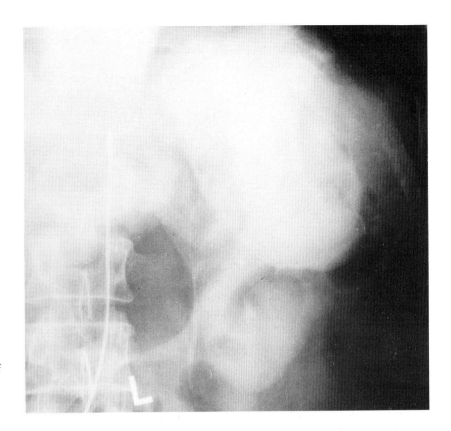

Fig. 29.37 Subcapsular haematoma demonstrated on the venous phase of coeliac axial angiography. Note that there is no demonstrable parenchymal defect.

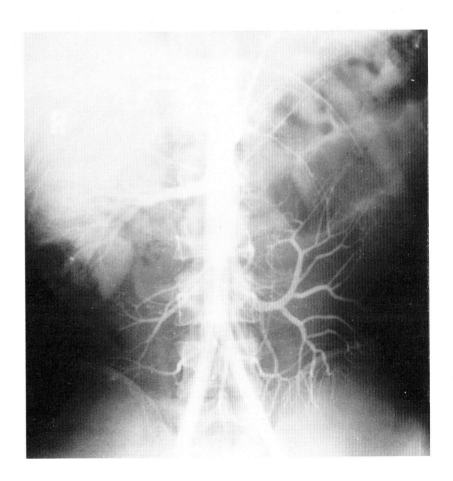

Fig. 29.38 Mainstream aortogram. Traumatic occlusions of the splenic and left renal arteries following a sports injury.

uncommon and abnormal findings in the pancreas are likely to be coincidental to conditions consequent to other major visceral injury (Figs 29.39, 29.40).

Digital vascular imaging

Intravenous angiography (DVSA) has no effective role in acute trauma. The hypovolaemic state will reduce the quality of the arterial phase images. The problems frequently associated with abdominal DVSA, that is, artefact produced by the diaphragm and cardiac movement, bowel activity, and super imposition of vascular structures, are relevant.

Intra-arterial imaging (DASA) is, however, a valuable complimentary method, combined with conventional angiography, in reducing the time taken to obtain a comprehensive examination and in the control of therapeutic embolization procedures.

ERCP

A small number of cases recording the use of this method of establishing the diagnosis of rupture of the pancreas have been reported (Vallon *et al.*, 1979, Bozymski *et al.*, 1981). It would appear to have limited value in those patients in whom CT or ultrasound have produced equivocal findings where clinical suspicion of pancreatic injury is high.

The late radiology of upper abdominal trauma

The complications of emergency surgery exceed those of elective procedures. While the main cause of death in the acute phase is haemorrhage, significant mortality later in the event is due to sepsis, and this may be associated with abscess formation and occasionally secondary haemorrhage. The presence of blood clot, necrotic, or ischaemic tissue

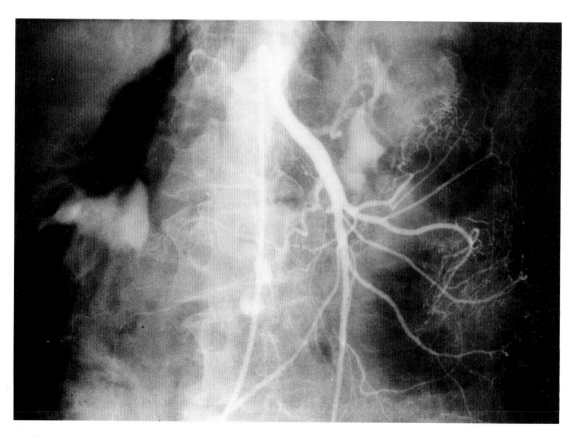

Fig. 29.39 Traumatic aneurysm of the inferior pancreatical duodenal artery following endoscopic sphincterotomy. Haemostasis was achieved by embolization.

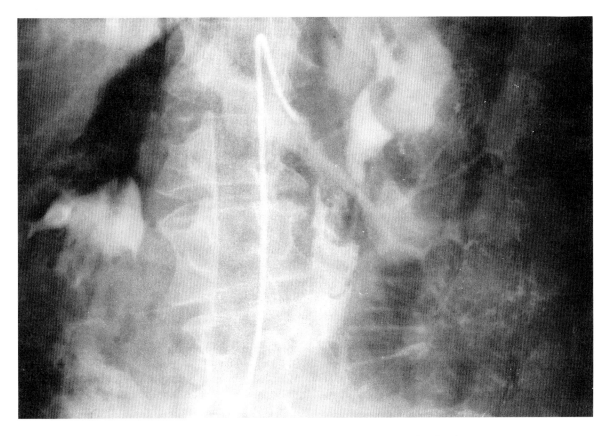

Fig. 29.40 Same traumatic aneurysm as in Fig. 29.39. Heavy staining is present in the duodenum.

provides a nidus for infection, and laparotomy in a sense converts a closed abdominal type into a penetrating type of injury.

Foreign bodies may be the result of missile injury, but abdominal drains are also alien to the peritoneal cavity. Surgery for life-threatening haemorrhage may cause accidental damage to the biliary or pancreatic duct systems with the sequela of fistula formation.

Major injury to other systems, particularly cranial and thoracic lesions, may mean that the investigation of the abdominal injury is delayed. High-velocity missiles tend to cause remote damage that is not discovered at emergency laparotomy and may not cause problems until 5–10 days after presentation.

The sequelae of upper abdominal trauma can be divided into four main groups:
1 Abscess or fluid collection
2 Fistula.
3 Haemorrhage.
4 Intestinal obstruction and ileus.

Abscess or fluid collection

The extent of peritoneal toilet will vary with the circumstances surrounding an emergency laparotomy, in particular the presence of injury to hollow organs such as the colon will increase the incidence of post-surgical sepsis.

Abscess formation will tend to occur either in those areas in which blood may be identified in the acute phase, i.e. the dependent peritoneal recesses and subphrenic spaces, or in devitalized tissue within a traumatized organ.

Both CT and ultrasound scanning are consistent and comprehensive methods of examining the contents of the peritoneal cavity. The examinations are performed as described previously, but it is important that an attempt should be made to quantify the volume of each collection and the thickness of the wall, and to assess the possibility for percutaneous drainage (Whitley et al., 1983) (Fig. 29.41).

A careful estimation of the character of the fluid content is required by either ultrasound or CT. The viscosity of the fluid or the presence of

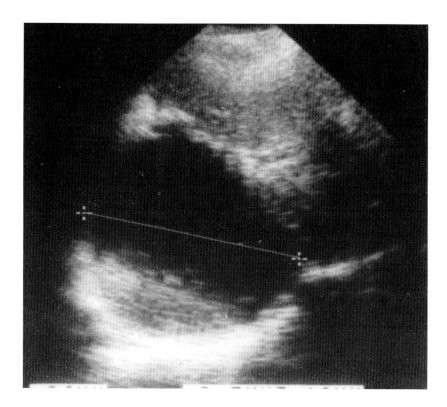

Fig. 29.41 A right posterior subphrenic abscess following partial hepatectomy for a gunshot wound to the liver.

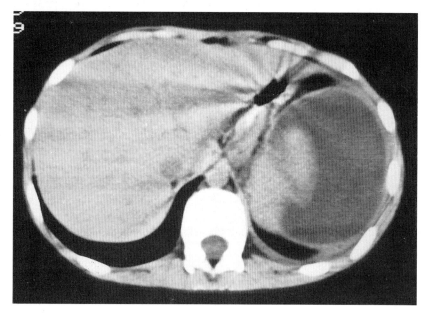

Fig. 29.42 A large left subphrenic abscess following attempted preservation of the spleen in a child.

sloughed material will influence the method of drainage (Fig. 29.42).

While purulent fluid is hyperechoic, with a pattern that varies with movement such as coughing, it must be remembered that extravasated blood passes through a hyperechoic phase during resolution. Similarly, in CT the attenuation values of clotted blood will gradually reduce as lysis occurs

but it may be possible to detect small amounts of gas within an abscess cavity.

It must be emphasized that careful examination of the pancreas is mandatory. Contrary to the paucity of findings in the immediate phase, pseudocysts, abscess, and retention may all be demonstrated at this later stage. Both pancreatic and splenic cysts may be found many years later as sequelae of trauma.

The technique of percutaneous drainage is potentially of great value, particularly in the postoperative patients, but requires an understanding of the principles of abscess drainage. These are that the abscess should be circumscribed, that the contents are fluid enough to be drained by the largest possible catheter available, and that drainage should be from the dependent aspect.

In all cases the fluid should be submitted for bacteriological examination and, if necessary, for biochemical assessment of urea or amylase content.

Conventional radiography

Intra-abdominal abscesses may occasionally be diagnosed directly on abdominal or chest radiographs by the presence of a gas in an inappropriate situation. More frequently the signs are indirect such as a soft-tissue mass displacing bowel, or elevation and paralysis of the diaphragm with basal pleural exudate, and non-specific lung signs of either atelectasis or consolidation.

CONTRAST STUDIES

Apart from proving the integrity of the gastrointestinal tract, conventional contrast studies are of little value in the diagnosis of intraperitoneal abscess. Displacement of the hollow organs may, however, offer indirect evidence of a subphrenic, lesser sac, pelvic, or paracolic collection.

SINOGRAPHY

This examination may give information fundamental to the management of an intra-abdominal abscess. The primary requirement is to make certain that contrast medium fills all ramifications of the sinus. This requires that the cutaneous opening should be completely sealed. Of various methods, the vacuum cannula by Malmstrom–Thoren, is recommended (Figs 29.43, 29.44).

Estimation of the size, the anatomical relationships of the cavity, the position of the tip of any drainage tube and, in particular, any fistulous communication is required.

SCINTIGRAPHY

Conventional radioisotope studies are primarily of use in the liver and spleen. Displacement of these organs or 'cold' areas indicating possible abscess or haematoma can be detected. CT or ultrasound have, however, virtually replaced combined lung/liver scintigraphy as a method of examining the right subphrenic space.

Gallium citrate offered a method of directly imaging inflammatory tissue but lacks total

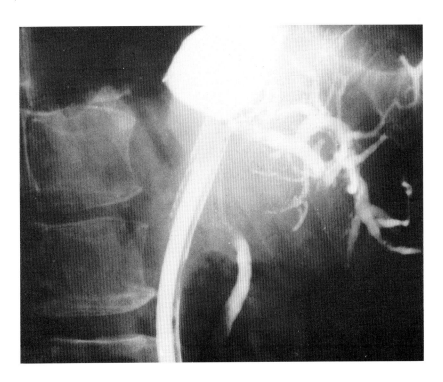

Fig. 29.43 Persistent biloma demonstrated by sinography following a partial hepatectomy for gunshot wound.

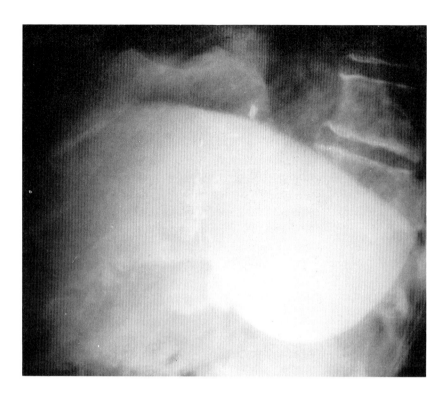

Fig. 29.44 Same biloma as in Fig. 29.43. A fistulous connection to the biliary tract is well demonstrated.

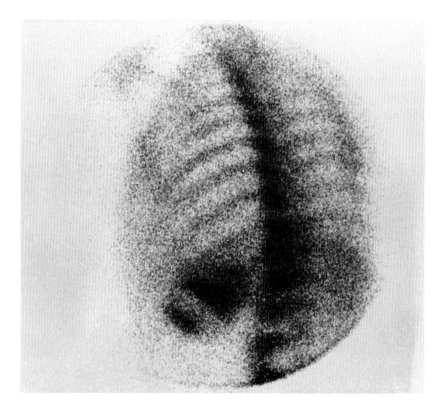

Fig. 29.45 Perisplenic abscess following attempted splenic preservation demonstrated by Indium-labelled white blood cells. (This is the same patient illustrated in Fig. 29.42.)

specificity and has poor ratio between the uptake in the inflammatory tissue and the background level.

The introduction of indium-labelled white blood cells (^{111}indium-WBC; 18 MBq), however, overcame the major disadvantages of gallium citrate. Thus, abscesses in which active WBC migration is occurring, either within the peritoneal cavity or in the liver, spleen, or pancreas, can be directly imaged utilizing this technique (Fig. 29.45).

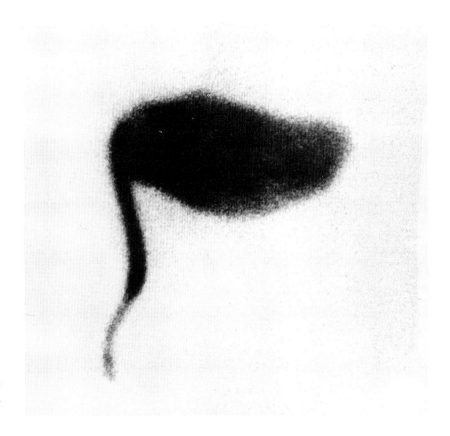

Fig. 29.46 After partial hepatectomy; biliary fistula demonstrated by HIDA scanning.

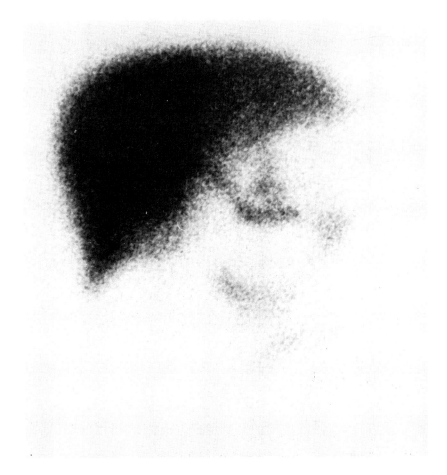

Fig. 29.47 Extravasation of HIDA from a delayed rupture of the common bile duct. The abnormal accumulation of isotope can be seen lying just medial to the common hepatic duct.

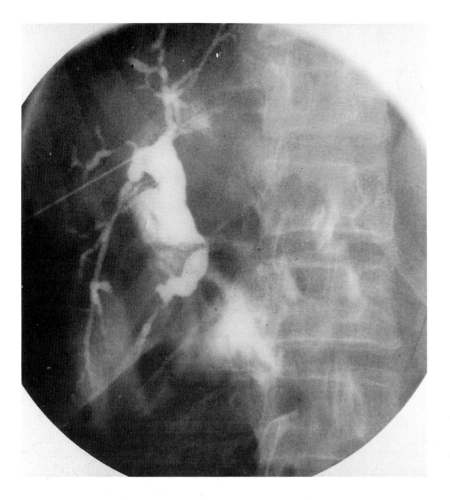

Fig. 29.48 Leakage of contrast medium from the bile duct during trans-hepatic cholangiography for sclerosing cholangitis was followed by the development of marked ascites.

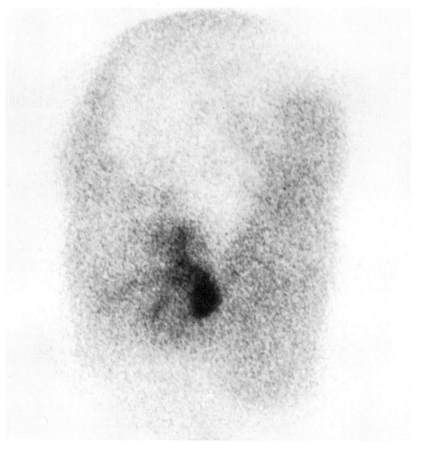

Fig. 29.49 HIDA scan, 1 week after Fig. 29.48, shows abnormal aggregation of isotope within the general peritoneal cavity as evidence of bilous ascites.

Indium-labelled WBCs have, however, been reported to aggregate in areas of fat necrosis subsequent to pancreatitis, and care is required in interpretation following trauma.

The use of the HIDA (^{99m}technetium; 74 MBq) biliary scan is an accurate method of assessing biliary fistula and is suitable for use in the postoperative patient (Figs 29.46—29.49).

Secondary haemorrhage that is not acutely life-threatening but which may be repeated can be investigated utilizing technetium-labelled RBCs (^{99m}technetium RBC; 370 MBq). This technique, however, requires active extravasation, and care must be exercised in localization of the extravasated blood as it enters the intestinal tract and before it passes distally.

Fistulae

Fistula may be associated with both abscess and fluid collections. Transient leakage of bile or pancreatic content is not an unusual complication following emergency surgery for trauma. Nevertheless, persistent fistula must arouse the suspicion that there is obstruction to the normal course of drainage via either the bile or pancreatic duct systems. While CT, and more particularly, ultrasound are capable of showing biliary or pancreatic duct dilatation, they play a secondary role to more direct methods (Fig. 29.50).

Sinography may demonstrate a connection to the biliary or pancreatic duct systems but may not show the more distal areas of the duct systems adequately.

ERCP offers the best available method of demonstrating the integrity of the major pancreatic ducts, but care should be exercised in the presence of pancreatic inflammation. PTC or ERCP may be required to demonstrate the degree of disruption of the biliary tract (Fig. 29.51). Free passage of contrast medium into the duodenum may prevent adequate visualization of the fistula and it should be noted that the intravenous injection of 5 mg of morphine sulphate will cause rapid closure of the sphincter of Oddi. Fistulous connections to the bowel may require a combination of oral contrast studies and sinography.

Haemorrhage

Secondary haemorrhage can occur as a single fulminant episode or as a series of subacute episodes. On occasions the latter may be demon-

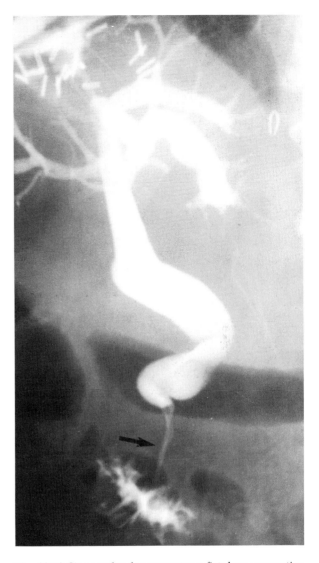

Fig. 29.50 Sinography demonstrates a fistulous connection between a right posterior subphrenic biloma and the bile ducts. (Same patient as in Figs 29.42 and 29.43.) Following several surgical interventions the fistula had failed to close. A stricture of the lower common bile duct is demonstrated. It was felt that this represents the type of remote injury encountered in high-velocity gunshot wounds.

strated with indium-labelled RBCs but in the former, rapid recourse to angiography is advised.

Haemorrhage can occur intraperitoneally either in an occult manner or evidenced via undwelling drains. It may also present as bleeding into the gastrointestinal tract directly by erosion or via the bile duct in haemobilia. The techniques of angiography and therapeutic embolization are similar to those described during the intermediate phase.

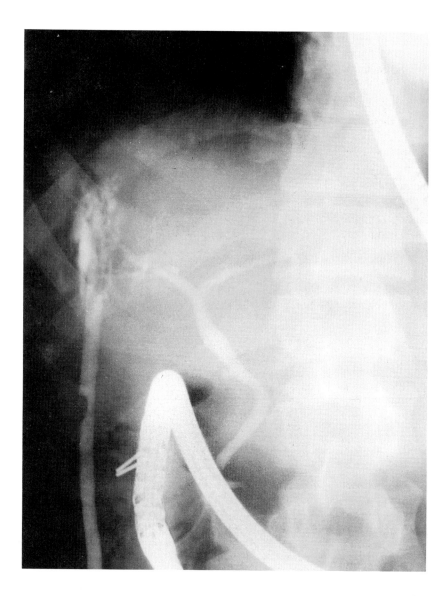

Fig. 29.51 ERCP demonstrates a fistula between the biliary tract and the right lateral subphrenic area following a gunshot wound to the liver.

Obstruction

Intestinal obstruction is a recognized complication of laparotomy, as is postoperative ileus. Particular care, however, should be taken in the later stage of upper abdominal trauma to exclude direct injury to the duodenum or duodenojejunal flexure (seat-belt injuries).

The late onset of intestinal ileus may be the presenting manifestation of pancreatic injury or abscess formation elsewhere in the upper abdomen.

Summary

In the small proportion of traumatized patients requiring intermediate and late stage radiology, the emphasis now lies on non-invasive studies. CT scanning, if available, represents the most consistent and comprehensive method of diagnosis (Fuchs & Robotti, 1983).

Ultrasound is more operator-dependent but can be brought to the bedside. Scintigraphy has a high specificity and sensitivity in the liver and spleen and is most useful in assessing viability for splenic preservation. Angiography is indicated only where haemorrhage is the predominant symptom, and can be combined with therapeutic embolization.

Other investigations are of limited value, mainly because of their lack of specificity.

References

American College of Surgeons (1976) *Early Care of the Injured Patient*, pp. 1–12, W.B. Saunders Company, Philadelphia.

Asher, W.M., Parvin, S., Virgillo, R.W. & Haber, K. (1976) Echographic evaluation of splenic injury after blunt trauma. *Radiology*, 118, 411–415.

Babcock, D.S. & Kaufman, R.A. (1983) Ultrasonography and computed tomography in the evaluation of the acutely ill paediatric patient. *Radiology Clinics of North America*, 21(3), 527–550.

Ben Menachem, Y. (1981) *Angiography in Trauma — a Work Atlas*, pp. 25–108. W.B. Saunders Company, Philadelphia.

Berg, B.C. (1983) Complementary roles of radionuclide and computed tomographic imaging in evaluating trauma. *Seminars in Nuclear Medicine*, 13, 86–103.

Bozymski, E.M., Orlando, R.C. & Holt, J.W. (1981) Traumatic disruption of the pancreatic duct demonstrated by endoscopic retrograde pancreatography. *Journal of Trauma*, 21(3), 244–245.

Bronfman, H.J., Konkel, B.K. & Rabin, H.S. (1981) Tc-99 m sulfur colloid scanning in blunt trauma: detection of abdominal bleeding. *Journal of Nuclear Medicine*, 22, 978–980.

Clark, R.A., Gallant, T.E. & Alexander, E.S. (1983) Angiographic management of traumatic arteriovenous fistulas: clinical results. *Radiology*, 147, 9–13.

Davis, J.J., Cohn, I. & Nance, F.C. (1976) Diagnosis and management of blunt, abdominal trauma. *Annals of Surgery*, 183, 672–677.

De Vincenti, F.C., Rives, J.D., Laborde, E.J., Fleming, I.D. & Cohn, I. (1968) Blunt abdominal trauma. *Journal of Trauma*, 8(6), 1004–1013.

Federle, M.P. (1983a) Computed tomography of abdominal trauma. *Critical Review of Diagnostic Imaging*, 19(4), 257–316.

Federle, M.P. (1983b) Computed tomography of blunt abdominal Trauma. *Radiology Clinics of North America*, 21(3), 461–476.

Federle, M.P. (1984) Computed tomography of upper abdominal trauma. *Seminars in Radiology*, 19(4), 269–279.

Fisher, R.G., Foucar, K., Estrada, R. & Ben Menachem, Y. (1981) Splenic rupture in blunt trauma. *Radiology Clinics of North America*, 19(1), 141–165.

Foley, L.E. & Teele, R.L. (1979) Ultrasound of epigastric injuries after blunt trauma. *American Journal of Roentgenology*, 132, 593–598.

Gelfand, M.J. (1984) Scintigraphy in upper abdominal trauma. *Seminars in Roentgenology*, 19(4), 296–307.

Gilday, D.L. & Alderson, P.O. (1974) Scintigraphic evaluation of liver and spleen injury. *Seminars in Nuclear Medicine*, 4, 357–370.

Haertel, M. & Fuchs, W.H. (1974) Angiography in pancreatic trauma. *British Journal of Radiology*, 47, 641–645.

Jander, H.P., Laws, H.L., Kogott, M.S. & Mihas, A.A. (1977) Emergency embolisation in blunt hepatic trauma. *American Journal of Roentgenology*, 129, 249–252.

Jones, R.G. (1978) Management of pancreatic trauma. *Annals of Surgery*, 187(5), 555–564.

Kaufman, R.A., Towbin, R., Babcock, D.S., Gerlfand, M.J., Guice, K.S., Oldham, K.T. & Noseworthy, J. (1984) Upper abdominal trauma in children: imaging evaluation. *American Journal of Roentgenology*, 142, 449–460.

Korobkin, M., Moss, A.A., Callen, P.W., Demartini, W.J. & Kaiser, J.A. (1978) Computed tomography of subcapsular splenic haematoma. *Radiology*, 129, 441–445.

Kuhn, J.P. & Berger, A.E. (1981) Computed tomography in the evaluation of blunt abdominal trauma in children. *Radiology Clinics of North America*, 19(3), 503–512.

Mindelzon, R.E. & McCort, J.J. (1984) Upper abdominal trauma: Conventional radiology. *Seminars in Roentgenology*, 19(4), 259–268.

Morayati, S., Sagar, V.V., Warsal, N.F. & Martenz, D. (1983) Rapid resolution of spleen scan changes after trauma. *Clinical Nuclear Medicine*, 8(9), 440.

Nebesar, R.A., Rabinov, K.R. & Potsaid, M.S. (1974) Radionuclide imaging of the spleen in suspected splenic injury. *Radiology*, 110, 609–614.

Odling-Smee, W. & Crockard, A. (1981) *Trauma Care*, pp. 527–548, Academic Press, London.

Roy, A.D. (1984) The spleen preserved. *British Medical Journal*, 289, 70–81.

Smith, F.W., Brown, R.G., Gilday, D.L., Ash, J.M. (1981) Bone marrow uptake of 99 m technetium — sulfur colloid after severe abdominal trauma in children. *Paediatric Radiology*, 10, 169–171.

Sonneberg, M.D., Simeone, J.F., Meuller, P.R., Wittenberg, J., Hall, D.A. & Ferrucci, J.T. (1983) Sonographic appearance of haematoma in liver, spleen and kidney: a clinical, pathologic, and animal study. *Radiology*, 147, 507–510.

Strauch, G.O. (1973) Clinical finding in abdominal trauma. *Radiology Clinics of North America*, 11, 555–560.

Strauch, G.O. (1979) Preservation of splenic function in adults and children with injured spleens. *American Journal of Surgery*, 137, 478–483.

Thompson, J.S., Moore, E.E., Van Duzer Moore, S., Moore, J.B., Galloway, A.C. (1980) The evolution of abdominal stab wound management. *Journal of Trauma*, 20(6), 478–484.

Toombs, B.D., Sandler, C.M., Rauschkolb, E.N., Strax, R. & Harle, T.S. (1982) Assessment of hepatic injuries with computed tomography. *Journal of Computed Tomography*, 6, 72–75.

Uthoff, L.B., Wyffels, P.L., Adams, C.S., Zwicky, G.F. & Berg, B.C. (1983) A prospective study comparing nuclear scintigraphy and computerised axial tomography in the initial evaluation of the trauma patient. *Annals of Surgery*, 198, 611–616.

Vallon, A.G., Lees, W.R., Cotton, P.B. (1979) Gray scale ultrasonography and endoscopic pancreatography after pancreatic trauma. *British Journal of Surgery*, 66, 169–172.

Wall, S.D., Federle, M.P., Jeffrey, R.B. & Brett, C.M. (1983) CT diagnosis of unsuspected pneumothorax after blunt abdominal trauma. *American Journal of Roentgenology*, 141, 919–921.

Wallace, S., Gianturco, C., Anderson, J.H., Goldstein, H.M., Davis, L.J. & Bree, R.L. (1976) Therapeutic vascular occlusion utilising steel coil technique: clinical application. *American Journal of Roentgenology*, 127, 381–387.

Whitley, N.O., Shatney, C.H. (1983) Diagnosis of abdominal abcesses in patients with major trauma: the use of computed tomography. *Radiology*, 147, 179–183.

30: An Approach to Abdominal Masses

A.K. DIXON

'So far as tumours are concerned, the abdomen is indeed a temple of surprise, and it is by our diagnostic humiliations when the abdomen is opened that we learn.' Hamilton Bailey.

Clinical considerations

Only a few years ago, the patient presenting with a palpable abdominal mass used to be referred directly to the surgeon. A 'diagnostic laparotomy' would often be performed with little or no further investigation. Nowadays the patient undergoes a wide variety of radiological tests in order to determine several key facts before embarking on the most suitable course of management. Indeed it should be possible to establish the precise diagnosis in most patients. But we would do well to beware of complacency in this 'temple of surprise'.

The first fact to establish beyond any reasonable doubt is whether a mass is present or not. The clinical examination of the abdomen is a far from precise art. Some clinicians are notoriously better than others in this respect; it is likely that experience plays a part here too. But even amongst experienced clinicians there is a tendency to 'invent' an abdominal mass at clinical examination and in up to 30% of patients no lesion will be found (Dixon et al., 1981a, Williams et al., 1984). The habitus of the patient will also affect the clinical appraisal. A mass may be easily palpated in a thin patient who can relax the anterior abdominal wall muscles, but a similar mass in an obese patient with a resistant abdominal wall may defy palpation.

Even when a mass is present there is a wide range of normal structures which may account for it (Bearn & Pilkington, 1959). The commonest of these is a loaded colon, where normally indentable faeces can mimic a fixed mass; repeat clinical examination after an interval of time should prevent this error. A pronounced lumbar lordosis can render the normal aorta unduly palpable, especially in the thin, elderly patient in whom the aorta is usually calcified and somewhat ectatic. Repeated palpation can cause discomfort and so a tender, palpable, pulsatile 'mass' develops; this frequently leads to the erroneous clinical diagnosis of an aneurysm. A Riedel's lobe (the caudal tongue-like projection of the anterior edge of the right lobe of the liver) is a potential cause for a mass in the right abdomen, although whether entirely normal liver parenchyma is firm enough to be palpable is debatable (Hobsley, 1979). However, the normal liver edge is considered to be rendered palpable in those with overinflated chests (namely emphysema). In a thin elderly patient a ptosed normal kidney can become palpable as it rides over the iliac crest. Similarly a malrotated, but otherwise normal kidney, is often palpable. The horseshoe kidney is the extreme example of such anomalies and one of great importance to the radiotherapist, who may be considering radiation treatment to the para-aortic nodes.

Having ascertained that a mass is definitely present and that it is indeed caused by a lesion rather than a normal variant, the next fact which the clinician will want to know is the likely organ of origin. An opinion as to the likely nature of the lesion will be expected, and for those lesions requiring surgery, radiotherapy, or chemotherapy an assessment as to whether the mass is solitary or whether there is evidence of disseminated disease (other lesions, liver secondaries, nodal deposits, etc.) is important. Furthermore an opinion as to the feasibility of biopsy or aspiration is helpful. In some institutions there is sufficient rapport between clinicians and radiologists for the biopsy to be directly performed whenever a suitable mass is demonstrated without waiting for further discussion.

Available tests

Because of the impact of modern imaging tests on clinical management and the seeming dependence of some clinicians on results, there is a tendency for such tests to be used at an increasingly earlier stage in the diagnostic process. This is despite the fact that many diagnoses can be reached on the basis of a good clinical history and examination (Hampton *et al.*, 1975). Even within radiology there is a tendency for many patients to undergo sophisticated investigations before plain film studies have been properly evaluated. This is to be avoided wherever possible. The presence of underlying bronchial carcinoma or disseminated lung metastases on the chest radiograph would substantially alter not only the list of possible causes for an abdominal mass, but also the diagnostic approach and subsequent management. The value of the plain abdominal radiograph is less clear-cut, but the presence of calcification (renal, tumefactive, infective, etc.) is a valuable clue which is sometimes overlooked. On occasions the plain abdominal radiograph can be diagnostic (e.g. aneurysm), and it is essential in children where associated congenital abnormalities may be demonstrated (e.g. anterior meningomyelocele) (Grossman *et al.*, 1983).

The potential range of imaging tests is wide. *Ultrasound* (US) is often used first as it is widely available, free from radiation risk, quick, cheap, and has been shown to have a very high diagnostic yield in abdominal masses (Holm *et al.*, 1982). It is certainly the best single test in children and thin patients. However, US may not demonstrate all the intra-abdominal organs at the site of the palpable mass in every patient because of obesity or overlying bowel gas. In these cases *computerized tomography* (CT), which is also very reliable in this clinical situation (Williams *et al.*, 1984), should be performed. There are many who now proceed directly to CT, arguing that if a malignant lesion is seen it will need to be staged as accurately as possible and that this is better done by CT. Furthermore CT is probably slightly more reliable at excluding an intra-abdominal lesion (see Fig. 30.12), particularly in the obese. So CT should be used in preference to US when the clinician is uncertain as to the presence of a mass. Ultrasound is particularly reliable in the right hypochondrium, where the liver acts as an acoustic window; indeed at this site there is some evidence that CT can sometimes be deceptively misleading (Frick & Feinberg, 1982). Allowing for such relative limitations the decision as to whether to embark on US or CT will often depend on the skill and confidence of the ultrasonographer and the availability of CT. In either case it is important to note that the initial imaging test of the mass should not be directed towards any one organ unless there is very strong evidence that one specific organ is responsible for the mass.

One possible danger of using an *organ-specific test* for a palpable abdominal mass is that an adjacent lesion may be missed (see Fig. 30.10). Furthermore, if the first test is negative, a sequence of organ-specific tests may develop that will be time consuming and expensive (Fig. 30.1), particularly if the 'mass' is non-existent and merely in the mind of the referring clinician. This is not to say that there is no place for the organ-specific test in the patient with a palpable mass, but there must be good evidence that one (or possibly one of two) particular organ is responsible. For example, if the patient is passing fresh blood *per rectum*, the mass is likely to be colonic in origin and a barium enema is the obvious initial test. There is often a real case for the definitive organ-specific test after a more generalized one; Fig. 30.2 shows an example where a barium study confirmed the CT findings and narrowed down a range of possible diagnoses to one probable contender. Many surgeons still require an IVU before performing nephrectomy in addition to US or CT evidence of a solid mass.

The use of *nuclear medicine* tests in the clinical setting of an abdominal mass is mainly limited to liver/spleen scintigraphy and tests for the localization of abscesses. These will be considered in the relevant sections below. The role of magnetic resonance imaging (MRI) for abdominal masses is not yet clear. The ability to image in any plane is valuable. Whether MRI will obviate the need for some biopsy procedures has yet to be answered.

The causes (Ellis, 1985)

Abdominal wall

Although it is usually easy to differentiate lesions arising from or involving the abdominal wall from true intra-abdominal masses on clinical grounds, difficulties can occur (Figs 30.1, 30.3). As many of these lesions contain fat (e.g. lipoma) or gas (e.g. hernia) CT is the optimal technique here. CT also gives good delineation of the relation of the lesion to the various abdominal wall muscles. The rectus abdominis muscle can be torn or suffer a direct blow (especially in windsurfing); the resulting haematoma may lead to a tender mass some weeks after a relatively minor incident. Inflammation of

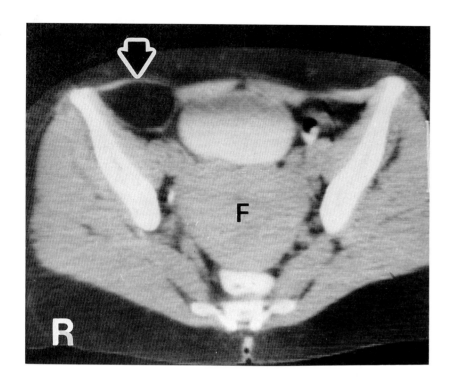

Fig. 30.1 Middle-aged lady with a palpable mass in the right iliac fossa. Barium enema was negative but it suggested a pelvic mass. Both US and a gynaecological opinion confirmed the presence of fibroids. IVU negative. CT (w 512, L + 45) shows a lipoma (*arrow*) in the anterior abdominal wall musculature to be responsible for the palpable mass (F = uterine mass of fibroids between bladder and rectum). This case illustrates well the value of a non-organ-specific test, such as CT. (Reproduced with permission from Dixon, 1983b.)

the abdominal wall is frequently secondary to an intraperitoneal abscess and thus a technique such as CT, which allows delineation of all the organs and fascial planes at one level, is optimal.

Generalized abdominal swelling

The clinical differentiation of obesity, ascites, and large intra-abdominal masses (especially ovarian cysts) can be difficult. Both US and CT will readily demonstrate ascites at a much earlier stage than a plain abdominal radiograph (Goldberg *et al.*, 1970, Jolles & Coulam, 1980). Pseudomyxoma peritonei is a rare alternative cause of generalized swelling and, when advanced, should be easily recognized by the scalloping it causes on the surface of the liver (Seshul & Coulam, 1981).

Because the clinical examination is so difficult in the very obese there is always a real fear that an abdominal mass may be overlooked. Men tend to deposit their excess fat within the abdomen; women tend to increase their subcutaneous stores with obesity (Dixon, 1983a). Accordingly, even in a relatively obese woman, the intra-abdominal organs may still be quite closely packed together, thereby allowing adequate US. However, CT is usually more reliable than US in the obese male. Very few patients (about 1 in 3000) are so obese that they cannot pass through the gantry aperture

of modern CT machines. It is always worth checking the appearances of the adrenal glands when there is marked central obesity; occasionally it may lead to a diagnosis of Cushing's syndrome. A lipo(sarco)ma within the mesenteric fat can also be overlooked in someone with apparent centralized obesity; displacement and crowding of bowel loops away from a localized region of fat may be the only clue to this condition.

Local intra-abdominal mass

Before considering lesions arising in particular organs, which tend to form masses localized to a particular part of the abdomen, some more general conditions that may be responsible for a mass arising in any part of the abdomen will be discussed. *Ascites* may loculate, especially in patients with multiple adhesions. Such a collection of encysted ascites may be found in any part of the peritoneal cavity and is especially common in patients who are being, or have been, treated by peritoneal dialysis. Loculated collections such as these may well become infected.

An *abscess* can develop in any part of the abdomen and can therefore be responsible for a mass at any site. The patient's clinical condition is usually indicative of the cause. However, in patients treated by immune suppression, steroids, or anti-

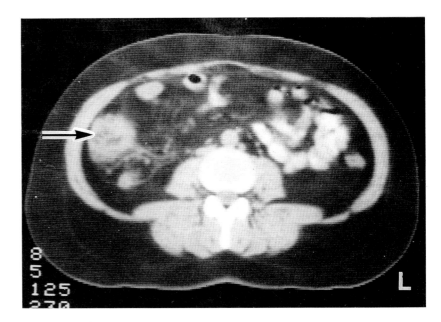

Fig. 30.2 Female patient with fullness in the lower part of the right abdomen. (a) CT (w 512, L + 45) shows the region of the caecum (*arrow*) to be poorly defined with abnormal fat medial to it. These appearances are non-specific but point to an abnormality around the terminal ileum and caecum.

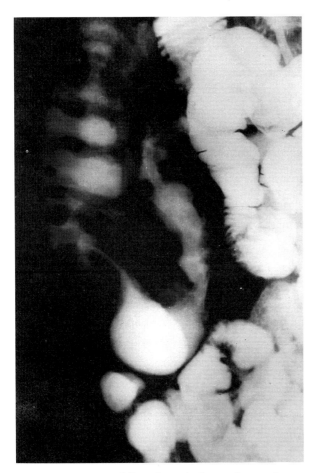

Fig. 30.2 (b) Barium follow-through shows abnormal terminal ileum with gross narrowing at ileocaecal junction. Crohn's disease correctly diagnosed.

biotics the classic clinical pointers may be absent or attenuated.

Hydatid cysts may similarly occur in any part of the abdomen although the right lobe of the liver is the most common single site. Hydatid cysts often have a classical configuration on both US and CT (Beggs, 1983), with the daughter cysts sometimes arranged in a spokewheel arrangement. However, this latter sign is not always present nor always specific; it can be simulated by necrotic *adeno-carcinoma* deposits. It is important that hydatid cysts should be considered whenever a fluid lesion is identified, because the treatment will be so very different. Hydatid cysts are either treated by chemotherapy or by formal surgery. Encysted ascites and abscesses are usually now referred for radiological intervention, a potentially hazardous procedure in a patient with a hydatid cyst.

Because most of the lesions described under this heading (loculated ascites, abscesses, etc.) are *fluid filled*, they should be well demonstrated by US. This will allow an US-guided drainage procedure to be performed. So long as a safe percutaneous route to the lesion can be identified, a pig-tail type catheter can be inserted into the abscess and this will allow drainage for some days. For smaller abscesses, more difficult sites, or just loculated ascites a fine/medium-gauge needle may be sufficient; those covered by a Teflon sheath which can then be left *in situ* for a few hours are especially valuable here.

Not all abscesses will be identified by US (Lundstedt *et al.*, 1983) although intrahepatic and

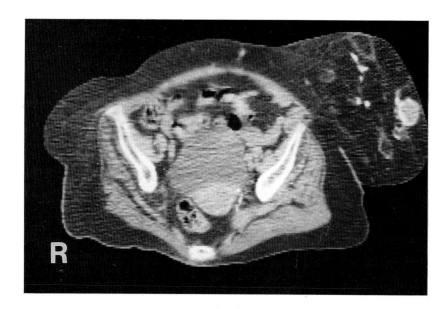

Fig. 30.3 Obese elderly lady with huge mass within the anterolateral part of the fatty apron. On clinical grounds a hernia was thought possible. CT (w 512, L + 45) shows a large mass of fat density with scattered calcification within. No communication with gut. No defect in anterior abdominal wall musculature.

subphrenic collections should be reliably identified and excluded. So if the clinical condition warrants, another test should be performed. There is debate as to whether CT or an isotope study (white cell scintigram, e.g. indium) is the ultimate test for the detection and exclusion of abscess formation (McNeil *et al.*, 1981, Lundstedt *et al.*, 1983, Martin *et al.*, 1984). They probably both carry roughly similar predictive values for positive and negative results of over 90% in each case. Much will depend on local availability and expertise. The white cell scintigram is extremely sensitive in detecting an abnormality and thus, when negative, is a very useful test of exclusion; such confident exclusion of an abscess requires multiple cuts at CT. However, the positive scintigram is not totally specific insofar that a healing wound or an area of colitis can both cause an area of increased uptake and thereby simulate an abscess. So limited CT may be needed to show the morphological features through the region of suspicion. Even when US has demonstrated an abscess, CT is still sometimes helpful to plan the optimal route for long-term catheter drainage; it is useful to be able to see all the organs and the relations of bowel loops before starting to approach a small deep-seated lesion (Haaga & Weinstein, 1980, Martin *et al.*, 1984).

Regional diagnosis of masses

Right hypochondrium

The liver is the predominant organ in this region and the one most commonly responsible for a mass. In the UK metastatic spread of carcinoma to the liver is the commonest cause of enlargement and this will often cause a characteristic hard and knobbly surface. If, on palpation, the focal enlargement is umbilicated, cancer is nearly always responsible. Although the surface of a cirrhotic liver can become hard and uneven, the irregularities here do not exceed 2—3 cm in diameter and do not become umbilicated. Primary carcinoma of the liver is relatively rare in the UK and usually follows cirrhosis; it is very common in some parts of Africa. Hydatid cysts and amoebic abscess should also be considered in patients from areas where these diseases are endemic.

If the liver is considered likely to be responsible for the palpable mass and there is a strong clinical indication as to the cause, such as metastases in a patient with known colonic cancer, then ultrasound seems the quickest and cheapest test. Occasionally interpretation can be difficult in some infiltrative processes (e.g. lymphoma); the features of cirrhosis may not be immediately evident. In these circumstances hepatic scintigraphy, an extremely sensitive test (Drum, 1982), can be helpful. Scintigraphy can provide some assessment of 'function' by the relative amount of hepatic and osseous uptake. However, scintigraphy cannot make much prediction as to the nature of an hepatic lesion, apart from the size and distribution of the defects in uptake. Thus it is less useful for a patient with a solitary large hepatic lesion with no known underlying cause, although more sophisticated nuclear tests can sometimes provide a precise diagnosis of hepatoma or abscess. Ultrasound is thus the ideal initial test, allowing differentiation of solid from cystic lesions and then guiding a suitable biopsy or aspiration which should give a definite diagnosis. It will also provide accurate information about the biliary and portal venous systems.

In hospitals with limited CT facilities, hepatic CT has to be mainly reserved for patients in whom ultrasound and scintigraphy have failed to resolve the problem. However, this rather belittles the usefulness of hepatic CT which, if performed carefully before and after i.v. contrast, will give very detailed information about hepatic masses. Indeed CT is increasingly being used as the initial test. Some would argue that CT should be performed before a biopsy of any solid liver mass in order to exclude the diagnosis of haemangioma; CT should show characteristic enhancement. Most surgeons considering resection of a hepatic tumour will want CT confirmation that the tumour is indeed confined to one lobe and that the major vessels at the porta hepatis are free of disease.

The liver also becomes palpable when an *adrenal* lesion or *right upper-pole renal mass* enlarges to such an extent as to produce hepatic displacement (Fig. 30.4). When such a lesion is 5–8 cm in diameter there is usually little difficulty in ascribing an organ of origin on either US or CT. However, the organ of origin of a very large lesion, especially if of reflectivity or attenuation close to hepatic and renal parenchyma, can be difficult to sort out. Could it be due to a large adrenal lesion displacing and distorting the right upper renal pole? Or could it be a predominantly extrarenal renal tumour, just connecting with the rest of the kidney by a relatively narrow pedicle? Such differentiation can be difficult on axial images and even on suitable parasagittal US images it can be difficult to establish the organ of origin. In the presence of a large upper-pole renal mass the normal adrenal will be grossly distorted and compressed against the liver, and may prove difficult to identify. Yet another possibility is a large localized hepatic tumour extending in an extrahepatic fashion at this site, although this is rare. Careful attention to the appearances of the capsule and retroperitoneal fat wedge may prevent errors here (Graif *et al.*, 1983). Very occasionally angiography may still prove to be the most valuable test for such differentiation. Such organ distinction is critical in a child presenting with a large solid mass, where the treatment for neuroblastoma and a Wilms' tumour will be very different and does not always include surgery at outset. Sometimes the clinical picture is obvious, with haematuria in a child with Wilms' tumour, or bone metastases and raised VMA levels in association with neuroblastoma. Ultrasound should accurately distinguish the vast majority,

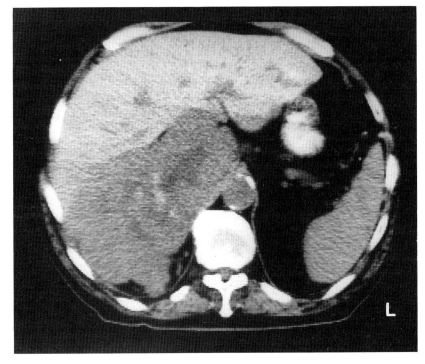

Fig. 30.4 Patient with clinical hepatomegaly. CT (w 300, L + 45) shows the liver displaced forwards. The huge lesion in the region of the right adrenal contains a few flecks of high attenuation — perhaps early calcification. Here there is a good line of cleavage between the lesion and the liver, as there was below with the kidney. An adrenal tumour was correctly diagnosed. (Reproduced with permission from Dixon, 1983b.)

but occasionally contrast-enhanced CT may be needed and even this can be difficult to interpret when the mass is very large.

The enlarged *gall bladder* is a common cause for a mass at this site; it often leads to very clear-cut clinical signs. When accompanied by jaundice, a carcinoma in the region of the pancreatic head is usually responsible. This is in keeping with Courvoisier's law, which states that: if in a jaundiced patient the gall bladder is palpably enlarged, it is probably *not* a case of stone impacted in the common bile duct. A mucocele is one of the possible causes for gall bladder enlargement without jaundice. Here a gall stone is impacted in the neck of the gall bladder and the gall bladder enlarges due to continued mucus secretion behind the stone. Just occasionally this can lead to jaundice should the neck of the gall bladder enlarge to such an extent, and the region of the cystic duct become so inflamed, that the common hepatic duct is compressed (Mirizzi's syndrome). The surgeon is usefully forewarned of this possibility (Htoo, 1983).

These two examples of gall bladder enlargement illustrate the importance of using an imaging technique which demonstrates the whole of the biliary system as well as the gall bladder itself; US is the obvious choice here. In obstructive jaundice due to a pancreatic tumour the distended gall bladder will be obvious, and so may the pancreatic mass at the distal end of the dilated common bile duct (Fig. 30.5). In Mirizzi's syndrome the distal common bile duct will be of normal calibre. The presence or absence of gall stones may be misleading in both conditions; in patients with carcinoma of the pancreas they are often discovered within the gall bladder as an incidental finding. Conversely it may be difficult to demonstrate the gall stone impacted within the neck of a mucocele.

Sometimes the level of obstruction in a *jaundiced* patient is not well seen at US because of bowel gas or obesity. The clinical setting may drive towards intervention (surgical or radiological) after percutaneous trans-hepatic cholangiography or ERCP. In some patients further information may be sought and CT will reliably demonstrate the level of obstruction (Pedrosa *et al.*, 1981). Although CT may also demonstrate a mass at the pancreatic head, the same difficulties that face the surgeon and pathologist occur, namely the difficult differentiation between carcinoma and focal pancreatitis. Even in experienced hands uncertainty about the diagnosis can still remain after laparotomy and

biopsy. The main use of CT is in assessing operability of the pancreatic mass and the detection of small liver metastases.

Returning to the gall bladder itself, US will also give valuable information about the gall bladder wall (Sanders, 1980), which will be thickened in both acute cholecystitis and an empyema. Ultrasound may also show high reflectivity in the gall bladder wall with distal reverberation indicative of emphysematous cholecystitis, which carries a grave prognosis (Blaquiere & Dewbury, 1982). It can also demonstrate perihepatic fluid, suggesting early peritonitis. Usually there is no difficulty in the clinical diagnosis of these inflammatory causes. Occasionally in ill or unconscious patients the gall bladder can become very distended, especially if there has been no oral feeding. This must be distinguished from an inflamed gall bladder; a normal gall bladder wall thickness is a useful discriminator here.

Carcinoma is a further potential cause for the gall bladder to develop into a palpable mass. It may be recognized by a bizarre echo pattern over and above the calculi that are almost inevitably present. As the tumour has often extended into the liver, loss of a clear line of cleavage between the two organs is a further sign (Yeh, 1979).

The *hepatic flexure of colon* can also be responsible for a palpable mass in the right hypochondrium. This portion of colon may become preferentially loaded with faeces. Alternatively a tumour may be present and this can be recognized at US by highly reflective central core surrounded by a peripheral mass of low reflectivity (Schwerk *et al.*, 1979). Similarly, CT should show bowel-wall thickening leading to a soft-tissue density mass although, as in barium studies, care must be taken to avoid misinterpreting faeces as tumour. Extension of the tumour to adjacent organs (e.g. liver) may also be evident, and such a finding might sway the surgeon away from operating in the very frail or elderly patient. Few surgeons will operate for colonic carcinoma on US or CT findings alone without confirmation by barium enema, colonoscopy or percutaneous cytological aspiration.

Epigastric region

The liver is again the commonest organ responsible for a mass at this site, especially when the left lobe is preferentially expanded. In this situation a left lobe biopsy should be performed and this can easily be done under US or CT control.

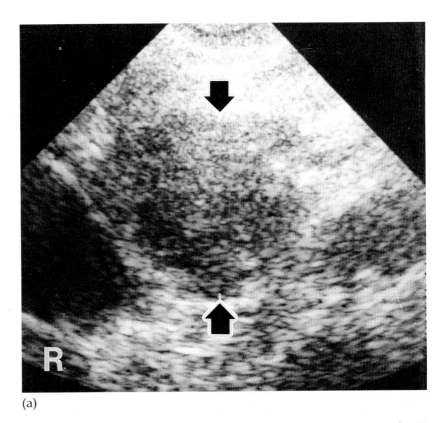

(a)

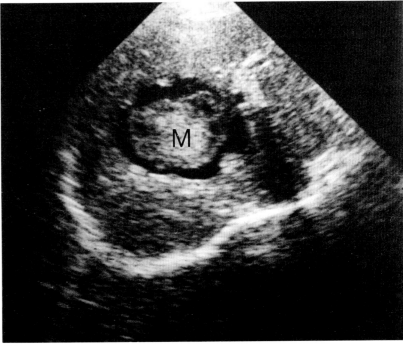

(b)

Fig. 30.5 Elderly male patient with clinical signs of obstructive jaundice. US showed dilated common bile duct ending in 5 cm diameter echogenic mass in the region of the head of the pancreas. Mass (*arrows*) well seen in (a) on transverse US. M = hepatic metastasis in oblique section (b), which made carcinoma the almost certain cause.

A *gastric* mass may cause fullness in this region and if the patient is vomiting, or has severe pain, a barium study or endoscopy may be performed at the outset (Fig. 30.6). Gastric dilatation alone can also lead to epigastric fullness. It may be necessary to aspirate the resting fluid by nasogastric tube in order to get good views of the antrum, which is the region of interest in outlet obstruction. Even then it can be difficult to distinguish between tumour around the pylorus and scarring secondary

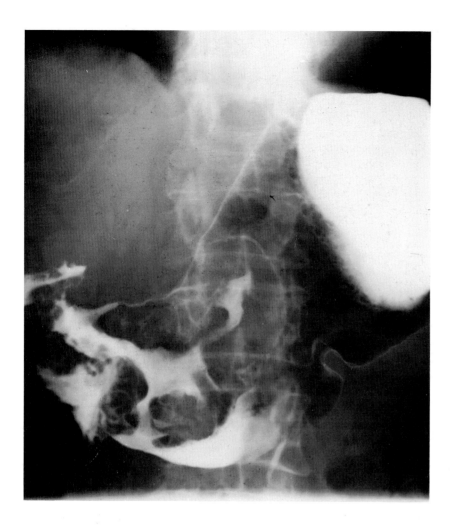

Fig. 30.6 Elderly female with epigastric mass, discomfort and vomiting. Barium meal shows an irregular antral filling defect caused by a gastric carcinoma. (Reproduced with permission of the editors of *Geriatric Medicine.*)

to an ulcer. When a distended stomach is seen at either US or CT, an attempt should be made to identify the cause. In children, the hypertrophied muscle of pyloric stenosis may either be palpated by skilled hands or demonstrated by US as a characteristic target sign just to the right of the midline (Pilling, 1983) (Fig. 30.7). In adults an antral carcinoma large enough to cause a palpable mass (namely Fig. 30.6) should be well demonstrated by CT, which can also demonstrate potential involvement of adjacent organs. Bezoars (usually trichobezoars) are rare nowadays; they are well demonstrated by a barium meal.

The transverse colon can harbour a lesion responsible for a palpable mass at this site. Again it may be demonstrated by US or CT but in order to confirm this diagnosis and assess the rest of the colon it is usually a wise precaution to perform a barium enema as well.

The *greater omentum* is a favoured site of metastatic involvement. Indeed, when studded with

tumour, it causes a characteristic CT appearance of heterogeneous omental fat which has been likened to a 'cake' (Whitley *et al.*, 1982). The clinical findings in this condition can be confusing, with fullness of the epigastric region extending to the umbilical and both hypochondrial regions. This can mimic more generalized abdominal swelling such as that caused by ascites; the patient may be subjected to several dry taps before imaging (usually CT) reveals the diagnosis. Biopsy will usually reveal adenocarcinoma but the hunt for the underlying primary may prove elusive, even at post-mortem (Stewart *et al.*, 1979). The greater omentum, regarded by some as the 'policeman' of the abdomen, will also become involved in tuberculous peritonitis, although this condition is rare in the UK.

Pancreatic lesions are commonly responsible for masses in the epigastric (and umbilical) regions. Some students have difficulty in appreciating how a retroperitoneal structure can push forwards from

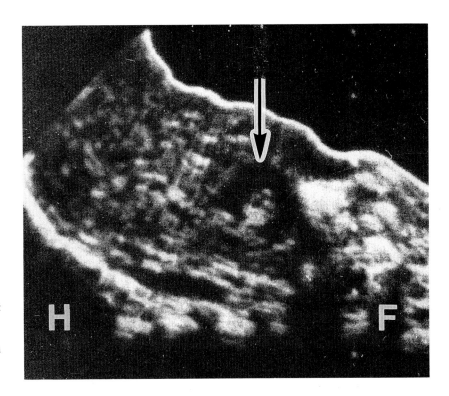

Fig. 30.7 Parasagittal US in an infant with forceful vomiting but no palpable epigastric mass. The characteristic target sign of the lumen within the hypertrophied pyloric muscle is well seen (*arrow*).

the depths of the abdominal cavity to cause an anterior mass. However, the body of the normal pancreas, albeit retroperitoneal, occupies a relatively anterior position on a cross-section of the torso. Indeed as it arches anterior to the aorta, the normal pancreas may only be a few centimetres beneath the anterior abdominal wall, and in some thin patients with a moderate lumbar lordosis it is possible to palpate the normal pancreas transmitting the aortic pulsation. Hence, the relatively easy anterior approach for fine-needle biopsy procedures of pancreatic lesions.

Cysts are the commonest lesions of the pancreas responsible for an abdominal swelling. True cysts form the minority and may develop in chronic pancreatitis (retention cysts) or be due to a cystic tumour (cystademona and cystadenocarcinoma). Most 'cysts' are in fact pseudocysts, fluid collections often separate from the pancreas, and most commonly sited within the lesser sac. Such a collection is a common sequel to acute pancreatitis and in this clinical setting US is obviously the best imaging test. It will confirm the suspected fluid nature of the lesion and, because it is both quick and cheap, it can readily provide serial follow-up.

Tumours of the body of the pancreas can be responsible for a palpable mass and will be well demonstrated by US (moderate reflectivity) or CT (soft-tissue density). Alas, such lesions are usually inoperable by the time the lesion has progressed to form a palpable mass, and confirmation of the diagnosis by fine-needle biopsy is all that can be done. Occasionally the patient presents earlier because of diabetes of recent onset. Lesions in the pancreatic head usually present at an even earlier stage because of biliary obstruction.

Other *retroperitoneal* lesions can present with a mass in the epigastric region, although by the time they have become palpable the mass often extends to other regions (especially umbilical or lumbar). A retroperitoneal cyst is a rare cause, but the fluid nature will readily be demonstrated by US. However when a cyst (or any mass) becomes very large, the precise site of origin may become more difficult to establish. Solid tumours originating in mesenchymal tissues are best demonstrated by CT and guided biopsy should also be possible. Enlargement of *para-aortic lymph nodes* can coalesce to form a large mass which can engulf the aorta; in an adult patient such massive enlargement is usually due to non-Hodgkin's lymphoma, and although US will show a characteristic mass of low reflectivity, the distribution is best demonstrated by CT. The aorta is characteristically lifted away from its neighbouring vertebral bodies; this sign is easy to recognize in middle-aged and elderly patients in whom the aortic wall will be partly calcified. As lymphoma is the likely cause in the absence of a known primary or other intra-abdominal mass, it is essential that a large histological biopsy is obtained wherever possible. This will usually necessitate a translumbar CT-guided biopsy.

The left hypochondrium

The *spleen* is a key organ in this region. Clinicians spend much time at the bedside deliberating over subtle signs of enlargement, although few of these are reliable until splenomegaly is marked. If possible splenic enlargement is the only question posed by the clinician, a liver–spleen scintigram is a quick and cheap test that will establish the relation of the splenic tip to the costal cartilage. It will also give useful information about the parenchyma of both liver and spleen. As poor liver function may be the cause of the splenomegaly, an increased uptake of the radionuclide by the bone marrow is a useful additional finding indicative of cirrhosis. Ultrasound will also quickly give the dimensions of the spleen and some information as to the homogeneity. Cysts will be confidently diagnosed and areas of tumour infiltration may be recognized. CT can also give useful information about splenic parenchyma, especially if rapid-sequence images are obtained after bolus enhancement. However, all tests have difficulty in distinguishing between lesions such as infarcts (very common), granulomata and metastatic deposits. Furthermore

lymphomatous infiltration is quite common in apparently homogeneous normal-sized spleens. For these reasons imaging of the spleen is difficult. However, splenic size and volume can be accurately documented.

The distended stomach may again be palpated in this region and must be considered before a fluid-filled lesion is diagnosed at US or CT. Similarly, colonic lesions may cause palpable abnormalities at this site.

Lesions of the *tail of the pancreas* have to be considerably larger than those of the body (see epigastric region above) to form a palpable mass because the tail is normally situated in a much more posterior position within the abdomen. Because of the overlying gas in the stomach and splenic flexure of colon, CT is usually the best test for the pancreatic tail. Furthermore it will accurately demonstrate adjacent organs, which are often involved (Fig. 30.8).

As in the right hypochondrium, massive enlargement of the *left adrenal* may occasionally be difficult to separate from an 'extrarenal' renal tumour. However, small and medium-sized adrenal masses are usually easily recognized as such. With the advent of US and CT, adrenal masses are often found by serendipity. Nonfunctioning adenomata and metastatic involvement are the commonest causes. But haemorrhage and infection should also be considered. Adrenal function tests and fine-needle aspiration biopsy

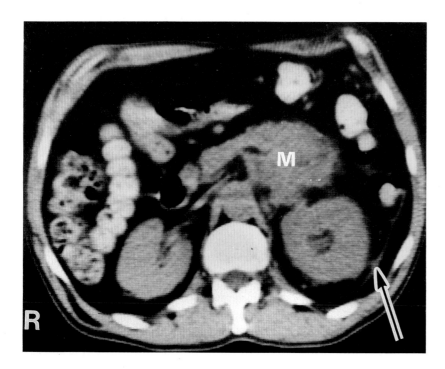

Fig. 30.8 Middle-aged male with weight loss and a mass in the left hypochondrium. CT (w 512, L + 45) shows a soft-tissue density mass (M) in the region of the tail of the pancreas. This has extended posteriorly into the anterior perirenal fat and left renal vein. Note Gerota's fascia thickened posterolaterally (*arrow*).

should be performed as appropriate to management (Gross *et al.*, 1983).

Lumbar regions

Many of the potential lesions in these sites have already been considered. On the right the enlarged liver or distended gall bladder can extend into these regions, especially a Riedel's lobe of the liver; on the left the spleen is a common culprit. Masses arising in the colon have similarly been considered above. Intussusception is an especial cause in a child with a right-sided colonic mass. This may lead to characteristic plain-film appearances with a soft-tissue density mass and proximal dilated loops of small bowel. The clinical history is usually straightforward but occasionally the patient is referred for US, which may yield diagnostic clues. However, an enema should be performed whenever intussusception is a diagnostic possibility both to confirm the diagnosis and in an attempt to effect hydrostatic reduction. An exception is the shocked child with signs of peritonitis in whom early surgery is indicated for possible bowel resection; an enema is contraindicated here because of the risk of perforation.

Lesions in the *kidneys* are responsible for most masses in the lumbar regions. Although *simple cysts* are very common in patients past middle age (Lauks & McLachlan, 1981) and frequently reach huge proportions, it is surprising that they only rarely feature as a cause for a *palpable* mass. Maybe this is because they are not under great pressure. Indeed, when they do cause a palpable mass, it is often the residual normal kidney which is palpated, the axis and position having been altered by the cyst. This is in contrast to the tense dilated renal pelvis caused, say, by a *pelviureteric obstruction*, often palpable in a child. Ultrasound should readily differentiate between these two fluid-filled lesions by recognition of distended calyces in the case of pelviureteric obstruction. A large parapelvic cyst is a potential pitfall as it can simulate a distended renal pelvis; an IVU will readily resolve this problem and will probably be required in any case of pelviureteric junction obstruction in order to give better anatomical delineation. This is another example of how the organ-specific test (IVU) may still be required when the site of the lesion has been narrowed down to one particular organ.

More complex cystic lesions often lead to a palpable mass. In the neonate, multicystic disease is a common cause for a unilateral palpable loin mass (Kyaw, 1973); US will demonstrate a bizarre pattern of multiple cysts that are usually of variable size — unlikely in a grossly hydronephrotic kidney where the dilated calyces tend to be of uniform size clustered around the larger renal pelvis. As ever in paediatric renal US, care must be taken not to confuse the prominent regions of medullary tissue (low reflectivity) with cysts (zero reflectivity). Infantile type polycystic disease, a very rare condition, will lead to palpable bilateral renal enlargement at birth or soon afterwards; US will show large, highly reflective kidneys with reduced corticomedullary differentiation but no cysts. In adult type polycystic disease the kidneys may not become palpable unless the disease is very advanced and the patient thin, but the cysts should be reliably recognized at US in patients over 20 years of age.

Sadly, a *renal neoplasm* is an all too common cause for a loin mass (usually a Wilms' tumour in the infant, adenocarcinoma in the adult). Again US is the optimal initial test and will show a mass of moderate reflectivity. This will usually prove to be due to a malignant neoplasm, but xanthogranulamatous pyelonephritis (characteristically associated with a calculus) and angiomyolipoma (very bright echoes due to the fat component) are two of the benign lesions that should be considered. Although the literature is replete with reports of the accuracy of CT in staging of renal carcinoma, all the surgeon really needs to know before nephrectomy is that the opposite kidney is normal and that the renal vein and inferior vena cava are free of thrombus or tumour extension. In thin patients US is often a satisfactory test for venous involvement, and normality of the cava can sometimes be better demonstrated by US than CT; streaming artefacts can cause problems at CT. Nevertheless, in centres with CT, most patients with renal-cell carcinoma do undergo CT for a further check on the opposite kidney and venous patency. CT is the best method of demonstrating tumour extension outside Gerota's fascia, to adjacent organs (e.g. psoas), or lymph nodes. In the elderly or frail patient such findings may sway the initial treatment towards radiologically controlled embolization.

Umbilical region

Most lesions which account for masses characteristically found at this site have already been described. The stomach, the transverse colon and the omentum should again be considered. Large lesions in the kidney, discussed above under the lumbar regions, may extend towards the midline. Para-aortic lymph node enlargement is also a common cause and will be well demonstrated by CT. CT is especially good at demonstrating enlarged *mesenteric nodes* that tend to accumulate on either side of the plane of the mesenteric vessels to form a characteristic appearance (Fig. 30.9), which when advanced has been likened to a 'sandwich' and a 'hamburger' (Mueller *et al.*, 1980). Meticulous attention to small-bowel opacification must be paid in order to differentiate between nodes of soft-tissue density and loops of bowel. A *mesenteric cyst* can develop into a large periumbilical mass. On clinical examination this may be ballotted and it is said that there will be maximal freedom of movement at right angles to the root of the mesentery (i.e. from right hypochondrium to left iliac fossa). On imaging, the cyst will be of low reflectivity on US and of fluid density on CT. In some patients its relation to the mesentery will be evident, with small bowel loops draped around it. However, when such cysts become large the organ of origin can become obscure and a pancreatic pseudocyst (the commonest intra-abdominal cyst lesion) is often thought to be responsible.

The bifurcation of the aorta is usually closely related to the umbilicus. Most *aneurysms of the abdominal aorta* begin below the renal arteries and end immediately above the bifurcation. So an aneurysm is likely to be palpable in both the epigastric and umbilical regions. Accentuated normal pulsation in a thin patient must be distinguished from aneurysmal dilatation proper. Ultrasound is the pivotal test here. In thin patients it is usually possible to demonstrate the whole length of the abdominal aorta; the calibre can be assessed accurately and aneurysm confidently excluded. When an aneurysm is found, US will give an accurate maximal diameter which will help determine both the need for and the urgency of surgery. When surgery is contemplated it is important to know whether the renal arteries are involved in the aneurysm; this is difficult to determine on clinical grounds. In some patients the renal arteries can be clearly demonstrated by US but in the majority CT will be required for evaluation of the longitudinal extent of the aneurysm (Dixon *et al.*, 1981b) (Fig. 30.10). Using thin cuts at contiguous intervals the main renal arteries can be demonstrated in all but the thinnest patient; patients with aneurysms are often quite obese. Anomalous lower-pole vessels may not be identified by CT but failure to do so will not greatly alter management; during surgery it is relatively straightforward to insert them into the graft as

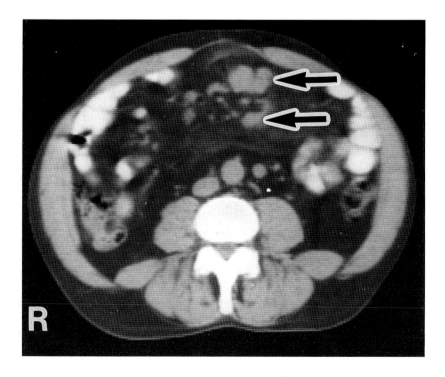

Fig. 30.9 Male, 65 years old, with non-Hodgkin's lymphoma. Probable mass on clinical examination. CT (w 512, L + 45) shows nodal masses (*arrows*) on either side of the plane of the superior mesenteric vessels. (Reproduced with permission from Dixon & Nightingale, 1984.)

appropriate. Although angiography will show such anomalous vessels, this test is no longer considered necessary in the evaluation of an abdominal aortic aneurysm. Apart from being invasive, it can severely underestimate both the maximal diameter and longitudinal extent, as only the lumen will be opacified. CT has the added advantage of demonstrating leakage and any perianeurysmal fibrosis (inflammatory aneurysm). This latter complication may engulf the ureters and hydronephrosis should always be excluded in patients with an abdominal aneurysm.

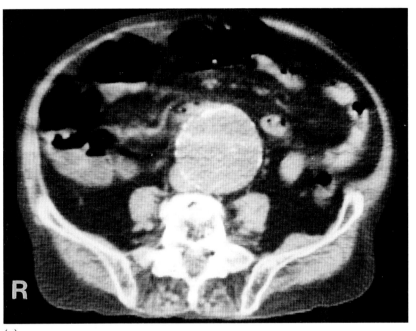

(a)

Fig. 30.10 Elderly man referred because of back pain, weight loss, and probable abdominal mass. US proved difficult due to obesity and copious bowel gas. (a) CT (w 512, L + 45) shows a large abdominal aortic aneurysm (maximal diameter 7 cm). Sharp margins — no leak; no perianeurysmal fibrosis. This aneurysm ended at the bifurcation. (b) CT (w 512, L + 45) 2 cm below renal arteries showing an aorta of much more normal calibre. CT also shows a large calculus within the right renal pelvis and hydronephrosis secondary to prostatic enlargement on the left. It also shows a large mass in the head of pancreas (*arrow*). Abnormal liver function tests developed soon afterwards but no tissue diagnosis was obtained. This is a good example of the benefits gained from a non-organ-specific test, especially one such as CT which shows all the intra-abdominal structures.

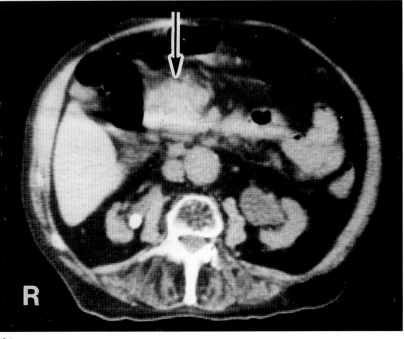

(b)

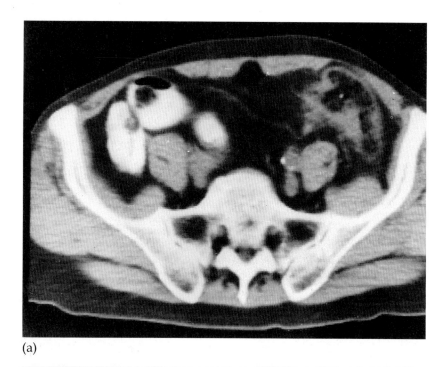

(a)

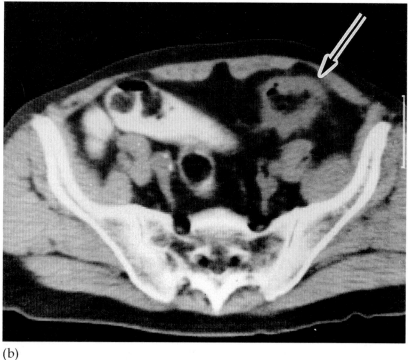

(b)

Fig. 30.11 (a, b) Three sequential CT images (w 512, L + 45) in a patient referred with a mass in the left iliac fossa. (a) There is some faecal accumulation above the thick wall stenosing lesion at the junction of descending and sigmoid colon, better seen in (b) (*arrow*).

Iliac fossae

The caecum on the right and the sigmoid colon on the left account for most masses in these regions (Fig. 30.11). Again faeces can often simulate a lesion (Fig. 30.12).

A mass of inflammatory tissue around a resolving inflamed appendix is an especial cause on the right. Sometimes a discrete collection of pus may be seen at US or CT, but more often resolving appendicitis merely leads to alterations in CT attenuation in the adjacent fat planes (Dixon & Nightingale, 1984). Similar subtle alterations in the CT attenuation of fat around the terminal ileum and caecum can be seen in the wide variety

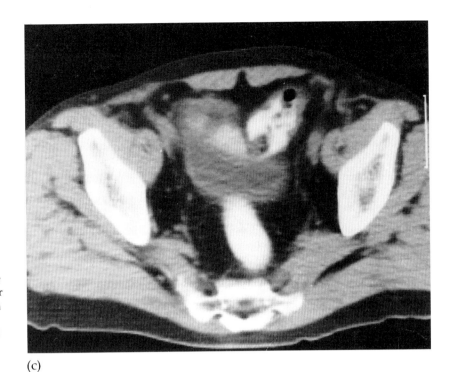

(c)

Fig. 30.11 (c) Rectally administered contrast medium is seen in (c) in the sigmoid colon just below the annular carcinoma shown in (b). Note how a gastrointestinal tract lesion *large enough to cause a palpable mass* should be shown by CT.

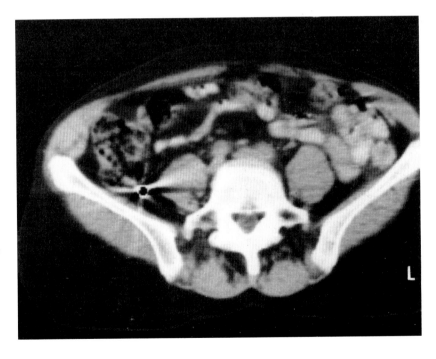

Fig. 30.12 Middle-aged lady referred on account of an ill-defined mass in the right iliac fossa. Barium enema had been negative. CT (w 512, L + 45) shows no abnormality through the level of the possible mass. Faeces within ascending colon. Artefacts from barium in appendix. Mass no longer palpable at clinical follow-up. (Reproduced with permission from Dixon, 1983b.)

of lesions that can affect this region (Crohn's disease, lymphoma, etc.) (see Fig. 30.2).

On the left, inflammation in association with *diverticular disease* is probably the commonest cause of a mass in the UK. CT, with early oral or rectal contrast medium preparation, can be quite specific here in so far that the long segment of thickened bowel wall can be well demonstrated with diverticula extending throughout the length of the abnormality; again the adjacent fat will often show increased attenuation. Barium enema may be needed to exclude a concomitant lesion (carcinoma or Crohn's disease). In thin patients, bowel-wall thickening in long standing colitis may lead to the sigmoid colon becoming unduly palpable.

In both iliac fossae the *psoas and iliacus muscles* can lead to palpable masses. These muscles are particularly well demonstrated by CT. Sarcomatous lesions can arise within or around these muscles and form solid local masses. Abscess formation within the psoas muscle classically presents with a mass in the groin, but occasionally such abscesses become more localized within the iliac fossae. Although spinal tuberculosis is still the commonest world-wide cause of psoas abscess, non-tuberculous causes are now commoner in the UK. Such non-tuberculous lesions may arise from other forms of spinal infection but they more commonly develop from adjacent renal or gastrointestinal lesions (appendicitis, Crohn's disease, recent surgery, etc.). Such spread from adjacent lesions seems to cause a more localized psoas abscess than

the classical 'cold' abscess caused by spinal tuberculosis. Spontaneous retroperitoneal haemorrhage in patients with coagulation disorders characteristically follows tissue planes around and within these muscles. This clinical diagnosis is usually obvious and CT is only used for confirmation, although sometimes the CT finding of a high-attenuation mass enveloping and distorting these muscles may be the first clue of such an event.

Suprapubic region

In women *gynaecological lesions* account for most masses here. In men the distended bladder is usually responsible for such a mass; prostatic outflow obstruction is the common underlying cause. Ultrasound is the optimal test for lesions at this site.

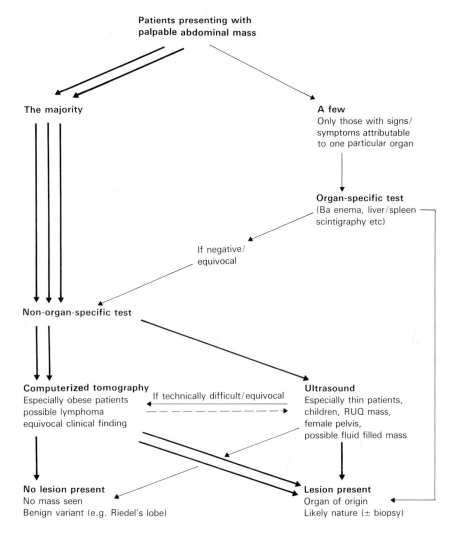

Fig. 30.13 Flow chart for tests on an abdominal mass.

It is important to remember that the *bladder* can become very large indeed and can simulate centrally placed cystic lesions. Even with all the advances in imaging techniques, simple catheterization can resolve some unusual abdominal 'masses'!

Conclusions

In many centres CT is increasingly being used as the first imaging test for an abdominal mass of unknown cause. A possible flow chart is shown in Fig. 30.13. Much will depend on locally available equipment and expertise.

Although the organ of origin and likely nature of the mass can be predicted with fair confidence, the ultimate diagnosis will rest on biopsy and aspiration. Radiologists are becoming increasingly involved with such interventional procedures (Isler *et al.*, 1981, Martin *et al.*, 1984). There is probably little to choose between the use of US and CT in obtaining such biopsies although CT carries advantages for deep-seated lesions, especially when a large cutting needle is needed (e.g. lymphoma) (Haaga & Weinstein, 1980, van Sonnenberg *et al.*, 1981, Pelaez *et al.*, 1983, Gross *et al.*, 1983).

References

Bearn, J.G. & Pilkington, T.R.E. (1959) Organs palpable in the normal adult abdomen. *Lancet*, **ii**, 212–213.

Beggs, I. (1983) The radiological appearances of hydatid disease of the liver. *Clinical Radiology*, **34**, 555–563.

Blaquiere, R.M. & Dewbury, K.C. (1982) The ultrasound diagnosis of emphysematous cholecystitis. *British Journal of Radiology*, **55**, 114–116.

Dixon, A.K., Kelsey Fry, I., Kingham, J.G.C., McLean, A.M. & White, F.E. (1981a) Computed tomography in patients with an abdominal mass: effective and efficient? A controlled trial. *Lancet*, **i**, 1199–1201.

Dixon, A.K., Springall, R.G., Fry, I.K. & Taylor, G.W. (1981b) Computed tomography (CT) of abdominal aortic aneurysms: determination of longitudinal extent. *British Journal of Surgery*, **68**, 47–50.

Dixon, A.K. (1983a) Abdominal fat assessed by computed tomography: sex difference in distribution. *Clinical Radiology*, **34**, 189–191.

Dixon, A.K. (1983b) *Body CT: A Handbook*. Churchill Livingstone, Edinburgh.

Dixon, A.K. & Nightingale, R.C. (1984) Abnormal fat: a useful marker of intra-abdominal disease at computed tomography. *Clinical Radiology*, **35**, 469–473.

Drum, D.E. (1982) Current status of radiocolloid hepatic scintiphotography for space-occupying disease. *Seminars in Nuclear Medicine*, **12**, 64–74.

Ellis, H. (1985) Abdominal swelling. In Dudley Hart, F. (ed) *French's Index of Differential Diagnosis* pp. 9–15. Wright, Bristol.

Frick, M.P. & Feinberg, S.B. (1982) Deceptions in localizing extrahepatic right-upper-quadrant abdominal masses by CT. *American Journal of Roentgenology*, **139**, 501–504.

Goldberg, B.B., Goodman, G.A. & Clearfield, H.R. (1970) Evaluation of ascites by ultrasound. *Radiology*, **96**, 15–22.

Graif, M., Manor, A. & Itzchak, Y. (1983) Sonographic differentiation of extra- and intrahepatic masses. *American Journal of Roentgenology*, **141**, 553–556.

Gross, B.H., Goldberg, H.I., Moss, A.A. & Harter, L.P. (1983) CT demonstration and guided aspiration of unusual adrenal metastases. *Journal of Computer Assisted Tomography*, **7**, 98–101.

Grossman, Z.D., Ellis, D.A. & Brigham, S.C. (eds) (1983) Abdominal mass in the infant or child. In *The Clinician's Guide to Diagnostic Imaging*, pp. 196–208. Raven Press, New York.

Haaga, J.R. & Weinstein, A.J. (1980) CT-guided percutaneous aspiration and drainage of abscesses. *American Journal of Roentgenology*, **135**, 1187–1194.

Hampton, J.R., Harrison, M.J.G., Mitchell, J.R.A., Prichard, J.S. & Seymour, C.A. (1975) Relative contributions of history-taking, physical examination, and laboratory investigation to diagnosis and management of medical outpatients. *British Medical Journal*, **2**, 486–489.

Hobsley, M. (ed) (1979) Palpable abdominal mass. In *Pathways in Surgical Management*, pp. 89–102. Arnold, London.

Holm, H.H., Gammelgaard, J., Jensen, F., Smith, E.H. & Hillman, B.J. (1982) Ultrasound in the diagnosis of a palpable abdominal mass. A prospective study of 107 patients. *Gastrointestinal Radiology*, **7**, 149–151.

Htoo, M.M. (1983) Surgical implications of stone impaction in the gall bladder neck with compression of the common hepatic duct (Mirizzi's syndrome). *Clinical Radiology*, **34**, 651–655.

Isler, R.J., Ferruci, J.T., Wittenberg, J., Mueller, P.R., Simeone, J.F., van Sonnenberg, E. & Hall, D.A. (1981) Tissue core biopsy of abdominal tumours with a 22 gauge cutting needle. *American Journal of Roentgenology*, **136**, 725–728.

Jolles, H. & Coulam, C.M. (1980) CT of ascites: differential diagnosis. *American Journal of Roentgenology*, **135**, 315–322.

Kyaw, M.M. (1973) Roentgenologic triad of congenital multicystic kidney. *American Journal of Roentgenology*, **119**, 710–719.

Lauks, S.P. & McLachlan, M.S.F. (1981) Ageing and simple cysts of the kidney. *British Journal of Radiology*, **54**, 12–14.

Lundstedt, C., Hederstrom, E., Holmin, T., Lunderquist, A., Navne, T. & Owman, T. (1983) Radiological diagnosis in proven intraabdominal abscess formation: A comparison between plain films of the abdomen, ultrasonography and computerized tomography. *Gastrointestinal Radiology*, **8**, 261–266.

Martin, E.C., Fankuchen, E.I. & Neff, R.A. (1984) Percutaneous drainage of abscesses: a report of 100 patients. *Clinical Radiology*, **35**, 9–11.

McNeil, B.J., Sanders, R., Alderson, P.O. *et al.* (1981) A prospective study of computed tomography, ultrasound and gallium imaging in patients with fever. *Radiology*, **139**, 647–653.

Mueller, P.R., Ferrucci, J.T. Harbin, W.P., Kirkpatrick, R.H.,

Simeone, J.F. & Wittenberg, J. (1980) Appearance of lymphomatous involvement of the mesentery by ultrasonography and body computed tomography: the 'sandwich' sign. *Radiology*, **134**, 467–473.

Pedrosa, C.S., Casanova, R. & Rodriguez, R. (1981) Computed tomography in obstructive jaundice. Part 1: The level of obstruction. *Radiology*, **139**, 627–634.

Pelaez, J.C., Hill, M.C., Dach, J.L., Isikoff, M.B. & Morse, B. (1983) Abdominal aspiration biopsies; sonographic v. computed tomographic guidance. *Journal of the American Medical Association*, **250**, 2663–2666.

Pilling, D.W. (1983) Infantile hypertrophic pyloric stenosis: a fresh approach to the diagnosis. *Clinical Radiology*, **34**, 51–53.

Sanders, R.C. (1980) The significance of sonographic gallbladder wall thickening. *Journal of Clinical Ultrasound*, **8**, 143–146.

Schwerk, W., Braun, B. & Dombrowski, H. (1979) Real-time ultrasound examination in the diagnosis of gastrointestinal tumours. *Journal of Clinical Ultrasound*, **7**, 425–431.

Seshul, M.B. & Coulam, C.M. (1981) Pseudomyxoma peritonei: computed tomography and sonography. *American Journal of Roentgenology*, **136**, 803–806.

Stewart, J.F., Tattersall, M.H.N., Woods, R.L. & Fox, R.M. (1979) Unknown primary adenocarcinoma: incidence of overinvestigation and natural history. *British Medical Journal*, **1**, 1530–1533.

van Sonnenberg, E., Wittenberg, J., Ferrucci, J.T., Mueller, P.R. & Simeone, J.F. (1981) Triangulation method for percutaneous needle guidance: The angled approach to upper abdominal masses. *American Journal of Roentgenology*, **137**, 757–761.

Whitley, N.O., Bohlman, M.E. & Baker, L.P. (1982) CT patterns of mesenteric disease. *Journal of Computer Assisted Tomography*, **6**, 490–496.

Williams, M.P., Scott, I.H.K. & Dixon, A.K. (1984) Computed tomography in 101 patients with a palpable abdominal mass. *Clinical Radiology*, **35**, 293–296.

Yeh, H.C. (1979) Ultrasonography and computed tomography of carcinoma of the gall bladder. *Radiology*, **133**, 167–173.

Index

Abbreviations used in this index: CT = computerized tomography: ERCP = endoscopic retrograde cholangiopancreatography; i.a. = intra-arterial; i.v. = intravenous; MRI = magnetic resonance imaging; PTC = percutaneous transhepatic cholangiography; RI = radionuclide imaging (scintigraphy); US = ultrasound. Page references in *italic* indicate figures or tables.